Neonatal Hematology

Third Edition

Edited by

Pedro A. de Alarcón

Eric J. Werner

Robert D. Christensen

Martha C. Sola-Visner

Neonatal Hematology

Pathogenesis, Diagnosis, and Management
of Hematologic Problems

Third Edition

Edited by

Pedro A. de Alarcón
University of Illinois College of Medicine

Eric J. Werner
Children's Specialty Group, Children's Hospital of
The King's Daughters and Eastern Virginia Medical School

Robert D. Christensen
University of Utah Health and Intermountain Healthcare

Martha C. Sola-Visner
Boston Children's Hospital and Harvard University

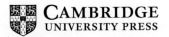

CAMBRIDGE
UNIVERSITY PRESS

CAMBRIDGE
UNIVERSITY PRESS

University Printing House, Cambridge CB2 8BS, United Kingdom

One Liberty Plaza, 20th Floor, New York, NY 10006, USA

477 Williamstown Road, Port Melbourne, VIC 3207, Australia

314–321, 3rd Floor, Plot 3, Splendor Forum, Jasola District Centre, New Delhi – 110025, India

79 Anson Road, #06–04/06, Singapore 079906

Cambridge University Press is part of the University of Cambridge.

It furthers the University's mission by disseminating knowledge in the pursuit of education, learning, and research at the highest international levels of excellence.

www.cambridge.org
Information on this title: www.cambridge.org/9781108488983
DOI: 10.1017/9781108773584

First edition published 2005
Second edition published 2013
Third edition published 2021

Printed in the United Kingdom by TJ Books Limited, Padstow Cornwall

A catalogue record for this publication is available from the British Library.

ISBN 978-1-108-48898-3 Hardback

Contents

Contents

Color plates are to be found between pages 242 and 243.

Foreword

Previous editions of *Neonatal Hematology: Pathogenesis, Diagnosis, and Management of Hematologic Problems* have included a chapter by Dr. Howard Pearson on the history of pediatric hematology. Sadly, Dr. Pearson passed away in 2016. The editors of this third edition have once again chosen to include Dr. Pearson's Historical Review as the opening chapter of this text. Its relevance to the practice of hematology remains undiminished. We honor the memory of Dr. Pearson in this Foreword by sharing some insights on his life, as he was one of the truly iconic figures in the discipline of pediatric hematology.

Howard Allen Pearson, one of seven children, was born in Panama just six days after the stock market crash of 1929. The Canal Zone was an American possession, isolated from the country of Panama, in a sense a totally socialistic system run by the US government and relatively immune from the financial impact of the great depression. His father was an accountant with the Panama Canal Company, which managed the affairs of the Panama Canal. Except for contracting malaria at age one, Howard had what for the time was a healthy early childhood. His experiences, at times comical, growing up in Panama were shared with his grandson, Matthew, who prepared his grandfather's Oral History which is archived at the American Academy of Pediatrics History Center [1]. His sense of humor shines through in that oral history where it is recorded that he once remarked: "Since the Canal Zone was an American possession, it was officially American soil. So, if I really wanted to, I could have become President; but I decided not to."

The Pearson family returned to their origins in Lynn, Massachusetts in 1939. Howard quickly became a standout among his peers. In his own words he was something of a leader in high school, doing very well academically. He was president of his graduating class of some 500 students, a member of the National Honor Society, and a winner of the Harvard Book Award. He was also an Eagle Scout with more than 40 merit badges, gaining skills that likely served him well many years later when he was Medical Director of The Hole in the Wall Gang Camp for children with serious diseases. After graduation from high school, it was off to college, in Howard's case, Dartmouth, a school he selected mostly because a close friend was headed there. He worked his way through Dartmouth babysitting for 25 cents an hour and getting free meals by hiring on to open the college dining room each morning at 6:00 a.m. Howard's $200/year academic scholarship fell far short of Dartmouth's $600/year tuition.

During Howard's first week as an undergraduate, the Dean of Dartmouth Medical School, Dr. Rolf Syversten, interviewed Howard as a possible candidate for later admission to the medical school. In those days, one could start medical school with only 36 months of college credits. Because of that interview, Howard was guaranteed an acceptance to Dartmouth Medical School to start three years hence. He ultimately graduated Dartmouth College magna cum laude and elected to Phi Beta Kappa while in medical school.

Howard entered Dartmouth Medical School in the fall of 1950. The school, now named the Audrey and Theodor Geisel School of Medicine at Dartmouth, was quite small at the time. His matriculating class consisted of just 24 students, almost all of whom had been Dartmouth undergrads. Shortly after starting medical school, Howard married Anne Livingston. He had met his future wife when they were both working at the Craigville Inn on Cape Cod. A year after they were married, the couple's first child was born. As Dartmouth was only a 2-year medical school, Howard, along with 20 of his classmates, transferred to Harvard Medical School to complete his

MD degree. In his Oral History, Howard recalls the family's struggles with finances. With two children to be cared for, there was little regular income. He would donate blood every 2 to 3 months for $25 and worked filing X-rays for 75 cents an hour in the radiology department at Peter Bent Brigham Hospital.

Graduating from Harvard Medical School in 1954, and with a family to support, Dr. Pearson chose to take a rotating internship and pediatric residency as a naval officer at the National Naval Medical Center in Bethesda. Unlike those in civilian residencies, those training as military officers received a reasonable salary. While still a resident, his first manuscript as a senior author was published. This was a report of a child with Diamond–Blackfan syndrome. The patient was the first child in the United States to be successfully treated with adrenocorticotropin hormone.

Howard received permission from the navy to accept a fellowship with Dr. Louis Diamond, Chief of Hematology at the Children's Hospital in Boston. He had met Dr. Diamond when he was a medical student at Harvard. Dr. Diamond is considered the "Father of Pediatric Hematology." The first generation of his trainees have been called "Diamond Chips." Howard was one of these "chips," along with Frank Oski, Lawrence Naiman and many others. If there were a 23andMe™ profile of pediatric hematologists in the United States, several score would find their training heritage linked back to Dr. Diamond in some way, including many contributors to this book.

Following his fellowship in Boston, Dr. Pearson returned to Bethesda, and for 4 years was Assistant Chief of the pediatric service under Dr. Thomas Cone, a consummate academic pediatrician, geneticist, historian and author. Much of Howard's later interests in the history of medicine likely can be traced to his relationship with Dr. Cone. When his military obligation was completed in 1962, Howard accepted a faculty position at the recently completed University of Florida Medical School in Gainesville where he established the Pediatric Department's first Division of Pediatric Hematology. He developed an interest in sickle cell disease and in animal models of human disorders. He was the first to show that dwarf cows with snorter's disease have the animal equivalent of the human Hurler's syndrome. Unfortunately, there are no videos of him performing a bone marrow on an affected cow, or

later a lion suspected of having the same disorder. His early years in Gainesville were extraordinarily productive and his efforts were recognized by moving from the rank of assistant professor to full professor in just 6 years. During his time in Florida, Howard became the perennial author of the chapter on hematology in Nelson's *Textbook of Pediatrics*. Dr. Waldo Nelson would later claim that by selecting Howard at such a young age to author that chapter, he had made him world famous.

By 1969, the Pearson family was ready to return to New England. Dr. Pearson was offered and accepted the opportunity to establish the first Division of Pediatric Hematology and Oncology at Yale. He later said that he never expected to stay in New Haven forever, but he remained on faculty well into his 80s and along the way, became chair of the Yale University School of Medicine's Department of Pediatrics. He won teaching awards and much kudos for establishing a truly collegial interaction with the community pediatricians in New Haven, an interaction that had fallen along the wayside over the years at Yale. Although his publications can be numbered in the many scores, perhaps the ones that have received much attention are his descriptions of the entity called functional asplenia (1969) and the "born again spleen" (1978), both of which were published in the *New England Journal of Medicine*. These and similar clinical reports cemented his reputation as one of the keenest minds in clinical research. It was he who also recognized that subjects with thalassemia could be identified and screened for simply by looking at their red blood cell indices. It is said that this single observation resulted in a marked reduction in the numbers of children being born with thalassemia major.

As his 12-year tenure as Chair of Pediatrics at Yale was ending, a friend of Paul Newman's stopped in to see Dr. Pearson to talk about a project Mr. Newman had envisioned, a summer camp for children with cancer. The camp was to be called "The Hole in the Wall Gang Camp" after the bunch of outlaws in Newman's film, *Butch Cassidy and the Sundance Kid*. Howard subsequently convinced Newman that the camp should also accept children with thalassemia, sickle cell disease, hemophilia, and other serious blood diseases. With a US$10 million gift from Paul Newman, along with other contributions, the camp opened within a year. Howard became its medical director. Reflecting on his work with Newman, years later Howard commented "I never dreamed in 1986 that the Camp would become such an important place in my life for such a long time" [1]. More than 1,000 youngsters were served each year during his time as medical director. Following his retirement as the camp's medical director in 2005, Howard remained as its medical consultant, volunteer physician, and member of its board of directors.

Dr. Pearson's influence and prominence extended well beyond New Haven. He held leadership positions in many professional societies. In 2002, he was named the recipient of the prestigious Howland Award. He was the President of the American Academy of Pediatrics during the important period when the Academy's statement on the relationship between sleep position and sudden infant death was published. Because of his long-standing interest in medical history he was called upon to write the histories of the American Pediatric Society, the American Academy of Pediatrics, and the American Board of Pediatrics. Howard was a key figure in establishing an historical archive for the American Academy of Pediatrics, an archive now called the Pediatric History Center.

Only at age 84 did Dr. Pearson turn over the keys to his office at Yale, devoting his time to writing and The Hole in the Wall Gang Camp (see Fig. 0.1). He remarked that:

> As I look back from the perspective of having far more time behind me than ahead of me, I probably spent too much time, including nights and weekends, on my own work and my career rather than my family. I really have no hobbies except an obsession with crossword puzzles. I do at least one crossword a day, and when I finish, I say to myself, "Another day without Alzheimer's!"

He also said that he came from a generation that emphasized time commitment and hard work as the essential ingredients for success and that he could not remember many days when he had gone to work reluctantly. That's a pretty good epitaph.

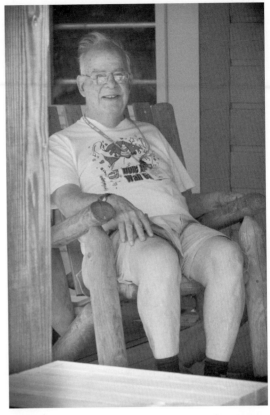

Fig. 0.1 Dr. Howard Pearson at the Hole in the Wall Gang Camp (Source: Hole in the Wall Gang Camp News, available at https://bit.ly/2YWnyKG)

Within the pages of this edition of *Neonatal Hematology* you will recognize how Dr. Pearson's commitment to hard work produced a voluminous quantity of clinical studies that form the basis for much of how we now provide care to infants and children with serious blood disorders. Read on.

James A. Stockman III MD

Reference

1. American Academy of Pediatrics. Pediatrics History Center: Oral history. Howard A. Pearson MD. Available online at https://bit.ly/2Yrgy9A.

Preface

Since the last edition of this book, there have been many advances on the diagnosis and management of neonatal hematological and oncological conditions. Particularly, the ability to perform genomic analysis continues to improve and it has become more and more affordable. This ability has made possible the diagnosis of many rare disorders that prior to these advances were difficult or impossible to diagnose. Technological advances have also made it possible for physicians caring for the newborn to provide care to smaller and smaller newborns. The growth of information technology has made it possible to have an immense amount of data, literally at your fingertips. In the chapters that follow we have attempted to bring this complex matrix of information to the practicing physicians caring for newborns, and yet, remain true to the purpose of this book to provide practical information, to be a "how-to" more than a "why" book. We have continued with the order of chapters from the second edition, beginning with introduction and historical perspective. We follow with the two chapters on the development of the hematopoietic system, specifically the pathophysiology of the hematopoietic and immunological systems, the essence of blood. The remainder of the book presents practical approach to white cell disorders, red cell disorders, platelet disorders, coagulation abnormalities, transfusion medicine, neonatal oncology and manifestations of systemic disorders. Each section devoted to one of the major three cell lines begins with a practical algorithms-driven approach to the disturbance of that particular cell line. We have brought together immunologists, infectologists, hematologist/oncologists, transfusion medicine experts, and neonatologists from both sides of the Atlantic to provide you with up-to-date yet practical information for the care of our smallest of patients. We have brought along a new generation of authors so that we can continue the devotion and enthusiasm

for this field of our mentors Doctors Frank A. Oski, J. Laurence Naiman, and Gerald Rothstein who helped us develop a passion for the field.

As in the previous edition, we asked Dr. James A. Stockman III to provide a foreword for the book. For this edition, we asked him to highlight the contributions to our field made by Dr. Howard A. Pearson a giant in pediatric hematology who recently died. Dr. Pearson was a contributor to the book as author and mentor. He always shared his knowledge; he was a true gentleman and a friend. He will be sorely missed. As Dr. Pearson had written the chapter on the historical perspective of the field of neonatal blood disorders in our previous edition, we asked Dr. Stockman to provide such a chapter for this edition. Attesting to the breadth of Dr. Pearson's knowledge, after reviewing the chapter in the previous edition, Dr. Stockman told us, "I cannot add any meaningful information to Howard's chapter. Can you just reprint the chapter?" Thus, after asking permission from our publisher, we elected to print, unchanged, the historical perspective authored by Dr. Howard A. Pearson.

For this edition, we have also added our colleague Dr. Martha Sola-Visner to the editorial group and brought in many new generation authors. Lastly, we thank our families who have supported us during the countless hours of editing the book, specifically our spouses (Alice, Jill, Wendy, and Gary), our children and grandchildren (Alessandro and Katie, Tessa and Travis, Lucas, Audrey, Jacob and Caroline, Abby and Josh, Andrew and Henry, Elizabeth, Grant, Amelia, Elsa, Ansel, Louisa, Atticus and Cosette, and Veronica and José). Without their understanding we could never have completed this text. We hope that you find the book helpful in your day-to-day practice.

Contributors

James A. Stockman III, MD
Retired President
American Board of Pediatrics
Chapel Hill, NC

Pedro A. de Alarcón, MD
William H. Albers
Professor and Head, Department of Pediatrics,
University of Illinois College of Medicine, Peoria,
IL, USA

Eric J. Werner, MD
Division of Pediatric Hematology/Oncology,
Children's Specialty Group, Children's Hospital
of The King's Daughters, Professor of Pediatrics,
Eastern Virginia Medical School, Norfolk, VA,
USA

**Robert D. Christensen is Director of
Neonatology**
Research at Intermountain Healthcare and
Professor of Pediatrics, University of Utah
HEALTH, Salt Lake City, UT, USA.

Martha C. Sola-Visner, MD
Associate Professor of Pediatrics,
Division of Newborn Medicine, Boston Children's
Hospital and Harvard University School of
Medicine, Boston, Massachusetts, USA

Howard A. Pearson, MD
deceased

Amber M. D'Souza
Assistant Professor, Department of Pediatrics,
University of Illinois College of Medicine, Peoria,
IL, USA

Mervin C. Yoder, MD
Professor of Pediatrics, Indiana University
School of Medicine, Indianapolis, IN,
USA

Amy E. O'Connell, MD, PhD
Instructor in Pediatrics, Harvard Medical School
Attending Neonatologist, Boston Children's
Hospital Boston, MA, USA

Angela E. Rivers MD, PhD
Assistant Professor of Pediatrics, University of
Illinois, Chicago

William B. Slayton, MD
Associate Professor of Pediatrics, Division of
Pediatric Hematology/Oncology, Stop Children's
Cancer of Palm Beach Country Endworld Chair,
University of Florida, Gainesville, FL, USA

Amy E. Geddis, MD PhD
Professor of Pediatrics, University of Washington
Director, Bone Marrow Failure Program Seattle
Children's Hospital, Cancer and Blood Disorders
Clinic

Meera Srikanthan, MD
Acting Instructor of Pediatrics, University of
Washington Seattle Children's Hospital, Cancer
and Blood Disorders Clinic

**Katie Bergstrom, LGC, Licensed Genetics
Counselor**
Seattle Children's Hospital, Cancer and Blood
Disorders Clinic

Julie J. Kim-Chang
Division of Pediatric Allergy, Immunology, and
Pulmonary Medicine, Department of Pediatrics,
Duke University School of Medicine, DUMC Box
2644, Durham, NC 27710

James L. Wynn, MD
Assistant Professor of Pediatrics, Division of
Neonatal-Perinatal Medicine, Department of
Pediatrics, Vanderbilt University Medical Center,
Nashville, TN, USA

Matthew A. Saxonhouse, MD
Division of Neonatology, Atrium Health Levine
Children's Hospital, 1000 Blythe Blvd. Charlotte,
NC 28203

John W. Sleasman, MD
Robert A. Good
Professor and Chief Medical Instructor,
University of South Florida, Department of
Pediatrics, all Children's Hospital, 801 6th St.
South, St Petersburg, FL

Parul Rai, MD
Instructor Department of Hematology St. Jude
Children's Research Hospital Memphis, TN

Ewelina K. Mamcarz, MD
Assistant Member Department of Bone Marrow
Transplantation and Cellular Therapy St. Jude
Children's Research Hospital Memphis,
TN

Jane S. Hankins, MD, MS
Associate Member Department of Hematology
St. Jude Children's Research Hospital Memphis,
TN

Pamela J. Kling, MD
Professor, University of Wisconsin, Madison, WI,
USA

Mary Elizabeth Ross, MD, PhD
Assistant Professor of Pediatrics, Division of
Pediatrics Hematology/Oncology, University of
Illinois College of Medicine, Peoria, IL, USA (no
email)

Stephen P. Emery, MD
Associate Professor
Divisions of Ultrasound and Maternal-Fetal
Medicine
Department of Obstetrics, Gynecology, and
Reproductive Sciences
University of Pittsburgh School of Medicine
Pittsburgh, PA

Jon F. Watchko, MD
Associate Professor
Professor Emeritus
Division of Newborn Medicine
Department of Pediatrics
University of Pittsburgh School of Medicine
Pittsburgh, PA.

Bertil Glader, MD, PhD
Lucile Packard Children's Hospital Stanford, Palo
Alto, CA Stanford University School of Medicine,
Stanford, CA, USA

Aditi Kamdar, MD
Lucile Packard Children's Hospital Stanford, Palo
Alto, CA Stanford University School of Medicine,
Stanford, CA, USA

Ted S. Rosenkrantz, MD
Professor of Pediatrics and Obstetrics, Division of
Neonatal–Perinatal Medicine, University of
Connecticut School of Medicine, Farmington, CT,
USA

William Oh, MD
Professor of Pediatrics, Warren Alpert Medical
School of Brown University, Attending
Neonatologist, Women and Infants' Hospital,
Providence, RI, USA

Emöke Deschmann, MD, MMSc, PhD
Attending Neonatologist, Department of
Women's and Children's Health, Division of
Neonatology, Karolinska Institutet Department
of Neonatology, Karolinska University Hospital,
Stockholm, Sweden

Patricia E. Davenport, MD
Instructor of Pediatrics, Division of Newborn
Medicine, Boston Children's Hospital and
Harvard University School of Medicine, Boston,
MA, USA.

W. Beau Mitchell, MD
Associate Professor of Pediatrics, Icahn School of
Medicine at Mount Sinai, New York

James B. Bussel, MD
Emeritus Professor of Pediatrics, Professor of
Pediatrics in Obstetrics and Gynecology, Weill
Cornell Medical College, New York

Kurt R. Schibler, MD
Division of Neonatology, Children's Hospital
Medical Center, Cincinnati, OH, USA

Thomas F. Michniacki, MD
Clinical Assistant Professor of Pediatric
Hematology/Oncology, Department of Pediatrics,
University of Michigan Medical School, Ann
Arbor, MI

Kelly Walkovich, MD
Clinical Associate Professor of Pediatric
Hematology/Oncology, Department of Pediatrics,
University of Michigan Medical School, Ann
Arbor, MI

Manuela Albisetti, MD
Division of Hematology, University Children's
Hospital, Zurich, Switzerland

**Paul Monagle, MBBS, MD, M.Sc, FRACP, FRCPA,
FCCP**
Department of Haematology Royal Children's
Hospital Flemington Rd. Melbourne Victoria,
Australia, 3052

Gary Woods, MD
Clinical Director, Pediatric Thrombosis Program
Aflac Cancer and Blood Disorders Center,
Children's Healthcare of Atlanta Emory
University School of Medicine, Atlanta, GA

Cyril Jacquot
Center for Cancer and Blood Disorders, Children's
National Hospital, Washington, DC, USA;
Department of Pediatrics and Pathology, George
Washington University School of Medicine and
Health Sciences, Washington, DC

Yunchuan D. Mo
Center for Cancer and Blood Disorders,
Children's National Hospital, Washington, DC,
USA; Department of Pediatrics and Pathology,
George Washington University School of
Medicine and Health Sciences, Washington, DC

Naomi L. C. Luban, MD, FAAP
Division Chief, Laboratory Medicine, Children's
National Hospital, Professor of Pediatrics and
Pathology, George Washington University School
of Medicine and Health Sciences, Washington,
DC, USA

Erin M. Guest, MD
Division of Hematology/Oncology Director,
Cancer Genomics Program, Children's Mercy
Hospital, 2401 Gillham Road, Kansas City MO
64108

Catherine Garnett, MD
PhD. Clinical Research Fellow, MRC Molecular
Haematology Unit, Weatherall Institute of

Molecular Medicine, Headington, Oxford, OX3
9DS, United Kingdom

Irene Roberts, MD
Professor of Paediatric Haematology Oxford
University Department of Paediatrics, Children's
Hospital and MRC Molecular Haematology Unit,
Weatherall Institute of Molecular Medicine,
Headington, Oxford, OX3 9DS, United Kingdom

Alan S. Gamis, MD, MPH Professor
Division of Hematology/Oncology Associate
Division Director, Children's Mercy Cancer
Center Children's Mercy Hospital, 2401 Gillham
Road, Kansas City MO 64108

Kevin F. Ginn MD, Assistant Professor
Division of Hematology/Oncology Director,
Pediatric Brain Tumor Program Children's Mercy
Hospital, 2401 Gillham Road, Kansas City MO
64108

Jaszianne A. Tolbert, Assistant Professor
Division of Hematology/Oncology and Clinical
Pharmacology Director, Experimental
Therapeutics in Pediatric Cancer Program
Children's Mercy Hospital, 2401 Gillham Road,
Kansas City MO 64108

Glenson Samuel, Assistant Professor
Division of Hematology/Oncology Children's
Mercy Hospital, 2401 Gillham Road, Kansas City
MO 64108

J. Allyson Hays, Assistant Professor
Division of Hematology/Oncology
Director, Histiocytosis Program Children's Mercy
Hospital, 2401 Gillham Road, Kansas City MO
64108

Nancy C. Chescheir, MD Clinical Professor
Department of Obstetrics and Gynecology,
Division of Maternal–Fetal Medicine, University
of North Carolina School of Medicine, Chapel
Hill, NC, USA

Randall G. Fisher, MD Medical Director
Division of Pediatric Infectious Diseases,
Children's Specialty Group; Children's Hospital
of the King's Daughters, Eastern Virginia Medical
School, Norfolk, VA, USA

Chapter 1

A Historical Review

Howard A. Pearson

Ancient concepts of the blood were described by Hippocrates and Galen 2000 years ago in their doctrine of "humors." It was believed that the body was made up of four humors – blood, phlegm, black bile, and yellow bile – and that these four components had the qualities of heat (hot-blooded!), cold, moist, and dry. The Galenic concept of the blood prevailed through the Middle Ages. Health or disease were a result of an imbalance, between these humors. This was the basis of the practice of therapeutic bloodletting (which, fortunately, was performed infrequently on children) through the mid nineteenth century as a way to rid the body of the imbalance of humors believed to cause a wide variety of diseases.

The hematology of the fetus and newborn is a relatively recent area of study whose development depended upon the evolution of the science of hematology and, especially, upon methods to study the blood and its elements. As Wintrobe has pointed out, the development of the field of hematology has been driven by technology. He divided the evolution of hematology into two general areas: *morphology*, which relied on the development of microscopy, and *quantitation* of the elements of the blood, which came later [1].

The invention of the microscope enabled identification of the blood cells. Antonie van Leeuwenhoek, working in Delft, Holland, constructed a primitive microscope from the minute biconcave lens mounted between two metal plates attached to a screw that permitted focusing. Leeuwenhoek's publication in 1674 contained the first accurate description of the red blood corpuscles [2]:

The blood is composed of exceedingly small particles, named globules, which in most animals are red in color ... These particles are so minute that 100 of them placed side by side would not equal the diameter of a common grain of sand.

In the centuries following, the development of compound microscopes with two lenses greatly increased magnification and minimized spherical aberration, permitting more accurate descriptions of the blood cells. Dr. William Hewson, who has been designated as one of the "fathers of hematology," noted that the red cells were flat rather than globular and also described the leukocytes for the first time [3]. The last of the formed elements of the blood, the platelet, was recognized independently by several investigators. The most definitive early work on the platelet was done by Giulio Bizzozero. His monograph, published in 1882, clearly recognized these cells as being distinct from red and white blood cells, and suggested that they should be called *Blutplättchen*. He also assigned a hemostatic function to the platelet [4]. Dr. William Osler, early in his illustrious career, also described platelets accurately, although he believed that they may be infectious agents, perhaps analogous to bacteria [5].

With improvements in microscopy, the morphology of the fixed blood cells began to be examined using thin films of blood, spread and dried on glass slides, which were then stained with aniline dyes that stained differentially the nuclei and granules of the leukocytes. Staining of peripheral blood smears was developed by Paul Ehrlich in 1877, while he was still a medical student [6], and became practical in the early twentieth century by the work of Dr. James Homer Wright of Boston, who formulated the polychromatic Wright stain that is still used today for morphologic examination of the blood and bone marrow. The

Neonatal Hematology, Pathogenesis, Diagnosis, and Management of Hematologic Problems, 3rd edition, ed. Pedro A. de Alarcón, Eric J. Werner, Robert D. Christensen, and Martha C. Sola-Visner. Published by Cambridge University Press. © Cambridge University Press 2021.

development of supravital dyes provided a method for assessment of erythropoiesis by reticulocyte counts. These techniques permitted the flowering of morphologic hematology, and many blood diseases such as the leukemias and the various types of anemia were described on the basis of typical morphological findings.

Hematology as a quantitative discipline began with the development of practical and reliable methods to quantify accurately the numbers of the various blood cells. These methods used gridded chambers of uniform depth (hematocytometers) into which precisely diluted suspensions of blood were placed. The numbers of cells in the chamber were counted and, when combined with the known dilutions, the actual numbers of cells per cubic milliliter in the patient's blood could be calculated. Hemoglobin levels were estimated by comparing the density of color in fixed dilutions of hemolyzed blood with colorometric standards and, later, by spectroscopy. For many years, hemoglobin values were reported as "% of normal"; and because the definition of "normal" was often different there was considerable variability from study to study. In 1929, Dr. Maxwell Wintrobe described his method for obtaining the hematocrit or packed red-cell volume (PCV) by centrifugation of blood in a glass tube [7]. He then defined so-called red-cell indices, the mean corpuscular volume (MCV), mean corpuscular hemoglobin (MCH), and mean corpuscular hemoglobin concentration (MCHC), which proved of enormous value in classifying the various forms of anemia [8]. The latest advance in blood-cell quantitation began in the 1950s with the introduction of increasingly more complicated and sophisticated computer-driven electronic instruments that measure hemoglobin very accurately, the numbers of all the blood cells, as well as the red-cell indices and the red-cell distribution width (RDW). Some instruments now also provide automated differential counts of the leukocytes.

Most of the pre-twentieth century American pediatric textbooks gave scant attention to hematologic problems of the neonate. Dr. W.P. Dewees's 1825 *A Treatise on the Physical and Medical Treatment of Children,* arguably the first American pediatric textbook, and Dr. Job Lewis Smith's 1869 *A Treatise on the Diseases of Infancy and Childhood* gave only passing notice to blood conditions of the neonate, such as neonatal jaundice and hemorrhage from improper ligature of the umbilical cord [9, 10]. However, the monumental pediatric text of

Dr. L. Emmett Holt, *The Diseases of Infancy and Childhood,* first published in 1897, contained a section on "the Diseases of the Newly-Born," including the hemorrhagic disease, and a 17-page section on "the Diseases of the Blood," which included the normal blood findings in the newborn [11]. Holt was obviously familiar with the many studies published in the German literature, and his descriptions are reasonably consistent with modern findings:

> The percentage of hemoglobin is highest in the blood of the newly born ... At this time the number of red blood corpuscles is from 4,350,000 to 6,500,000 in each cubic millimeter ... In size, a much greater variation is seen in the red cells of the neonate. In the blood of the foetus there are present nucleated red corpuscles or erythroblasts. These diminish in number toward the end of pregnancy. These are always found in the blood of prematures, but in infants born at term, they are seen only in small numbers. The number of leukocytes in the blood of the newly born is three or four times that of the adult, being on the average 18,000 per cubic millimeter.

In 1921, Dr. W.P. Lucas and associates from the University of California Medical School in San Francisco described their extensive studies of the blood of 150 infants at birth and during the first 2 months of life [12]. Their samples were obtained from serial punctures of the longitudinal sinus! The polycythemia of the newborn and changes in the leukocytes were defined clearly.

In 1924, Dr. H.S. Lippman from the University of Minnesota published detailed studies of the blood of newborn infants [13]. He noted (without further details) that "Denis published the first observations on the subject in 1831." Lippman's review of the literature cited 70 previous articles on the hematology of the newborn. Most of these studies were published in European, especially German, journals. Although there was considerable variability because of different methods and standards, the consensus of these early studies was that "Hemoglobin values at birth are higher than at any other period in the children's life." Some of these studies described reticulocytosis and normoblastemia in the first day of life, which declined rapidly in the first week of life. Lippman conducted serial studies of capillary blood over the first 48 hours of life in 71 normal newborns as well as changes in the leukocytes during this period.

It has been known for 100 years that the red-blood cells (RBC) of the fetus and newborn are large compared with those of adults, as determined by microscopic measurement of red-cell diameter. Newer electronic cell-sizing techniques have demonstrated that the mean MCV of the neonate's red blood cells averages 110 fl, compared with the 90 fl of adults. The red cells of midgestational fetuses are even larger [14].

In 1856, E. Korber, in his doctoral dissertation, is reported to have described his experiments that showed that solutions of the hemoglobin of newborn infants resisted denaturation by strong alkaline solutions and maintained a red color, while hemoglobin solutions from adults treated in the same way were rapidly denatured and decolorized [15]. The property of alkali resistance became the basis of the Singer one-minute alkali denaturation test for quantitation of fetal hemoglobin (HB F), as well as the Apt test, used to differentiate fetal from swallowed maternal blood in infants with gross blood in the gastrointestinal tract [16, 17]. Fetal hemoglobin is also resistant to acid denaturation, which is the basis for the red-cell acid elution staining procedure of Drs. C. Kleihauer, H. Braun, and K. Betke that is used widely to quantitate the magnitude of fetomaternal transfusions [18].

The understanding of the protein structure of hemoglobin advanced rapidly in the 1950s when it was shown that adult hemoglobin, Hb A ($\alpha_2 \beta_2$), is a tetramer of alpha (α) and beta (β) polypeptide chains and that Hb F ($\alpha_2 \gamma_2$) contains a different pair of polypeptide chains designated as gamma (γ) chains [19, 20]. During fetal development, synthesis of γ chains predominates, but with approaching term there is a fall-off of γ-chain synthesis and a simultaneous reciprocal increase in β-chain synthesis. The regulatory mechanisms that govern this "β/γ switch" remain to be elucidated. The blood of the newborn contains large amounts of Hb F, averaging 60%–80%. The affinity of Hb F for oxygen is greater than that of Hb A because of poor binding of 2,3-diphosphoglycerate. This results in a shift of the oxygen dissociation curve to the left, which is favorable for oxygen transport to the fetus in the relative hypoxia of intrauterine existence but which may be disadvantageous after birth [21]. The high level of Hb F at birth offers temporary protection from β hemoglobinopathies, such as sickle cell anemia, and may hamper their diagnosis in the newborn.

Roland Scott, using the relatively insensitive "sickle cell prep," demonstrated a much lower frequency of "sicklemia" in black newborns than was found in older children from the same community [22]. The development of techniques such as acid agar gel electrophoresis and high pressure liquid chromatography have permitted genotypic diagnosis of most hemoglobinopathies at birth, and neonatal testing for hemoglobinopathies is now performed routinely in all 50 states of the USA [23].

The only somewhat common hemoglobinopathy that produces symptoms in the newborn is homozygous alpha-thalassemia resulting from deletion of four alpha-globin genes [24]. In parts of Southeast Asia, fetal hydrops is caused much more frequently by alpha-thalassemia than by Rh immunization. The recent immigrations of large numbers of Southeast Asian people into the USA have resulted in increasing numbers of affected infants. Some of these have survived after intrauterine transfusions but are transfusion dependent [25].

Other inherited conditions such as hereditary spherocytosis, a defect in RBC spectrin, may be associated with non-immune hemolysis, both in utero and in the neonatal period, resulting in anemia and hyperbilirubinemia. Inherited deficiency of RBC enzymes such as glucose 6-phosphate dehydrogenase combined with exposure to oxidant substances, perhaps fava beans, causes epidemic neonatal hyperbilirubinemia in Greek infants.

Since the turn of the twentieth century, a large number of studies of the hematology and blood diseases of the newborn have been reported. Much of this information has been incorporated into textbooks of hematology. Dr. Maxwell Wintrobe's monumental *Clinical Hematology*, which was first published in 1943, contained sections on normal blood values, anemias, and hemorrhagic diseases of the newborn. Neonatal thrombocytopenia in infants born of mothers with immune thrombocytopenic purpura (ITP) was also mentioned briefly. In subsequent editions of Wintrobe's text, many more neonatal hematological conditions were described. In 1960, Dr. Carl Smith published *Blood Diseases of Infancy and Childhood,* the first American textbook of pediatric hematology/oncology. This had several chapters devoted to normal values and hematologic problems in the neonatal period.

In 1966, Drs. Frank Oski and Laurie Naiman published *Hematological Problems in the Newborn,* the first text devoted solely to the hematology and hematological problems of the neonate [26]. The authors' stated purpose was

> ... to provide in a single source much of what is known concerning both the normal and abnormal hematologic processes of the first month of life and the effects of prenatal factors on them ... And to provide a useful guide to all who care for the newborn infant – those who are continually confronted with infants who are bleeding, anemic or jaundiced.

The Oski–Naiman text had two subsequent editions in 1972 and 1982. Subsequently, there have been a plethora of texts and handbooks on pediatric hematology, most of which devote chapters to the newborn.

The history of neonatal hematology and the process of understanding hematologic diseases based on clinical and laboratory observations that stimulate investigation of basic mechanisms and then therapeutic interventions are illustrated well by three quintessential neonatal blood conditions: *erythroblastosis fetalis; hemorrhagic disease of the newborn;* and *physiological anemia of infancy.*

Erythroblastosis Fetalis

As recently as 1946, erythroblastosis fetalis, or hemolytic disease of the newborn, affected between 0.5% and 1.0% of fetuses and newborns in the USA. It had a 50% mortality as well as significant neurologic morbidity in many survivors [27]. Prior to 1936, three seemingly distinct neonatal syndromes had been identified: *fetal hydrops, icterus gravis neonatorum,* and *anemia of the newborn.* Based on histological and hematological similarities, Drs. L.K. Diamond, K. Blackfan, and J. Baty advanced a unifying hypothesis that these three syndromes were manifestations of a single underlying disease process. They designated all of these neonatal syndromes "erythroblastosis fetalis" because of massive nucleated RBC proliferation in the organs and blood [28].

Dr. Ruth Darrow was a pathologist who had several of her own children die of erythroblastosis. In 1938, she advanced a brilliant inductive hypothesis about its cause. Assembling all of the available information, as well as drawing on her tragic personal experiences, she noted the usual sparing of the first child and the progressive involvement of most subsequently born children. She recognized that the clinical, hematologic, and histopathologic findings in these infants could be best explained by severe hemolysis. She concluded that the disease results because [29]:

> The mother is actively immunized against fetal red cells or some component of them ... The antibodies formed in the maternal organism may then pass to the child through the placenta.

The elusive offending red-cell antigen and its antibody were discovered in 1940 by Drs. Karl Landsteiner and Alexander Weiner. It was given the name Rh (rhesus factor) because the antibody was produced by injection of red-blood cells of rhesus monkeys into rabbits. This antibody agglutinated the red cells of 85% of normal individuals [30]. Interestingly, Landsteiner's discovery of the Rh blood group was accomplished almost 40 years after he had discovered the ABO blood groups [31]. In 1941, Dr. Philip Levine and associates described a severe transfusion reaction in a postpartum woman who received a transfusion of her husband's blood shortly after delivering a stillborn baby with hydrops fetalis. Levine was able to demonstrate Rh antibodies in the mother's circulation, defining clearly the pathophysiology of erythroblastosis fetalis [32, 33].

Effective treatment for erythroblastosis progressed slowly. The treatment of icterus gravis by "exsanguination transfusion" was first reported in 1925 by Dr. A.P. Hart at the Toronto Hospital for Sick Children [34]. With the discovery of the Rh factor, exchange transfusion evolved rapidly as a way to remove circulating antibodies, sensitized red-blood cells, and bilirubin; Drs. Harry Wallerstein and Alexander Weiner in New York and Louis K. Diamond in Boston spearheaded this treatment. Wallerstein's method involved aspiration of the neonate's blood from the sagittal sinus and infusion of Rh negative blood into a peripheral vein [35]. Weiner's method employed heparinization and surgical cannulation of the radial artery and saphenous vein. Interestingly, at a time long before institutional review boards for research, he first evaluated the technique in a nonerythroblastic "Mongolian idiot" [36]. Diamond's much more practical method utilized the umbilical vein to alternately remove and infuse blood, and this rapidly became the accepted method around the world [37]. Drs. Diamond and F. Allen developed practical guidelines for the prenatal and postnatal management of Rh-sensitized mothers and their erythroblastotic newborns. These reduced neonatal mortality from 50% to 5% and intrauterine death from 20% to less than 10%.

Kernicterus associated with severe hyperbilirubinemia was virtually eliminated [38]. Implicit in the pathogenesis of Rh erythroblastosis is that small numbers of fetal erythrocytes gain entrance into the maternal circulation, particularly during labor, where they evoke maternal immunization and Rh antibody formation. The possibility of large fetomaternal transfusion was first hypothesized by Dr. A. Weiner and proven definitively by Dr. Bruce Chown, who used differential agglutination to demonstrate and quantitate fetal red cells in the maternal circulation in a case of neonatal anemia [39, 40]. It is now recognized that acute, massive fetomaternal transfusion during labor can result in severe anemia, neonatal pallor and hypovolemic shock resembling asphyxia pallida. Chronic fetal/maternal hemorrhage during pregnancy may be associated with a well-compensated congenital microcytic hypochromic anemia due to iron deficiency because of chronic blood loss by the fetus [41].

Two penultimate important developments in erythroblastosis fetalis were provided by Dr. A.W. Liley of New Zealand, who devised a method of spectroscopic analysis of amniotic fluid to determine increase in fetal bilirubin as a result of hemolysis. This enabled identification of immunized fetuses who were at high risk of intrauterine death. Liley showed that these severely affected infants could be given intrauterine intraperitoneal transfusion of Rh negative RBC to carry them to delivery [42, 43]. Development of percutaneous umbilical blood sampling under ultrasonographic guidance has enabled perinatologists to directly diagnose and assess the severity of anemia in immunized fetuses and to treat them with simple or exchange transfusion in utero.

In 1967, Drs. C.A. Clark in Liverpool and V.J. Freda and associates in New York showed independently that primary isoimmunization of Rh-negative mothers by the Rh-positive red cells of their fetuses could be largely prevented by immediate postnatal administration of potent anti-Rh gamma globulin to the mother [44, 45]. In most of the developed world, erythroblastosis fetalis has become a rare disease of largely historical interest, and exchange transfusion has become a lost skill [46].

Hemorrhagic Disease of the Newborn

Newborn infants may bleed seriously from several causes. More than 2000 years ago, the familial occurrence of severe bleeding following ritual circumcision of boys, who doubtless had hemophilia, was recognized [47]:

> It has been reported of four sisters at Sepphoris, the first one circumcised her son, and he died, the second, and he died; the third and he died. The fourth came before R. Simeon b. Ganaliel who said to her abstain from circumcision ... for there are families whose blood is loose; while in others it coagulates.
> (Babylonian Talmud, Tracate Yevamoth, fol. 64b)

Dr. Armand Quick, in a 1942 review of the history of coagulation, noted that possible cases of a neonatal hemorrhagic disease, distinct from hemophilia, had been reported as far back as 1682. Quick also postulated that the delay of ritual circumcision by Jews until the eighth day of life may have been based on their empirical observations that neonatal bleeding symptoms have largely waned by that time [48].

However, the first definitive description of "the haemorrhagic disease of the newborn" was provided by Dr. C.W. Townsend in Boston in 1894. Townsend described a generalized, not local, bleeding disorder beginning on the second or third day of life. About 0.6% of newborns were affected with clinical hemorrhage, chiefly into the skin, gastrointestinal tract, and central nervous system. There was a 62% mortality rate, but if not fatal, the disease was self-limited, with most cases recovering within 5 days. The sexes were affected equally [49]. The onset of transient bleeding only in the first few days of life, as well as the involvement of girls, clearly differentiated hemorrhagic disease of the newborn from hemophilia.

Dr. W.P. Lucas and associates performed serial clotting times, a measure of the entire coagulation mechanism, in newborns and showed that during the first four days of life "there is a definite and fairly consistent prolongation of the coagulation time which favors the so called hemorrhagic condition of the newborn" [12]. Dr. G.H. Whipple in 1912 showed that the plasma of infants with hemorrhagic disease was deficient in prothrombin [50], and this deficiency was corroborated and expanded by Drs. K.M. Brinkhaus and associates in 1937 [51].

Treatment of hemorrhagic disease of the newborn was essentially limited to supportive measures, including local compression when possible [11: p. 104]. More than half of affected babies died of intracranial hemorrhage or hemorrhagic shock. Dr. S.W. Lambert in 1908 was able to rapidly reverse the bleeding of an affected baby by a transfusion in which the father's radial artery was anastomosed to the baby's popliteal vein [52]. In 1923, Dr. J.B. Sidbury, a practicing pediatrician in North Carolina, successfully treated the hypovolemic shock as well as the bleeding disorder of an affected newborn by giving a blood transfusion through the umbilical vein. Sidbury stated that "human whole blood has acted as a specific in this condition" [53]. In the 1920s, and continuing into the 1940s, the standard treatment of hemorrhagic disease of the newborn, and in some centers the prophylaxis of the condition, was the intramuscular injection of adult blood, often obtained from the father. This was before the discovery of the Rh factor, and this led to the Rh immunization of some girls and subsequent erythroblastosis fetalis in their offspring [54].

Understanding of the pathogenesis of hemorrhagic disease of the newborn was made possible in 1929 when Dr. H. Dam and associates showed that chicks fed an ether-extracted diet developed a severe bleeding tendency that could be prevented by feeding material they extracted and purified from cereals or seeds. They named the correcting factor "Koagulations-vitamin," or vitamin K [55, 56]. The nature of the bleeding defect in vitamin K-deficient chicks was soon localized to a deficiency of prothrombin and defined clearly by Brinkhaus and colleagues and Dam and colleagues in normal babies and those with hemorrhagic disease [57, 58]. Dr. W.W. Waddell and associates showed that vitamin K administration could prevent coagulation abnormalities in newborns [59]. Synthesis of vitamin K was accomplished in 1939 [60]. Routine vitamin K prophylaxis (0.5–1.0 mg given subcutaneously) for all newborns was recommended by the Committee on Nutrition of the American Academy of Pediatrics in 1961, and hemorrhagic disease of the newborn has virtually disappeared in the developed world [61]. It should be mentioned, however, that the incidence of hemorrhagic disease of the newborn had decreased markedly in the USA even before vitamin K prophylaxis became routine. This decrease was probably a consequence of the declining incidence of breast feeding from the 1930s through the 1960s. The vitamin K content of breast milk is much lower than that of cows' milk and hemorrhagic disease of the newborn occurs almost exclusively in breast-fed infants who, deliberately or inadvertently, do not receive prophylactic vitamin K [62, 63]. The biochemical basis of the action of vitamin K has been shown to relate to the gamma-carboxylation of glutamine acid residues in the vitamin K-dependent coagulation factors, including prothrombin [64].

Physiological Anemia of Infancy and the Early Anemia of Prematurity

At birth, the concentration of hemoglobin of full-term infants averages 16.4 gm/dL, higher than it will ever be during a lifetime. This relative polycythemia of the newborn is attributable to the low arterial PaO_2 in utero that stimulates erythropoietin (EPO) production with a consequent high rate of erythropoiesis. In the fetus and neonate, most EPO production occurs in the liver rather than in the kidney. After birth and the establishment of respiration, the arterial PaO_2 rises, triggering sharp declines both in EPO production and the rate of erythropoiesis. The dampened red-cell production is reflected in the disappearance of circulating nucleated RBCs and a fall in the reticulocyte count that continues for 6–8 weeks. During this period, the red-cell life span is only about 90 days, compared with 120 days in adults [65]. As a consequence of continuing RBC destruction and lack of production, hemoglobin levels in the term baby fall steadily from about 16.4 gm/dL to about 11.0 gm/DL at 6–8 weeks of age. This fall, which reflects the physiologic transition from the relatively hypoxic intrauterine environment to the oxygen replete extrauterine state, is appropriately called the *physiological anemia of infancy* [66].

After 6–8 weeks, red cell production resumes as indicated by a rise in reticulocyte count, resulting in stabilization of the hemoglobin level, and then an increase in hemoglobin level that plateaus at an average of 12.5 gm/dL for the first 5–6 years of life. The rate of RBC production is sufficient to maintain a stable hemoglobin level during childhood despite the increase in blood volume that occurs in the first years of life because of the expanding blood volume that accompanies growth.

In the preterm infant, the postnatal fall in hemoglobin concentration is more marked and occurs sooner than in the full-term infant – the smallest infants having the greatest decline in hemoglobin concentration. This is called the *early anemia of prematurity*, which is in part an exaggerated physiological anemia. Premature infants have inappropriately low EPO levels for the severity of the anemia, perhaps because hepatic EPO production is less sensitive to reduced oxygen concentrations relative to the renal production mechanism [67]. It was thought that administration of EPO might be specific therapy that would modify the degree of anemia and reduce the need for RBC transfusion. However, the possible clinical benefit of EPO therapy is controversial and today the drug is not usually routinely administered to small premature infants [68]. Other factors that contribute to the early anemia of prematurity include a very large expansion of blood volume (so-called "bleeding into the circulation!"), a red-cell life span that is even shorter than in term infants, and especially the relatively large amounts of blood often removed for laboratory studies in sick, premature infants.

Epilog

This review of the history of neonatal hematology shows clearly that the study of the blood of the fetus and newborn has captured the attention of pediatricians and hematologists over many years. It is surprising how large their contributions were and that "there is nothing new under the sun." The sagas of erythroblastosis fetalis and hemorrhagic disease of the newborn and the understanding of the physiological anemia of infancy illustrate the progress from clinical recognition and description, to definition of pathogenesis, to empiric and then specific therapy, and finally in many instances to prevention.

The majority of work and investigation in neonatal hematology has been performed by pediatric hematologists. However, there is now an emerging generation of neonatologists who have been trained in clinical and investigational hematology, who work in newborn special care units, and who have made hematology their clinical and research focus.

As we examine neonatal hematology today, the morphological and quantitative studies of earlier eras of hematology have been succeeded by a modern era of genetic, biochemical, and molecular investigations of the processes that regulate the fetal and neonatal blood and may result in diseases when they go awry. Discoveries in these areas will revolutionize neonatal hematology and, hopefully, lead to ever more effective interventions in this vulnerable population.

References

1. Wintrobe MM (ed.). *Blood, Pure and Eloquent* (New York: McGraw-Hill, 1980), pp. 1–31.

2. Leeuwenhoek A. Microscopical observations concerning blood, milk, bones, the brain, cuticula and spittle. *Philos Trans (London)* 1674;**9**:121–8.

3. Hewson W. On the figure and configuration of the red particles of the blood, commonly called the red globules. *Philos Trans* 1963;**63**(part 2):303–23.

4. Bizzozero G. Uber einen neuen Formbestandtheil des Blutes und dessen Rolle bei der Thrombose und der Blutgerinnung. *Virch Archiv Pathol Anat Physiol* 1882; **90**:261–332.

5. Osler W. An account of certain organisms occurring in the liquor sanguinis. *Proc R Soc Lond* 1874;**22**:391–8.

6. Ehrlich P. Beitrag zur Kenntnis der Amilinfarbungen und ihrer Verwendung in der mikroscopischen Technik. *Arch Mikr Anat* 1877;**13**:263–77.

7. Wintrobe MM. A simple and accurate hematocrit. *J Lab Clin Med* 1929;**15**:287–9.

8. Wintrobe MM. Anemia: Classification and treatment on the basis of differences in the average volume and hemoglobin content of the red corpuscles. *Arch Intern Med* 1934;**54**:256–80.

9. Dewees WP. *A Treatise on the Physical and Medical Treatment of Children* (Philadelphia, PA: B.C. Carey & L. Lea, 1825).

10. Smith JL. *A Treatise on the Diseases of Infancy and Childhood* (Philadelphia PA: H.C. Lea, 1869).

11. Holt LE. *The Diseases of Infancy and Childhood* (New York: D. Appleton and Co, 1897).

12. Lucas WP, Dearing BF, Hoobler HR, Cox A, Smythe F. Blood studies in the new-born:

Morphological chemical coagulation, urobilin and bilirubin. *Am J Dis Child* 1921;**22**:524–58.

13. Lippman HS. A morphologic and quantitative study of the blood corpuscles in the new-born period. *Am J Dis Child* 1924;**27**:473–526.

14. Mattoth Y, Zaizov R, Varsano L. Postnatal changes in some red cell parameters. *Acta Paediatr* 1971;**60**:317–23.

15. Korber E. Inaugural dissertation; Dorpet, 1866. Cited by Bischoff H. Untersuchungen uberdie Resistenz des Hamoglobins des menschenblutes mit besonderer beruchsichtigung des Sauglingalters. *Z Gesante Exp Med* 1926;**48**:472–89.

16. Singer K, Chernoff AI, Singer L. Studies on abnormal hemoglobins 1. Their demonstration in sickle cell anemia and other hematologic disorders by means of alkali denaturation. *Blood* 1951;**6**:413–28.

17. Apt L, Downey WS. Melena neonatorum: the swallowed blood syndrome; a simple test for the differentiation of adult and fetal hemoglobin in bloody stools. *J Pediatr* 1955;**47**:6–12.

18. Kleihauer E, Braun H, Betke K. Demonstration von fetalen Haemoglobin in den Erythrocyten eines Blutaustrichs. *Klin Wochenschr* 1957;**35**:637–8.

19. Rhinesmith HS, Schroeder WA, Pauling LA. A quantitative study of hydrolysis of human dinitrophenyl (DNP) globin: the number and kind of polypeptide chains in normal adult human hemoglobin. *J Am Chem Soc* 1957;**79**:4682–6.

20. Schroeder WA. N-terminal residues of human fetal hemoglobin. *J Am Chem Soc* 1958;**80**:1521.

21. Bensch R, Bensch RE, Yu CI. Reciprocal binding of oxygen and diphosphoglycerate by human hemoglobins. *Proc Natl Acad Sci USA* 1968;**59**:526–32.

22. Scott RB. Screening for sickle cell in newborn infants. *Am J Dis Child* 1948;**75**:842–6.

23. Pearson HA, O'Brien RT, McIntosh S, Aspenes GT, Yang MM. Routine screening of umbilical cord blood for sickle cell diseases. *J Am Med Assoc* 1974;**227**:420–2.

24. Benz EJ, Forget BG. The molecular genetics of the thalassemia syndromes. *Prog Hematol* 1975;**129**:107–55.

25. Singer ST, Styles L, Bojanski J, Vinchinsky E. Changing outcomes of homozygous alpha-thalassemia: cautious optimism. *J Pediatr Hematol Oncol* 2000;**22**:539–42.

26. Oski FA, Naiman JL. *Hematologic Problems in the Newborn* (Philadelphia, PA: W.B. Saunders Co., 1966).

27. Diamond LK, Forward. In Miller D, Pearson HA, McMillan CW, eds. *Smith's Blood Diseases of Infancy and Childhood* (St. Louis, MO: C.V. Mosby Co., 1978).

28. Diamond LK, Blackfan ED, Baty JM. Erythroblastosis fetalis, and its association with universal edema of the fetus, icterus gravis neonatorum and anemia of the newborn. *J Pediatr* 1932;**1**:269–309.

29. Darrow RR. Icterus gravis neonatorum: an examination of etiologic considerations. *Arch Pathol* 1938;**25**:378–417.

30. Landsteiner K, Weiner P. An agglutinable factor in human blood recognized by human sera for rhesus blood. *Proc Soc Exp Biol Med* 1940;**43**:223.

31. Landsteiner K. Uber Agglutinationsercheiunungen normalen menschlichen Blutes. *Wein Klin Wocheschr* 1901;**14**:1132–4.

32. Levine P, Katzin EM, Burnham L. Isoimmunization in pregnancy; its possible bearing on the etiology of erythroblastosis fetalis. *J Am Med Assoc* 1941;**116**:825–8.

33. Levine P, Burnham L. The role of isoimmunization in the pathogenesis of erythroblastosis fetalis. *Am J Obstet Gyneocol* 1941;**42**:825–7.

34. Hart AP. Familial icterus gravis of the newborn and its treatment. *Can Med Assoc J* 1925;**15**:1008–19.

35. Wallerstein H. Treatment of severe erythroblastosis by simultaneous removal and replacement of the blood of the new born infant. *Science* 1946;**103**:583–4.

36. Weiner AS, Wexler IB. The use of heparin in performing exchange transfusions in newborn infants. *J Lab Clin Med* 1946;**31**:1016–19.

37. Diamond LK. Replacement transfusion as a treatment of erythoblastosis fetalis. *Pediatrics* 1948;**2**:520–4.

38. Allen FH, Diamond LK. *Erythroblastosis Fetalis* (Boston, MA: Little, Brown Co., 1957).

39. Weiner AS. Diagnosis and treatment of anemia of the newborn caused by occult placental hemorrhage. *Am J Obstet Gynecol* 1948;**56**:717–22.

40. Chown B. Anemia from bleeding of the fetus into the mother's circulation: proof of bleeding. *Lancet* 1954;**1**:1213–15.

41. Pearson HA, Diamond LK. Fetomaternal transfusion. *Am J Dis Child* 1959;**97**:267–73.

42. Liley AW. Liquor amni analysis in the management of the pregnancy complicated by

rhesus sensitization. *Am J Obst Gynecol* 1961;**82**:1359–70.

43. Liley AW. Intrauterine transfusion of foetus in haemolytic disease. *Br Med J* 1963;**2**:1107–11.

44. Clarke CA. Prevention of Rh hemolytic disease. *Br Med J* 1967;**4**:7–12.

45. Freda VJ, Gorman JG, Pollack WI. Prevention of Rh immunization. *J Am Med Assoc* 1967;**199**:390–4.

46. Ross ME, Waldron PE, Cashore WJ, de Alarcón PA. Hemolytic disease of the fetus and newborn. In de Alarcón PA, Werner EJ, Christensen RD eds. *Neonatal Hematology* 2nd ed. (Cambridge: Cambridge University Press, 2013), pp. 80–81.

47. Garrison EH. *An Introduction to the History of Medicine*, 4th ed. (Philadelphia, PA: Saunders, 1929).

48. Quick AJ. *The Hemorrhagic Diseases and the Physiology of Hemostasis* (Springfield: IL: C.C. Thomas, 1942).

49. Townsend CW. The haemorrhagic disease of the newborn. *Arch Pediatr* 1894;**11**:559–65.

50. Whipple GH. Hemorrhagic disease. *Arch Intern Med* 1912;**9**:363–99.

51. Brinkhaus KM, Smith HP, Warner ED. Plasma protein level in normal infancy and in hemorrhagic disease of the newborn. *Am J Med Sci* 1937;**193**:475–80.

52. Lambert SW. Melena neonatorum with report of a case cured by transfusion. *Med Record* 1908;**73**:885–7.

53. Sidbury JB. Transfusion through the umbilical vein in hemorrhage of the newborn. *Am J Dis Child* 1923;**25**:290–6.

54. Zuelzer WW. Pediatric hematology in historical perspective. In Nathan DG, Orkin SH, eds. *Nathan and Oski's Hematology of Infancy and Childhood*, 5th ed. (Philadelphia, PA: W.R. Saunders, 1998).

55. Dam H, Dyggve H, Larsen H. Cholesterolstoffwechsel in Huhneriern und Huhnchen. *Biochem J* 1929;**215**:475–92.

56. Dam H, Dyggve H, Larsen H, Schonheyder F, Tage-Hansen E. Studies on the mode of action of Vitamin K. *Biochem J* 1936;**30**:1275–9.

57. Brinkhaus KM, Smith HP, Warner ED. Plasma protein level in normal infancy and in hemorrhagic disease of the newborn. *Am J Med Sci* 1937;**193**:475–80.

58. Dam H, Dyggve H, Larsen H. The relationship of vitamin K deficiency to hemorrhagic disease of the newborn. *Adv Pediatr* 1952;**5**:129–53.

59. Waddell WW, Jr., Guerry DP III, Bray WE, Waddell Kelley OR. Possible effects of vitamin K on prothrombin and clotting time in the newly born infant. *Proc Soc Exp Biol Med* 1937;**40**:432–4.

60. Almquist HJ, Klose AA. Synthetic and natural antihemorrhagic compounds. *Am J Chem Soc* 1939;**61**:2557–8.

61. Committee on Nutrition of the American Academy of Pediatrics. Vitamin K in the newborn. *Pediatrics* 1961;**28**:501–7.

62. Dam H, Glavind J, Larsen H, Plum P. Investigations into the cause of physiological hypoprothrombinemia in newborn children. IV. The vitamin K content of women's milk and cow's milk. *Acta Med Scand* 1942;**112**:210–16.

63. Sutherland JM, Glueck HL, Gleser G. Hemorrhagic disease of the newborn: breast feeding as a necessary factor in the pathogenesis. *Am J Dis Child* 1967;**113**:524–33.

64. Stentlo J, Fernlund P, Egan W, Raestorff P. Vitamin K dependent modifications of glutamic acid residues in prothrombin. *Proc Natl Acad Sci USA* 1974;**71**:2730–3.

65. Pearson HA. Life span of the fetal red blood cell. *J Pediatr* 1967;**70**:166–171.

66. O'Brien RT, Pearson HA. Physiological anemia of the new-born infant. *J. Pediatr* 1971;**79**:132–8.

67. Gallagher PG, Ehrenkranz RA. Erythropoietin therapy for anemia of prematurity. *Clin Perinatol* 1993;**20**:169–91.

68. Von Kohorn I, Ehrenkranz RA. Anemia in the preterm infant: Erythropoietin versus erythrocyte transfusion – It's not that simple. *Clin Perinatol* 2009;**36**:111–23.

Chapter

2

Hematopoiesis

Amber M. D'Souza, Pedro A. de Alarcón, and Mervin C. Yoder

Hematopoiesis refers to the continuous production and release of blood cells into the circulation. As blood cells become old or injured, self-renewing hematopoietic stem cells (HSC) proliferate and differentiate to replenish multiple hematopoietic lineages. This process produces nearly 200 billion red blood cells, 10 billion white blood cells, and 400 billion platelets every day. In addition to the requirement for high cell production, the concentration of individual blood cell lineages is precisely regulated in the peripheral blood and tissues. The production and use of circulating blood cells increase during periods of altered homeostasis such as defense against infection or replenishment of circulating red cells after hemorrhage. When the tightly regulated production of blood cells fails, the host may encounter life-threatening anemia or other cytopenias or suffer from excessive neoplastic growth of blood cells manifesting as leukemia.

During embryogenesis, hematopoiesis occurs in tightly regulated, tissue specific sites, including the extraembryonic yolk sac, para-aortic mesonephric area, fetal liver, and the preterm marrow. A harmonious relationship between hematopoietic stem cells, neighboring tissue stromal components, and hematopoietic growth factors promotes the evolution of red cell production throughout human development. This chapter will briefly review the cellular model of hematopoiesis starting in the human embryo. Although human hematopoiesis is the focus of this chapter, certain concepts gathered from murine studies will be presented to demonstrate some basic hematopoietic principles [1].

Overview of Hematopoiesis

Early Blood Cell Investigators

With the invention of the microscope came the identification of the first blood cell in the late 1600s: erythrocytes. Dutch scientist Antonie van Leeuwenhoek described red blood cells as "sanguinous globules" that were "flexible and pliant" in order to pass through small vessels [2]. Colorless white blood cells were not identified for nearly 200 more years, when a medical student named Paul Ehrlich devised a triacid stain that allowed for the identification of different white blood cell lineages based on size, nuclear shape, and cytoplasmic elements. Platelets were first described in the mid 1800s as small globules derived from plasma [3], and later established as the third element of blood, distinct from white and red cells, by Giulio Bizzozero [4]. With additional improvements in microscopes and triacid stains, the field of hematology began to expand, and changes in blood cell number, morphology, and function were correlated with specific human diseases. Further progress in studying hematopoiesis was largely limited to conjecture and opinion derived from morphologic studies of blood cell-containing tissues until the middle of the twentieth century, when hematologists began to examine the hematopoietic consequences of animal exposure to ionizing radiation [2].

Methods of Identifying Hematopoietic Stem Cells and Progenitor Cells

Assays of hematopoietic stem and progenitor cell (HSPC) potential were first developed in the 1950s–1960s. After discovering that whole-body

Neonatal Hematology, Pathogenesis, Diagnosis, and Management of Hematologic Problems, 3rd edition, ed. Pedro A. de Alarcón, Eric J. Werner, Robert D. Christensen, and Martha C. Sola-Visner. Published by Cambridge University Press. © Cambridge University Press 2021.

irradiation of animals led to significant pancyto-penia (i.e. reduction in blood cell counts), scientist Lo Jacobson discovered that mice were protected from hematopoietic effects of radiation if their spleens were shielded or if irradiated mice were subsequently infused with blood cells from a healthy mouse [5]. Confirmation that hemato-poietic cells, not plasma, conferred radiation pro-tection was reported by Ford and colleagues in 1956 [6]. In 1961, Till and McCulloch provided evidence that single, multipotent hematopoietic precursors (i.e. cells giving rise to more than one lineage of blood cells) could be identified in vivo by injecting the donor marrow cells into the spleen of a lethally irradiated recipient animal and examining the recipient spleen for hemato-poietic colonies 8 to 12 days later ([7]; Fig. 2.1). Each colony of hematopoietic cells in the spleen arose from a single precursor cell, the colony-forming unit in the spleen cell (CFU-S) [7]. Although this method advanced the study of hematopoietic stem cell biology, little was known in the early 1960s of the mechanisms that caused or permitted stem cells to differentiate into mature cells.

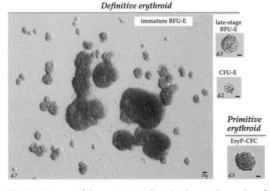

Fig. 2.1 Image of the various erythroid colonies. Examples of colonies derive from murine definitive and primitive erythroid progenitors. Immature BFU-E derived colonies, counted at day 7 of culture, typically consist of one or more large colonies surrounded by smaller colonies, which constitute a "burst." Late-stage BFU-E derived colonies, counted at day 3 of culture, consist of smaller single colonies. CFU-E derived colonies, counted at day 2 of culture, consist of a single small colony containing 16–64 hemoglobinizing cells. Primitive erythroid progenitors (EryP-CFC) derived from the mouse embryo or from differentiating mouse embryonic stem cells generate single compact grape-like colonies of large primitive erythroblasts at 5 days of in vitro culture. Abbreviations: d, day. (From Joyce A. Lloyd (ed): *Erythropoiesis: Methods and Protocols*, Methods in Molecular Biology, vol 1698, Springer, 2018, p. 119.)

In the mid 1960s, several groups demon-strated that murine hematopoietic cells could be cultured in vitro [8, 9]. Additionally, these single precursor cells, called colony-forming unit in culture (CFU-C), could differentiate into myeloid colonies when grown in the presence of soluble fluid from murine organs (i.e. urine or pregnant uterine extracts), which became known as colony-stimulating activity (CSA). Later work revealed that these colonies were composed of granulocytes, macrophages, or both (CFU-GM), and that the specific cell type formed was based on the type of CSA added. Later, using anemic mouse serum as a growth factor, Axelrad and coworkers demonstrated that red blood cell colo-nies were clonally derived in vitro, and they called the most primitive red cell precursors the erythroid burst-forming unit (BFU-E) and the most committed erythroid precursors colony-forming unit-erythroid (CFU-E) cells ([10]; see Fig. 2.1). Multipotent progenitor cells were also identified and called colony-forming unit-mix (CFU-Mix). These assays, developed for studying murine hematopoiesis, were rapidly adapted for human studies and continue to be sensitive assays for detecting human hematopoietic pro-genitor cells [11].

Because the frequency of human and murine hematopoietic stem cells is estimated to be 1 of 10^4 to 10^5 marrow cells [12, 13], the primary obstacle in studying human hematopoietic stem cell biology is that few methods can identify these rare cells. As such, results of studies of murine hematopoietic stem cells were essential to advan-cing our understanding of human hematopoi-esis. In fact, it was murine bone marrow transplantation experiments that provided the evidence to reliably identify hematopoietic stem cells, which were defined as cells that self-renew in vivo, proliferate, and differentiate into all lineages of circulating peripheral blood cells for more than 4 months after transplantation into recipient animals [14]. Because of ethical con-straints, similar in vivo reconstitution assays in human patients are not possible, and several alternative in vitro and in vivo estimates of hematopoietic precursors have been developed.

In vitro studies have identified two types of hematopoietic progenitor cells. Lineage-committed hematopoietic progenitor cells form colonies in vitro in response to one or two recombinant growth factors. In contrast, more primitive multipotent hematopoietic cells form in vitro colonies only when cultured with multiple recombinant growth factors. These results have been interpreted as evidence that the more primitive hematopoietic stem and progenitor cells (HSPC) require complex growth factor combinations to fuel or support lineage commitment and progenitor cell differentiation. Plating hematopoietic stem cells in special double-layer agar cultures with multiple recombinant cytokines permits identification of blood progenitors that are highly proliferative (i.e., high proliferative potential colony-forming cells (HPP-CFC)). High proliferative potential colony-forming cells produce colonies containing more than 50,000 cells that are visible without magnification (most CFU-Cs are less than 50,000 and microscopic) and are considered to be the most primitive progenitor cell grown in semisolid medium without added stromal cells.

Additionally, complex in vitro cultures of hematopoietic stem cells with a monolayer of bone marrow or fetal liver stromal cells (includes macrophages, endothelial cells, fibroblasts, and preadipocytes) results in sustained hematopoiesis for several months [15]. The most primitive hematopoietic cells (i.e. those giving rise to hematopoietic progenitors) reside beneath the stromal monolayers, whereas the mature blood cells produced are released into the tissue culture medium as nonadherent cells [16]. Using limiting dilution analysis, the number of such murine or human long-term culture-initiating cells (LTC-IC) that give rise to multipotent and committed progenitors for 3 to 4 weeks in vitro can be calculated [17]. As such, LTC-IC are considered to be the most primitive hematopoietic precursor detectable by means of in vitro assays.

In attempts to develop an in vivo system for detection of human hematopoietic stem cells, several groups developed xenotransplantation models. Enriched populations of human hematopoietic stem cells from human bone marrow, cord blood, or fetal liver have been observed to engraft in the pre-immune sheep fetus (<60 days of gestation) with long-term evidence of multilineage peripheral human blood cell chimerism in the transplanted animals [18]. Nonobese diabetic (NOD) mice bred with severe combined immunodeficient (SCID) mice produce NOD/SCID mice that accept human hematopoietic grafts [19]. This NOD/SCID model permits calculation of the frequency of human repopulating cells in a donor sample, but it remains unclear whether this assay is robust and can accurately identify the same hematopoietic stem cells that repopulate the blood system of a larger animal such as a nonhuman primate [20]. More recent immunodeficient murine models apparently permit higher levels of human cell engraftment and even full lymphoid reconstitution under certain circumstances, but these models have not yet been compared to the nonhuman primate models for detection of engrafting long-term repopulating human stem cells [21–24].

Stem Cell Model of Hematopoiesis

The stem cell theory of hematopoiesis posits that the hematopoietic system comprises a continuum of functionally distinct hematopoietic cell compartments. Stem cells are rare, self-renewing, relatively quiescent cells (Fig. 2.2). In the mouse, hematopoietic stem cells have a half-life (i.e., time to 50% of stem cells cycled) of approximately 19 days [25], though slower rates may be identified in a subset [26]. Stem cells can divide to give rise to a daughter cell that retains all of the pluripotentiality of the parent (i.e., self-renewal) or can proliferate into daughter cells that have lost some multipotentiality and have become committed to producing progenitor cells [27]. After the commitment decision is made, the progenitor cell gives rise to progressively more lineage-committed hematopoietic progenitor cells and eventually to mature blood cells (see Fig. 2.2). It remains unclear how hematopoietic stem cells become committed to follow a certain lineage, but thought to be regulated by multiple environmental factors including tissue specific growth factors, cytokines, metabolic products, oxygen levels, extracellular matrix molecules, or cell-cell interaction and feedback loops [28–32].

With the development of flow cytometry, monoclonal antibodies to cell-surface antigens, and in vivo and in vitro assays for primitive hematopoietic cells, investigators succeeded in identifying enriched populations of human hematopoietic stem cells and provided evidence that a single murine hematopoietic stem cell is sufficient to restore multilineage hematopoiesis in an irradiated host [33, 34]. Purification of hematopoietic stem cells permitted investigators to pursue basic investigations of stem cell biology that translated into new methods for human hematopoietic transplantations and improved

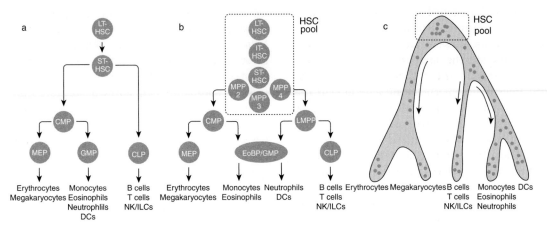

Fig. 2.2 Timeline of hierarchical models of hematopoiesis. (a) Visualization based on cutting-edge research around the year 2000: HSC are represented as a homogeneous population, downstream of which the first lineage bifurcation separates the myeloid and lymphoid branches via the common myeloid progenitor (CMP) and common lymphoid progenitor (CLP) populations. (b) During the years 2005–2015, this visualization incorporates new findings: The HSC pool is now accepted to be more heterogeneous both in terms of self-renewal (vertical axis) and differentiation properties (horizontal axis), the myeloid and lymphoid branches remain associated further down in the hierarchy via the lymphoid-primed multipotential progenitor (LMPP) population, the GMP compartment is shown to be fairly heterogeneous. (c) From 2016 onwards, single-cell transcriptomic snapshots indicate a continuum of differentiation. Each red dot represents a single cell and its localization along a differentiation trajectory. Abbreviations: DCs, dendritic cells; EoBP, eosinophil–basophil progenitor; GMP, granulocyte–monocyte progenitors; LT, long-term; ILCs, innate lymphoid cells; MEP, megakaryocyte–erythrocyte progenitors; NK, natural killer cells; ST, short-term. (From Laurenti E, Göttgens B. From haematopoietic stem cells to complex differentiation landscapes. *Nature* 2018; **553**(7689):418–26.) (See plate section for color version.)

methods of somatic gene transfer. Further studies to examine hematopoietic stem cell function in patients with bone marrow failure syndromes and hematologic malignancies will also probably translate into clinical therapies.

A significant challenge to the in vitro study of hematopoietic stem cells is the realization that many of the growth factors required to stimulate the in vitro proliferation and differentiation of hematopoietic progenitor cells are associated with measurable declines in the concentrations of functional hematopoietic stem cells. Although certain stromal cell lines and primary human or murine stromal cells can maintain hematopoietic stem cell function in vitro, only in the last several decades have tissue culture conditions been developed that permit expansion of murine hematopoietic cell numbers with retention of individual hematopoietic stem cell self-renewal and reconstituting ability [35–37]. The conditions to support in vitro expansion of adult human and murine bone marrow hematopoietic progenitor cells indicate that the proliferative potential and growth factor requirements for survival in vitro differ among hematopoietic cells during ontogeny [36, 38].

Embryonic Hematopoiesis

Studies of Murine Embryonic Hematopoiesis

The murine visceral yolk sac is composed of visceral endoderm and mesoderm cells that proliferate, differentiate, migrate, and co-localize during gastrulation. The endoderm cells face the yolk sac cavity and are highly active in the absorption of material from the maternal circulation and in the biosynthesis and secretion of numerous nutrients [39]. In the mouse, yolk sac endoderm cells are also the primary route for transporting maternal immunoglobulins into the embryo. The mesoderm cells of the yolk sac give rise to blood islands containing blood cells and endothelial cells [40–42]. The simultaneous appearance of endothelial and hematopoietic cells in the blood islands, the apparent intimate cell-to-cell contact of the blood island endothelial and hematopoietic cells, and the shared requirements for certain growth factors and growth factor receptors support the idea that blood island endothelial cells and hematopoietic cells must be derived from a common precursor, called the hemangioblast [41–43]. Study of the hemangioblast remains elusive, although some reports have suggested that isolating the cell is feasible in the murine or chick embryo [43–46].

The precise temporal and spatial origins of the first hematopoietic stem cells in the murine embryo remain unknown. Studies using chicks and frogs indicate that the mesoderm cells that become committed to the formation of blood cells migrate from the posterior primitive streak and into the embryo and the extraembryonic yolk sac [40]. The mesoderm cells contributing to the formation of murine blood cells are also restricted to the posterior primitive streak at 6.75 days postconception (DPC). Some mesoderm cells fated to become blood cells migrate along the extraembryonic endoderm cells and participate in forming the extraembryonic yolk, sac blood islands [40]. Presumably, certain mesoderm cells are acted on by local factors to undergo differentiation into endothelial and hematopoietic stem and progenitor cells. Although little is known about the factors that induce murine mesodermal cell commitment to blood and endothelial differentiation, some evidence suggests that certain transcription factors and growth factor receptors are required for this process [28, 47]. Because blood cells arise from different sites at different times during murine embryogenesis, the site of origin of

hematopoietic stem cells remains a vital question in experimental hematology. Hematopoietic stem cells may arise de novo in each hematopoietic site during ontogeny [48, 49]. Alternatively, all hematopoietic stem cells may arise in the embryonic yolk sac and/or the para-aortic splanchnopleura (PS) and migrate to all other sites during development [50–53]. Several groups of investigators have identified hematopoietic stem cell activity in the mouse that appears to originate from the ventral wall of the embryonic paired dorsal aorta and/or from the subendothelial mesenchyme of the PS [54–58]. The most recent data suggest that all murine hematopoietic stem and progenitor cells that reside in the bone marrow compartment are derived from hemogenic endothelium present in embryonic and extraembryonic vessels [57, 59, 60]. It is also apparent that biomechanical forces generated by flowing blood promote the emergence of the first blood cells [61–63].

Differentiated blood cells are first recognizable in the murine yolk sac at 7 DPC. The primary cells observed are nucleated red blood cells expressing embryonic forms of hemoglobin [64]. Hematopoiesis peaks in the murine yolk sac at 11 DPC, and the liver becomes the predominant site of hematopoiesis at 12 DPC. The murine fetal

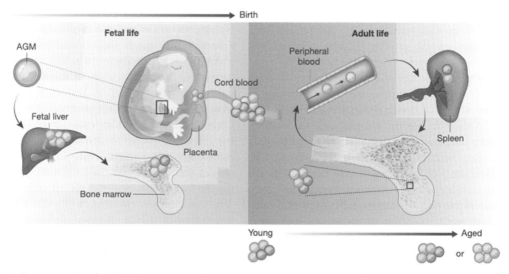

Fig. 2.3 The composition of the HSPC compartment changes in space and time. HSPCs are found in many organs in the body across a lifetime. Cells of different colors represent distinct HSPC subsets. It is unclear whether all HSPC subsets and differentiation trajectories are present in the same proportion in each of the organs. Current evidence suggests that age-related changes result from a combination of shifts in the composition of the HSPC pool, as well as phenotypic changes in particular cell types driven by intrinsic genetic or epigenetic changes and systemic alterations of the microenvironment. Abbreviation: AGM, aorta gonad mesonephros. (From Laurenti E, Göttgens B. From haematopoietic stem cells to complex differentiation landscapes. *Nature* 2018;**553** (7689):418–26.) (See plate section for color version.)

liver remains the primary site of hematopoiesis until the time of birth, when the bone marrow and to some extent the spleen provide lifelong provision of circulating blood cells (Fig. 2.3). Although red blood cell production predominates in the liver and spleen, white blood cell production predominates in the bone marrow compartment [64].

The pattern of hematopoietic cell differentiation also varies greatly in the yolk sac and PS. Primitive red blood cells, macrophages, and megakaryocytes are produced in the early yolk sac. The red blood cells are called primitive because they are large, nucleated cells that contain forms of hemoglobin expressed only during the embryonic phase of development. Other hematopoietic progenitors emerging in the yolk sac include BFU-E (expressing primitive and adult-type hemoglobins), CFU-GM, and CFU-Mix that vary with the age of the donor embryo [65]. Culture of hematopoietic progenitors from the PS gives rise to BFU-E and CFU-GM that are composed of cells with definitive features; red blood cells are enucleated and synthesize adult-type hemoglobins, and granulocytes predominate over macrophages in the CFU-GM. Of interest, more recent data suggest that all of the circulating definitive progenitor cells that seed the fetal liver at 10 DPC and differentiate into mature elements by 12 DPC are derived from the yolk sac and not the embryo proper [66].

Studies of Human Embryonic Hematopoiesis

The inability to use transplantation methods for identification of hematopoietic stem cells in human patients has limited the analysis of stem cell function during human embryonic hematopoiesis. However, much of the ontogeny of blood cell production in the human embryo has been described using morphologic approaches and some in vitro hematopoietic progenitor cell assays. Human hematopoiesis occurs in a sequential process throughout the embryonic and fetal period: the yolk sac, the aorta–gonad–mesonephros region (AGM), the fetal liver, and finally the bone marrow (see Fig. 2.3). This section reviews the formation and function of the human yolk sac, determination of the site and kinetics of blood cell appearance, and determination of the number and behavior of cultured human embryonic hematopoietic progenitor cells.

The human yolk sac develops in three stages: a formative period, a period of yolk sac function, and a period of yolk sac regression [67]. The first phase of yolk sac formation can be further subdivided into formation of the primary and secondary yolk sacs. The primary yolk sac is formed after implantation (7 to 8 DPC) by proliferation and differentiation of primitive endoderm cells into visceral endoderm adjacent to the developing embryonic disk and parietal endoderm projecting into the uterine lumen. This simple bilaminar structure has no identifiable function, but the endoderm cells lining the primary yolk sac give rise to mesodermal precursors (i.e. intermediate cells) that colonize the space between the yolk sac cavity and the surrounding trophoblast cells. The primary yolk sac then appears to collapse, with heterogeneous foci of re-expansion breaking up the primary yolk sac into smaller vesicles. The secondary yolk sac is formed (12 to 15 DPC) from the remnants of the primary yolk sac (i.e. parietal endoderm and mesoderm) that are contiguous with the visceral endoderm underlying the embryonic disk.

The secondary yolk sac is an active site of protein biosynthesis, nutrient transport, and hematopoiesis. A variety of proteins are synthesized including albumin, alpha–fetoprotein, prealbumin, apolipoproteins, insulin-like growth factor, transferrin, vascular endothelial growth factor, and colony-stimulating factor 1 (i.e. macrophage colony-stimulating factor) [67]. The endodermal component of the secondary yolk sac is a transporter of proteins and vitamins [68]. Another primary function of the secondary yolk sac is to produce hematopoietic cells. The first primitive red blood cells in the yolk sac adhere to surrounding endothelial cells, and these hematopoietic-endothelial masses are called blood islands [69]. Commensurate with blood island formation, the mesenchymal layer in the secondary yolk sac thickens, but the endoderm layer is not affected.

Macroscopically, the secondary yolk sac begins as a small structure (<0.4 mm) but steadily increases in size to 2 mm by day 19, to 4–5 mm by 7 weeks, and 6–6.5 mm by the end of week 10. As the yolk sac matures, an extensive network of superficial capillaries is formed as the blood island endothelial cells migrate toward one another and form vascular channels. The secondary yolk sac circulation is fed and drained by the vitelline arteries and veins, which connect the embryonic to the extraembryonic circulation. Initially, the vitelline vessels empty into the sinus venosus of the liver, establishing a preportal-type circulation. Later in gestation, the yolk sac regresses, new capillaries arising from the developing gut contribute to the vitelline circulation, and as the liver cords proliferate, the portal circulation is established [70, 71]. Although evident until week 12 of development, the yolk sac begins regressing around week 10, with progressive evidence of tissue degeneration and with loss of blood flow through the yolk sac vascular network [67, 72].

Many twentieth century investigators using microscopic analysis of tissue sections of human embryonic tissues described the sequence of hematopoietic development that occurs in the human embryo and fetus [73–75]. During human development in utero, blood cells first arise in the yolk sac between days 16 and 19, followed sequentially by fetal liver hematopoiesis by weeks 5 to 6 and engraftment and expansion of hematopoietic cells in developing long bones by weeks 8 to 19 (e.g., most bones become hematopoietic between weeks 11 and 12) [76, 77]. The liver functions as the primary site of hematopoiesis from weeks 6 through 22 of gestation until the bone marrow becomes the lifelong predominant site of blood cell production. Distinct patterns of blood cell differentiation and proliferation occur in each specific site of hematopoiesis during ontogeny [78, 79].

The most extensive morphologic analysis of hematopoiesis in the developing human was reported in a 1979 monograph by Kelemen and colleagues [76]. These investigators studied tissue sections from 190 human embryos of between 3 and 28 weeks of gestation. Hematopoietic cells were first observed in the human embryo at day 18 in the mesenchymal layer of the secondary yolk sac. Most blood islands were composed of hematopoietic cells completely surrounded by endothelial cells, but some extravascular free aggregates of blood cells were present in the mesenchyme close to the visceral endoderm. The 3- to 4-week embryo had more defined vessels, many of which were empty of hematopoietic cells. Frequently, small clusters of undifferentiated cells called hemocytoblasts (equivalent to the hemangioblast in the mouse) associated with the endothelium protruded into the vessel lumen. Concomitantly, clusters of primitive erythroblasts

(>20 μm cells with central to eccentric nucleus and orthochromatic cytoplasmic staining) began to fill capillaries and larger vessels (e.g., vitelline, umbilical, chorionic, and amniotic). Wherever the number of primitive erythroblasts predominated in vessels, few hemocytoblasts were detectable. This was a surprising finding, because the erythroblasts had previously been thought to originate from the hemocytoblasts [48]. At the sixth week of development, intraembryonic and extraembryonic blood vessels became macroscopically visible, and definitive erythroblasts (<20 μm cells with condensed nuclei and abundant hemoglobin cytoplasmic staining) and primitive erythroblasts could be identified in the yolk sac vessels. The only other mature blood cell in the yolk sac was the macrophage. In contrast to normal fetal liver and bone marrow patterns of differentiation, macrophages in the yolk sac arose without evidence of a monocytic precursor. An overall decline in hematopoiesis was observed in the human yolk sac after the eighth week of gestation.

Hematopoiesis occurred in the liver by the fifth to sixth week of gestation. The establishment of the systemic circulation (weeks 4 to 5) had just commenced before liver hematopoiesis at week 5. The predominant blood cell observed in the large vessels and in developing liver sinusoids was the primitive erythroblast. Over the next 4 weeks, there was a shift away from the primitive to the definitive erythroblast. Mature enucleated red blood cell production in the fetus was associated with a 40-fold increase in the total liver mass, with hematopoietic cells comprising 60% of the total cell number (weeks 11 to 12). Macrophages, megakaryocytes, granulocytes, and lymphocytes also were identifiable during weeks 5 through 22. Macrophages were the predominant mature blood cell type identified early in liver hematopoiesis (weeks 5 to 6), but the concentration of macrophages diminished thereafter. Megakaryocytes were present throughout the liver phase of hematopoiesis, but a notable shift from megakaryocytes with one to two nuclei to megakaryocytes with four or more nuclei occurred as liver hematopoiesis diminished (weeks 18 to 21) and bone marrow hematopoiesis began to flourish. The few granulocytes were restricted to the connective tissue of the hepatic portal area from weeks 5 through 15. A significant increase in granulocytes was observed beyond week 21 of development, coinciding with enhanced hematopoiesis in the bone marrow. Lymphocytes were sparse until week 7 of development, and even through week 13, they remained a minor population (1% of blood cells) in the liver. It was not evident whether these lymphocytes were of the B or T cell lineage, but the thymus did not have lymphocytes until week 9. The percentage of hemocytoblasts (presumed stem cells) was high (10% of blood cells) in the 5- to 6-week embryo liver but declined for the remainder of the liver phase of hematopoiesis.

The earliest bone marrow sample in which hematopoietic cells were present was taken from an embryo at week 8 of development. The predominant cell type at 8 to 9 weeks was the primitive erythroblast. Definitive erythroblast production increased greatly from weeks 11 through 14, and by 14 weeks, nearly all erythroblasts were definitive types. It was speculated that primitive erythroblasts were presented to the marrow by means of the systemic circulation and that only definitive erythroblasts were produced in the marrow. Erythrocytic cells constituted about 35% of total marrow cells by week 12 and 20% to 30% thereafter. At weeks 8 to 9 of embryonic development, granulocytes were observed in the marrow of long bones. Neutrophilic granulocytes composed 30% to 40% of total marrow cells between weeks 10 and 13. By 21 weeks, neutrophilic granulocytes were the major blood cell produced, representing nearly 60% of hematopoietic cells in the marrow. Eosinophilic granulocytes (1%) were present in the marrow of embryos at week 10 and gradually increased to nearly 5% of total marrow cells by week 21. Basophilic granulocytes were few in the 10-week embryo and remained low (0.3%) even in the 28-week embryo. Macrophages were most numerous in the embryonic marrow at weeks 10 through 16, whereas monocytes peaked between weeks 12 and 16. Lymphocytes increased from 12% of total marrow cells at week 12 to 20% to 30% in older embryos. Megakaryocytes were present in all samples examined. The percentage of immature "blast cells," which probably represented hematopoietic stem and progenitor cells, varied from 15% at weeks 12 through 13 to 1% to 4% at weeks 21 through 23. Whereas erythropoiesis exceeded granulocytopoiesis in the 10- to 11-week-old embryo (erythropoiesis/granulopoiesis ratio of 0.8), granulopoiesis predominated by week 12 and reached a nearly adult ratio of 3 (1.8 to 3.3) by the twenty-first week of human development.

Splenic hematopoiesis in the human embryo has been difficult to prove. At 8 weeks of gestation, the spleen is composed primarily of a meshwork of mesenchymal cells with some primitive erythroblasts contained in the blood vessels [76]. Few macrophage and neutrophil precursors were present in the spleen at 8 weeks. The hematopoietic cells in the spleen were dispersed throughout, but most erythroblasts were confined to the vascular system. This distribution of hematopoietic cells in the spleen contrasted with the same-stage embryo liver in which the developing blood cells were confined to focal sites of hematopoiesis. Similar observations were made by other investigators [80], and these results raised the question of whether the hematopoietic cells observed in the embryonic spleen were circulating blood cells or were cells produced in the spleen [80].

Calhoun and coworkers used several methods to determine whether the human mid-gestation spleen (13 to 22 weeks' gestation) was an active site of hematopoiesis [81]. Liver, spleen, and bone marrow samples were examined by histology, and cell suspensions from each site were prepared for enumeration of mature blood cells and their immediate precursors. Lymphocytes, macrophages, and erythroid cells predominated at 13 weeks' gestation. Neither mature nor immature neutrophils were identified in the spleen until 16 weeks' gestation. Throughout the study period, active foci of hematopoiesis were present in the liver and bone marrow but never in the spleen. Because the distribution of blood cells observed for the splenic suspensions was similar to the blood cell concentrations previously reported after fetal blood sampling [82], these results in total suggest that the mid-gestation human spleen is not normally an active hematopoietic organ [81].

Numerous investigators extended these morphologic observations by examining the onset of human hematopoiesis by means of functional assays of hematopoietic CFU-C formation and by using cell-surface antigen detection to identify specific hematopoietic lineages (i.e. monoclonal antibodies with immunohistochemical or FACS analysis). Although many studies have focused on human fetal liver and marrow hematopoiesis, little is known about the biology of hematopoietic stem and progenitor cells that arise in the human yolk sac. The data reviewed indicate that the transient population of yolk sac hematopoietic cells differs in many aspects from hematopoietic cells produced within the embryo proper or in the liver or bone marrow.

Migliaccio and colleagues performed a careful examination of the kinetics of yolk sac CFU-C in human embryos from 4.5 to 10 weeks' gestation [83]. This stage encompassed the period of yolk sac hematopoietic decline and initiation of liver hematopoiesis. CFU-E and BFU-E were abundant in the yolk sac of the 4.5-week embryos. CFU-GMs were also present in high concentration. At 5 weeks, the liver contained abundant primitive erythroblasts and some macrophages in the hepatic sinusoids. The concentrations of CFU-E, BFU-E, and CFU-GM in the liver rose rapidly over the next 3 weeks and reached a plateau by 8 to 9 weeks of gestation. Although definitive erythropoiesis (i.e. CFU-E and BFU-E) predominated for the remainder of the fetal liver phase of hematopoiesis, CFU-GMs increased from week 8 through 12 and remained stable until almost 20 weeks, when the number of myeloid progenitor cells declined [84]. Concomitant with the changes in progenitor cell concentrations, the percentage of circulating and tissue-restricted mature blood cells of the myeloerythroid lineages changed as hematopoiesis shifted from the yolk sac to the liver. A gradual shift from primarily embryonic to primarily fetal and adult hemoglobin molecules also occurred in yolk sac and liver BFU-E-derived red blood cells respectively, during the fifth through eighth weeks of gestation [85].

Investigators have also attempted to isolate and enrich populations of hematopoietic stem and progenitor cells from the developing human embryo. Through the use of monoclonal antibodies and FACS, a stem cell-surface "phenotype" has emerged that is useful in isolating hematopoietic progenitor and putative hematopoietic stem cells [86]. Because numerous monoclonal antibodies may recognize the same cell-surface antigen, an international classification is assigned to each monoclonal antibody; all monoclonal antibodies reacting with a single blood cell-surface antigen are given a cluster of differentiation (CD) number designation [87].

The CD34 antigen is one that has been used extensively in the positive selection of human adult hematopoietic stem and progenitor cells [88]. CD34, a cell-surface sialomucin, is also expressed on human fetal liver hematopoietic cells; more CD34 is expressed on the fetal hematopoietic progenitor cells than on adult hematopoietic progenitor cells [89]. The cell-surface phenotype that permits the highest enrichment of committed and primitive hematopoietic progenitor cells is found in embryonic and fetal hematopoietic cells that do not express any mature blood cell lineage antigens (lin−), CD38 (a transmembrane glycoprotein), or CD71 (transferrin receptor) but express CD4, CD34, CD117 (KIT tyrosine kinase receptor), and CD90 (Thy-1 antigen) [89–91]. Other antigens that are more controversial with regard to enriching for hematopoietic stem and progenitor cell activity in the embryo and fetus include expression of CD15 (3-fucosyl-N-acetyl-lactosamine), and human major histocompatibility complex class II antigen (HAD-DR)[90].

The CD34+ hematopoietic progenitor cells have been identified as early as day 23 of human gestation in the yolk sac and within the embryo proper [92]. The intraembryonic CD34+ cells were localized to the ventral aspect of the dorsal aorta around the peri-umbilical region, or the AGM. The hematopoietic clusters were in the luminal side in tight association with the endothelial cells [92]. When tissue explants of the peri-umbilical aortic region, liver, heart, limbs, blood, and umbilical cord of embryos at days 30 through 40 of gestation were co-cultured in vitro with a murine bone marrow stromal cell line, fivefold more hematopoietic progenitors were derived from the peri-umbilical aortic region than from all other sites combined [92]. Additionally, long-term hematopoietic engraftment was achieved by transplanting cells from the AGM into immuno-deficient mice [93]. These results confirmed the presence of hematopoietic progenitor cells in the human embryo at sites distinct from the yolk sac and liver and more recently have defined vascular endothelium as the cells giving rise to the hematopoietic clusters [94, 95]. Huyhn and coworkers isolated yolk sac, liver, and embryonic tissues from 25 to 40-day-gestation embryos and plated the enzyme-disaggregated samples in methylcellulose cultures for detection of hematopoietic progenitor cells [96]. Although the concentration of BFU-E in the yolk sacs and embryo proper were similar, 7–12-fold higher numbers of CFU-GM were present in the embryo proper than in the yolk sac. These results were interpreted as evidence that intraembryonic hematopoietic precursors occur in high concentrations when the liver is initiating hematopoiesis.

In addition to differences in progenitor cell concentration in the 25- to 50-day yolk sac, liver, and embryo samples, distinct differences in the biology of the hematopoietic progenitors were also observed. Yolk sac BFU-Es were distinct from liver and embryo proper-derived BFU-Es by being larger and containing dispersed myeloid cells on microscopic examination. It appeared that the yolk sac BFU-Es were more primitive (i.e. containing erythroid and myeloid progenitor activity) than typical adult marrow-derived BFU-Es [12]. Dose-response curves analyzing the in vitro growth factor responsiveness of the progenitor cells did not indicate any difference in the growth factor sensitivity of progenitors from these sites [96]. The CFU-E concentrations were low in the yolk sac and embryo proper but were abundant in the liver. These CFU-E results contrast with the findings of Migliaccio and coworkers, who observed high numbers of yolk sac CFU-Es in the 4.5- to 5-week human embryonic yolk sac [83]. The discrepant results have not been resolved.

The yolk sac and embryo proper are known to be composed of hematopoietic cells demonstrating HPP-CFC activity. The CD34$^+$ hematopoietic cells recovered from the yolk sac and embryo yielded 45 HPP-CFC and 20 HPP-CFC, respectively, with 10,000 CD34$^+$ cells were plated with specific combinations of growth factors [96]. All CD34$^+$ progenitors and HPP-CFC in the yolk sac and embryo proper failed to express CD38 or CD33, consistent with the pattern of expression observed for adult marrow hematopoietic stem cells.

The LTC-IC concentration is reported to be higher in fetal liver CD34$^+$CD38$^-$ cells than in phenotypically similar adult marrow cells, and the number of secondary colonies derived from cultured LTC-IC was sevenfold higher in fetal liver compared with adult marrow CD34$^+$CD38$^-$ cells [97]. Hematopoietic stem cells from the livers of 12- to 15-week gestation human fetuses can engraft and produce circulating blood cell progeny for more than 2 years after in utero transplantation into preimmune fetal sheep [18, 98]. Human fetal liver cells can also engraft and repopulate blood cell lineages in human patients with a variety of hematopoietic disorders [99, 100].

No published reports have characterized the biology of hematopoietic stem and progenitor cells in the human late embryonic and early fetal bone marrow. Several groups have isolated enriched populations of hematopoietic cells from the bone marrow (e.g. tibias and femurs) of human fetuses at 12 to 24 weeks' gestation. Turner and colleagues compared in vivo repopulating ability of CD34$^+$ cells isolated from fetal bone marrow, adult bone marrow, and mobilized peripheral blood cells (e.g. patients treated for 5 to 7 days with recombinant growth factors and blood cells collected by apheresis)[101]. The fetal marrow cells expanded to constitute 23% of the total number of marrow and spleen cells in 15% of the recipient mice, whereas adult marrow cells only engrafted in 2% of the recipients. Human peripheral blood cells engrafted in 3% of the mice but only in the T lymphocyte lineage. The investigators concluded that fetal marrow appears superior to adult marrow and mobilized peripheral blood in engrafting in this xenograft model and that human hematopoiesis can occur in this model without the administration of human cytokines to recipient mice. One factor that may have contributed to the high level of fetal marrow engraftment in the mice was that 18- and 9-fold more CD34$^+$ cells were recovered in the fetal marrow than in the mobilized peripheral blood and adult bone marrow, respectively.

While the use of human embryonic hematopoietic stem cells has not been widely applied for therapeutic transplantation, human umbilical cord blood has emerged as an effective alternative to adult bone marrow as a source of transplantable stem cells [102–106]. Human embryonic stem (hES) cell-derived hematopoietic stem cells has been proposed as an emerging hopeful inexhaustible alternative to all current sources of stem cells, though progress in defining full multilineage engraftment from a hES cell has been elusive [107–110]. Most encouraging are the increasing amounts of literature on reprogramming human somatic cells to pluripotent stem cells [111–113]. Indeed, recent work has demonstrated that human pluripotent stem cells can be differentiated into human hematopoietic stem and progenitor cells and that adult murine endothelial cells may be directly programmed into hematopoietic stem cells [114, 115]. These exciting developments may provide novel approaches to treating human disease, but more work is needed to understand the molecular regulation of hematopoietic stem cell development, and as such, both great challenges and life-altering opportunities lie ahead.

References

1. Purton LE, Scadden DT. Limiting factors in murine hematopoietic stem cell assays. *Cell Stem Cell* 2007;**1**:263–70.

2. Wintrobe, M. Milestones on the path of progress. *In* Wintrobe, M. ed. *Blood, Pure, and Eloquent* (New York: McGraw-Hill, 1980), p. 1.

3. Donne, A. De I-oringe des gloubles du sang, de leur mode de formation et de leur fin. *C R Seances Acad Sci* 1842;366–8.

4. Bizzozero, G. Uber einen Formbestandteil des Blutes und dessen Rolle bei der Thrombose und der Blutgerinnung. *Virch Archiv Pathol Anat Physiol* 1882; **90**:261–332.

5. Jacobson LO, Marks EK, et al. The role of the spleen in radiation injury. *Proc Soc Exp Biol Med* 1949;**70**:740–2.

6. Ford CE, Hamerton JL, Barnes DW, Loutit JF. Cytological identification of radiation-chimaeras. *Nature* 1956;**177**:452–4.

7. Becker AJ, McCulloch EA, Till JE. Cytological demonstration of the clonal nature of spleen colonies derived from transplanted mouse marrow cells. *Nature* 1963;**197**:452–4.

8. Pluznik DH, Sachs L. The cloning of normal "mast" cells in tissue culture. *J Cell Physiol* 1965;**66**:319–24.

9. Bradley TR, Metcalf D. The growth of mouse bone marrow cells in vitro. *Aust J Exp Biol Med Sci* 1966;**44**:287–99.

10. Stephenson JR, Axelrad AA, McLeod DL, Shreeve MM. Induction of colonies of hemoglobin-synthesizing cells by erythropoietin in vitro. *Proc Natl Acad Sci USA* 1971;**68**:1542–6.

11. Spangrude GJ. Biological and clinical aspects of hematopoietic stem cells. *Annu Rev Med* 1994;**45**:93–104.

12. Harrison DE. Competitive repopulation: a new assay for long-term stem cell functional capacity. *Blood* 1980;**55**:77–81.

13. Sutherland HJ, Eaves CJ, Eaves AC, Dragowska W, Lansdorp PM. Characterization and partial purification of human marrow cells capable of initiating long-term hematopoiesis in vitro. *Blood* 1989;**74**:1563–70.

14. Orlic D, Bodine DM. What defines a pluripotent hematopoietic stem cell (PHSC): will the real PHSC please stand up! *Blood* 1994;**84**:3991–4.

15. Dexter TM, Allen TD, Lajtha LG. Conditions controlling the proliferation of haemopoietic stem cells in vitro. *J Cell Physiol* 1977;**91**:335–44.

16. Ploemacher RE, van der Sluijs JP, Voerman JS, Brons NH. An in vitro limiting-dilution assay of long-term repopulating hematopoietic stem cells in the mouse. *Blood* 1989;**74**:2755–63.

17. Verfaillie CM, Miller JS. A novel single-cell proliferation assay shows that long-term culture-initiating cell (LTC-IC) maintenance over time results from the extensive proliferation of a small fraction of LTC-IC. *Blood* 1995;**86**:2137–45.

18. Zanjani, ED. Pallavicini MG, Ascensao JL, et al. Engraftment and long-term expression of human fetal hemopoietic stem cells in sheep following transplantation in utero. *J Clin Invest* 1992:**89**;1178–88.

19. Shultz, LD. Schweitzer PA, Christianson SW, et al. Multiple defects in innate and adaptive immunologic function in NOD/LtSz-scid mice. *J Immunol* 1995;**154**:180–91.

20. Mezquita P, Beard BC, Kiem H-P. NOD/SCID repopulating cells contribute only to short-term repopulation in the baboon. *Gene Ther* 2008;**15**:1460–2.

21. Park YS, Lee CH, Kim JW, Shin S, Park CM. Differentiation of hepatocellular carcinoma from its various mimickers in liver magnetic resonance imaging: What are the tips when using hepatocyte-specific agents? *World J Gastroenterol* 2016;**22**:284–99.

22. Okada S, Harada H, Ito T, Saito T, Suzu S. Early development of human hematopoietic and acquired immune systems in new born NOD/Scid/Jak3null mice intrahepatic engrafted with cord blood-derived CD34+ cells. *Int J Hematol* 2008;**88**:476–82.

23. Traggiai, E. Chicha L, Mazzucchelli L, et al. Development of a human adaptive immune system in cord blood cell-transplanted mice. *Science* 2004;**304**:104–7.

24. Ishikawa F, Yasukawa M, Lyons B, et al. Development of functional human blood and immune systems in NOD/SCID/IL2 receptor {gamma} chain(null) mice. *Blood* 2005;**106**:1565–73.

25. Bradford GB, Williams B, Rossi R, Bertoncello I. Quiescence, cycling, and turnover in the primitive hematopoietic stem cell compartment. *Exp Hematol* 1997;**25**:445–53.

26. Foudi A, Hochedlinger K, van Buren D, et al. Analysis of histone 2B-GFP retention reveals slowly cycling hematopoietic stem cells. *Nat Biotechnol* 2009;**27**:84–90.

27. Ogawa M. Differentiation and proliferation of hematopoietic stem cells. *Blood* 1993;**81**:2844–53.

28. Watowich SS, Wu H, Socolovsky M, et al. Cytokine receptor signal transduction and the control of hematopoietic cell development. *Annu Rev Cell Dev Biol* 1996;**12**:91–128.

29. Enver T, Pera M, Peterson C, Andrews PW. Stem cell states, fates, and the rules of attraction. *Cell Stem Cell* 2009;**4**:387–97.

30. Golan K, Kumari A, Kollet O, et al. Daily onset of light and darkness differentially controls hematopoietic stem cell differentiation and maintenance. *Cell Stem Cell* 2018;**23**:572–85, doi:10.1016/j.stem.2018.08.002.

31. Wang C, Cheng L. Gankyrin as a potential therapeutic target for cancer. *Invest New Drugs* 2017;**35**:655–6, doi:10.1007/s10637-017-0474-8.

32. Okawa S, Nicklas S, Zickenrott S, Schwamborn JC, Del Sol AA. Generalized gene-regulatory network model of stem cell differentiation for predicting lineage specifiers. *Stem Cell Rep* 2016;**7**:307–15.

33. Osawa M, Hanada K, Hamada H, Nakauchi H. Long-term lymphohematopoietic reconstitution by a single CD34-low/negative hematopoietic stem cell. *Science* 1996;**273**:242–5.

34. Kent DG, Copley MR, Benz C, et al. Prospective isolation and molecular characterization of hematopoietic stem cells with durable self-renewal potential. *Blood* 2009;**113**:6342–50.

35. Fraser CC, Eaves CJ, Szilvassy SJ, Humphries RK. Expansion in vitro of retrovirally marked totipotent hematopoietic stem cells. *Blood* 1990;**76**:1071–6.

36. Miller CL, Eaves CJ. Expansion in vitro of adult murine hematopoietic stem cells with transplantable lympho-myeloid reconstituting ability. *Proc Natl Acad Sci USA* 1997;**94**:13648–53.

37. Wineman J, Moore K, Lemischka I, Müller-Sieburg C. Functional heterogeneity of the hematopoietic microenvironment: rare stromal elements maintain long-term repopulating stem cells. *Blood* 1996;**87**:4082–90.

38. Bowie MB, Kent DG, Copley MR, Eaves CJ. Steel factor responsiveness regulates the high self-renewal phenotype of fetal hematopoietic stem cells. *Blood* 2007;**109**:5043–8.

39. Jollie WP. Ultrastructural studies of protein transfer across rodent yolk sac. *Placenta* 1986;**7**:263–81.

40. Zon LI. Developmental biology of hematopoiesis. *Blood* 1995;**86**:2876–91.

41. Shalaby F, Ho J, Stanford WL, et al. A requirement for Flk1 in primitive and definitive hematopoiesis and vasculogenesis. *Cell* 1997;**89**:981–90.

42. Choi K, Kennedy M, Kazarov A, Papadimitriou JC, Keller G. A common precursor for hematopoietic and endothelial cells. *Development* 1998;**125**:725–32.

43. Kabrun N, Buhring HJ, Choi K, et al. Flk-1 expression defines a population of early embryonic hematopoietic precursors. *Development* 1997;**124**:2039–48.

44. Huber TL, Kouskoff V, Fehling HJ, Palis J Keller, G. Haemangioblast commitment is initiated in the primitive streak of the mouse embryo. *Nature* 2004;**432**:625–30.

45. Teixeira V, Arede N, Gardner R, Rodríguez-León J, Tavares, AT. Targeting the hemangioblast with a novel cell type-specific enhancer. *BMC Dev Biol* 2011;**11**:76.

46. Serrado Marques J, Teixeira V, Jacinto A Tavares AT. Identification of novel hemangioblast genes in the early chick embryo. *Cells* 2018;**7**:9.

47. Shivdasani RA, Orkin SH. The transcriptional control of hematopoiesis. *Blood* 1996;**87**:4025–39.

48. Maximow, A. Relation of blood cells to connective tissues and endothelium. *Physiol Rev* 1924;**4**:533–63.

49. Rhodes KE, Gekas C, Wang Y, et al. The emergence of hematopoietic stem cells is initiated in the placental vasculature in the absence of circulation. *Cell Stem Cell* 2008;**2**:252–63.

50. Moore MA, Metcalf D. Ontogeny of the haemopoietic system: yolk sac origin of in vivo and in vitro colony forming cells in the developing mouse embryo. *Br J Haematol* 1970;**18**:279–96.

51. Samokhvalov IM, Samokhvalova NI, Nishikawa S. Cell tracing shows the contribution of the yolk sac to adult haematopoiesis. *Nature* 2007;**446**:1056–61.

52. Mikkola HKA, Gekas C, Orkin SH, Dieterlen-Lievre F. Placenta as a site for hematopoietic stem cell development. *Exp Hematol* 2005;**33**:1048–54.

53. Gekas C, Dieterlen-Lièvre F, Orkin, SH, Mikkola HKA. The placenta is a niche for hematopoietic stem cells. *Dev Cell* 2005;**8**:365–75.

54. Müller AM, Medvinsky A, Strouboulis J, Grosveld F, Dzierzak E. Development of hematopoietic stem cell activity in the mouse embryo. *Immunity* 1994;**1**:291–301.

55. Medvinsky A, Dzierzak E. Definitive hematopoiesis is autonomously initiated by the AGM region. *Cell* 1996;**86**:897–906.

56. Cumano A, Dieterlen-Lievre F, Godin I. Lymphoid potential, probed before circulation in mouse, is restricted to caudal intraembryonic splanchnopleura. *Cell* 1996;**86**:907–16.

57. Chen MJ, Yokomizo T, Zeigler BM, Dzierzak E, Speck NA. Runx1 is required for the endothelial to haematopoietic cell transition but not thereafter. *Nature* 2009;**457**:887–91.

58. Bertrand JY, Giroux S, Golub R, et al. Characterization of purified intraembryonic hematopoietic stem cells as a tool to define their site of origin. *Proc Natl Acad Sci USA* 2005;**102**:134–9.

59. Lis R, Karrasch CC, Poulos MG, et al. Conversion of adult endothelium to immunocompetent haematopoietic stem cells. *Nature* 2017;**545**:439–45.

60. Zovein AC, Hofmann JJ, Lynch M, et al. Fate tracing reveals the endothelial origin of hematopoietic stem cells. *Cell Stem Cell* 2008;**3**:625–36.

61. Adamo L, Naveiras O, Wenzel PL, et al. Biomechanical forces promote embryonic haematopoiesis. *Nature* 2009;**459**:1131–5.

62. North TE, Goessling W, Peeters M, et al. Hematopoietic stem cell development is dependent on blood flow. *Cell* 2009;**137**:736–48.

63. Diaz MF, Li N, Lee HY, et al. Biomechanical forces promote blood development through prostaglandin E2 and the cAMP-PKA signaling axis. *J Exp Med* 2015;**212**:665–80.

64. Tavassoli M. Embryonic and fetal hemopoiesis: an overview. *Blood Cells* 1991;**17**:269–81; discussion 282–6.

65. Rich IN. The developmental biology of hemopoiesis: effect of growth factors on the colony formation by embryonic cells. *Exp Hematol* 1992;**20**:368–70.

66. Lux CT, Yoshimoto M, McGrath K, et al. All primitive and definitive hematopoietic progenitor cells emerging before E10 in the mouse embryo are products of the yolk sac. *Blood* 2008;**111**:3435–8.

67. Enders A, King B. Development of the human yolk sac. In Nogales F, *ed. The Human Yolk Sac and Yolk Sac Tumors* (Berlin: Springer-Verlag, 1993) pp. 33–47.

68. Brent RL, Beckman DA, Jensen M, Koszalka TR. Experimental yolk sac dysfunction as a model for studying nutritional disturbances in the embryo during early organogenesis. *Teratology* 1990;**41**:405–13.

69. Pereda J, Niimi G. Embryonic erythropoiesis in human yolk sac: two different compartments for two different processes. *Microsc Res Tech* 2008;**71**:856–62.

70. Bremer J. The earliest blood vessels in man. *Am J Anat* 1914;**16**:447–76.

71. Pereda J, Monge JI, Niimi G. Two different pathways for the transport of primitive and definitive blood cells from the yolk sac to the embryo in humans. *Microsc Res Tech* 2010;**73**:803–9.

72. Freyer C, Renfree MB. The mammalian yolk sac placenta. *J Exp Zoolog B Mol Dev Evol* 2009;**312**:545–54.

73. Gilmour J. Normal hematopoiesis in intra-uterine and neonatal life. *J Path* 1941;**52**:25–55.

74. Thomas DB, Yoffey JM. Human foetal haemopoiesis. I. The cellular composition of foetal blood. *Br J Haematol* 1962;**8**:290–5.

75. Thomas DB, Yoffey JM. Human foetal haemopoiesis. Ii. Hepatic haematopoiesis in the human foetus. *Br J Haematol* 1964;**10**:193–7.

76. Kelemen E, Calvo W, Fliedner TM. *Atlas of Human Hemopoietic Development* (New York: Springer-Verlag, 1979).

77. Charbord P, Tavian M, Humeau L, Péault B. Early ontogeny of the human marrow from long bones: an immunohistochemical study of hematopoiesis and its microenvironment. *Blood* 1996;**87**:4109–19.

78. Tavassoli M. Ontogeny of hempoiesis. In Meisami E, Timiras P, eds. *Handbook of Human Growth and Developmental Biology* (Boca Raton: CRC Press, 1988), pp. 101–12.

79. Kelemen E, Gulya E, Vass K. Ontogeny of human neutrophil granulocyte alkaline phosphatase. *J Cell Physiol* 1978;**95**:353–4.

80. Wolf BC, Luevano E, Neiman RS. Evidence to suggest that the human fetal spleen is not a hematopoietic organ. *Am J Clin Pathol* 1983;**80**:140–4.

81. Calhoun DA, Li Y, Braylan RC, Christensen RD. Assessment of the contribution of the spleen to granulocytopoiesis and erythropoiesis of the mid-gestation human fetus. *Early Hum Dev* 1996;**46**:217–27.

82. Forestier F, Daffos F, Galacteros F, et al. Hematological values of 163 normal fetuses between 18 and 30 weeks of gestation. *Pediatr Res* 1986;**20**:342–6.

83. Migliaccio G, Migliaccio AR, Petti S, et al. Human embryonic hemopoiesis. Kinetics of progenitors and precursors underlying the yolk sac–liver transition. *J Clin Invest* 1986;**78**:51–60.

84. Porcellini A, Manna A, Manna M. Ontogeny of granulocyte-macrophage progenitor cells in the human fetus. *Int J Cell Cloning* 1983;**1**:92–104.

85. Peschle C, Migliaccio AR, Migliaccio G, et al. Embryonic–fetal Hb switch in humans: studies on

erythroid bursts generated by embryonic progenitors from yolk sac and liver. *Proc Natl Acad Sci USA* 1984;**81**:2416–20.

86. Park CY, Majeti R, Weissman IL. In vivo evaluation of human hematopoiesis through xenotransplantation of purified hematopoietic stem cells from umbilical cord blood. *Nat Protoc* 2008;**3**:1932–40.

87. Barclay A Birkeland M, Brown M, et al. *The Leucocyte Antigen Facts Book* (London: Academic Press, 1993).

88. Krause DS, Fackler MJ, Civin CI, May WS. CD34: structure, biology, and clinical utility. *Blood* 1996;**87**:1–13.

89. Gilles JM, Divon MY, Bentolila E, et al. Immunophenotypic characterization of human fetal liver hematopoietic stem cells during the midtrimester of gestation. *Am J Obstet Gynecol* 1997;**177**:619–25.

90. Muench MO, Roncarolo MG, Namikawa R. Phenotypic and functional evidence for the expression of CD4 by hematopoietic stem cells isolated from human fetal liver. *Blood* 1997;**89**:1364–75.

91. Emerson SG. The regulation of hematopoiesis in the human fetal liver. *Prog Clin Biol Res* 1990;**352**:21–8.

92. Tavian M, Coulombel L, Luton D, et al. Aorta-associated CD34+ hematopoietic cells in the early human embryo. *Blood* 1996;**87**:67–72.

93. Ivanovs A, Rybtsov S, Welch L, et al. Highly potent human hematopoietic stem cells first emerge in the intraembryonic aorta-gonad-mesonephros region. *J Exp Med* 2011;**208**:2417–27.

94. Oberlin E, Tavian M, Blazsek I, Péault B. Blood-forming potential of vascular endothelium in the human embryo. *Development* 2002;**129**:4147–57.

95. Zambidis ET, Oberlin E, Tavian M, Péault B. Blood-forming endothelium in human ontogeny: lessons from in utero development and embryonic stem cell culture. *Trends Cardiovasc Med* 2006;**16**:95–101.

96. Huyhn A, Dommergues M, Izac B, et al. Characterization of hematopoietic progenitors from human yolk sacs and embryos. *Blood* 1995;**86**:4474–85.

97. Nicolini FE, Holyoake TL, Cashman JD, et al. Unique differentiation programs of human fetal liver stem cells shown both in vitro and in vivo in NOD/SCID mice. *Blood* 1999;**94**:2686–95.

98. Zanjani ED, Flake AW, Rice H, Hedrick M, Tavassoli M. Long-term repopulating ability of xenogeneic transplanted human fetal liver hematopoietic stem cells in sheep. *J Clin Invest* 1994;**93**:1051–5.

99. Touraine J. Transplantation of fetal hematopoietic and lymphopoietic cells in humans, with special reference to in utero transplantation. In Edwards R, ed. *Fetal Tissue Transplants in Medicine* (Cambridge: Cambridge Univeristy Press, 1992), pp. 155–76.

100. Kochupillai V, Sharma S, Sundaram KR, Ahuja RK. Hemopoietic improvement following fetal liver infusion in aplastic anemia. *Eur J Haematol* 1991;**47**:319–25.

101. Turner CW, Yeager AM, Waller EK, Wingard JR, Fleming WH. Engraftment potential of different sources of human hematopoietic progenitor cells in BNX Mice. *Blood* 1996;**87**:3237–44.

102. Kumar P, Defor TE, Brunstein C, et al. Allogeneic hematopoietic stem cell transplantation in adult acute lymphocytic leukemia: impact of donor source on survival. *Biol Blood Marrow Transplant* 2008;**14**:1394–1400.

103. Atsuta Y, Suzuki R, Nagamura-Inoue T, et al. Disease-specific analyses of unrelated cord blood transplantation compared with unrelated bone marrow transplantation in adult patients with acute leukemia. *Blood* 2009;**113**:1631–8.

104. Sauter C, Barker JN. Unrelated donor umbilical cord blood transplantation for the treatment of hematologic malignancies. *Curr Opin Hematol* 2008;**15**:568–75.

105. Brunstein CG. Umbilical cord blood transplantation for the treatment of hematologic malignancies. *Cancer Control J Moffitt Cancer Cent* 2011;**18**:222–36.

106. Chen Y, Xu LP, Liu DH, et al. Comparative outcomes between cord blood transplantation and bone marrow or peripheral blood stem cell transplantation from unrelated donors in patients with hematologic malignancies: a single-institute analysis. *Chin Med J (Engl)* 2013;**126**:2499–503.

107. McKinney-Freeman SL, Daley GQ. Towards hematopoietic reconstitution from embryonic stem cells: a sanguine future. *Curr Opin Hematol* 2007;**14**:343–7.

108. Vodyanik MA, Slukvin II. Hematoendothelial differentiation of human embryonic stem cells. *Curr Protoc Cell Biol* 2007;Chapter 23:Unit 23.6.

109. Tian X, Woll PS, Morris JK, Linehan JL, Kaufman DS. Hematopoietic engraftment of human embryonic stem cell-derived cells is regulated by recipient innate immunity. *Stem Cells* 2006;**24**:1370–80.

110. Li Z, Han Z, Wu JC. Transplantation of human embryonic stem cell-derived endothelial cells for vascular diseases. *J Cell Biochem* 2009;**106**:194–9.

111. Gomes KMS, Costa IC, Santos JF, et al. Induced pluripotent stem cells reprogramming: Epigenetics and applications in the regenerative medicine. *Rev Assoc Med Bras(1992)* 2017;**63**:180–9.

112. van den Hurk M, Kenis G, Bardy C, et al. Transcriptional and epigenetic mechanisms of cellular reprogramming to induced pluripotency. *Epigenomics* 2016;**8**:1131–49.

113. Hu C, Li L. Current reprogramming systems in regenerative medicine: from somatic cells to induced pluripotent stem cells. *Regen Med* 2016;**11**:105–32.

114. Sugimura R, Jha DK, Han A, et al. Haematopoietic stem and progenitor cells from human pluripotent stem cells. *Nature* 2017;**545**:432–8.

115. Barcia Durán JG, Lis R, Lu TM, Rafii S. In vitro conversion of adult murine endothelial cells to hematopoietic stem cells. *Nat Protoc* 2018;**13**:2758–80.

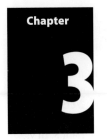

Chapter

3

The Development of the Human Immune System

Amy E. O'Connell, Angela E. Rivers, and William B. Slayton

Introduction

Neonates frequently suffer from life threatening infections. Immaturity of the immune system increases the vulnerability to infection, and the preterm and term neonatal immune system has specific deficiencies relative to that of an older child or adult [1, 2]. During pregnancy, the physical barrier of the placenta and the maternal immune system protect the developing human fetus from infection. However, maternal infections such as rubella, almost eradicated in developed nations through vaccination [3], or the zika virus, an emerging pathogen [4, 5], can ravage the developing embryo and fetus, leading to life-long disabilities. Furthermore, immaturity of natural barrier systems such as skin, bronchial epithelium, and the lining of the gastrointestinal tract compound the weaknesses of the immune system of the premature infant [6, 7]. The importance of interactions between the developing immune system, epithelial barriers, and the microbiome to protect the preterm neonate from infection and promote health is increasingly recognized [8, 9]. Ethical concerns limit our ability to study the embryological development of the human immune system to the same depth [10, 11].

At the earliest stages of human development, the immune system consists of cells and molecules that are nonspecific in their action and do not have the ability to produce amplified responses with repeat exposure to pathogens [12]. The natural, innate immune system functions during the embryonic stage (first 8 weeks post-conception) and consists of macrophages, granulocytes, dendritic, and natural killer cells. The adaptive immune system, consisting of T- and B-cells, begins to function by the second trimester, but is

not at full capacity at birth [13, 14]. This chapter reviews how elements of the innate and adaptive immune system develop, how these elements function together as a whole, and relates immune deficiencies that are present in premature and term neonates to development.

The Evolution of Immunity

The ability to recognize self versus non-self as a way to identify and eliminate invading organisms is a basic requirement of survival. Even the simplest single cell organisms such as bacteria have mechanisms such as the CRISPR/Cas system to fend against invading viruses [15]. In more complex organisms such as mammals, the development of epithelial barriers such as skin, mucosal barriers such as gastrointestinal mucosa, and bioactive substances such as pulmonary surfactant, play an integral role in a newborn evading pathogens. However, organisms that penetrate these barriers have the potential to weaken or even kill a host without functional immune effector cells. Furthermore, organisms have evolved the ability to coexist with commensals, bacteria that also can provide protection against potential invading organisms [16].

The time at which various immune cells appear during fetal development mimics the evolutionary order of the appearance of various immune mechanisms. In the late 1800s, Carl van Beer noted that the common features of the simplest to the most complex organisms were present at the earliest stages of fetal development. Development of the blood is no exception. Blood cells have specific developmental stages that are similar to and related to our evolutionary past. For instance, hemoglobin progresses through larval (embryonic and fetal hemoglobin) and adult

Neonatal Hematology, Pathogenesis, Diagnosis, and Management of Hematologic Problems, 3rd edition, ed. Pedro A. de Alarcón, Eric J. Werner, Robert D. Christensen, and Martha C. Sola-Visner. Published by Cambridge University Press. © Cambridge University Press 2021.

stages, through mechanisms that evolved in jawed vertebrates [17].

To better understand the embryological development of the human immune system, scientists have studied the evolution of the immune system studying organisms from the most primitive invertebrates to humans. Systems of natural (innate) immunity are present in primitive invertebrates, whereas adaptive mechanisms first appear in the vertebrates, specifically jawless fish [18]. Phagocytic cells first appeared in invertebrate animals and perform many of the functions that macrophages perform in humans. Phagocytic cells in the starfish produce interleukin-1 [19].

Invertebrate phagocytic cells kill bacteria by producing superoxide via an enzymatic reaction. In humans, absence or reduced function of the homologous NADPH oxidase subunit gp91-phox is the cause of X-linked chronic granulomatous disease [20–22]. Aggregates of immune tissue that are directly associated with epithelial tissues such as the skin, gill regions, and gut tissue in echinoderms and tunicates, are similar to the location of lymphatic tissue in mammals [23].

The ability to discriminate self from non-self in multicellular organisms is important for basic nutrition as well as successful reproduction. Mechanisms to discriminate self from non-self are seen in invertebrate animals such as the primitive cnidarian *Hydracinia* [24]. Furthermore, the colonial tunicate *Botryllus schlosseri* achieves allo-recognition and rejection through a protein homologous to heat shock protein [25, 26]. The major histocompatibility complex (MHC), required in the human adaptive immune responses, has a common ancestral origin traced to early chordates. In humans, self-recognition is accomplished by the major histocompatibility system MHC. However, the MHC is found in some fishes, amphibians, birds, and mammals [23].

Adaptive immunity first appears in vertebrates. The most primitive lymphocytes, innate lymphoid cells that defend against infection and contribute to wound healing, but do not express rearranged receptors, have been identified in mammals. This group includes natural killer (NK) cells, and cells similar to NK cells that are present in tunicates, the most primitive of chordates [27]. Lymphocytes that rearrange their receptors are thought to have appeared first in the jawless fishes, ancestors to lampreys, and the more specialized T- and B-cells

in ancestors of sharks [23]. Both jawed and jawless vertebrates have prototypic T- and B-like lymphocytes which suggest that their origin comes from a common ancestor [28].

Origin of Hematopoietic Stem Cells during Fetal Development in the Mouse

Much of what is known about the biology of the earliest embryological development of the immune system is inferred from the studies in mice. Three waves of hematopoiesis occur in mammals, including humans. The first wave, also described as primitive hematopoiesis, produces primitive erythrocytes, megakaryocytes, and macrophages [29]. Blood cell formation originates in multiple sites in the mouse embryo from "hemogenic endothelium." The earliest production of blood arises from mesoderm in several sites, including the yolk sac, allantois, vitelline artery and lateral plate [30]. Transcription factors such as SCL/Tal1 [31–33], LMO2/RBTN-2, [34, 35], and AML-1/Runx 1 [30], are critical for the differentiation of hematopoietic cells from primitive mesoderm.

Primitive hematopoiesis results in the production of erythrocytes which are larger than definitive erythrocytes, contain more hemoglobin and are nucleated when they first circulate [36, 37]. These erythrocytes are very well suited for capturing and carrying oxygen in an oxygen poor environment. In addition, primitive megakaryocytes small diploid are produced that are morphologically distinct from adult, bone marrow-derived megakaryoctyes which are polyploid [29].

Macrophages are the sole immunocyte produced in the yolk sac as a result of primitive hematopoiesis [38]. Interestingly, in the mouse, the yolk sac is the common origin of Kupffer cells in the liver, microglia, and dendritic cells, and these persist into adulthood. In contrast, alveolar macrophages in the lungs are progressively replaced by bone marrow-derived macrophages [39]. Recently, a subset of B-cells called innate like atypical B-cells have been described. They have highly restricted immunoglobulin repertoires and reside in epithelial lined cavities such as the peritoneum. The production of these cells, which are critical to neonatal immune responses, occurs from stem cells developmentally restricted to the fetal liver [40, 41].

While able to contribute to the short-term production of primitive erythropoiesis, hematopoietic stem cells (HSCs) from the yolk sac are unable to provide for hematopoiesis long term in the fetal liver or bone marrow, and are unable to reconstitute irradiated mice. The question whether HSCs arise within a given site and colonize other sites or arise independently in each hematopoietic site is controversial. The fact that HSCs from the yolk sac are unable to produce lymphocytes supports the second model; specifically, that the yolk sac and bone marrow independently produce HSCs [42]. However, the ability to track HSCs in mice indicates that definitive HSCs are present in both the yolk sac and intraembryonically in the splanchno pleura/aorta, gonads, and mesonephros (P-Sp/AGM), named for the structures which these areas differentiate into. After generation, these HSCs migrate to and successively colonize the fetal liver, spleen, and bone marrow (Fig. 3.1) [43–47]. The Runx1/AML-1 gene, a proto-oncogene involved with terminal erythroid and megakaryocyte development also plays a crucial role in establishing definitive hematopoiesis [48–50].

The second wave of hematopoiesis begins with the appearance of "definitive" hematopoietic cells. This term initially referred to the adult form of erythrocytes. The first adult like polyploid megakaryocytes are seeing during this phase [29]. More recently some have defined wave two as hematopoiesis derived from stem cells and multilineage progenitors that can reconstitute neonatal animals but not adult animals following lethal irradiation [51]. Cells destined to be lymphocytes arise during wave two in the yolk sac and are present in the para-aortic splancnopleura, placenta, and vitelline vessels [52–55].

The third wave of blood formation is defined by the emergence of self-renewing stem cells that can provide long-term, high level multilineage engraftment when transplanted into adult mice. Adult repopulating stem cells appear in the aorto/gonado/mesonephros, vitelline and umbilical arteries, placenta and the head of mice prior to engrafting in the fetal liver and bone marrow [30, 56, 57]. Wave 2 and Wave 3 HSCs colonize the fetal liver and bone marrow and are the source of all blood in the adult mouse [51], with the exception of some tissue specific macrophages that derive from wave 1 [39].

Studies focused on gene expression and epigenetic changes in single hematopoietic stem and progenitor cells have suggested that epigenetic changes lead to differences in fate determination in fetal and adult stem cells are derived from interactions that occur between hematopoietic stem cells and surrounding cells during embryological development. In the mouse aorto–glomerulo–mesenephros (AGM) region, studies using single pre-hematopoietic stem cells from the AGM region were cultured with endothelial cells from the

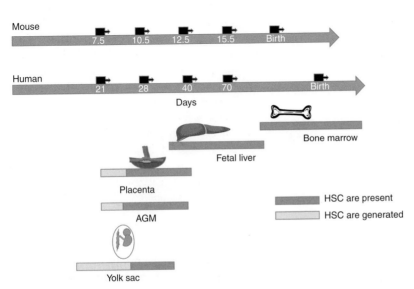

Fig. 3.1 Establishment of hematopoietic stem cells. Abbreviations: AGM, aorta gonad mesonephros, HSC, hematopoietic stem cells. (See plate section for color version.)

AGM. The progeny of these single cells were able to re-populate all the B-cell populations, including B1a cells. Adult stem cells cultured with AGM cells repopulated B-cell populations excluding B1a cells [58]. The changes in stem cells that allow yolk sac derived stem cells to produce certain tissue specific macrophages but not adult stem cells may be related to specific epigenetic changes that occur in hematopoietic stem cells based on cell–cell interactions in the developing embryo [59]. In fact, when fetal liver or cord blood derived stem cells are transplanted into adult hosts, stem cells initially produce immature low ploidy megakaryocytes [60, 61] and immature T-cells [62]. This leads to delayed engraftment and slow immune recovery after cord blood transplant in humans.

Development of the Human Immune Cells and Organs

In the human fetus, hematopoiesis first begins in the yolk sac (weeks 2–5 post-conception), then moves to the liver (weeks 5–24 post-conception), and finally to the bone marrow (week 11 to adult) [63]. The yolk sac phase begins with blood cells developing from mesodermal cells and adjacent to endothelial cells that later become blood vessels. The yolk sac mainly produces large, nucleated erythrocytes with some primitive megakaryocytes and macrophages [64, 65].

The factors that induce changes in sites of hematopoiesis during embryologic development in humans are largely unknown. Five to six weeks post-

conception, CD34 positive hematopoietic stem cells appear in the human placenta, and the placenta becomes a major site of erythropoiesis [66, 67]. Simultaneously, macrophages appear in the liver [68]. It is not clear whether these Kupffer cells are derived from yolk sac stem cells as they are in the mouse [39]. Kupffer cells line the sinusoidal spaces and initially account for approximately 70% of the hematopoietic cells in the liver. These macrophages may be involved in remodeling the hepatic structure to make space for hematopoiesis (which will follow). By 6–7 weeks post-conception, erythrocytes outnumber macrophages. The placenta and fetal liver provide an environment that allows for a massive expansion of hematopoiesis that can provide for the needs of the fetus prior to the development of the bony skeleton as the yolk sac recedes in importance. The fetal liver contains precursor cells that produce the full repertoire of immune cells [69, 70]. The common lymphoid progenitors (CLP) generate a full spectrum of lymphoid cells, including T-, B-, and natural killer cells [71–74].

Eight weeks post-conception, the bone marrow space begins to develop. Hematopoiesis begins in the bone marrow between the tenth and eleventh week. (See Fig. 3.2 for hematopoietic stem cell development of mouse and human.) The bone marrow is colonized by HSCs from three separate sources: the yolk sac, P-Sp/AGM, and fetal liver [71–74]. As in the fetal liver, the first hematopoietic cells to appear in the bones in greatest numbers are macrophages, which appear to carve out the marrow space

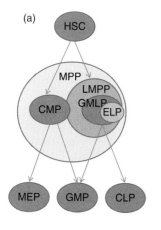
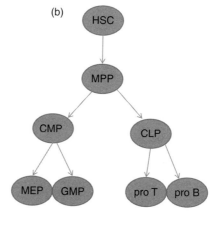

Fig. 3.2 Hematopoietic stem cell development. (a) Mouse hematopoietic hierarchy. (b) Human hematopoietic hierarchy. HSC, hematopoietic stem cell; MPP, multipotent progenitor; LMPP, lymphoid primed multipotent progenitor; CMP, common myeloid progenitor; GMLP, granulocyte monocyte lymphoid progenitor; GMP, granulocyte monocyte progenitor; CLP, common lymphoid progenitor; ELP, early lymphoid progenitor; MEP, megakaryocyte erythrocyte progenitor; pro T, pro T-cell; pro B, pro B-cell. (See plate section for color version.)

through chondrolysis 8–9 weeks post-conception [71, 74]. By weeks 10–11 neutrophils are the predominant leukocyte in the bone marrow [73, 74].

At the same time hematopoiesis appears in the bone marrow, the thymus begins to develop. Rudiments of the thymus appears 8 weeks post-conception. The function of the thymus is to support the differentiation of T-lymphocytes. Progenitors of the T-cells originating in the fetal liver and later from the bone marrow migrate to the thymus beginning 8–9 weeks post-conception [75, 76]. By the tenth week, lymphocytes constitute 95% of the cells present in the thymus. Granulocyte precursors and macrophages are also present in the developing thymus.

B-cell precursors appear simultaneously in the omentum and fetal liver at 8 weeks post-conception. By 11 weeks, lymphocytes appear in the spleen. By week 22, 70% of splenocytes are lymphocytes [72]. Lymph nodes first appear around 11 weeks post-conception, and lymphocytes appear within the lymph nodes approximately 1 week later. Gut-associated lymphatic tissue also begins to develop 11–12 weeks post-conception. By 19 weeks, structurally mature but immunologically naive Peyer's patches appear in the intestines [77].

Innate Immunity

As stated earlier, all organs and cell types of the immune system are present by the eleventh week post-conception, but the function and interaction of these cells are poorly understood. In its earliest stages the immune system consists of cells and molecules that are nonspecific in their action. At 8 weeks post-conception, macrophages, granulocytes, and NK cells are the cellular component of the immune system. The noncellular humoral component consists of complement and passively acquired maternal immunoglobulin. Figure 3.3 provides a pictorial summary of the hyporeactive cellular neonatal innate immunity.

Monocytes/Macrophages

Macrophages play a critical role in the morphogenesis of the fetus. Macrophages are highly mobile, even in their most primitive form. Although a primitive circulatory system is present at 4–5 weeks, there is evidence to suggest that macrophages move through mesenchymal stroma and loose connective tissue. Macrophages shape organs and scavenge debris from apoptotic cells during embryogenesis [78, 79]. They are present in the urogenital ridges where they engulf degenerated cells of the Mullerian duct in the male and the Wolffian duct in the female. They play a similar role in the retina and brain. Fetal hepatic macrophages express Fc receptors and are capable of immune-mediated phagocytosis [80]. In the embryo, Kupffer cells may detoxify circulating endotoxins through their lipopolysaccharide receptor [73].

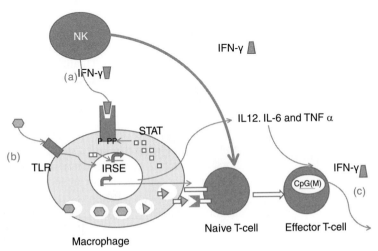

Fig. 3.3 Defects in neonatal innate immune signaling system. (See plate section for color version.) (a). Hypoactive response of nenonatal macrophages to activation by IFN-γ may be related to defective STAT posphorylation (b). Impaired response by neonatal monocytes to multiple TLR ligands (c). Diminished IFN-γ by neonatal lympocytes may be secondary to hypermethylationof IFN-γ promoter.

Toll-like receptor (TLR)

⬯ Antigen

▫ STAT

Macrophages derived from the fetal yolk sac have been shown to constitute the majority of adult tissue-resident macrophages in the liver, brain, lung, and epidermis, demonstrating the importance of these fetal cells over the lifetime of the organism [39, 81]. These fetal-derived cells do not require myb expression for their development in contrast to hematopoietic stem cell-derived macrophages [82]. Lineage tracing experiments showed that fetal yolk sac derived macrophages later give rise to microglia in the brain, while yolk sac monocytes go on to generate the other lineages of tissue-specific macrophages [83].

Studies based mainly on cord-blood derived macrophages demonstrate that neonatal macrophages have diminished immunogenic potential compared to adult cells. Neonatal macrophages have reduced expression of the co-stimulatory molecules CD86 and CD40 leading to poor response to interferon gamma (IFN-γ) and the CD40 ligand [84, 85]. This impaired response leads to an impaired ability for neonatal macrophages to phagocytose pathogens and to activate T cells. Neonatal macrophages also have elevated production of IL-27, which is mainly an immunosuppressive cytokine that blunts the immune response [86]. Neonatal monocytes have been demonstrated to have lower phagocytosis of *Escherichia coli* when compared to adult monocytes and this is believed to be due to a defect in the toll-like receptor (TLR) activation cascade. In addition, signaling via TLR4 seems to have different requirements in neonates versus adults, where neonates require activity of the TRIF pathway in contrast to adults, who require MyD88 for TLR4 signaling [87]. Neonatal monocytes produce low levels of pro-inflammatory cytokines such as tumor neurosis factor alpha (TNF-α), IL-1 β, or IL-12 in response to lipopolysaccharide (LPS) [88]. Despite the functional immaturity of the macrophage lineage in neonates at birth, the macrophages population in neonates is one of the quickest cellular immune components to mature and approximates adult function within a few weeks [89].

Neutrophils

Neutrophils are also phagocytes. In the adult they internalize and kill microbes. Neutrophils contain granules with reactive oxygen species and hydrolytic enzymes. Neutrophils appear after macrophages in the human fetus. Scattered neutrophil precursors appear in the liver as early as 5 weeks [68, 72, 73]. Neutrophils are also present in small nests in mesenchymal areas prior to onset of hematopoiesis in the bone marrow [72]. Neutrophils first appear in scattered clusters in the bone marrow at the onset of hematopoiesis 10–11 weeks post-conception. By 14 weeks post-conception, neutrophils comprise up to 40% of the hematopoietic cells in the bone marrow [72, 74]. At the time of their appearance in the bone marrow, fetal neutrophils contain myeloperoxidase, an enzyme produced by promyelocytes that is present within the azurophilic granules of neutrophils.

The cycling rates of neonatal neutrophils are elevated compared with adults which suggest an incapacity of precursors to respond to sepsis [90, 91]. Therefore, in the neonate and fetus there is a quantitative defect in neutrophils, discussed in greater detail in Chapter 16. In addition to their quantitative defect, neutrophils have a number of qualitative impairments: transendothelial migration, endothelial adherence, chemotaxis, phagocytosis, intracellular killing, and delayed apoptosis. However, some of these impaired functions may be due more to an increased presence of precursor neutrophils than to impaired function of maturely differentiated neonatal neutrophils [92, 93]. Adhesion and chemotactic defects may be due to the fact that the neonatal neutrophils have lower levels of L-selectin, CD18/CD11b, and CD18/CD11a, which are molecules involved in neutrophil adherence and movement across the vascular endothelium. Chemotactic defects of neonatal neutrophils are caused by a poor response to inflammatory stimuli. Defects in neutrophil phagocytosis are due to reduced levels of serum immunoglobulins. Qualitative neutrophil defects are discussed in Chapter 17.

Natural Killer Cells

Natural killer (NK) cells are phylogenetically primitive lymphocytes that lack specific T-cell receptors, that contain numerous cytoplasmic granules. Natural killer cells develop in secondary lymphoid tissue. Natural killer cells can secrete cytokines and chemokines (IFN-γ, GM-CSF, and TNF-α), and/or kill infected or transformed cells via perforin/granzyme or death receptor. Natural killer cells produce IFN-γ. And IFN-γ triggers the Th1 immune response, activates antigen presenting cells (APC) to upregulate MHC class I expression, activates macrophage killing, and has antiproliferative effects on viral and/or malignant transformed cells. Natural killer cells kill by releasing granules containing esterase and perforin onto the plasma membrane of target cells [94]. They are triggered by the loss of MHC I. Natural killer cells express CD56 on their cell surface but do not express CD3ε, a marker for T-cells.

Natural killer cells appear in the human fetal liver 5 weeks post-conception. As early as 6 weeks, 5%–8% of cells in the fetal liver are NK cells, and by 18 weeks, these increase to 15%–25% of cells. Approximately 10%–15% of cord blood lymphocytes are NK cells. Little is known about the function of NK during the developmental and neonatal period. However, even at birth, NK function is impaired relative to adults [95]. Impaired NK function leads to susceptibility to viral infections [96].

Innate Lymphoid Cells

Innate lymphoid cells (ILC) are lymphoid cells that target conserved pathogen epitopes rather than specific antigens like classic lymphocytes [97]. This lack of recombination-driven antigen recognition makes them ready to respond quickly to infectious insults and classifies ILC as innate even though they are lymphoid in lineage, similar to NK cells. Rather than having directly microbicidal functions like other innate cells including neutrophils and macrophages, ILC function to release cytokines and other bioactive factors that propagate and enhance the immune response. Three categories of ILC have been delineated [98]. The first, ILC1, express the transcription factor T-bet and produce cytokines such as IFNγ that are associated with type 1 immune responses targeting intracellular pathogens [99, 100]. The second, ILC2, generate IL-4 and IL-13 along with other type 2 cytokines that are involved in anti-helminth and allergic responses [101, 102]. The third, ILC3, express RORγt and IL-17A and IL-22 in a type 3 cytokine response which can be involved in extracellular immunity and fibrosis [103–106]. Innate lymphoid cells are active in the fetus and the neonate [107]. And ILC3 in particular are important for gut development and interactions with the microbiota. Innate lymphoid cells also help to prevent homeostatic expansion of T cells in the developing neonatal niche [108].

Complement

The complement system was discovered almost a century ago and is composed of a family of over 25 serum proteins and cell surface receptors that act in an amplifying cascade. The complement system protects against a variety of fungal, bacterial, and viral organisms. The complement system mediates the inflammatory response, serves as a link between the innate and adaptive immunity by increasing B-cell memory, and is important in antibody-dependent killing of micro-organisms. The alternative pathway, which is the more primitive pathway, is initiated without antibodies by endotoxin or other polysaccharides. Complement increases B-cell memory function by: (1) lowering the threshold for activation and maintenance of B-cell survival within the germinal center, (2) causing retention of antigen by the follicular dendritic cell (FDC), and, (3) causing the transport of the immune complex to the FDC by B-cells via complement receptors. There are three general pathways to complement activation: classical, lectin mediated, and the alternative pathway. Typically, the classical pathway requires the binding of the first component of complement (C1) to IgM or IgG antibodies bound to their target antigen. Each pathway activates C3, which causes the terminal cascade to form the membrane attack complex, which lyses invading cells by inserting into the cell membrane.

Various components of the complement cascade appear early in fetal development. C2 and C4 are synthesized in the fetal liver as early as 8 weeks after conception [109]. At 11 weeks post-conception, the receptor for C3B is present on macrophages and neutrophils in the bone marrow, suggesting that neutrophils at this stage have the ability to respond to this chemokine and mediator of inflammation [73]. By 13 weeks, C1, C3, and C5 appear, and by 18 weeks, C7 and C9 are present in the fetal liver. Serum complement levels are low until the third trimester, when they begin to rise and correlate with birth weight and gestational age. At term, complement enzyme levels are approximately 50% of their adult levels [110, 111].

Adaptive Immunity

The last system to mature is the adaptive immune system [89]. These immune components are unique in that they utilize DNA rearrangements to produce unique cell surface receptors that are specific for a certain small amino acid sequence. Other cells that produce major histocompatibility (MHC) molecules use the MHC to present antigenic epitopes to the T and B cells, which causes activation of those T or B cells that are specific to that antigen. The adaptive immune system thus typically takes longer to respond to an infectious insult, because the small number of T or B cells that recognize the antigen then must not only find their cognate antigen but must also clonally expand to generate a cellular immune response. Meanwhile, the B cells in particular can also adapt to the antigen by making small rearrangements to their receptors in a process called somatic hypermutation (SHM), which enhances the avidity of the receptor for the antigen. Figure 3.4 provides a pictorial summary of the neonatal adaptive immune system.

T-lymphocytes

The thymus develops from the endoderm of the third pharyngeal pouch through epithelial mesenchymal signaling and Notch interaction. Lymphoid commitment has been reported to precede thymic development. Haynes described the presence of CD7+ T-cell precursors that are negative for all other T-cell markers in the yolk sac, liver, and thoracic mesenchyme in a fetus 7 weeks post-conception [76]. By 8.5 weeks, cells co-expressing CD7 and CD2, which are progenitors committed to the T-lymphocyte lineage, are present within the thymus. One week later, cells expressing both CD4 and CD8 were present. Progenitor T (pT) cells are found in the circulation and in the fetal liver at 11–12 weeks post-conception, which coincides with their thymic colonization. T-cell maturation depends on the rearrangement and expression of the antigen recognition molecule, the T-cell receptor (TcR). Two types of TcR exist: one composed of a heterodimer called "gamma/delta" and the other called "alpha/beta." The δ chain is rearranged prior to the β chain [35, 36], and γ/δ T-cells appear prior to the α/β cells during fetal development. However, in the adult the α/β receptor is the most predominant T-cell receptor. The antigen-specific T-cell receptor is complexed to a signal transduction complex called CD3. This complex, when stimulated with a specific antigen, causes the activation and clonal proliferation of T-cells bearing that receptor.

As T-cells mature in the thymus, they progress through three developmental stages: (1) T-cell precursors that do not express CD4 or CD8 antigens; these are called "double negative T-cells," (2) Cells then become "double positive," by expressing both CD4 and CD8 antigens, and finally

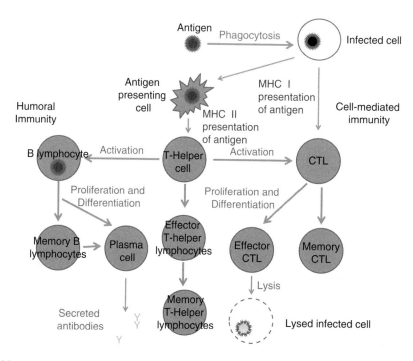

Fig. 3.4 Defects in the neonatal adaptive immune system. (See plate section for color version.)

(3) cells then express either CD4 or CD8 and are now mature T-cells [112]. Stage 2 cells exhibit low level surface expression of the TcR–CD3 complex and are positively selected for a rearranged T-cell receptor that recognizes MHC molecules expressed by thymic stromal cells. Stage 3 thymocytes are located in the thymic medulla, with small numbers located within the inner cortex. These cells now express either CD4 or CD8. Cells expressing receptors that recognize "self" MHC or other endogenous antigens presented by the medullary thymic epithelial cells (mTEC) with high affinity undergo apoptosis within the thymus via a process termed "negative selection" [113].

After completing thymic differentiation, mature T-cells enter the bloodstream and migrate to secondary lymphoid organs including the spleen, peripheral lymph nodes, and mucosa-associated lymphoid tissue (MALT). Within the parenchyma of the secondary lymphoid organ, they can be activated after encountering processed antigen. Mature T-cells are able to recognize foreign antigens presented in the context of the MHC. Major histocompatibility class I molecules are expressed by most cells and display mainly intracellular peptides to CD8 positive T-cells. Infected B cells, lymphocytes, macrophages, DC, and other antigen-presenting cells (APCs) express pathogenic antigens in the context of MHC class II molecules. Antigens presented by these cells, which are mainly extracellular in origin, are recognized by the CD4-expressing helper T-cells [114]. Compared with adults, most of the T-cells in the fetus and neonate are CD45RA+, which indicates an immunologically naive state [115]. Fetal T-cells are able to respond to infection, though not at the level found in a newborn or adult. In the congenitally infected fetuses T-cells expressed CD45RO+, a phenotype consistent with previous antigenic activation, as early as 20 weeks after conception [116, 117]. They also expressed the IL-2 receptor-α, another marker of activation. T-cells express CD40 ligand, which is necessary for B-cell activation and class-switching during the second trimester. Durandy found CD40-ligand expression in fetuses from 19 to 28 weeks, but not from 31 weeks to 10 days after birth. CD40-ligand was again detectable 3 weeks after birth [118].

Peripheral blood lymphocytes are capable of cell-mediated lympholysis from 18 weeks post-conception [119, 120]. CD4 to CD8 ratios and alpha–beta to gamma–delta T-cell ratios in cord blood of fetuses from 18 to 34 weeks were similar to newborn and adult levels, suggesting that the altered immune responses are due to intrinsic immaturity in the signaling system of the T-cells [117]. Neonates have higher levels of regulatory T-cells [121], which express CD25 and the transcription factor Foxp3 and are crucial in preventing autoimmunity. Regulatory T-cells (Tregs) may impair the ability of the neonatal immune system to control infections, in particular through inhibition of the activity of antigen presenting cells, however, there is additional evidence that neonatal Tregs may be less functionally competent than adult Tregs [122, 123].

Neonatal susceptibility to many types of infections including enterovirus, *Herpes simplex* virus, *Candida albicans*, and *Toxoplasma gondii* are due in part to impairment of T-cell function. Immaturity of other elements of the immune system and reduced cytokine production contribute to T-cell dysfunction in human neonates. Neonatal antigen presenting cells such as dendritic cells (DC) have been shown to have decreased function compared to adult DC [124]. T cell-derived cytokines control the immune responses in the neonate. Compared with the adult, they have decreased production of certain lymphokines, such as interferon-gamma, IL-4, and IL-5 [125].

B-Lymphocytes

Humoral immunity begins to develop around the same time as cellular immunity. B-cell precursors appear in the fetal liver around 8 weeks post-conception. Recent studies in mice demonstrate that HSC and progenitor B-cells or progenitor B-cells and macrophage cells (pBM) migrate from the AGM and YS. pBM are believed to retain their ability to differentiate into macrophages by maintaining lower Pax 5 levels. The chemokine stromal-derived factor 1 has been implicated in promoting migration of B-cell progenitor cells. In the liver, B-cell precursors expand and differentiate. Mature B-cells expressing surface immunoglobulin appear at 10 weeks post-conception [126]. By 18 weeks post-conception, the absolute number of circulating and splenic B-cells nears the level found in adults [126, 127]. Though B-cells begin to differentiate in the fetal liver and bone marrow independently of T-cells, the final developmental step of becoming an antigen-producing plasma cell requires functional T-cells [128].

The first fully mature B-cells produced are CD5 positive B-1 cells. CD5 expressing B-cells are located predominantly in the omentum and later in the intestines. In the fetus, B-1 cells produce IgM in response to a variety of common bacterial products including phosphatidyl choline, lipopolysaccharide, and phosphocholine. Rather than being antigen specific, these antibodies are broadly reactive and can react to host tissue [129]. The reasons for this are: (1) the lack of N regions and (2) the predominance of specific junctional sequences. Thus, the immune system first creates a small repertoire of predictable immunoglobulin sequences.

Mouse studies have shown that γ/δ T-cells, also present in the intestines, may interact with B-1 cells and cause them to produce antibody. This interaction may be how "helper" activity evolved in vertebrates. Immunoglobulin production in the fetus and neonate is normally very low. Adult levels of IgG, IgA, and IgE are not reached until several months to years after birth [130, 131]. Infected fetuses can produce IgG and IgA [131]. Newborns are relatively IgA deficient unless supplied with IgA from the mother's milk.

Cytokines

Cytokines are small peptides that control the proliferation, expansion, and homing of the cells that make up the various components of the immune system. The primary role of cytokines is cell-to-cell interaction. The major classes of cytokines are interleukins (IL) (Table 3.1), interferons (INF), tumor necrosis factor (TNF), transforming growth factor (TGF), hematopoietic growth factors, and chemokines. Cytokines support hematopoiesis in the fetus and modulate maternal–fetal homeostasis by altering maternal immunity so that the fetus is not rejected. Cytokines can be categorized into two groups based on the types of helper T-cells that produce them: Th1 cells produce pro-inflammatory cytokines including IFN-gamma, IL-2, IL-12, and tumor necrosis factor, and favor a strong cellular immune response. These cytokines are associated with intracellular infections, tumor suppression, organ rejection, and spontaneous abortion. Th2 cytokines include IL-4, IL-5,

Table 3.1 Interleukins

Interleukin	Function
IL-1	• Increases the proliferative responses of fetal thymocyte progenitors to IL-2 [78] • Upregulates production of G-CSF by monocytes in human fetuses from 14 to 24 weeks post-conception • Upregulates production of GM-CSF by tracheal and bronchial epithelial cells [80] • Increases the antibody production induced by IL-2 [11] • A mediator of an acute phase response in inflammation [82]
IL-2	• Stimulates the proliferation of T-cells • A pleiotropic activator of T- and B-lymphocytes and NK cells [83] • Stimulates CD8 positive T-cell-mediated cytotoxicity and delayed hypersensitivity • IL-2 promotes proliferation of mature B-cells [84] • IL-2 drives immunoglobulin production by primed B-1 and mature B cells
IL-3	• Promotes the differentiation of human basophils and other hematopoietic progenitor cells [87–89] • Maximizes the development of BFU-Es of fetal mouse liver cells grown in culture with erythropoietin [90]
IL-4	• Stimulates the proliferation and differentiation of B-cells • Induces production of immunoglobulin IgM, IgG, and IgE, but not IgA by pre-B cells from the liver, spleen and bone marrow as early as 12 weeks post-conception [93]
IL-5	• Promotes the growth of activated B-cells and eosinophils [95] • Necessary for the mobilization of eosinophils from the bone marrow during allergic inflammation, and regulation of the homing and migration of eosinophils in response to chemotactic stimuli [96]
IL-6	• Supports hematopoietic progenitor growth, promotes T- and B-cell function • Mediates the acute phase response of hepatocytes to inflammation [98] • Promotes the final differentiation of activated B-cells to plasma cells [99] • Induces hepatocytes to produce acute phase reactants [101]

Table 3.1 (cont.)

Interleukin	Function
IL-7	• Important regulator for the earliest stages of T-cell development [104] • Essential for B-lymphopoiesis in mice [105] • Promotes γδ chain formation and the expression of CD8 in fetal mouse thymocytes
IL-8	• Chemotactic effects on neutrophils at inflammatory sites, and acts as a chemokine • Promotes softening and dilatation of the cervix in rabbits
IL-10	• Prevents antigen-specific T-cell activation • Inhibits T-cell expansion by directly inhibiting IL-2 production by these cells • Inhibits the lethal effects of lipopolysaccharide and staphylococcal enterotoxin B in mice [120] • Enhances immunoglobulin production and causes plasma cells to increase in number
IL-11	• Stimulates megakaryopoiesis and production of macrophages
IL-12	• Stimulates CD8+ cells to become cytotoxic lymphocytes [42] • Potent inducer of interferon-gamma production • Promotes antitumor immunity and influences antiviral responses [125]
IL-13	• Inhibits production of proinflammatory cytokines and chemokines by monocytes • Promotes B cell proliferation and differentiation • Induces expression of IgE by pre-B cells from the marrow and spleen
IL-14	B-cell growth factor [129]
IL-15	• Activates T-cell and NK cells • Promotes immunoglobulin production from B-cells
IL-16	• Activates helper T-cells • Strong chemoattractant for lymphocytes and eosinophils
IL-17	Induces IL-6 secretion from mouse stromal cells
IL-18	• Inducer of IFN-gamma production by helper T cells • Increases the production of GM-CSF • Decreases production of IL-10 • Activates NK cells and cytotoxic T lymphocytes
IL-22	• Produced primarily by T cells, ILC, and NKT cells • Expressed in many inflammatory conditions • Important activity in the gut

IL-6, IL-10, IL-13; these favor a strong humoral response, mast cell, and eosinophil production [132]. Th2 cytokines are associated with allergic and autoimmune disorders with increased antibody production. Th17 cells are characterized by production of IL-17 and IL-22 and are associated with pro-fibrotic responses [133].

Cytokine production is generally reduced in neonates with some exceptions [134]. Levels of IL-1 are similar to adults. Levels of IL-2 and IL-6 are variable, but can be low compared to adults, whereas levels of IL-4, IL-8, IL-10, and IL-12 and IFN-γ are low relative to adults. Low cytokines contribute to impaired cellular and humoral immunity. Decreased IL-6 levels contribute to lower levels of secretory IgA relative to adults. Lower IL-8 levels lead to decreased neutrophil chemotaxis in neonates. Interferon α and β activate NK cells, which secrete IFN-γ. Increased levels of IFN-γ have been demonstrated in cord blood of neonates living in areas endemic for schistosomiasis, filariasis, and tuberculosis [135].

Conclusions

The embryological development of the human immune system is poorly studied and understood. The neonatal immune system is immature in almost all levels of functioning. This immaturity leads to impaired ability to fight infection. Understanding the responses of neonatal immune cells to various cytokines and chemokines may lead to decreased morbidity and improved survival in premature and term neonates with infection (Table 3.2).

Table 3.2 Growth factors

Growth factor	Action	Developmental facts
G-CSF	Promotes the differentiation of neutrophils	Present in the developing fetal bone as early as six weeks post-conception [38], and in the fetal liver at least as early as eight weeks post-conception Monocytes in the fetal liver produced less G-CSF in response to IL-1 than monocytes in the marrow
GM-CSF	Stimulates phagocytosis, chemotaxis, adhesion, and tumor lysis	Produced by endothelial cells, T lymphocytes, macrophages, endothelial cells, trophoblasts and decidua, and the epithelial lining of the bronchi, trachea, and amnion A large amount produced in the fetal lungs
SCF	Selectively promotes the growth and differentiation of mast cells Plays a role in the early stages of lymphocyte development and the normal fetal development of gut associated lymphoid tissue	During embryogenesis, SCF and *c-kit* are expressed along the migratory pathways and destinations of primordial germ cells, melanocytes, hematopoietic cells, the gut, and the central nervous system Absence of either SCF in mice leads to intra-uterine death or death shortly after birth from severe macrocytic anemia
M-CSF	Essential growth factor for monocytes and macrophages	M-CSF is present in the human fetal liver and developing fetal bone as early as 6 weeks post-conception Mice that are deficient in M-CSF lack osteoclastic activity, and consequently develop osteopetrosis

References

1. Collins A, Weitkamp JH, Wynn JL. Why are preterm newborns at increased risk of infection? *Arch Dis Child Fetal Neonatal Ed* 2018;**103**:F391–F394.

2. Simon AK, Hollander GA, McMichael A. Evolution of the immune system in humans from infancy to old age. *Proc Biol Sci* 2015;**282**:20143085.

3. Meissner HC, Reef SE, Cochi S. Elimination of rubella from the United States: a milestone on the road to global elimination. *Pediatrics* 2006;**117**:933–5.

4. May M, Relich RF. A comprehensive systems biology approach to studying zika virus. *PLoS One* 2016;**11**:e0161355.

5. Mehta R, Soares CN, Medialdea-Carrera R, et al. The spectrum of neurological disease associated with Zika and chikungunya viruses in adults in Rio de Janeiro, Brazil: A case series. *PLoS Negl Trop Dis* 2018;**12**:e0006212.

6. Narendran V, Visscher MO, Abril I, et al. Biomarkers of epidermal innate immunity in premature and full-term infants. *Pediatr Res* 2010;**67**:382–6.

7. Whitsett JA. Review: The intersection of surfactant homeostasis and innate host defense of the lung: lessons from newborn infants. *Innate Immun* 2010;**16**:138–42.

8. Collado MC, Cernada M, Neu J, et al. Factors influencing gastrointestinal tract and microbiota immune interaction in preterm infants. *Pediatr Res* 2015;**77**:726–31.

9. Tamburini S, Shen N, Wu HC, et al. The microbiome in early life: implications for health outcomes. *Nat Med* 2016;**22**:713–22.

10. Cefalo RC, Berghmans RL, Hall SP. The bioethics of human fetal tissue research and therapy: moral decision making of professionals. *Am J Obstet Gynecol* 1994;**170**:12–19.

11. Reardon S. Trump administration launches sweeping review of fetal-tissue research. *Nature* 2018;**562**:16–17.

12. Dudley DJ, Wiedmeier S. The ontogeny of the immune response: perinatal perspectives. *Semin Perinatol* 1991;**15**:184–95.

13. Haddad R, Guimiot F, Six E, et al. Dynamics of thymus-colonizing cells during human development. *Immunity* 2006;**24**:217–30.

14. Zlotoff DA, Schwarz BA, Bhandoola A. The long road to the thymus: The generation, mobilization, and circulation of T-cell progenitors in mouse and man. *Semin Immunopathol* 2008;**30**:371–82.

15. Westra ER, Swarts DC, Staals RH, et al. The CRISPRs, they are a-changin': How prokaryotes generate adaptive immunity. *Annu Rev Genet* 2012;**46**:311–39.

16. Dishaw LJ, Cannon JP, Litman GW, et al. Immune-directed support of rich microbial communities in the gut has ancient roots. *Dev Comp Immunol* 2014;**47**:36–51.

17. Rohlfing K, Stuhlmann F, Docker MF, et al. Convergent evolution of hemoglobin switching in jawed and jawless vertebrates. *BMC Evol Biol* 2016; **16**:30.

18. Buchmann K. Evolution of innate immunity: Clues from invertebrates via fish to mammals. *Front Immunol* 2014;**5**:459.

19. Beck G, Habicht GS. Immunity and the invertebrates. *Sci Am* 1996;**275**:60–3, 66.

20. Orkin SH. Molecular genetics of chronic granulomatous disease. *Annu Rev Immunol* 1989;**7**:277–307.

21. Segal AW, Jones OT, Webster D, et al. Absence of a newly described cytochrome b from neutrophils of patients with chronic granulomatous disease. *Lancet* 1978;**2**:446–9.

22. Yoshida LS, Saruta F, Yoshikawa K, et al. Mutation at histidine 338 of gp91(phox) depletes FAD and affects expression of cytochrome b558 of the human NADPH oxidase. *J Biol Chem* 1998;**273**:27879–86.

23. Sharp JG, Crouse DA, Purtilo DT. Ontogeny and regulation of the immune system. *Arch Pathol Lab Med* 1987;**111**:1106–13.

24. Dishaw LJ, Litman GW. Invertebrate allorecognition: The origins of histocompatibility. *Curr Biol* 2009;**19**:R286–8.

25. Fagan MB, Weissman IL. Sequence and characterization of two HSP70 genes in the colonial protochordate Botryllus schlosseri. *Immunogenetics* 1996;**44**:134–42.

26. Fagan MB, Weissman IL. Linkage analysis of HSP70 genes and historecognition locus in botryllus schlosseri. *Immunogenetics* 1998;**47**:468–76.

27. Parrinello N. Cytotoxic activity of tunicate hemocytes. *Prog Mol Subcell Biol* 1996;**15**:190–217.

28. Hirano M, Guo P, McCurley N, et al. Evolutionary implications of a third lymphocyte lineage in lampreys. *Nature* 2013;**501**:435–8.

29. Potts KS, Sargeant TJ, Markham JF, et al. A lineage of diploid platelet-forming cells precedes polyploid megakaryocyte formation in the mouse embryo. *Blood* 2014; **124**:2725–9.

30. Tober J, Maijenburg MW, Speck NA. Taking the leap: runx1 in the formation of blood from endothelium. *Curr Top Dev Biol* 2016;**118**:113–62.

31. Bockamp EO, McLaughlin F, Gottgens B, et al. Distinct mechanisms direct SCL/tal-1 expression in erythroid cells and CD34 positive primitive myeloid cells. *J Biol Chem* 1997;**272**:8781–90.

32. Endoh M, Ogawa M, Orkin S, et al. SCL/tal-1-dependent process determines a competence to select the definitive hematopoietic lineage prior to endothelial differentiation. *EMBO J* 2002;**21**:6700–8.

33. Robertson SM, Kennedy M, Shannon JM, et al. A transitional stage in the commitment of mesoderm to hematopoiesis requiring the transcription factor SCL/tal-1. *Development* 2000;**127**:2447–59.

34. Stanulovic VS, Cauchy P, Assi SA, et al. LMO2 is required for TAL1 DNA binding activity and initiation of definitive haematopoiesis at the haemangioblast stage. *Nucleic Acids Res* 2017;**45**:9874–88.

35. Zhu H, Traver D, Davidson AJ, et al. Regulation of the lmo2 promoter during hematopoietic and vascular development in zebrafish. *Dev Biol* 2005;**281**:256–69.

36. Kingsley PD, Malik J, Fantauzzo KA, et al. Yolk sac-derived primitive erythroblasts enucleate during mammalian embryogenesis. *Blood* 2004;**104**:19–25.

37. Palis J. Primitive and definitive erythropoiesis in mammals. *Front Physiol* 2014;**5**:3.

38. Enzan H. Electron microscopic studies of macrophages in early human yolk sacs. *Acta Pathol Jpn* 1986;**36**:49–64.

39. Gomez Perdiguero E, Klapproth K, Schulz C, et al. Tissue-resident macrophages originate from yolk-sac-derived erythro-myeloid progenitors. *Nature* 2015;**518**:547–51.

40. Beaudin AE, Boyer SW, Perez-Cunningham J, et al. A transient developmental hematopoietic stem cell gives rise to innate-like B and T cells. *Cell Stem Cell* 2016;**19**:768–83.

41. Beaudin AE, Forsberg EC. To B1a or not to B1a: Do hematopoietic stem cells contribute to tissue-resident immune cells? *Blood* 2016;**128**:2765–9.

42. Dieterlen-Lievre F. On the origin of haemopoietic stem cells in the avian embryo: an experimental approach. *J Embryol Exp Morphol* 1975;**33**:607–19.

43. Bertrand JY, Giroux S, Golub R, et al. Characterization of purified intraembryonic hematopoietic stem cells as a tool to define their site of origin. *Proc Natl Acad Sci USA* 2005;**102**:134–9.

44. Choi K, Kennedy M, Kazarov A, et al. A common precursor for hematopoietic and endothelial cells. *Development* 1998;**125**:725–32.

45. Cumano A, Dieterlen-Lievre F, Godin I. Lymphoid potential, probed before circulation in mouse, is restricted to caudal intraembryonic splanchnopleura. *Cell* 1996;**86**:907–16.

46. Cumano A, Godin I. Ontogeny of the hematopoietic system. *Annu Rev Immunol* 2007; **25**:745–85.

47. Tavian M, Robin C, Coulombel L, et al. The human embryo, but not its yolk sac, generates lympho-myeloid stem cells: Mapping multipotent hematopoietic cell fate in intraembryonic mesoderm. *Immunity* 2001;**15**:487–95.

48. de Bruijn M, Dzierzak E. Runx transcription factors in the development and function of the definitive hematopoietic system. *Blood* 2017;**129**:2061–9.

49. Draper JE, Sroczynska P, Tsoulaki O, et al. RUNX1B expression is highly heterogeneous and distinguishes megakaryocytic and erythroid lineage fate in adult mouse hematopoiesis. *PLoS Genet* 2016;**12**:e1005814.

50. Kamikubo Y. Genetic compensation of RUNX family transcription factors in leukemia. *Cancer Sci* 2018;**109**:2358–63.

51. Yoder MC. Inducing definitive hematopoiesis in a dish. *Nat Biotechnol* 2014;**32**:539–41.

52. Boiers C, Carrelha J, Lutteropp M, et al. Lymphomyeloid contribution of an immune-restricted progenitor emerging prior to definitive hematopoietic stem cells. *Cell Stem Cell* 2013;**13**:535–48.

53. Gekas C, Dieterlen-Lievre F, Orkin SH, et al. The placenta is a niche for hematopoietic stem cells. *Dev Cell* 2005;**8**:365–75.

54. Gordon-Keylock S, Sobiesiak M, Rybtsov S, et al. Mouse extraembryonic arterial vessels harbor precursors capable of maturing into definitive HSCs. *Blood* 2013;**122**:2338–45.

55. Lin Y, Yoder MC, Yoshimoto M. Lymphoid progenitor emergence in the murine embryo and yolk sac precedes stem cell detection. *Stem Cells Dev* 2014;**23**:1168–77.

56. Medvinsky A, Dzierzak E. Definitive hematopoiesis is autonomously initiated by the AGM region. *Cell* 1996;**86**:897–906.

57. Muller AM, Medvinsky A, Strouboulis J, et al. Development of hematopoietic stem cell activity in the mouse embryo. *Immunity* 1994;**1** 291–301.

58. Hadland BK, Varnum-Finney B, Mandal PK, et al. A common origin for B-1a and B-2 lymphocytes in clonal pre-hematopoietic stem cells. *Stem Cell Reports* 2017;**8**:1563–1572.

59. Zhang Y, Gao S, Xia J, et al. Hematopoietic hierarchy: An updated roadmap. *Trends Cell Biol* 2018;**28**:976–86.

60. Ignatz M, Sola-Visner M, Rimsza LM, et al. Umbilical cord blood produces small megakaryocytes after transplantation. *Biol Blood Marrow Transplant* 2007;**13**:145–50.

61. Slayton WB, Wainman DA, Li XM, et al. Developmental differences in megakaryocyte maturation are determined by the microenvironment. *Stem Cells* 2005;**23**:1400–8.

62. Hiwarkar P, Hubank M, Qasim W, et al. Cord blood transplantation recapitulates fetal ontogeny with a distinct molecular signature that supports CD4(+) T-cell reconstitution. *Blood Adv* 2017;**1**:2206–16.

63. Tavassoli M. Embryonic and fetal hemopoiesis: an overview. *Blood Cells* 1991;**17**:269–81; discussion 282–6.

64. Fukuda T. Fetal hemopoiesis. I. Electron microscopic studies on human yolk sac hemopoiesis. *Virchows Arch B Cell Pathol* 1973;**14**:197–213.

65. Luckett WP. Origin and differentiation of the yolk sac and extraembryonic mesoderm in presomite human and rhesus monkey embryos. *Am J Anat* 1978;**152**:59–97.

66. Barcena A, Kapidzic M, Muench MO, et al. The human placenta is a hematopoietic organ during the embryonic and fetal periods of development. *Dev Biol* 2009;**327**:24–33.

67. Barcena A, Muench MO, Kapidzic M, et al. A new role for the human placenta as a hematopoietic site throughout gestation. *Reprod Sci* 2009;**16**:178–87.

68. Kelemen E, Janossa M. Macrophages are the first differentiated blood cells formed in human embryonic liver. *Exp Hematol* 1980;**8**:996–1000.

69. Fomin ME, Beyer AI, Muench MO. Human fetal liver cultures support multiple cell lineages that can engraft immunodeficient mice. *Open Biol* 2017;**7**:170108.

70. Yurasov S, Kollmann TR, Kim A, et al. Severe combined immunodeficiency mice engrafted with human T cells, B cells, and myeloid cells after transplantation with human fetal bone marrow or liver cells and implanted with human fetal thymus: a model for studying human gene therapy. *Blood* 1997;**89**:1800–10.

71. Charbord P, Tavian M, Humeau L, et al. Early ontogeny of the human marrow from long bones: an immunohistochemical study of hematopoiesis and its microenvironment. *Blood* 1996;**87**:4109–19.

72. Kelemen E, Calvo W, Fliedner TM. *Atlas of Human Hematopoietic Development* (New York: Springer-Verlag, 1979).

73. Slayton WB, Juul SE, Calhoun DA, et al. Hematopoiesis in the liver and marrow of human fetuses at 5 to 16 weeks post-conception:

quantitative assessment of macrophage and neutrophil populations. *Pediatr Res* 1998;**43**:774–82.

74. Slayton WB, Li Y, Calhoun DA, et al. The first-appearance of neutrophils in the human fetal bone marrow cavity. *Early Hum Dev* 1998;**53**:129–44.

75. Haynes BF, Denning SM, Singer KH, et al. Ontogeny of T-cell precursors: A model for the initial stages of human T-cell development. *Immunol Today* 1989;**10**:87–91.

76. Haynes BF, Martin ME, Kay HH, et al. Early events in human T cell ontogeny. Phenotypic characterization and immunohistologic localization of T cell precursors in early human fetal tissues. *J Exp Med* 1988;**168**:1061–80.

77. MacDonald TT, Spencer J. Ontogeny of the gut-associated lymphoid system in man. *Acta Paediatr Suppl* 1994;**83**:3–5.

78. Hinchliffe D. *Development of the Vertebrate Limb* (Oxford: Clarendon Press, 1980).

79. Hofman FM, Danilovs J, Husmann L, et al. Ontogeny of B cell markers in the human fetal liver. *J Immunol* 1984;**133**:1197–201.

80. Naito K, Takahashi H, Kojima M. *Ontogenic Development of Kupffer Cells* (Amsterdam: Elsevier Biomedical Press, 1982).

81. Guilliams M, De Kleer I, Henri S, et al. Alveolar macrophages develop from fetal monocytes that differentiate into long-lived cells in the first week of life via GM-CSF. *J Exp Med* 2013;**210**:1977–92.

82. Schulz C, Gomez Perdiguero E, Chorro L, et al. A lineage of myeloid cells independent of Myb and hematopoietic stem cells. *Science* 2012;**336**:86–90.

83. Hoeffel G, Chen J, Lavin Y, et al. C-Myb(+) erythro-myeloid progenitor-derived fetal monocytes give rise to adult tissue-resident macrophages. *Immunity* 2015;**42**:665–78.

84. Orlikowsky TW, Spring B, Dannecker GE, et al. Expression and regulation of B7 family molecules on macrophages (MPhi) in preterm and term neonatal cord blood and peripheral blood of adults. *Cytometry B Clin Cytom* 2003;**53**:40–7.

85. Marodi L. Deficient interferon-gamma receptor-mediated signaling in neonatal macrophages. *Acta Paediatr Suppl* 2002;**91**:117–9.

86. Kraft JD, Horzempa J, Davis C, et al. Neonatal macrophages express elevated levels of interleukin-27 that oppose immune responses. *Immunology* 2013;**139**:484–93.

87. Cuenca AG, Joiner DN, Gentile LF, et al. TRIF-dependent innate immune activation is critical for survival to neonatal gram-negative sepsis. *J Immunol* 2015;**194**:1169–77.

88. Chelvarajan RL, Collins SM, Doubinskaia IE, et al. Defective macrophage function in neonates and its impact on unresponsiveness of neonates to polysaccharide antigens. *J Leukoc Biol* 2004;**75**:982–94.

89. Olin A, Henckel E, Chen Y, et al. Stereotypic immune system development in newborn children. *Cell* 2018;**174**:1277–92 e14.

90. Christensen RD, Hill HR. Rothstein G: granulocytic stem cell (CFUc) proliferation in experimental group B streptococcal sepsis. *Pediatr Res* 1983;**17**:278–80.

91. Christensen RD. Rothstein G: Pre- and postnatal development of granulocytic stem cells in the rat. *Pediatr Res* 1984;**18**:599–602.

92. Makoni M, Eckert J, Anne Pereira H, et al. Alterations in neonatal neutrophil function attributable to increased immature forms. *Early Hum Dev* 2016;**103**:1–7.

93. Prosser A, Hibbert J, Strunk T, et al. Phagocytosis of neonatal pathogens by peripheral blood neutrophils and monocytes from newborn preterm and term infants. *Pediatr Res* 2013;**74**:503–10.

94. Henkart P, Yue CC: The role of cytoplasmic granules in lymphocyte cytotoxicity. *Prog Allergy* 1988;**40**:82–110.

95. Strauss-Albee DM, Liang EC, Ranganath T, et al. The newborn human NK cell repertoire is phenotypically formed but functionally reduced. *Cytometry B Clin Cytom* 2017;**92**:33–41.

96. Lopez C. *Immunology and Pathogenesis of Persistent Virus Infections* (Washington, DC: American Society of Microbiology, 1988).

97. Yu JC, Khodadadi H, Malik A, et al. Innate immunity of neonates and infants. *Front Immunol* 2018;**9**:1759.

98. Eberl G, Colonna M, Di Santo JP, et al. Innate lymphoid cells. Innate lymphoid cells: a new paradigm in immunology. *Science* 2015;**348**: aaa6566.

99. Bernink JH, Peters CP, Munneke M, et al. Human type 1 innate lymphoid cells accumulate in inflamed mucosal tissues. *Nat Immunol* 2013;**14**:221–9.

100. Fuchs A, Vermi W, Lee JS, et al. Intraepithelial type 1 innate lymphoid cells are a unique subset of IL-12- and IL-15-responsive IFN-gamma-producing cells. *Immunity* 2013;**38**:769–81.

101. Moro K, Yamada T, Tanabe M, et al. Innate production of T(H)2 cytokines by adipose tissue-associated c-Kit(+)Sca-1(+) lymphoid cells. *Nature* 2010;**463**:540–4.

102. Neill DR, Wong SH, Bellosi A, et al. Nuocytes represent a new innate effector leukocyte that mediates type-2 immunity. *Nature* 2010;**464**:1367–70.

103. Cella M, Fuchs A, Vermi W, et al. A human natural killer cell subset provides an innate source of IL-22 for mucosal immunity. *Nature* 2009;**457**:722–5.

104. Luci C, Reynders A, Ivanov, II, et al. Influence of the transcription factor RORgammat on the development of NKp46+ cell populations in gut and skin. *Nat Immunol* 2009;**10**:75–82.

105. Sanos SL, Bui VL, Mortha A, et al. RORgammat and commensal microflora are required for the differentiation of mucosal interleukin 22-producing NKp46+ cells. *Nat Immunol* 2009;**10**:83–91.

106. Satoh-Takayama N, Vosshenrich CA, Lesjean-Pottier S, et al. Microbial flora drives interleukin 22 production in intestinal NKp46+ cells that provide innate mucosal immune defense. *Immunity* 2008;**29**:958–70.

107. Miller D, Motomura K, Garcia-Flores V, et al. Innate lymphoid cells in the maternal and fetal compartments. *Front Immunol* 2018;**9**:2396.

108. Bank U, Deiser K, Finke D, et al. Cutting edge: Innate lymphoid cells suppress homeostatic T cell expansion in neonatal mice. *J Immunol* 2016;**196**:3532–6.

109. Colten HR, Goldberger G. Ontogeny of serum complement proteins. *Pediatrics* 1979;**64**:775–80.

110. Ballow M, Fang F, Good RA, et al. Developmental aspects of complement components in the newborn. The presence of complement components and C3 proactivator (properdin factor B) in human colostrum. *Clin Exp Immunol* 1974;**18**:257–66.

111. Grumach AS, Ceccon ME, Rutz R, et al. Complement profile in neonates of different gestational ages. *Scand J Immunol* 2014;**79**:276–81.

112. Adkins B, Mueller C, Okada CY, et al. Early events in T-cell maturation. *Annu Rev Immunol* 1987;**5**:325–65.

113. Haynes BF. The role of the thymic microenvironment in promotion of early stages of human T cell maturation. *Clin Res* 1986;**34**:422–31.

114. Germain RN, Margulies DH. The biochemistry and cell biology of antigen processing and presentation. *Annu Rev Immunol* 1993;**11**:403–50.

115. Kingsley G, Pitzalis C, Waugh AP, et al. Correlation of immunoregulatory function with cell phenotype in cord blood lymphocytes. *Clin Exp Immunol* 1988;**73**:40–5.

116. Bruning T, Daiminger A, Enders G. Diagnostic value of CD45RO expression on circulating T lymphocytes of fetuses and newborn infants with pre-, peri- or early post-natal infections. *Clin Exp Immunol* 1997;**107**:306–11.

117. Paganelli R, Cherchi M, Scala E, et al. Activated and "memory" phenotype of circulating T lymphocytes in intrauterine life. *Cell Immunol* 1994;**155**:486–92.

118. Durandy A, De Saint Basile G, Lisowska-Grospierre B, et al. Undetectable CD40 ligand expression on T cells and low B cell responses to CD40 binding agonists in human newborns. *J Immunol* 1995;**154**:1560–8.

119. Granberg C, Hirvonen T. Cell-mediated lympholysis by fetal and neonatal lymphocytes in sheep and man. *Cell Immunol* 1980;**51**:13–22.

120. Granberg C, Manninen K, Toivanen P: Cell-mediated lympholysis by human neonatal lymphocytes. *Clin Immunol Immunopathol* 1976;**6**:256–63.

121. Hayakawa S, Ohno N, Okada S, et al. Significant augmentation of regulatory T cell numbers occurs during the early neonatal period. *Clin Exp Immunol* 2017;**190**:268–79.

122. Xu L, Tanaka S, Bonno M, et al. Cord blood CD4(+)CD25(+) regulatory T cells fail to inhibit cord blood NK cell functions due to insufficient production and expression of TGF-beta1. *Cell Immunol* 2014;**290**:89–95.

123. Prince LR, Maxwell NC, Gill SK, et al. Macrophage phenotype is associated with disease severity in preterm infants with chronic lung disease. *PLoS One* 2014;**9**:e103059.

124. Charrier E, Cordeiro P, Cordeau M, et al. Post-transcriptional down-regulation of Toll-like receptor signaling pathway in umbilical cord blood plasmacytoid dendritic cells. *Cell Immunol* 2012;**276**:114–21.

125. Wilson CB, Penix L, Melvin A, et al. Lymphokine regulation and the role of abnormal regulation in immunodeficiency. *Clin Immunol Immunopathol* 1993;**67**:S25–32.

126. Lawton AR, Cooper MD. B cell ontogeny: Immunoglobulin genes and their expression. *Pediatrics* 1979;**64**:750–7.

127. Gathings WE, Lawton AR, Cooper MD. Immunofluorescent studies of the development of pre-B cells, B lymphocytes and immunoglobulin isotype diversity in humans. *Eur J Immunol* 1977;**7**:804–10.

128. Coffman RL, Seymour BW, Lebman DA, et al. The role of helper T cell products in mouse B cell differentiation and isotype regulation. *Immunol Rev* 1988;**102**:5–28.

129. Waddick KG, Uckun FM. CD5 antigen-positive B lymphocytes in human B cell ontogeny during fetal development and after autologous bone marrow transplantation. *Exp Hematol* 1993;**21**:791–8.

130. Cooper MD. Current concepts. B lymphocytes. Normal development and function. *N Engl J Med* 1987;**317**:1452–6.

131. Gathings WE, Kubagawa H, Cooper MD. A distinctive pattern of B cell immaturity in perinatal humans. *Immunol Rev* 1981;**57**:107–26.

132. Lucey DR, Clerici M, Shearer GM. Type 1 and type 2 cytokine dysregulation in human infectious, neoplastic, and inflammatory diseases. *Clin Microbiol Rev* 1996;**9**:532–62.

133. Ghilardi N, Ouyang W. Targeting the development and effector functions of TH17 cells. *Semin Immunol* 2007;**19**:383–93.

134. Nesin M, Cunningham-Rundles S. Cytokines and neonates. *Am J Perinatol* 2000;**17**:393–404.

135. Malhotra I, Ouma J, Wamachi A, et al. In utero exposure to helminth and mycobacterial antigens generates cytokine responses similar to that observed in adults. *J Clin Invest* 1997;**99**:1759–66.

Bone Marrow Failure Syndromes

Amy E. Geddis, Meera Srikanthan, and Katie Bergstrom

Introduction

Inherited bone marrow failure syndromes (IBMFS) are a rare but important consideration in the differential diagnosis of cytopenias in childhood [1]. However, diagnosis of IBMFS in the newborn period can be challenging because many of the manifestations considered typical for a specific disorder may not yet be present, and in many cases children will not be recognized until later in life. Young children with IBMFS may have one or more cytopenias, congenital anomalies, both, or neither. A high index of suspicion for an IBMFS is required in order to establish the correct diagnosis, determine appropriate clinical management and follow up plans, and provide the family with genetic counseling. Some IBMFS predispose to leukemia or solid tumors; while the development of cancer is uncommon in the newborn period, this risk is an important determinant of subsequent follow up for the child and any affected family members.

A comprehensive review of IBMFS is beyond the scope of this chapter; instead, we will focus on disorders most likely to present in the newborn period. We will discuss the clinical findings, diagnostic work up, implications for treatment in the first year of life, and general prognosis. In particular, we will discuss congenital anemia, neutropenia, and thrombocytopenia syndromes, as well as Fanconi anemia (FA), and dyskeratosis congenita (DC), with a brief mention of miscellaneous disorders that may be considered in the differential of bone marrow failure during infancy.

Approach to Evaluation for an IBMFS in the Neonate

The initial approach to evaluation for an IBMFS in the neonate starts with a careful history and physical examination. Additional laboratory and radiographic studies will depend on the index of suspicion. A general algorithm is proposed in Fig. 4.1, acknowledging that a variation to this approach may be appropriate in individual situations.

Physical Examination

Findings on physical exam that may raise suspicion for an IBMFS may include those associated with anemia (pallor, difficulty feeding, tachycardia, in rare cases hydrops), thrombocytopenia (bruising, petechiae, hematoma), or leukopenia (infection of the skin or umbilical cord, recurrent thrush or diaper rash). Alternatively, findings may be limited to physical anomalies such as low birth weight or short stature, dysmorphism, microcephaly, café au lait spots, nail dystrophy, urogenital malformations, or skeletal abnormalities, particularly involving the radial ray and thumbs (Table 4.1). Some findings that are considered to be characteristic of specific diagnoses may not be apparent in the newborn period.

Family History

A detailed family history should be obtained with regard to congenital anomalies, unexplained cytopenias, stillbirths, or spontaneous abortions, and unusual infections in siblings or close relatives [2]. A family history of cancer, particularly at a young age, or excessive toxicity from chemotherapy or radiotherapy could suggest an IBMFS. If the information is available, three generations should

Neonatal Hematology, Pathogenesis, Diagnosis, and Management of Hematologic Problems, 3rd edition, ed. Pedro A. de Alarcón, Eric J. Werner, Robert D. Christensen, and Martha C. Sola-Visner. Published by Cambridge University Press. © Cambridge University Press 2021.

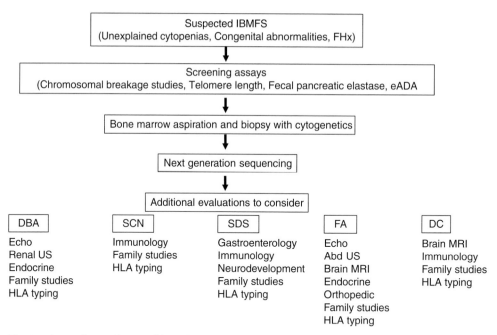

Fig. 4.1 Approach to evaluation of the child with a suspected inherited bone marrow failure syndrome

be included as some associated conditions such as malignancies, may not develop until an older age. Consanguinity within the family increases the likelihood of an autosomal recessive disorder. Some genetic variants may be present at higher frequency in certain ethnic groups; for example, a variant in *FANCC* is unique to FA patients of Ashkenazi Jewish ancestry, and has a carrier frequency of greater than 1/100 in this population [3].

Laboratory Evaluation

The general laboratory evaluation of a child suspected of having an IBMFS should include a complete blood count with differential, peripheral smear, and reticulocyte count. It is important to be aware of gestation- and age-specific normal ranges for hematopoietic parameters (see Chapter 24 for reference ranges in neonatal hematology). For example, the lower limit of normal for absolute neutrophil count in a >36 week gestation newborn is 2,700/microliter, whereas for a 28–36 week gestation newborn it is 1,000/microliter. An elevation of the red cell mean corpuscular volume (MCV) is suggestive of a marrow failure disorder, but again one must take into account that some degree of macrocytosis is normal in the newborn period. Additional factors that may affect red cell size include

reticulocytosis (because reticulocytes are larger than other red cells), trisomy 21 (associated with an elevated MCV), or concomitant thalassemia (causes red cell microcytosis). Recent transfusion will also affect interpretation of the MCV. Bone marrow aspiration and biopsy are generally required in the evaluation of an IBMFS. However, in the absence of clinically significant cytopenias, this study may in some cases reasonably be delayed until an age where sedation can be performed more safely. Important diagnostic findings from the marrow include paucity or abnormal maturation of specific precursors, generalized hypocellularity or cytogenetic changes. More specific diagnostic studies are reviewed in conjunction with individual disorders below.

Additional Studies

Radiographic studies can be useful to document congenital abnormalities not obvious on external exam. In the setting of suspected IBMFS an echocardiogram, abdominal ultrasound, brain MRI, or plain x-rays may be appropriate.

Counseling

Available genetic testing approaches are discussed in Chapter 15. Once an IBMFS is suspected, involvement of a genetic counselor can

Table 4.1 Comparison of frequent congenital anomalies in inherited bone marrow failure syndromes

Frequency of any anomaly	Fanconi anemia	Diamond–Blackfan anemia	Shwachman–Diamond syndrome	Telomere biology disorder	Thrombocytopenia absent radius
	75%	40%–50%	55%	75%	100%
Head and face	Microcephaly Micro-ophthalmia Hypotelorism Ear abnormalities Hearing loss	Microcephaly Hypertelorism Epicanthus Micro-ophthalmia Broad nasal bridge Micrognathia Cleft lip/palate		Microcephaly Lacrimal duct stenosis Exudative retinopathy Leukoplakia	Macrocephaly Micrognathia Hypotelorism Posteriorly rotated low-set ears
Central nervous system	Small pituitary Hydrocephalus Abnormal corpus callosum Developmental delay		Developmental delay	Cerebellar hypoplasia Intracranial calcification Developmental delay	
Skeletal	Short stature Absent or abnormal thumbs Absent or hypoplastic radii Congenital hip dislocation Vertebral anomalies	Short stature Triphalangeal, bifid or hypoplastic thumbs Vertebral anomalies	Short stature Metaphyseal dysplasia of long bones and costochondral junctions Narrow thorax	Short stature	Short stature Absent radii Hypoplastic thumbs Ulnar or humeral hypoplasia Phocomelia Congenital hip dislocation Small patella Bowed legs
Cardiac	ASD VSD PDA Coarctation Pulmonary stenosis	ASD VSD Coarctation	ASD VSD PDA		ASD VSD PDA TOF
Pulmonary	Tracheoesophageal fistula			Pulmonary fibrosis	
Gastrointestinal	Imperforate anus Esophageal and duodenal atresia Malrotation		Exocrine pancreatic insufficiency Fatty pancreatic changes Hepatomegaly Transaminitis	Esophageal stenosis Hepatic fibrosis	Cow's milk intolerance

Table 4.1 (cont.)

Frequency of any anomaly	Fanconi anemia 75%	Diamond–Blackfan anemia 40%–50%	Shwachman–Diamond syndrome 55%	Telomere biology disorder 75%	Thrombocytopenia absent radius 100%
Urogenital	Ectopic, horseshoe, absent, or dysplastic kidney Duplex ureters Cryptorchidism Hypospadias Small or absent testes Cryptorchidism Uterine abnormalities	Horseshoe or absent kidney Hypospadias			Horseshoe kidney Duplex ureter
Dermatologic	Café au lait spots Hypo or hyperpigmentation		Eczema	Lacy pigmentation of the neck and chest Dysplastic nails Sparse hair	
Endocrine	Growth hormone deficiency Hypothyroidism Abnormal glucose Osteopenia	Hypothyroidism Abnormal glucose Osteopenia	Hypothyroidism Osteopenia		

Abbreviations: FA (Fanconi anemia), DBA (Diamond–Blackfan anemia), SDS (Shwachman–Diamond syndrome), TBD (telomere biology disorder), TAR (thrombocytopenia absent radius), ASD (atrial septal defect), VSD (ventricular septal defect), PDA (patent ductus arteriosus), TOF (tetralogy of fallot) facilitate pre- and post-test counseling for the family. A genetic counselor can ensure appropriate testing is being performed, educate the family about the implications and limitations of testing, help to interpret results, identify additional family members who should be tested as well as discuss options for planning future pregnancies. Appropriate counseling is particularly important when evaluating families for disorders that carry a significant risk for malignancy. Family members who are found to be affected should be referred for appropriate follow up.

Specific Disorders

Congenital Anemias

Diamond–Blackfan Anemia

The incidence of Diamond–Blackfan anemia (DBA) is 6–7 per million live births with no ethnic or gender predilection. DBA is an important consideration in the evaluation of neonatal anemia, commonly presenting with macrocytic, hypoproliferative anemia in infants less than 1 year of age. Congenital anomalies are frequent, occurring in 40%–50% of patients (Table 4.1), and may include growth failure, microcephaly, facial dysmorphism (hypertelorism, flat nasal bridge, micrognathia), cleft palate, cardiac, and genitourinary malformations, and abnormal thumbs (triphalangeal, bifid, hypoplastic) [4]. Non-classical presentations of DBA, with a later onset of anemia, other cytopenias or even normal blood counts may be more common than is recognized. The phenotype may vary considerably even within the same family [5]. Registry studies have demonstrated a predisposition to cancer in adult patients, including myelodysplasia and solid tumors such as osteosarcoma and colon cancer, and patients with unrecognized DBA may experience unexpected hematologic toxicity with chemotherapy [6, 7].

Pathophysiology

DBA is a ribosomopathy, resulting from a pathogenic variant or deletion of one of several known ribosomal genes, with *RPS19* and *RPL5* being the most common [8–10]. Inheritance is autosomal dominant, with approximately 55% of cases being sporadic. There are rare cases of the DBA phenotype associated with pathogenic variants of non-ribosomal genes including *GATA1*, *TSR2*, *ADA2*

and *EPO* [11–13]. There is no clear relationship between phenotype and genotype, although cleft palate may be associated with abnormalities in *RPL5*.

Diagnostic Evaluation

A diagnosis of classical DBA can be made if all of the following criteria are present: age less than 1 year, macrocytic anemia, reticulocytopenia, and normocellular bone marrow with a paucity of erythroid precursors [14]. While other cytopenias are not considered classical, neutropenia and thrombocytopenia are sometimes present. Additional criteria can be used to make a diagnosis of non-classical DBA if the above clinical criteria are not met. A family history of DBA or of symptoms suspicious for DBA increases the likelihood of this diagnosis; if there is a known familial mutation then testing of the child is straightforward. The finding of congenital abnormalities commonly seen in patients with DBA supports the diagnosis and should be sought by a careful exam as well as an echocardiogram and abdominal ultrasound. Erythrocyte adenosine deaminase (eADA) is elevated in approximately 80% of patients with DBA [15]. Hemoglobin F is frequently elevated in children with DBA, though it is not specific and in children less than 6 months of age elevation of hemoglobin F can be physiologic. Interpretation of eADA and hemoglobin F results will be confounded by red cell transfusion. Genetic studies are an increasingly important diagnostic tool, particularly in the patient who does not meet classical criteria. It is important to note that the features of many of the IBMFS overlap, thus the screening approach should include chromosomal breakage studies, telomere length and fecal pancreatic elastase to rule out an alternative diagnosis (see Fig. 4.1). Unless there is a known familial mutation, the most efficient approach to genetic testing is to use a next-generation sequencing panel with coverage of the known genes associated with DBA, including copy number analysis of deletions and duplications, as well as other IBMFS. With such a panel, testing will identify a pathogenic variant in about 70% of cases [16].

Management

The cornerstone of therapy in infants with DBA involves the use of red cell transfusions as needed in order to maintain the hemoglobin above 9 g/dl

[17]. Additional supportive care in the newborn period includes referral to endocrinology and nutrition for children with poor growth, as well as management of associated cardiac or other congenital defects [18]. Although about 80% of children with DBA will have improvement of anemia in response to glucocorticoids, it is recommended to delay institution of this treatment until after 1 year of age, to minimize adverse effects on growth and neurocognitive development [14]. An earlier trial of steroid therapy can be considered if vascular access or other factors are making transfusions difficult. Children who are transfusion-dependent are at risk for iron overload. Chelation is generally required after 10–15 transfusions or when the liver iron content as measured by MRI exceeds 6–7 mg/g dry tissue weight, usually occurring after 1–2 years of age [17, 19]. Ultimately, bone marrow transplantation may be considered for children who are transfusion-dependent and non-responsive to steroids and who have suitable donors. Decisions around the timing of transplant are complicated by the natural history of the disease which can include spontaneous remission. Approximately 20% of patients experience a remission by the age of 25 years, with 72% of those remitting in the first year of life, irrespective of the severity of their phenotype [19]. While incompletely understood, the mechanisms of remission may include somatic revertant mosaicism, whereby spontaneous correction of the pathogenic allele and subsequent clonal expansion of the revertant cell leads to hematologic improvement [20–22]. Other indications for transplant include the development of myelodysplastic syndrome (MDS) which is most commonly a complication of adulthood. Data from the North American Diamond–Blackfan Anemia Registry indicate a median survival of patients with DBA to be 56 years [6].

Additional Congenital Anemias

While DBA is the most common congenital anemia, additional rare anemias that may be present in the newborn period include deficiency of adenosine deaminase 2 (DADA2), Pearson marrow-pancreas syndrome, and congenital dyserythropoietic anemia (CDA).

Deficiency of adenosine deaminase 2 is an autosomal recessive disorder that typically presents as a vasculitis syndrome, with early onset of fevers,

rash and stroke, but patients with a phenotype resembling DBA have been reported [23, 24]. Additional hematologic findings may include neutropenia or thrombocytopenia, marrow aplasia, lymphadenopathy, and immunodeficiency [25]. DADA2 can be diagnosed by measurement of ADA2 enzyme activity in plasma or genetic testing. Patients are usually managed by immunology or rheumatology with therapies such as TNF-alpha inhibitors.

Pearson marrow-pancreas syndrome results from single large scale deletions of mitochondrial DNA (mtDNA) and presents during infancy with sideroblastic anemia, exocrine pancreatic dysfunction, and acidosis [26–28]. Though most cases are sporadic, transmission of mutated mtDNA from an affected mother has been described [29]. Anemia is hypoproliferative and macrocytic. Bone marrow findings include vacuolization of erythroid and myeloid precursors and ringed sideroblasts. Muscle weakness, cataract, renal Fanconi syndrome with organic aciduria and cardiac dysfunction may be present, highlighting this as a disorder of multiorgan dysfunction [30]. Treatment is supportive. More than half of patients with Pearson marrow-pancreas syndrome die before 4 years of age due to complications of infection, marrow failure, metabolic acidosis, or liver and renal failure; those who survive may exhibit hematologic improvement and evolution to Kearns-Sayre syndrome [31].

Congenital dyserythropoietic anemia (CDA) is a heterogeneous group of inherited anemias characterized by ineffective erythropoiesis and morphologic abnormalities in bone marrow erythroblasts [32]. Several types of CDA can be distinguished based on the morphologic findings in bone marrow erythroblasts and identification of the causative genes [33]. CDA type I is most likely to be diagnosed in infancy. Infants may present with normocytic or macrocytic anemia, reticulocytopenia, and persistent jaundice; rarely hydrops may develop in utero [34–37]. Review of the peripheral smear may reveal anisocytosis, poikilocytosis, and occasional nucleated red blood cells. In addition to jaundice, manifestations of ineffective erythropoiesis include splenomegaly, frontal bossing, pulmonary hypertension, cholelithiasis, and iron overload [38–40]. Non-hematologic features in CDA-I may be present in 10%–20% of cases and include missing distal

Table 4.2 Summary of genes associated with inherited marrow failure syndromes

	Genes	Location	Inheritance
Congenital anemias			
Diamond–Blackfan anemia	RPS19	19q13.2	Autosomal dominant
	RPL5	1p22.1	
	RPS26	12q13.2	
	RPL11	1p36.11	
	RPL35a	3q29	
	RPS10	6p21.31	
	RPS24	10q22.3	
	RPS17	15q25.2	
	RPL15	3p24.2	
	RPS28	19p13.2	
	RPS29	14q21.3	
	RPS7	2p25.3	
	RPS15	19p13.3	
	RPS27a	2p16.1	
	RPS27	1q21.3	
	RPL9	4p14	
	RPL18	19q13.33	
	RPL26	17p13.1	
	RPL27	17q21.31	
	RPL31	2q11.2	
	TSR2	Xp11.22	X-linked
	GATA1	Xp11.23	
	EPO	7q22.1	Autosomal recessive
	ADA2	22q11.1	
Adenosine deaminase deficiency	ADA2	22q11.1	Autosomal recessive
Pearson marrow-pancreas syndrome	Multi-gene deletion	mtDNA	Mitochondrial
Congenital dyserythropoietic anemia	CDAN1	15q15.2	Autosomal recessive
	C15ORF41	15q14	
	SEC23B	20p11.23	
	CDAN3	15q21	
	KLF1	19p13.13	Autosomal dominant
Congenital neutropenias			
Congenital neutropenia	ELANE	19p13.3	Autosomal dominant
	GFI1	1p22.1	
	HAX1	1q21.3	Autosomal recessive
	CSF3R	1p34.3	
	G6PC3	17q21.31	
	JAGN1	3p25.3	
	WAS	Xp11.23	X-linked
Familial platelet disorder with associated myeloid malignancy	RUNX1	21q22.12	Autosomal dominant
Shwachman–Diamond syndrome	SBDS	7q11.21	Autosomal recessive
	DNAJC21	5p13.2	
	EFL1	15q25.2	
	SRP54	14q13.2	Autosomal dominant
Cohen syndrome	VPS13B	8q22.2	Autosomal recessive
Glycogen storage disease 1B	SLC37A4	11q23.3	Autosomal recessive
WHIM syndrome	CXCR4	2q22.1	Autosomal dominant

Table 4.2 (cont.)

	Genes	Location	Inheritance
Congenital thrombocytopenias			
Congenital amegakaryocytic thrombocytopenia	MPL	1p34.2	Autosomal recessive
Thrombocytopenia with absent radii	RBM8A	1q21.1	Autosomal recessive
Radioulnar synostosis amegakaryocytic thrombocytopenia	HOXA11	7p15.2	Autosomal dominant
	MECOM	3q26.2	
Wiscott–Aldrich syndrome	WAS	Xp11.23	X-linked
Fanconi anemia			
	FANCA	16q24.3	Autosomal recessive
	FANCC	9q22.32	
	FANCG	9p13.3	
	BRCA2	13q13.1	
	FANCD2	3p25.3	
	FANCE	6p21.31	
	BRIP1	17q23.2	
	FANCF	11p14.3	
	FANCI	15q26.1	
	PALB2	16p12.2	
	FANCL	2p16.1	
	ERCC4	16p13.12	
	MAD2L2	1p36.22	
	RFWD3	16q23.1	
	UBE2T	1q32.1	
	XRCC2	7q36.1	
	RAD51C	17q22	
	FANCM	14q21.2	
	SLX4	16p13.3	
	RAD51	15q15.1	Autosomal dominant
	FANCB	Xp22.2	X-linked
Dyskeratosis congenita			
	DKC1	Xq28	X-linked
	TINF2	14q12	Autosomal dominant
	TERC	3q26.2	
	RTEL1	20q13.33	Autosomal dominant/ autosomal recessive
	TERT	5p15.33	
	PARN	16p13.12	
	ACD	16q22.1	
	CTC1	17p13.1	Autosomal recessive
	NHP2	5q35.3	
	WRAP53	17p13.1	
	NOP10	15q14	

Note: Comprehensive listing of the conditions described in the text, including the associated gene utilizing Human Genome Organization's Gene Nomenclature Committee approved gene symbols, chromosomal location, and inheritance pattern.

phalanges, syndactyly, and absence of nails [41]. Bone marrow morphology is notable for erythroid hyperplasia and a range of dyserythropoietic changes including binucleation, internuclear bridging, and megaloblastic changes [35]. If available, scanning electron microscopy can confirm the presence of nuclear abnormalities in erythroid cells and may show additional widening of nuclear pores, 'spongy' heterochromatin, and invagination of the cytoplasm into the nucleus. Genetic testing can confirm the diagnosis and may obviate the need for electron microscopy. Homozygous or compound heterozygous pathogenic variants in CDAN1 or C15ORF41 are identified in approximately 90% of patients [42, 43]. Treatment of CDA-I is generally supportive, including transfusions and management of iron overload which may develop even in the absence of transfusion due to ineffective erythropoiesis [44]. Interferon-alpha may result in stabilization of the hemoglobin and reduction of ineffective erythropoiesis [45–47], and is recommended in the setting of transfusion dependent anemia. While CDA type I is most likely to be recognized in infancy, CDA type II is the most frequent overall. Bone marrow findings in CDA type II include binucleated erythroblasts and, if electron microscopy is available, the appearance of a double membrane in erythroid nuclei. Abnormalities of band 3 expression on erythrocytes may lead to the misdiagnosis of hereditary spherocytosis [48]. CDA type II is caused by homozygous or compound heterozygous variants in the *SEC23B* gene. Type III CDA is the rarest subtype, with most patients described belonging to a single Swedish kindred and associated with a heterozygous variant in *KIF23*; bone marrow findings include multinucleated erythroblasts and gigantoblasts. Additional subgroups have been described and include genetic variants in the erythroid transcription factors *KLF1* and *GATA1* (CDA type IV), or dyserythropietic anemia as part of a broader syndrome (Majeed syndrome, mevalonate kinase deficiency) [49]. Hematopoietic stem cell transplantation has been successfully performed in patients with CDA but the experience is limited [50].

Congenital Neutropenias

Congenital neutropenia syndromes are a heterogeneous group of disorders, both clinically and genetically. They may be categorized according to bone marrow findings, the presence of extrahematopoietic manifestations and the associated risk for leukemia. Now that molecular diagnosis is available, it is more precise to discuss them according to the affected gene, when known (Table 4.2).

Severe Congenital Neutropenia

Severe congenital neutropenia (SCN) includes neutropenia syndromes that are associated with a maturational arrest of myelopoiesis. Neutropenia is present at birth, with absolute neutrophil counts less than 500/microliter and often less than 200/microliter. Infections, including pneumonia, cellulitis, skin

or liver abscesses and gastrointestinal infections, are common and may be life threatening [51, 52]. Gingivitis and stomatitis are frequently seen by 2 years of age but may not be present in the newborn period. Children with SCN are also at a significantly increased risk to develop myelodysplasia and leukemia (see below) [53].

Pathophysiology

Heterozygosity for a pathogenic variant in the *ELANE* gene, encoding neutrophil elastase, is present in about 50% of patients with SCN in European and North American registries [54, 55]. Pathogenic variants in *ELANE* trigger the unfolded protein response in myeloid precursors, resulting in apoptosis of promyelocytes and myelocytes just as they are starting to produce the aberrant protein [56, 57]. It is notable that complete abrogation of *ELANE* expression is not associated with neutropenia [58]. Variants involving additional genes have been described in patients with the SCN phenotype including *HAX1* (Kostmann's syndrome, autosomal recessive), *WAS* (Wiskott–Aldrich syndrome, X-linked recessive), as well as others (*CSF3R, G6PC3, JAGN1, GFI1*) [59]. There are population differences in the frequency of these mutations; for example, data from a Turkish registry found pathogenic variants in *HAX1* to be the most common cause of SCN, reflecting a higher rate of consanguinity in that cohort [60].

Diagnostic Evaluation

In addition to neutropenia, a relative monocytosis and eosinophilia may also be present. Bone marrow examination is remarkable for a maturational arrest of myelopoiesis at the level of the promyelocyte or myelocyte. Promyelocytes may exhibit atypical nuclei and vacuolization of the cytoplasm. Overall bone marrow cellularity is either normal or slightly decreased. Because multiple variants may be associated with the phenotype of SCN, in the absence of a known molecular etiology in the family, the most efficient approach to genetic testing is to use a next-generation panel with coverage of all the genes known to be associated with congenital neutropenia.

Management

The availability of granulocyte colony stimulating factor (G-CSF) treatment has led to improved survival for children with SCN, as in the pre-cytokine era more than 40% of reported patients with SCN died from infection before age 2 years [61]. In general, dosing is adjusted to maintain an absolute neutrophil count (ANC) >500–1,000/microliter with the goal of preventing severe infections. However, even if they are better protected from infection, patients with SCN remain at increased risk for leukemic transformation, with a cumulative incidence of death due to MDS or acute myeloid leukemia (AML) in 22% of patients after 15 years of G-CSF therapy in contrast to 10% of death due to infection [53]. The leukemic risk is highest in patients who require doses of G-CSF greater than 8 mcg/kg per day to maintain a protective ANC. Surveillance with annual bone marrow evaluations is recommended to detect morphologic or molecular changes associated with leukemic progression. Bone marrow transplant should be strongly considered for patients who require G-CSF doses greater than 8–10 mcg/kg per day, have significant infections despite G-CSF, have syndromes known to confer a high risk of AML, or who develop somatic mutations associated with leukemic progression (e.g. *CSF3R*, *RUNX1* or development of monosomy 7) [62], on surveillance bone marrow evaluations [52]. Transplant outcomes are better if transplant is performed prior to the development of overt leukemia [63].

Cyclic Neutropenia

Cyclic neutropenia is an enigmatic congenital neutropenia syndrome in which neutrophil counts fluctuate with a regular periodicity [64]. Frequency is estimated at 1 per 10^6 in the general population. Children usually present prior to 1 year of age with recurrent fevers, mouth ulcers, adenopathy, and bacterial infections, associated with severe neutropenia. Life threatening infections may occur. In between episodes, patients are typically asymptomatic and this can result in a delay in the diagnosis.

Pathophysiology

Intriguingly, the genetic cause of cyclic neutropenia in most cases can be traced to pathogenic variants in *ELANE*, the same gene that is affected in SCN. Inheritance is autosomal dominant, and a careful history may reveal an affected parent with a history of mouth sores in childhood that abated as they got older, as longitudinal studies have shown that in some cases the amplitude of cycling decreases with age. The reason for cycling remains unclear but the 21 day periodicity is thought to reflect the kinetics of granulopoiesis.

Diagnostic Evaluation

The hallmark of cyclic neutropenia is a pattern of severe neutropenia occurring every 21 days with recovery in between. Blood counts are obtained 2–3 times a week for at least 6 weeks in order to capture 2 nadirs and define the cycle length. At the nadir, an ANC of near 0 typically persists for 3–5 days and is associated with clinical symptoms. Upon recovery, ANC may approach the normal range. Monocytes can be seen to cycle in an opposite pattern; red cell and platelet counts may also fluctuate. A bone marrow evaluation is important to rule out alternative diagnoses.

Management

As in SCN, treatment of symptomatic patients with cyclic neutropenia includes G-CSF to prevent the episodes of oral ulcers and reduce their risk of infection. Relatively low doses of G-CSF are required, with most patients responding to less than 3 mcg/kg per day. Importantly, unlike SCN, patients with cyclic neutropenia are not at significantly increased risk for leukemia and surveillance bone marrow evaluation is not routinely required. Bone marrow transplant is not generally indicated.

Shwachman–Diamond Syndrome

The incidence of Shwachman–Diamond syndrome (SDS) is estimated at 1/76,000 births, with a slight predominance in males [65, 66]. In contrast to SCN, SDS is a multisystem disorder in which extrahematopoietic symptoms such as failure to thrive, exocrine pancreatic insufficiency and skeletal dysplasia may dominate the clinical picture, especially in the newborn period [67] (see Table 4.1). Neutropenia is usually less severe than in SCN, and neutrophil counts may even be intermittently in the normal range. Other cytopenias including anemia (normocytic or macrocytic), thrombocytopenia or even pancytopenia may be seen, and a variety of immunologic abnormalities are also described. Additional findings relevant to the newborn period may include intrauterine growth retardation, immunologic abnormalities, recurrent infections, hepatomegaly with transaminitis, and developmental delay. Significant phenotypic variability may occur, even within the same family. Shwachman–Diamond syndrome carries a risk for later development of MDS or AML, seen in about 30% of patients over time. Those at highest risk for malignant transformation are children who are less than 3 months old at diagnosis who have persistent severe cytopenias (ANC <500/microliter, Hgb <9 g/dl, and/or platelets <100 K/microliter) [51, 59].

Pathophysiology

Shwachman–Diamond syndrome is considered a ribosomopathy, with approximately 90% of patients having pathogenic variants in the *SBDS* gene on chromosome 7q11 [68]. The most common pathogenic variants are p.Lys62X and Cys84fs, resulting from conversion events between the *SBDS* gene and its highly homologous pseudogene. The SBDS protein cooperates with elongation factor 1 (EFL1) to catalyze the release of eIF6 from the 60S subunit of the ribosome [69]. Recently, variants in additional genes involved in this pathway, including *SRP54*, *DNAJC21*, and *EFL1*, have been identified in patients who have the SDS phenotype but lack identifiable *SBDS* mutations [70–72].

Diagnostic Evaluation

Diagnostic criteria for SDS include any cytopenia (though neutropenia is most common) in combination with exocrine pancreatic dysfunction [73]. Additional findings that may support the diagnosis include persistent elevation of hemoglobin F, macrocytosis, bony dysplasia, or a family history of SDS in a first degree relative. Evidence of pancreatic exocrine insufficiency may include excess fecal fat, abnormal fecal pancreatic elastase, deficiency of fat soluble vitamins, or fatty replacement of the pancreas assessed by ultrasound. Serum pancreatic isoamylase activity is not useful for diagnosis in children less than 3 years old, given that expression is not yet at adult levels. Bony abnormalities may include skeletal dysplasia, particularly involving the long bones and costochondral junctions, which may be elucidated by x-ray. Thoracic dystrophy may be severe enough to lead to a narrow or bell-shaped chest and respiratory distress [74]. Bone marrow findings are variable and may include hypocellularity, single-lineage hypoplasia, left-shifted granulopoiesis, and dysgranulopoeitic features [73]. If the diagnosis of SDS is strongly suspected based on the clinical picture, then it is reasonable to send single gene testing for *SBDS* rather than a multigene next generation sequencing panel that includes other genes associated with congenital neutropenia; however, if the

picture is unclear, then sending broader testing or utilizing a reflex strategy is more efficient.

Management

Affected children should be referred to a pediatric gastroenterologist for ongoing management of pancreatic insufficiency and monitoring of pancreatic enzyme and fat-soluble vitamin supplementation. Additional referrals may be indicated for orthopedic, endocrinologic, neurodevelopmental, or other concerns. Neutropenia may not require specific management; G-CSF can be given in the setting of infection or severe persistent neutropenia and does not appear to confer an increased risk for malignancy [75]. Routine hematologic monitoring includes peripheral blood counts every 3–4 months and bone marrow evaluation to evaluate for changes that suggest progression to MDS or AML. The appropriate frequency of bone marrow evaluation is controversial but at minimum should be performed at diagnosis, with persistent change in blood counts and annually in patients who are maintained on G-CSF [73]. Interpretation of cytogenetic changes on serial marrows can be challenging. Acquired variants such as i(7)(q10) and del(20q) are frequently observed in SDS and are not always associated with an increased risk for malignancy; in the absence of other severe cytopenias they can usually be monitored [59]. However, acquisition of monosomy 7 or multilineage dysplasia is worrisome for malignant progression. Additionally, acquisition of *TP53* mutations is associated with MDS/AML in patients with SDS and may be an early marker of malignant progression [76]. Indications for bone marrow transplant include severe infections not responding to G-CSF, severe cytopenias or development of MDS or AML [73]. SDS is associated with a high rate of transplant-related toxicities, making it challenging to determine the appropriate timing of transplant [77]; however, outcomes are best if transplant is performed prior to the onset of MDS or AML [59].

Other Congenital Neutropenias

A growing number of genes have been associated with congenital neutropenia (see Table 4.2) [59]. Clinically, the syndromes associated with each gene may be distinguished based on their pattern of inheritance, presence, or absence of extrahematopoietic features, or predisposition to malignancy;

however, a high degree of phenotypic variability and overlap between disorders are seen and provide a rationale for the early use of genetic testing as the most expedient way to establish the correct diagnosis. Children with mild neutropenia may be asymptomatic and may not present until later in life. A few disorders that deserve mention due to findings that may be present in infancy are Cohen syndrome, glycogen storage disease type IB, and WHIM (warts, hypogammaglobulinemia, immunodeficiency, and myelokathexis) syndrome.

Cohen syndrome is due to pathogenic variants in *VPS13B* and is inherited in an autosomal recessive manner [78]. In addition to neutropenia, infants may have feeding difficulties, laryngomalacia, hypotonia, microcephaly and psychomotor retardation. As children get older, typical facial features, truncal obesity with slender extremities, joint laxity, and ophthalmologic changes including retinochoroidal dystrophy and myopia, become more prominent. Neutropenia with infections and gingivitis is a variable finding and responds to G-CSF.

In **glycogen storage disease type IB** (GSD1B), homozygous or compound heterozygous pathogenic variants in the *SLC37A4* gene, which encodes glucose-6-phosphate translocase (G6PT), lead to a block in glycogenolysis and gluconeogenesis, with a resultant accumulation of glycogen and fat in the liver, kidney, and intestine [79]. While the disease occurs in all populations, prevalence is high in individuals of Ashkenazi Jewish descent. Children most commonly develop hypoglycemia and hepatomegaly at 3–6 months, as the interval between feeds gets longer, though hypoglycemic episodes may occur in the newborn period. G6PT is normally expressed in all cells but, given the high glucose demands of neutrophils, deficiency results in neutropenia, neutrophil dysfunction, and frequent infections. In addition, children with GSD1B are at increased risk for the development of hepatic adenomas, renal dysfunction, and inflammatory bowel disease. GSD1B can be diagnosed by liver biopsy and confirmed with genetic studies. Management requires intensive nutritional support to avoid hypoglycemia and G-CSF to reduce infections; liver transplant may be performed but will not correct neutropenia.

WHIM syndrome is a rare autosomal dominant immunodeficiency disorder due to heterozygous gain of function pathogenic variants in CXCR4 [80]. Approximately 100 cases have been reported in the literature. CXCR4 and its ligand CXCL12 (also known as SDF-1) regulate trafficking of neutrophils between the bone marrow and peripheral blood; in WHIM syndrome, mature neutrophils are retained in the bone marrow where they undergo apoptosis (myelokathexis). Similarly, CXCR4/CXCL12 regulate trafficking of developing B-cells within the peripheral lymphoid organs and the release of mature lymphocytes from the bone marrow, resulting in lymphopenia and immunodeficiency. While warts and HPV infections are distinctive, children frequently have pneumonias, sinusitis, cellulitis, abscesses, and urinary tract infections [81]. Once the diagnosis is suspected, a bone marrow will show the distinctive finding of myelokathexis and should prompt investigation of *CXCR4*. Common treatments include G-CSF and IVIG; however, Plerixafor, a CXCR4 antagonist, offers more targeted therapy and has shown efficacy in this rare syndrome [82].

Congenital Thrombocytopenias

As with neutropenia syndromes, congenital thrombocytopenias are heterogeneous, both clinically and genetically, and they may vary as to the presence of extrahematopoietic manifestations and risk for marrow failure or leukemia. Disorders that are most frequently diagnosed in infancy include congenital amegakaryocytic thrombocytopenia (CAMT), thrombocytopenia with absent radii (TAR), radioulnar synostosis amegakaryocytic thrombocytopenia (RUSAT), and Wiskott–Aldrich syndrome (WAS). These disorders are discussed in Chapter 15 and will not be further reviewed here.

Fanconi Anemia

Fanconi anemia (FA) is a rare hereditary disorder associated with defective DNA repair, bone marrow failure, congenital anomalies, and cancer predisposition. FA has an estimated incidence of 1 in 360,000 live births and a carrier frequency of 1 in 200 [83]. While FA is best known as a marrow failure syndrome, cytopenias may be absent in the newborn period, and thus the diagnosis may be initially suspected on the basis of characteristic congenital findings (see Table 4.1). Congenital anomalies are present in approximately 75% of patients with FA and may affect almost every organ system [84]. Important associations with FA to recognize include VACTERL-H (vertebral anomalies, anal atresia, cardiac anomalies, tracheoesophageal fistula, esophageal atresia, renal structural anomalies, limb anomalies, and hydrocephalus), and PHENOS (skin pigmentation, small head, small eyes, nervous system, otology, short stature) [85]. Additional findings may include cleft palate, developmental delay, and urogenital malformations such as hypogenitalia, undescended testes, and hypospadias in males, and bicornate uterus, aplasia, or hypoplasia of the vagina and uterus in females. Endocrinopathies such as growth hormone deficiency, abnormal glucose metabolism, hypothyroidism, and poor growth are common [86].

Bone marrow failure in FA typically presents in the first decade of life, with the average age of onset reported as 7.6 years; some patients may present earlier with cytopenias whereas others may preserve relatively normal blood counts [87]. Cytopenias are thought to be secondary to increase in accrual of DNA damage in hematopoietic stem cells (HSCs) and a pro-inflammatory state leading to apoptosis [88]. Red cell macrocytosis is often the first presenting hematologic abnormality, with thrombocytopenia typically preceding other cytopenias. Importantly, FA is a cancer predisposition syndrome, with an increased risk for both hematologic malignancies and solid tumors. Patients with FA have 67% risk of developing clonal cytogenetic abnormalities by the age of 30 and a 52% risk of MDS or AML by the age of 40 [87]. Notably in adults with FA, the incidence of squamous cell carcinomas of the head and neck, esophagus, and genitourinary tract is increased 600-fold [89, 90]. Individual subtypes of FA are associated with an especially high risk of malignancy in children, particularly BRCA2 (FANCD1) and PALBE (FANCN). The cumulative probability of any cancer, including AML, Wilm's tumor, neuroblastoma, and medulloblastoma, has been reported to be as high as 97% by 5.2 years of age in children with FA due to biallellic pathogenic variants in BRCA2 [91]. Pathogenic variants in PALB2, a BRCA2-interacting protein, confer a similar cancer risk [92].

Pathophysiology

The hallmark of FA is a defect in the repair of DNA interstrand cross links. The FA pathway includes more than 20 genes which, when mutated, lead to increased rates of chromosomal breakage [93]. In particular, FA patients are exquisitely sensitive to oxidative stress, DNA cross-linking agents and radiation. Pathogenic variants in FANCA constitute the most common subtype, whereas FANCC mutations are frequent in the Ashkenazi Jewish population [3]. The majority of FA subtypes are inherited in an autosomal recessive manner with the exception of FA associated with variants in FANCB, which are X-linked. Genetic heterogeneity is thought to contribute to the variation in clinical presentation found in FA patients, with null mutations causing a more severe phenotype [84]. Similar to DBA, somatic mosaicism has been described which may modulate the severity of the hematologic phenotype in FA. In somatic mosaicism, the spontaneous reversion of one of the inherited germ-line mutations leads to a genetically distinct population of hematopoietic stem cells which are resistant to genotoxic agents and have a proliferative advantage over the defective FA stem cells [94, 95]. Additionally, variations in non-FA genes may affect the clinical expression of the disease; for example, the coinheritance of FANCA pathogenic variants and ALDH2 variants associated with decreased detoxification of acetaldehyde leads to earlier onset of marrow failure [96].

Diagnostic Evaluation

Fanconi anemia is diagnosed by the finding of increased chromosomal breakage in an in vitro cytogenetic assay in which patient cells are exposed to a DNA cross-linking agent such as diepoxybutane (DEB) or mitomycin C (MMC) and resultant chromosomal breaks and radials are scored. The test is typically performed on peripheral blood lymphocytes, however, it is important to note that FA patients with somatic mosaicism may have indeterminate results due to the presence of revertant cells [94]. Breakage studies can be performed on cultured skin fibroblasts for a definitive result. Genetic testing should be performed in an attempt to identify the specific FA subtype. Understanding the specific FA genotype is important in order to predict the clinical phenotype and to guide the plan for cancer screening, as well as to aid in genetic counseling for families. Results of genetic studies can be used for prenatal diagnosis and pre-implantation testing, if parents are planning to have additional children. Most importantly, if a bone marrow transplant is considered, family members must be screened to ensure they do not have FA before they are used as donors [97].

Management

Management of FA includes supportive care for bone marrow failure and congenital abnormalities if present, as well as screening for malignancies [98]. Bone marrow failure is the major cause of early morbidity and mortality and frequently presents in the first decade of life. Standard recommendations are to monitor peripheral blood counts approximately every three months to detect changes indicative of marrow failure, and to evaluate the bone marrow annually to screen for dysplasia or cytogenetic abnormalities that may herald the development of leukemia. Allogeneic bone marrow transplantation is the current standard of care for the management of symptomatic bone marrow failure in FA. Androgens may improve cytopenias but are associated with complications such as virilization, abnormal growth, and hepatic toxicity, including the development of liver adenomas. They also do not prevent malignant transformation, and thus are usually reserved for patients who are not candidates for transplant [99, 100]. Gene therapy is being investigated currently in clinical trials, with some early promising results [101]. Novel treatment approaches are being explored on an investigational basis.

Additional investigations for potential extra-hematological manifestations of FA should include evaluation for immunologic, hepatic, renal, cardiac, auditory, visual, and endocrinologic abnormalities. Furthermore, patients with *BRCA2* mutations should have an abdominal US and brain MRI as a screen for neuroblastoma and medulloblastoma. Given the high risk of squamous cell carcinomas, all patients should have regular dental evaluations and older children and adults receive additional screening for squamous cell cancers [90].

Dyskeratosis Congenita

The phenotype of dyskeratosis congenita (DC) is generally defined by the diagnostic triad of lacy reticulated pigmentation, dysplastic nails and oral leukoplakia, also known as the "mucocutaneous triad". Additional clinical findings include pulmonary or hepatic fibrosis,

esophageal stricture and bone marrow failure, and patients are at risk for myeloid as well as squamous cell malignancies. This phenotype, however, is rarely seen in young children. Hoyeraal–Hreidarsson syndrome (HHS), Resvesz syndrome (RS) and Coats plus are considered severe variants of DC that present in infancy [102–104]. Clinical findings in HHS are distinctive and include intrauterine growth retardation, developmental delay, microcephaly, cerebellar hypoplasia, immunodeficiency, and bone marrow failure; RS includes similar features with the addition of exudative retinopathy (see Table 4.1) [105]. The more classical mucocutaneous findings of DC may be present or develop later in life. A variety of other manifestations, including seizures, spastic hemiparesis, intracranial calcifications, esophageal stricture, lacrimal duct stenosis, colitis, or other enteropathy, premature graying, taurodontism, hypogonadism, and urinary tract abnormalities have been reported [102].

Pathophysiology

Telomere biology disorders including DC, HHS, and RS are caused by defects that result in very short telomeres [106]. To date, X-linked pathogenic variants in *DKC1* (dyskerin), autosomal dominant pathogenic variants in *TINF2*, and autosomal recessive pathogenic variants in *TERT*, *ACD*, *PARN*, and *RTEL1*, have been reported in patients with HHS and RS [102]. Genetic anticipation, in which a disease phenotype becomes more severe or presents at an earlier age with successive generations, has been observed in DC and has been proposed a possible mechanism for the severe phenotype in HHS [107].

Diagnostic Evaluation

The hallmark of a telomere biology disorder is the finding of telomere lengths that are less than the first percentile for age in multiple subsets of peripheral blood leukocytes. Short telomeres may be seen in other marrow failure disorders, so obtaining chromosomal breakage studies, eADA and stool studies for pancreatic elastase can help to eliminate FA, DBA, and SDS, respectively, as alternative diagnoses [108]. Genetic studies, typically utilizing multigene panels, may confirm the diagnosis of DC in patients with very short telomeres; however, genetic testing fails to identify the causative mutation in about 40% of cases or, conversely, may identify genetic variants without clear clinical significance. In infants in whom a telomere biology disorder is suspected, an MRI of the brain should be performed to assess for cerebellar hypoplasia, seen in HHS, or intracranial calcifications, seen in RS, and an ophthalmologic exam should be done to look for exudative retinopathy. Laboratory studies include a complete blood count to assess for peripheral cytopenias, as well as an evaluation of immune function. A variable pattern of immunodeficiency has been noted in HHS including lymphopenia, decreased B-lymphocytes, and hypogammaglobulinemia; a picture of severe combined immunodeficiency has less commonly been reported [102].

Management

Management during infancy depends on the organs involved and the severity of disease. In contrast to DC, where cancers contribute significantly to mortality, death in HHS and RS is primarily attributed to bone marrow failure and infection [102, 109]. Therefore, careful attention to monitoring of peripheral blood counts and supportive care to prevent infections is vital. If cytopenias are present, then surveillance bone marrow evaluations are recommended in order to evaluate for the development of aplastic anemia or myelodysplasia. Treatment of cytopenias is considered when hemoglobin is less than 8 mg/dl, platelets are lower than 30 K/µl, and absolute neutrophil count is less than 1,000/µl, or if myelodysplasia is present [106]. If a matched related donor, who has been tested and is unaffected, is available, then hematopoietic stem cell transplant is generally recommended in the setting of marrow failure. There is no consensus regarding the use of matched unrelated donors. While transplant should resolve the cytopenias, radiation therapy used in conditioning or GVHD may worsen risks for strictures, squamous cell cancers, or pulmonary and hepatic fibrosis later in life. Androgen therapy (oxymethalone or danazol) may improve hematologic parameters in DC and thus is considered in patients who are not candidates for transplant; adverse effects of therapy include hepatotoxicity (transaminitis, jaundice, pelosis hepatitis, liver tumors), virilization, lipid abnormalities, aggressive behavior, and growth changes [110, 111]. Additional supportive care includes referrals for nutritional and developmental support, ophthalmologic care, hearing screen, and dental follow up to optimize oral hygiene and monitor

for changes suggestive of malignancy. Assessment of pulmonary function should begin when children are old enough to participate in testing. All efforts should be undertaken to minimize toxic exposures such as smoking, unnecessary radiation, and excessive sun exposure.

Summary

Neonatal bone marrow failure disorders are an important consideration in the differential diagnosis for the newborn with unexplained cytopenias, failure to thrive, or congenital anomalies, and the increasing availability of genetic testing has made it easier to diagnose affected children. Early diagnosis can have important implications for management of the child, identification of appropriate referrals, and counseling of the family.

References

1. Khincha PP, Savage SA. Neonatal manifestations of inherited bone marrow failure syndromes. *Semin Fetal Neonatal Med* 2016;**21**(1):57–65.

2. Giri N, Reed HD, Stratton P, Savage SA, Alter BP. Pregnancy outcomes in mothers of offspring with inherited bone marrow failure syndromes. *Pediatr Blood Cancer* 2018;**65**(1).

3. Kutler DI, Auerbach AD. Fanconi anemia in Ashkenazi Jews. *Fam Cancer* 2004;**3**(3–4):241–8.

4. Vlachos A, Klein GW, Lipton JM. The Diamond–Blackfan Anemia Registry: Tool for investigating the epidemiology and biology of Diamond–Blackfan anemia. *J Pediatr Hematol Oncol* 2001;**23**(6):377–82.

5. Farrar JE, Dahl N. Untangling the phenotypic heterogeneity of Diamond Blackfan anemia. *Semin Hematol* 2011;**48**(2):124–35.

6. Vlachos A, Rosenberg PS, Atsidaftos E, Alter BP, Lipton JM. Incidence of neoplasia in Diamond–Blackfan anemia: A report from the Diamond–Blackfan Anemia Registry. *Blood* 2012;**119**(16):3815–9.

7. Vlachos A, Rosenberg PS, Atsidaftos E, et al. Increased risk of colon cancer and osteogenic sarcoma in Diamond–Blackfan anemia. *Blood* 2018;**132**(20):2205–8.

8. Boria I, Garelli E, Gazda HT, et al. The ribosomal basis of Diamond–Blackfan anemia: Mutation and database update. *Hum Mutat* 2010;**31**(12):1269–79.

9. Dianzani I, Loreni F. Diamond–Blackfan anemia: A ribosomal puzzle. *Haematologica* 2008;**93**(11):1601–4.

10. Da Costa L, Narla A, Mohandas N. An update on the pathogenesis and diagnosis of Diamond–Blackfan anemia. *F1000Res* 2018;7.

11. Ulirsch JC, Verboon JM, Kazerounian S, et al. The genetic landscape of Diamond–Blackfan anemia. *Am J Hum Genet* 2018;**103**(6):930–47.

12. Sankaran VG, Ghazvinian R, Do R, et al. Exome sequencing identifies GATA1 mutations resulting in Diamond–Blackfan anemia. *J Clin Invest* 2012;**122**(7):2439–43.

13. Parrella S, Aspesi A, Quarello P, et al. Loss of GATA-1 full length as a cause of Diamond-Blackfan anemia phenotype. *Pediatr Blood Cancer* 2014;**61**(7):1319–21.

14. Vlachos A, Ball S, Dahl N, et al. Diagnosing and treating Diamond–Blackfan anaemia: Results of an international clinical consensus conference. *Br J Haematol* 2008;**142**(6):859–76.

15. Fargo JH, Kratz CP, Giri N, et al. Erythrocyte adenosine deaminase: Diagnostic value for Diamond–Blackfan anaemia. *Br J Haematol* 2013;**160**(4):547–54.

16. Da Costa L, O'Donohue MF, van Dooijeweert B, et al. Molecular approaches to diagnose Diamond–Blackfan anemia: The EuroDBA experience. *Eur J Med Genet* 2018;**61**(11):664–73.

17. Bartels M, Bierings M. How I manage children with Diamond–Blackfan anaemia. *Br J Haematol* 2019;**184**(2):123–33.

18. Lahoti A, Harris YT, Speiser PW, et al. Endocrine dysfunction in Diamond–Blackfan anemia (DBA): A report from the DBA Registry (DBAR). *Pediatr Blood Cancer* 2016;**63**(2):306–12.

19. Vlachos A, Muir E. How I treat Diamond–Blackfan anemia. *Blood* 2010;**116**(19):3715–23.

20. Venugopal P, Moore S, Lawrence DM, et al. Self-reverting mutations partially correct the blood phenotype in a Diamond–Blackfan anemia patient. *Haematologica* 2017;**102**(12):e506–e9.

21. Garelli E, Quarello P, Giorgio E, et al. Spontaneous remission in a Diamond–Blackfan anaemia patient due to a revertant uniparental disomy ablating a de novo RPS19 mutation. *Br J Haematol* 2019;**185**(5):994–8.

22. Jongmans MCJ, Diets IJ, Quarello P, et al. Somatic reversion events point towards. *Haematologica* 2018;**103**(12):e607–e9.

23. Ben-Ami T, Revel-Vilk S, Brooks R, et al. Extending the clinical phenotype of adenosine deaminase 2 deficiency. *J Pediatr* 2016;**177**:316–20.

24. Hashem H, Egler R, Dalal J. Refractory pure red cell aplasia manifesting as deficiency of adenosine deaminase 2. *J Pediatr Hematol Oncol* 2017;**39**(5): e293–e6.

25. Meyts I, Aksentijevich I. Deficiency of adenosine deaminase 2 (DADA2): Updates on the phenotype, genetics, pathogenesis, and treatment. *J Clin Immunol* 2018;**38**(5):569–78.

26. Pearson HA, Lobel JS, Kocoshis SA, et al. A new syndrome of refractory sideroblastic anemia with vacuolization of marrow precursors and exocrine pancreatic dysfunction. *J Pediatr* 1979;**95** (6):976–84.

27. Rotig A, Colonna M, Bonnefont JP, et al. Mitochondrial DNA deletion in Pearson's marrow/pancreas syndrome. *Lancet* 1989;**1** (8643):902–3.

28. Rötig A, Cormier V, Blanche S, et al. Pearson's marrow-pancreas syndrome: A multisystem mitochondrial disorder in infancy. *J Clin Invest* 1990;**86**(5):1601–8.

29. Shanske S, Tang Y, Hirano M, et al. Identical mitochondrial DNA deletion in a woman with ocular myopathy and in her son with Pearson syndrome. *Am J Hum Genet* 2002;**71**(3):679–83.

30. Superti-Furga A, Schoenle E, Tuchschmid P, et al. Pearson bone marrow-pancreas syndrome with insulin-dependent diabetes, progressive renal tubulopathy, organic aciduria and elevated fetal haemoglobin caused by deletion and duplication of mitochondrial DNA. *Eur J Pediatr* 1993;**152** (1):44–50.

31. Tadiotto E, Maines E, Degani D, et al. Bone marrow features in Pearson syndrome with neonatal onset: A case report and review of the literature. *Pediatr Blood Cancer* 2018;**65**(4): 10.1002/pbc.26939.

32. Roy NBA, Babbs C. The pathogenesis, diagnosis and management of congenital dyserythropoietic anaemia type I. *Br J Haematol* 2019;**185**(3):436–49.

33. Moreno-Carralero MI, Horta-Herrera S, Morado-Arias M, et al. Clinical and genetic features of congenital dyserythropoietic anemia (CDA). *Eur J Haematol* 2018;**101**(3):368–78.

34. Heimpel H. Congenital dyserythropoietic anemias: Epidemiology, clinical significance, and progress in understanding their pathogenesis. *Ann Hematol* 2004;**83**(10):613–21.

35. Heimpel H, Matuschek A, Ahmed M, et al. Frequency of congenital dyserythropoietic anemias in Europe. *Eur J Haematol* 2010;**85**(1):20–5.

36. Parez N, Dommergues M, Zupan V, et al. Severe congenital dyserythropoietic anaemia type I: Prenatal management, transfusion support and alpha-interferon therapy. *Br J Haematol* 2000;**110** (2):420–3.

37. Kato K, Sugitani M, Kawataki M, et al. Congenital dyserythropoietic anemia type 1 with fetal onset of

severe anemia. *J Pediatr Hematol Oncol* 2001;**23** (1):63–6.

38. Chin HL, Lee LY, Koh PL. Fetal-onset congenital dyserythropoietic anemia type 1 due to a novel mutation with severe iron overload and severe cholestatic liver disease. *J Pediatr Hematol Oncol* 2019;**41**(1):e51–e3.

39. Liu S, Liu YN, Zhen L, Li DZ. Fetal-onset congenital dyserythropoietic anemia type 1 due to CDAN1 mutations presenting as hydrops fetalis. *Pediatr Hematol Oncol* 2018;**35**(7–8):447–50.

40. Shalev H, Moser A, Kapelushnik J, et al. Congenital dyserythropoietic anemia type I presenting as persistent pulmonary hypertension of the newborn. *J Pediatr* 2000;**136**(4):553–5.

41. Wickramasinghe SN. Congenital dyserythropoietic anaemias: Clinical features, haematological morphology and new biochemical data. *Blood Rev* 1998;**12**(3):178–200.

42. Dgany O, Avidan N, Delaunay J, et al. Congenital dyserythropoietic anemia type I is caused by mutations in codanin-1. *Am J Hum Genet* 2002;**71** (6):1467–74.

43. Babbs C, Roberts NA, Sanchez-Pulido L, et al. Homozygous mutations in a predicted endonuclease are a novel cause of congenital dyserythropoietic anemia type I. *Haematologica* 2013;**98**(9):1383–7.

44. Heimpel H, Schwarz K, Ebnöther M, et al. Congenital dyserythropoietic anemia type I (CDA I): Molecular genetics, clinical appearance, and prognosis based on long-term observation. *Blood* 2006;**107**(1):334–40.

45. Marwaha RK, Bansal D, Trehan A, Garewal G. Interferon therapy in congenital dyserythropoietic anemia type I/II. *Pediatr Hematol Oncol* 2005;**22** (2):133–8.

46. Bader-Meunier B, Leverger G, Tchernia G, et al. Clinical and laboratory manifestations of congenital dyserythropoietic anemia type I in a cohort of French children. *J Pediatr Hematol Oncol* 2005;**27**(8):416–9.

47. Rathe M, Møller MB, Greisen PW, Fisker N. Successful management of transfusion-dependent congenital dyserythropoietic anemia type 1b with interferon alfa-2a. *Pediatr Blood Cancer* 2018;**65** (3): e26866.

48. Bianchi P, Fermo E, Vercellati C, et al. Diagnostic power of laboratory tests for hereditary spherocytosis: A comparison study in 150 patients grouped according to molecular and clinical characteristics. *Haematologica* 2012;**97**(4):516–23.

49. Iolascon A, Heimpel H, Wahlin A, Tamary H. Congenital dyserythropoietic anemias: Molecular insights and diagnostic approach. *Blood* 2013;**122** (13):2162–6.

50. Ayas M, al-Jefri A, Baothman A, et al. Transfusion-dependent congenital dyserythropoietic anemia type I successfully treated with allogeneic stem cell transplantation. *Bone Marrow Transplant* 2002;**29**(8):681–2.

51. Donadieu J, Fenneteau O, Beaupain B, Mahlaoui N, Chantelot CB. Congenital neutropenia: Diagnosis, molecular bases and patient management. *Orphanet J Rare Dis* 2011;**6**:26.

52. Dale DC. How I manage children with neutropenia. *Br J Haematol* 2017;**178**(3):351–63.

53. Rosenberg PS, Zeidler C, Bolyard AA, et al. Stable long-term risk of leukaemia in patients with severe congenital neutropenia maintained on G-CSF therapy. *Br J Haematol* 2010;**150**(2):196–9.

54. Xia J, Bolyard AA, Rodger E, et al. Prevalence of mutations in ELANE, GFI1, HAX1, SBDS, WAS and G6PC3 in patients with severe congenital neutropenia. *Br J Haematol* 2009;**147**(4):535–42.

55. Donadieu J, Leblanc T, Bader Meunier B, et al. Analysis of risk factors for myelodysplasias, leukemias and death from infection among patients with congenital neutropenia: Experience of the French Severe Chronic Neutropenia Study Group. *Haematologica* 2005;**90**(1):45–53.

56. Nanua S, Murakami M, Xia J, et al. Activation of the unfolded protein response is associated with impaired granulopoiesis in transgenic mice expressing mutant Elane. *Blood* 2011;**117** (13):3539–47.

57. Nayak RC, Trump LR, Aronow BJ, et al. Pathogenesis of ELANE-mutant severe neutropenia revealed by induced pluripotent stem cells. *J Clin Invest* 2015;**125**(8):3103–16.

58. Nasri M, Ritter M, Mir P, et al. CRISPR/Cas9 mediated ELANE knockout enables neutrophilic maturation of primary hematopoietic stem and progenitor cells and induced pluripotent stem cells of severe congenital neutropenia patients. *Haematologica* 2020;**105**(3):598–609.

59. Donadieu J, Beaupain B, Fenneteau O, Bellanné-Chantelot C. Congenital neutropenia in the era of genomics: Classification, diagnosis, and natural history. *Br J Haematol* 2017;**179**(4):557–74.

60. Yılmaz Karapınar D, Patıroğlu T, Metin A, et al. Homozygous c.130−1 ins A (pW44X) mutation in the HAX1 gene as the most common cause of congenital neutropenia in Turkey: Report from the Turkish Severe Congenital Neutropenia Registry. *Pediatr Blood Cancer* 2019;**66**(10):e27923.

61. Dale DC, Bolyard AA, Schwinzer BG, et al. The Severe Chronic Neutropenia International Registry: 10-year follow-up report. *Support Cancer Ther* 2006;3(4):220–31.

62. Touw IP. Game of clones: The genomic evolution of severe congenital neutropenia. *Hematology Am Soc Hematol Educ Program* 2015;2015:1–7.

63. Fioredda F, Iacobelli S, van Biezen A, et al. Stem cell transplantation in severe congenital neutropenia: An analysis from the European Society for Blood and Marrow Transplantation. *Blood* 2015;126(16):1885–92; quiz 970.

64. Dale DC, Welte K. Cyclic and chronic neutropenia. *Cancer Treat Res* 2011;157:97–108.

65. Ginzberg H, Shin J, Ellis L, et al. Shwachman syndrome: Phenotypic manifestations of sibling sets and isolated cases in a large patient cohort are similar. *J Pediatr* 1999;135(1):81–8.

66. Goobie S, Popovic M, Morrison J, et al. Shwachman-Diamond syndrome with exocrine pancreatic dysfunction and bone marrow failure maps to the centromeric region of chromosome 7. *Am J Hum Genet* 2001;68(4):1048–54.

67. Myers KC, Bolyard AA, Otto B, et al. Variable clinical presentation of Shwachman–Diamond syndrome: update from the North American Shwachman–Diamond Syndrome Registry. *J Pediatr* 2014;164(4):866–70.

68. Boocock GR, Morrison JA, Popovic M, et al. Mutations in SBDS are associated with Shwachman-Diamond syndrome. *Nat Genet* 2003;33(1):97–101.

69. Finch AJ, Hilcenko C, Basse N, et al. Uncoupling of GTP hydrolysis from eIF6 release on the ribosome causes Shwachman-Diamond syndrome. *Genes Dev* 2011;25(9):917–29.

70. Carapito R, Konantz M, Paillard C, et al. Mutations in signal recognition particle SRP54 cause syndromic neutropenia with Shwachman–Diamond-like features. *J Clin Invest* 2017;127 (11):4090–103.

71. Dhanraj S, Matveev A, Li H, et al. Biallelic mutations in DNAJC21 cause Shwachman–Diamond syndrome. *Blood* 2017;129(11):1557–62.

72. Tan S, Kermasson L, Hoslin A, et al. EFL1 mutations impair eIF6 release to cause Shwachman-Diamond syndrome. *Blood* 2019;134 (3):277–90.

73. Dror Y, Donadieu J, Koglmeier J, et al. Draft consensus guidelines for diagnosis and treatment of Shwachman–Diamond syndrome. *Ann N Y Acad Sci* 2011;1242:40–55.

74. Keogh SJ, McKee S, Smithson SF, Grier D, Steward CG. Shwachman–Diamond syndrome: A complex case demonstrating the potential for misdiagnosis as asphyxiating thoracic dystrophy (Jeune syndrome). *BMC Pediatr* 2012;12:48.

75. Rosenberg PS, Alter BP, Bolyard AA, et al. The incidence of leukemia and mortality from sepsis in patients with severe congenital neutropenia receiving long-term G-CSF therapy. *Blood* 2006;107(12):4628–35.

76. Link DC. Mechanisms of leukemic transformation in congenital neutropenia. *Curr Opin Hematol* 2019;26(1):34–40.

77. Toiviainen-Salo S, Pitkänen O, Holmström M, et al. Myocardial function in patients with Shwachman–Diamond syndrome: Aspects to consider before stem cell transplantation. *Pediatr Blood Cancer* 2008;51(4):461–7.

78. Chandler KE, Kidd A, Al-Gazali L, et al. Diagnostic criteria, clinical characteristics, and natural history of Cohen syndrome. *J Med Genet* 2003;40(4):233–41.

79. Kishnani PS, Austin SL, Abdenur JE, et al. Diagnosis and management of glycogen storage disease type I: a practice guideline of the American College of Medical Genetics and Genomics. *Genet Med* 2014;16(11):e1.

80. Bachelerie F. CXCL12/CXCR4-axis dysfunctions: Markers of the rare immunodeficiency disorder WHIM syndrome. *Dis Markers* 2010;29 (3–4):189–98.

81. Kawai T, Malech HL. WHIM syndrome: Congenital immune deficiency disease. *Curr Opin Hematol* 2009;16(1):20–6.

82. McDermott DH, Pastrana DV, Calvo KR, et al. Plerixafor for the treatment of WHIM syndrome. *N Engl J Med* 2019;380(2):163–70.

83. Mamrak NE, Shimamura A, Howlett NG. Recent discoveries in the molecular pathogenesis of the inherited bone marrow failure syndrome Fanconi anemia. *Blood Rev* 2017;31(3):93–9.

84. Fiesco-Roa MO, Giri N, McReynolds LJ, Best AF, Alter BP. Genotype-phenotype associations in Fanconi anemia: A literature review. *Blood Rev* 2019;37:100589.

85. Alter BP, Giri N. Thinking of VACTERL-H? Rule out Fanconi Anemia according to PHENOS. *Am J Med Genet A* 2016;170(6):1520–4.

86. Petryk A, Kanakatti Shankar R, Giri N, et al. Endocrine disorders in Fanconi anemia: Recommendations for screening and treatment. *J Clin Endocrinol Metab* 2015;100(3):803–11.

87. Kutler DI, Singh B, Satagopan J, et al. A 20-year perspective on the International Fanconi Anemia Registry (IFAR). *Blood* 2003;101(4):1249–56.

88. Brosh RM, Bellani M, Liu Y, Seidman MM. Fanconi anemia: A DNA repair disorder characterized by accelerated decline of the hematopoietic stem cell compartment and other features of aging. *Ageing Res Rev* 2017;**33**:67–75.

89. Rosenberg PS, Alter BP, Ebell W. Cancer risks in Fanconi anemia: Findings from the German Fanconi Anemia Registry. *Haematologica* 2008;**93** (4):511–7.

90. Alter BP, Giri N, Savage SA, Rosenberg PS. Cancer in the National Cancer Institute inherited bone marrow failure syndrome cohort after fifteen years of follow-up. *Haematologica* 2018;**103**(1):30–9.

91. Alter BP, Rosenberg PS, Brody LC. Clinical and molecular features associated with biallelic mutations in FANCD1/BRCA2. *J Med Genet* 2007;**44**(1):1–9.

92. Reid S, Schindler D, Hanenberg H, et al. Biallelic mutations in PALB2 cause Fanconi anemia subtype FA-N and predispose to childhood cancer. *Nat Genet* 2007;**39**(2):162–4.

93. Gueiderikh A, Rosselli F, Neto JBC. A never-ending story: The steadily growing family of the FA and FA-like genes. *Genet Mol Biol* 2017;**40** (2):398–407.

94. Lo Ten Foe JR, Kwee ML, Rooimans MA, et al. Somatic mosaicism in Fanconi anemia: Molecular basis and clinical significance. *Eur J Hum Genet* 1997;**5**(3):137–48.

95. Gross M, Hanenberg H, Lobitz S, et al. Reverse mosaicism in Fanconi anemia: Natural gene therapy via molecular self-correction. *Cytogenet Genome Res* 2002;**98**(2–3):126–35.

96. Hira A, Yabe H, Yoshida K, et al. Variant ALDH2 is associated with accelerated progression of bone marrow failure in Japanese Fanconi anemia patients. *Blood* 2013;**122**(18):3206–9.

97. Ebens CL, MacMillan ML, Wagner JE. Hematopoietic cell transplantation in Fanconi anemia: Current evidence, challenges and recommendations. *Expert Rev Hematol* 2017;**10** (1):81–97.

98. Dufour C. How I manage patients with Fanconi anaemia. *Br J Haematol* 2017;**178**(1):32–47.

99. Calado RT, Clé DV. Treatment of inherited bone marrow failure syndromes beyond transplantation. *Hematology Am Soc Hematol Educ Program* 2017;**2017**(1):96–101.

100. Paustian L, Chao MM, Hanenberg H, et al. Androgen therapy in Fanconi anemia: A retrospective analysis of 30 years in Germany. *Pediatr Hematol Oncol* 2016;**33**(1):5–12.

101. Río P, Navarro S, Wang W, et al. Successful engraftment of gene-corrected hematopoietic stem cells in non-conditioned patients with Fanconi anemia. *Nat Med* 2019;**25**(9):1396–401.

102. Glousker G, Touzot F, Revy P, Tzfati Y, Savage SA. Unraveling the pathogenesis of Hoyeraal–Hreidarsson syndrome, a complex telomere biology disorder. *Br J Haematol* 2015;**170**(4):457–71.

103. Hoyeraal HM, Lamvik J, Moe PJ. Congenital hypoplastic thrombocytopenia and cerebral malformations in two brothers. *Acta Paediatr Scand* 1970;**59**(2):185–91.

104. Knight SW, Heiss NS, Vulliamy TJ, et al. Unexplained aplastic anaemia, immunodeficiency, and cerebellar hypoplasia (Hoyeraal–Hreidarsson syndrome) due to mutations in the dyskeratosis congenita gene, DKC1. *Br J Haematol* 1999;**107**(2):335–9.

105. Revesz T, Fletcher S, al-Gazali LI, DeBuse P. Bilateral retinopathy, aplastic anaemia, and central nervous system abnormalities: A new syndrome? *J Med Genet* 1992;**29**(9):673–5.

106. Niewisch MR, Savage SA. An update on the biology and management of dyskeratosis congenita and related telomere biology disorders. *Expert Rev Hematol* 2019;**12**(12):1037–52.

107. Vulliamy TJ, Marrone A, Knight SW, et al. Mutations in dyskeratosis congenita: Their impact on telomere length and the diversity of clinical presentation. *Blood* 2006;**107**(7):2680–5.

108. Alter BP, Giri N, Savage SA, Rosenberg PS. Telomere length in inherited bone marrow failure syndromes. *Haematologica* 2015;**100** (1):49–54.

109. Alter BP, Giri N, Savage SA, Rosenberg PS. Cancer in dyskeratosis congenita. *Blood* 2009;**113** (26):6549–57.

110. Islam A, Rafiq S, Kirwan M, et al. Haematological recovery in dyskeratosis congenita patients treated with danazol. *Br J Haematol* 2013;**162** (6):854–6.

111. Khincha PP, Wentzensen IM, Giri N, Alter BP, Savage SA. Response to androgen therapy in patients with dyskeratosis congenita. *Br J Haematol* 2014;**165**(3):349–57.

Immunodeficiency Diseases of the Neonate

Julie J. Kim-Chang, James L. Wynn, Matthew A. Saxonhouse, and John W. Sleasman

Understanding the development of specific components of the neonatal immune system is critical to the understanding of the susceptibility of the neonate to specific pathogens [1]. With the increasing survival of extremely premature infants, neonatologists and other physicians caring for these newborns need to be aware of the vulnerability of this population. Furthermore, it is important for neonatologists to be able to differentiate between immune immaturity and the manifestations of a true primary immunodeficiency that present during the neonatal period. Failure to properly identify primary or acquired immunodeficiency diseases can result in delayed diagnosis and treatment, adversely affecting outcomes. This chapter will briefly define the immune immaturity of the neonate and a diagnostic approach for primary immune deficiency diseases that may present in the neonatal period.

Immaturity of the Neonatal Immune System

The immaturity of a neonate's immune response places them at an increased risk for serious infection. An understanding of the development of the neonatal immune system is essential in order to be able to differentiate the clinical manifestations of infections associated with immaturity from those that identify a specific acquired or primary immunodeficiency disease. For further detail on the development of the immune system, the reader should refer to Chapter 3. The primary components of immunity are subdivided into innate and adaptive responses. Innate immunity is antigen non-specific and composed of barriers, phagocytic cells, the complement system, pattern recognition receptors (PRRs), and soluble components of inflammation. Adaptive immunity, composed of T cells and B cells, provides immunologic specificity and memory. Because adaptive immunity is not fully developed in term and preterm infants, innate immunity plays a critical role in protecting the newborns from infection.

Innate Immunity

Barriers

Barriers provide the first line of defense from microbial invasion. Neonates have two important barrier regions: the mucosa (gastrointestinal and respiratory) and the skin. Each barrier possesses elements that reduce attachment and propagation of pathogens. The skin's antimicrobial peptides are also present in high concentrations within vernix and amniotic fluid [2]. Lack of vernix and immature stratum corneum increases the risk of microbial invasion in premature infants. Medical procedures such as placement of intravenous lines breach cutaneous barriers and further raise the risk. Immediately after birth, the gastrointestinal (GI) microbiome is quickly established, providing barrier function based on the interaction between commensal organisms and host epithelium [3, 4]. Alteration of this homeostasis through hypoxic stress, sepsis, or use of antibiotics increases the risk for barrier dysfunction and resultant bacterial translocation [5].

Respiratory barrier defense include epithelial cells, resident phagocytes, mucociliary clearance, and the secretion of a number of proteins and peptides [6]. Surfactant proteins A and D play

Neonatal Hematology, Pathogenesis, Diagnosis, and Management of Hematologic Problems, 3rd edition, ed. Pedro A. de Alarcón, Eric J. Werner, Robert D. Christensen, and Martha C. Sola-Visner. Published by Cambridge University Press. © Cambridge University Press 2021.

a valuable immune function by increasing opsonization of inhaled pathogens [7]. Respiratory mucosal function can be disrupted through altered mucus production, mechanical ventilation, surfactant deficiency, and chemical injury. The respiratory barrier defense is compromised in premature infants due to impaired mucociliary clearance, often due to deficiency in surfactant proteins, especially in infants with respiratory distress syndrome [8]. Unfortunately, these proteins are absent in commercially available surfactants due to destruction during the purification process [9].

Pathogen Recognition

Once the barrier function is breached, local sentinel immune cells respond, such as tissue macrophages that recognize invading pathogens via the activation of pattern recognition receptors (PRRs), including the toll-like receptors (TLRs), nucleotide-binding oligomerization domain (NOD)-like receptors (NLRs), retinoic acid-inducible gene-I (RIG-I)-like receptors, and c-type lectin receptors (CLRs) [10, 11]. Present on multiple cell types, TLRs recognize extracellular and intracellular pathogens by their respective microbial products. The TLR ligand–receptor binding results in downstream production proinflammatory cytokines and chemokines that initiate antimicrobial effector mechanisms [12]. At present, there are 10 known TLRs in humans, and each receptor has a specific molecular activation trigger [12, 13]. Microorganisms often stimulate more than one TLR simultaneously with the result similar to a "molecular piano" playing "chords" signaling the presence of particular types of pathogens [13, 14]. TLRs play an essential role in pathogen recognition and response, thus alterations in their function can have consequences for host response. Most aspects of cytokine response are linked to TLR stimulation, which is diminished in neonates compared to children and adults [15–18].

The NOD-like receptors are involved in activating NF-κB and MAPK pathways, as well as in the formation of the inflammasome by mediating the activation of caspase-1 [19]. Mutation in the *NLRP3* (**N**ACHT domain-, **l**eucine-**r**ich **r**epeat- and **PYRIN** domain-containing protein 3), a type NLR, leads to an autoinflammatory condition neonatal-onset multisystem inflammatory disorder (NOMID) that present in the neonatal period [20].

Adaptive Immunity

Adaptive immunity provides memory and specificity to the immune system and is mediated by T and B lymphocytes that recognize antigens in the context of their antigen specific receptors. Lymphocyte development begins in the bone marrow where a common progenitor either develops into a B cell within the bone marrow or migrates to the thymus to undergo T cell development. Both the T cell receptor (TCR) and B cells receptor (BCR) form via rearrangement of genes to form the antigen binding domains (complementary determining region 3 or CDR3) composed of variable (V), diversity (D), and joining (J) segments. The rearrangement of multiple VDJ segments is the first step in the generation of receptor diversity [21]. Further diversity is generated by terminal deoxynucleotidyl transferase (TdT) which inserts or deletes nucleotides at gene junctions creating further amino acid and CDR3 length variability. TdT is developmentally regulated throughout gestation, being less active in the fetus and premature infants resulting in less junctional diversity and shorter CDR3 lengths [22]. The impact of immature antigen receptors on immune priming and the TCR and BCR repertoire in preterm infants is unclear but likely plays an important role in the severity of intrauterine infections such as toxoplasmosis and cytomegalovirus (CMV) [23].

T-Cell Development

The primordial thymus develops at 6 weeks gestational age, and CD4$^+$ and CD8$^+$ T cells can be detected in the thymic cortex by 10 weeks. Hassall's corpuscles in the thymic medulla, an indicator of T-cell selection, are evident by 14 weeks, and intact thymic architecture forms by 18 weeks. TCR rearrangement occurs during thymic development with the initial rearrangement of the D to J and then V to DJ segments of the TCRβ chain so that a naive T cell leaving the thymus have fully functional TCRs [24]. Naive T cells can be identified by distinct surface molecules, such as CD45RA, CCR7, CD31, and CD62L allowing their identification by flow cytometry [25]. In newborns, 80% to 90% of blood T cells express a naive phenotype. T-cell numbers and percentages are higher in newborns and infants compared to adults [26]. Normal newborn values for blood lymphocytes including T-cell subsets, B cells, and NK cells as measured by flow cytometry are shown in Table 5.1 [26].

63

Table 5.1 Normal ranges of lymphocyte subset count and percent from birth to adulthood

Subset	0–3 months	3–6 months	6–12 months	1–2 years	2–6 years	6–12 years	12–18 years	adult
ALC ($\times 10^3$/mm³)	3,400–7,600	3,900–9,000	3,400–9,000	3,600–8,900	2,300–5,400	1,900–3,700	1,400–3,300	1,000–2,800
CD3+ %	73 (53–84)	66 (51–77)	65 (49–76)	65 (52–75)	66 (56–75)	69 (60–76)	73 (56–84)	55–83
CD3+ ($\times 10^3$/mm³)	3.68 (2.50–5.50)	3.93 (2.50–5.60)	3.93 (1.90–5.90)	3.55 (2.10–6.20)	2.39 (1.40–3.70)	1.82 (1.20–2.60)	1.48 (1.00–2.20)	0.7–2.1
CD19+ %	15 (06–32)	25 (11–41)	24 (14–37)	25 (16–35)	21 (14–33)	18 (13–27)	14 (06–23)	28–57
CD19 ($\times 10^3$/mm³)	0.73 (0.30–2.00)	1.55 (0.43–3.00)	1.52 (0.61–2.60)	1.31 (0.72–2.60)	0.75 (0.39–1.40)	0.48 (0.27–0.86)	0.30 (0.11–0.57)	0.3–1.4
CD16+CD56+ %	8 (04–18)	6 (03–14)	7 (03–15)	7 (03–15)	9 (04–17)	9 (04–17)	9 (03–22)	10–39
CD16+CD56+ ($\times 10^3$/mm³)	0.42 (0.17–1.10)	0.42 (0.17–0.83)	0.40 (0.16–0.95)	0.36 (0.18–0.92)	0.30 (0.13–0.72)	0.23 (0.10–0.48)	0.19 (0.07–0.48)	0.2–0.9
CD3+CD4+ %	52 (35–64)	46 (35–56)	46 (31–56)	41 (32–51)	38 (28–47)	37 (31–47)	41 (31–52)	
CD3+CD4+ ($\times 10^3$/mm³)	2.61 (1.60–4.00)	2.85 (1.80–4.00)	2.67 (1.40–4.30)	2.16 (1.30–3.40)	1.38 (0.70–2.20)	0.98 (0.65–1.50)	0.84 (0.53–1.30)	
CD3+CD8+ %	18 (12–28)	16 (12–23)	17 (12–24)	20 (14–30)	23 (16–30)	25 (18–35)	26 (18–35)	
CD3+CD8+ ($\times 10^3$/mm³)	0.98 (0.56–1.70)	1.05 (0.59–1.60)	1.04 (0.50–1.70)	1.04 (0.62–2.00)	0.84 (0.49–1.30)	0.68 (0.37–1.10)	0.53 (0.33–0.92)	
CD4/45RA/62L+ %	89 (61–94)	88 (61–94)	83 (58–91)	79 (62–90)	70 (50–85)	58 (42–74)	51 (31–65)	7–31
CD4/45RA/62L+ ($\times 10^3$/mm³)	2.25 (1.20–3.60)	2.23 (1.30–3.60)	2.10 (1.10–3.60)	1.64 (0.95–2.80)	0.96 (0.42–1.50)	0.56 (0.31–1.00)	0.39 (0.21–0.75)	0.09–0.6
CD8/45RA/62L+ %	79 (56–88)	77 (53–88)	72 (47–87)	71 (46–85)	64 (42–81)	58 (39–73)	56 (42–73)	6–19
CD8/45RA/62L+ ($\times 10^3$/mm³)	0.73 (0.38–1.30)	0.74 (0.45–1.20)	0.70 (0.33–1.20)	0.76 (0.40–1.40)	0.54 (0.26–0.85)	0.41 (0.20–0.65)	0.30 (0.17–0.56)	0.1–0.5

Note: Normal T, B, and NK values are presented as the 10th and 90th percentiles.
Source: Modified from [26].

B-Cell Development and Immunoglobulin Production

As early as the 1st trimester, IgM+/IgD+ B cells develop and IgM antibody production begins. By the 15th week of gestation B cells are present in the spleen, blood, and lymph nodes. Immunoglobulin M responses to intrauterine infections occur by the 25th week. During mid-gestation, B cells exposed to antigen become anergic, as one mechanism of neonatal tolerance [23, 27]. Immunoglobulin production is dominated by polyreactive, low affinity, *natural* IgM [28]. Preterm and term infants can mount robust responses to proteins, known as T-dependent antigens, but cannot form protective antibody responses to T-independent polysaccharide bacterial antigens [29]. The majority of blood B cells are naïve, transitioning from the bone marrow to the germinal centers (GC). In the GC, they encounter antigen presenting cells and CD4$^+$ T cells expressing CD40 ligand which induce cognate interactions with CD40 on B cells, resulting in isotype class switch [30]. All neonates have underdeveloped germinal centers, which contributes to the delay in class switch from IgM to IgA, IgG, and IgE [31]. Normal neonates are deficient in IgA, which may last throughout infancy.

Infants acquire only IgG transplacentally. It is actively transported via the FcγRn in an energy dependent process primarily during the 3rd trimester, thus IgG levels are 10 to 20% higher in term infants compared to their mother [32]. Preterm infants have significantly lower IgG levels than their mothers due to insufficient/absent transplacental transport. IgG subclass distributions and pathogen specific antibody reflect maternal levels.

Maternal IgG has a half-life of approximately 28 days and maternal levels often decline faster than the infant's ability to generate their own IgG [33]. As a result, all infants have a transient hypogammaglobulinemia of infancy in which the IgG nadir occurs between 2 and 6 months of age. If an infant is premature, IgG levels can be less than 100 mg/dl. However, for the most part, these infants can mount robust IgM and IgG immune responses to pathogens or immunizations. The changes in IgG levels during the first year of life for preterm and term infants is illustrated in Fig. 5.1. Reference values for immunoglobulin isotypes for term and preterm (>28 weeks) infants are shown in Tables 5.2–5.4.

Specific Immune Deficiency Disorders Presenting in the Neonatal Period

Primary immune deficiency diseases (PIDDs) represent over 300 genetic defects with distinct clinical phenotypes including susceptibility to infection, malignancy, immune dysregulation, and inflammation. The International Union of Immunological Societies (IUIS) Expert Committee classification system categorizes these disorders into common groups based on their pathogenesis, genotype, and clinical phenotypes [34]. The majority of PIDDs are not clinically apparent during the neonatal period, but a number of these disorders may manifest in early infancy. Due to the intrinsic immaturity of the immune system in preterm and term infants, it can be difficult to distinguish primary immune deficiency disease with underlying genetic defect from

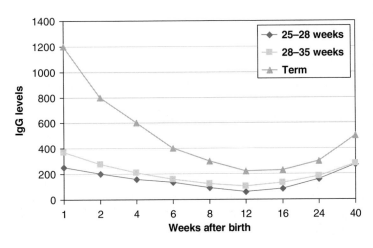

Fig. 5.1 Median IgG levels (*y*-axis) for term infants (triangle), preterm infants 28–35 weeks (square), and 25–28 weeks (diamond). Decay of maternal IgG over the first 40 weeks of life is shown on the *x*-axis. Modified from Ballow et al. [33]. (See plate section for color version.)

Table 5.2 Plasma immunoglobulin levels from birth to 3 years of age

Age	IgG (mg/dl)	IgA (mg/dl)	IgM (mg/dl)
Newborn	598–1672	0–5	5–15
1–3 months	218–610	20–53	11–51
4–6 months	228–636	27–72	25–60
7–9 months	292–816	27–73	12–124
10–18 months	383–1070	27–169	28–113
2 years	423–1184	35–222	32–131
3 years	477–1334	40–251	28–113

Reproduced with permission from Buckley, et al. [195].

Table 5.3 Plasma immunoglobulin levels in preterm infants 25–28 weeks' gesation

Age	IgG* (mg/dl)	IgM* (mg/dl)	IgA* (mg/dl)
1 week	251 (114–552)**	7.6 (1.3–43.3)	1.2 (0.07–20.8)
2 weeks	202 (91–446)	14.1 (3.5–56.1)	3.1 (0.09–10.7)
1 month	158 (57–436)	12.7 (3.0–53.3)	4.5 (0.65–60.9)
1.5 months	134 (59–307)	16.2 (4.4–59.2)	4.3 (0.9–20.9)
2 months	89 (58–136)	16.0 (5.3–36.1)	4.1 (1.5–11.1)
3 months	60 (23–156)	13.8 (5.3–36.1)	3.0 (0.6–15.6)
4 months	82 (32–210)	22.2 (11.2–43.9)	6.8 (1.0–47.8)
6 months	159 (56–455)	41.3 (8.3–205)	9.7 (3.0–31.2)
8–10 months	273 (94–794)	41.8 (31.1–56.1)	9.5 (0.9–98.6)

Reproduced with permission from Ballow M. et al. [33].
Notes: * Geometric mean.
** Normal ranges determined by taking antilog of (mean logarithm ±2 SD of the logarithms).

immune immaturity common to all newborns. Increased susceptibility to infections during the neonatal period is more likely the result of secondary immune deficiencies (immune immaturity, breakdown of innate barriers, and changes in microbial flora associated with prolonged use of antibiotics) and invasive medical procedures that compromise the barrier system (prolonged mechanical ventilation, indwelling urinary, venous, and arterial catheters) [35–37]. The IUIS classification system is shown in Table 5.5 and brief summary of disorders that present during the neonatal period are shown in Table 5.6. Specific conditions that often present during the neonatal period are described next.

Immunodeficiencies Affecting Cellular and Humoral Immunity

Cell-mediated immunity is pivotal to the neonatal immune response, but infants lack maternally acquired cellular immunity. T cell and combined immunodeficiency disorders commonly have their

Table 5.4 Plasma immunoglobulin levels in preterm infants 29–32 weeks' gestation

Age	IgG (mg/dl)*	IgM (mg/dl)*	IgA (mg/dl)*
1 week	368 (186–728)**	9.1 (2.1–39.4)	0.6 (0.04–1.0)
2 weeks	275 (119–637)	13.9 (4.7–41)	0.9 (0.01–7.5)
1 month	209 (97–452)	14.4 (6.3–33)	1.9 (0.3–12.0)
1.5 months	156 (69–352)	15.4 (5.5–43.2)	2.2 (0.7–6.5)
2 months	123 (64–237)	15.2 (4.9–46.7)	3.0 (1.1–8.3)
3 months	104 (41–268)	16.3 (7.1–37.2)	3.6 (0.8–15.4)
4 months	128 (39–425)	26.5 (7.7–91.2)	9.8 (2.5–39.3)
6 months	179 (51–634)	29.3 (10.5–81.5)	12.3 (2.7–57.1)
8–10 months	280 (140–561)	34.7 (17–70.8)	20.9 (8.3–53)

Reproduced with permission from Ballow M. et al. [33].

Notes: * Geometric mean.

** Normal ranges determined by taking antilog of (mean logarithm ±2 SD of the logarithms).

Table 5.5 International Union of Immunological Societies classification of primary immunodeficiencies seen in the newborn period

I. **Combined T- and B-cell deficiencies**
   a. SCID (based on T, B, NK phenotype)
   b. CID less profound than SCID

II. **CID with syndromic features**
   a. Wiskott–Aldrich syndrome
   b. DNA repair defects
   c. Thymic defects with congenital anomalies

III. **Predominantly antibody deficiencies**
   a. Congenital agammaglobulinemia
   b. Other antibody deficiencies (Hyper IgM)

IV. **Diseases of immune dysregulation**
   a. Hemophagocytic lymphohistiocytosis
   b. Syndromes with autoimmunity with regulatory T cell defects (IPEX)

V. **Congenital defects in phagocytes**
   a. Neutropenia
   b. Functional defects (LAD and CGD)

VI. **Defects in intrinsic and innate immunity**
   a. Bacterial and parasitic
   b. Mycobacterial and viral

VII. **Auto-inflammatory disorders**
   a. Neonatal onset multisystem inflammatory disease

VIII. **Complement deficiencies**

IX. **Phenocopies of PID**

Source: Modified from 2017 International Union of Immunological Societies (IUIS), Bousfiha et al. [34].

initial clinical manifestations during the neonatal period. Signs and symptoms suggestive of a disorder in cell-mediated immunity include opportunistic infections with organisms such as *Pneumocystis carinii* (*jirovecii*) pneumonia (PCP), *Mycobacterium tuberculosis*, fungal infections (most commonly due to *Candida*), disseminated viral infections, and graft-versus-host disease (GVHD) either due to maternally derived T cells or from transfusions with non-irradiated blood products. Manifestations of GVHD including macular erythematous rash, hepatitis, and chronic diarrhea can occur during the newborn period [38].

Severe Combined Immunodeficiency (SCID)

As implied in its name, without treatment, severe combined immunodeficiency (SCID) results in death due to infection or malignancy within the first few years of life. The condition is heterogeneous and are classified based on the relative impact on T, B, and natural killer (NK) cell numbers and function; (T^-, B^+, NK^+), (T^-, B^+, NK^-), $(T^-, B^- NK^+)$, or (T^-, B^-, NK^-). The implementation of newborn screening using T-cell receptor excision circles (TRECs) have shown that the overall incidence of SCID and other cellular

Table 5.6 Clinical and laboratory findings of primary immune deficiencies seen in the newborn period

Condition	Clinical/laboratory findings	Confirmation testing
Cellular immune deficiencies		
ZAP70 deficiency	Low T-cell numbers with elevated CD4/CD8 T cell ratio Normal TREC	Absent mitogen response corrected ex vivo by phorbol ester. Genetic testing shows mutation in ZAP70
MHC-I deficiency	Sinopulmonary infections, granulomatous skin lesions. CD8 lymphopenia Normal TREC	CD8 lymphopenia on flow cytometry
MHC-II deficiency	Diarrhea, hepatosplenomegaly, transaminitis, sclerosing cholangitis, pulmonary infections (PCP, encapsulated bacteria, herpesvirus), meningitis. CD4 T lymphopenia, hypogammaglobulinemia, absent germinal centers in lymph nodes Normal TREC	CD4 lymphopenia on flow cytometry
DOCK8 deficiency	Eczema, food allergies, refractory viral skin lesions (HPV, HSV, VZV, molluscum), mucocutaneous candidiasis, pneumonias. Lymphopenia, eosinophilia, IgE may be elevated Low TREC	DOCK8 mutation by genetic analysis
Ataxia–telangiectasia	Progressive cerebellar ataxia, oculocutaneous telangiectasia, recurrent sinupulmonary infections, low B and T cell numbers, elevated serum AFP and CEA, may have low IgA or IgG levels TREC may be low	ATM mutation by genetic analysis
DiGeorge syndrome	Thymic hypoplasia/aplasia, hypocalcemia (parathyroid deficiency), congenital heart disease (conotruncal defects) Complete: Naïve T cells < 50/mm^3 + low/no mitogen proliferation Partial: +/− low T cells, usually normal mitogen proliferation May have low immunoglobulins if T cell defect severe TREC may be low	Meeting 2 of 3 clinical criteria (thymic hypoplasia/ hypoparathyroidism/ congenital heart disease), or detection of 22q11 deletion on FISH or microarray, or identification of known gene mutations (such as TBX1, CHD7)
Cartilage hair hypoplasia (CHH)	Short-limbed dwarfism, sparse hair, bone marrow failure, autoimmunity, thymic hypoplasia, Hirschsprung's disease. Low to normal T cell numbers TREC may be low	RMRP mutation by genetic analysis
Netherton syndrome	Generalized scaly erythroderma, "bamboo hair" (short brittle spiky), atopy (severe atopic dermatitis), elevated IgE, IgA, hypernatremic dehydration, failure to thrive, bacterial infections Normal TREC	SPINK5 mutation by genetic analysis. Hair microscopy confirms the presence of *trichorrhexis invaginata* for quick diagnosis
Dyskeratosis congenita (DC)	Nail dystrophy, abnormal skin pigmentation, oral leukoplakia, severe enteropathy, recurrent infections, bone marrow failure. Lymphopenia, low B-cell numbers, hypogammaglobulinemia, decreased T-cell function possible TREC may be low	Telomere length analysis and genetic mutation identified in one of the multiple known mutations in addition to meeting clinical criteria
NEMO deficiency syndrome	Conical teeth, sparse scalp hair, frontal bossing, absent sweat glands, eczema, recurrent bacterial infections or MAI infection. Low IgG, specific antibody deficiency, poor NK cell function, variable T and B cell dysfunction Normal TREC	IKBKG mutation by genetic analysis

Antibody deficiency diseases

X-linked agammaglobulinemia	Recurrent bacterial infection, overwhelming enteroviral sepsis in newborn. Low or absent immunoglobulins Normal TREC	Lack of CD19 or CD20 on flow cytometry analysis. Genetic mutation in BTK
Hyper-IgM syndrome	Infections with encapsulated bacteria, peri-rectal abscesses, oral ulcers, PCP pneumonia, *Cryptosporidium* infections, diarrhea (*Salmonella, Giardia, Entamoeba*), generalized lymphadenopathy and splenomegaly. Low or absent IgG, IgA, IgE, with normal or elevated IgM Normal TREC	Identification of known genetic mutations: CD40L, CD40, UNG, AID

Diseases of immune dysregulation

Familial hemophagocytic lymphohistiocytosis (F-HLH)	Fever, splenomegaly, cytopenia, hypertriglyceridemia, hypofibrinogenemia, elevated sIL-2Rα, reduced NK cell function, evidence of HLH in BM or lymphoid tissues Normal TREC	Diagnostic criteria and/or Identification of known genetic mutations: PRF1, UNC13D, STX11, STXBP2
Wiskott–Aldrich syndrome	Eczema, thrombocytopenia, recurrent bacterial infections with low IgM, elevated IgA, normal IgG Normal TREC	WASP mutation by genetic analysis.
Chédiak–Higashi syndrome (CHS)	Recurrent bacterial infections, oculocutaneous albinism, coagulation defects, neurological deterioration. Enlarged azurophilic lysosomal granules in neutrophils, eosinophils. Absent NK cytotoxicity, decreased neutrophil chemotaxis, neutropenia. Progress to accelerated phase (HLH) Normal TREC	Peripheral blood smear examination for pathognomonic giant cytoplasmic granules in leukocytes and platelets. Mutation in *CHS/LYST* by genetic analysis
Griscelli syndrome type 2	Partial albinism, neutropenia, thrombocytopenia, progressive neurologic deterioration. Progress to accelerated phase (HLH) Normal TREC	Microscopic examination of hair shaft showing clumps of pigment. No giant granules on peripheral smear (DDx CHS)
XIAP deficiency	Recurrent splenomegaly, HLH triggered by virus, intractable IBD Normal TREC	Mutation in XIAP by genetic analysis
Immunedysregulation, polyendocrinopahty, enteropaty, X-linked (IPEX)	Type I Diabetes in infancy, chronic enteropathy, failure to thrive, eczema, elevated IgA, and IgE Normal TREC	Absent T regulatory cells by FoxP3 staining, or mutations in the FOXP3 gene

Defects in granulocyte function

Leukocyte adhesion deficiency (LAD)	LADI: Delayed separation of umbilical cord, impaired wound healing, serious/recurrent bacterial infections of skin and mucosal surfaces with absent pus formation. Persistent leukocytosis (>25,000 cells/uL) LADII: Milder infections, no delay in separation of umbilical cord. Intellectual disabilities, short stature LADIII: Similar to LADI plus life-threatening bleeding disorder Normal TREC	LADI: Absence of CD11a, b, c, and/or CD18 expression on leukocytes on flow cytometry. Mutation in *ITGB2* gene LADII: Absence of H antigen on myeloid cells (Bombay), absence of CD15a expression on flow cytometry. Mutation in *SLC35C1* gene LADIII: Mutation in *FERMT3* gene
Chronic granulomatous disease (CGD)	Recurrent bacterial and fungal infections with catalase positive organisms, inflammatory granuloma formation Normal TREC	Abnormal respiratory burst by DHR assay. Mutation in *CYBB, CYBA, NCF1, NCF2*, or *NCF4* on genetic analysis

Defects in Innate Immunity

Toll-like receptor signaling pathway deficiency (includes *TLR3, UNC93B1, TRIF, TRAF3, TBK1*)	HSV-1 encephalitis. Abnormal TLR function (performed when patient clinically well) Normal TREC	Mutation in *TLR3* and associated genes

Table 5.6 (cont.)

NOMID	Frontal bossing, protruding eyes, saddle-shaped nose, recurrent fevers, migratory erythematous rash, impaired growth, chronic aseptic meningitis, sensorineural hearing loss, cerebral atrophy, lymphadenopathy, hepatosplenomegaly Normal TREC	*NLRP3* mutation by genetic analysis
Acquired immune deficiency		
Pediatric AIDS	Opportunistic infections, inverted CD4/CD8 ratio, elevated IgA and IgM Normal TREC	Detection of HIV RNA in plasma or DNA in cells

Notes: Alpha-fetoprotein (AFP), Carcinoembryonic antigen (CEA), *Mycobacterium avium* (MAI), dihydrorhodamine 123 (DHR).

Table 5.7 Inheritance and distribution of lymphocyte subsets in different forms of SCID

Lymphocyte subsets	Defect	Inheritance
T⁻/B⁻/NK⁻	ADA deficiency	Autosomal recessive
	PNP deficiency (NK may be +)	Autosomal recessive
	Adenylate kinase 2 (Reticular Dysgenesis)	Autosomal recessive
T⁻/B⁻/NK⁺	RAG 1/2	Autosomal recessive
	Artemis	Autosomal recessive
	Cernunnos	Autosomal recessive
	Ligase IV	Autosomal recessive
T⁻/B⁺/NK⁻	Common γc (X-linked SCID)	X-linked
	Jak3 deficiency	Autosomal recessive
T⁻/B⁺ /NK⁺	IL-7Rα	Autosomal recessive
	IL-2Rα	Autosomal recessive
	CD45	Autosomal recessive
	Defects of CD3 chain (CD3δ, CD3ε, CD3ζ)	Autosomal recessive
	FOXN1	Autosomal recessive

immune deficiencies in the United States is 1 in 20,000 live births with variation in incidence and type [39]. The different cellular phenotypes of SCID are summarized in Table 5.7. Because of the high complexity and rapid changes in the management of infants with T-cell deficiency and SCID, rapid referral to a tertiary care center is recommended for early hematopoietic stem cell transplantation (HSCT) prior to infections [40].

T⁻, B⁺, NK⁺ SCID

Examples include IL-7Rα deficiency which results in intrathymic arrest in T-cell development and FOXN1 deficiency that results in abnormal thymic epithelia. Mutations in antigen receptor genes such as CD3δ, CD3ε, and CD3ζ, as well as CD45, a critical regulator of signaling thresholds, also lead to this phenotype [41]. In all cases, T cells fail to develop, but B cells and NK cells are spared [38].

T⁻, B⁺, NK⁻ SCID

This phenotype results from abnormal signaling through the interleukin receptor common γ chain (γc) or further downstream defects involving JAK/STAT pathway. The X-linked form impairs the common interleukin γc cell surface receptor required for signaling of multiple cytokines including IL-2, IL-4, IL-7, IL-21, and IL-15. JAK-3 deficiency results in an identical phenotype because it associates with the common γc receptor for cell signaling, but is inherited in an autosomal recessive pattern [42]. Taken together, all are critical components of T, B, and NK cell function. Infants with these forms of SCID lack circulating T cells because T-cell maturation arrests in the thymus [43]. B cells are present in normal or increased numbers but are deficient in function. NK cell numbers and function are low as well. Gene therapy trials are underway to treat X-linked SCID.

T⁻, B⁻, NK⁺ SCID

The most common form of this SCID subtype is defects in recombinase-activating gene (RAG), which plays a critical role in the formation of T- and B-cell antigen receptors, leading to failure of T- and B-cell development, with intact NK cells [44]. Other deficiencies with similar phenotypes include Artemis (DCLRE1C) deficiency and DNA ligase IV deficiency (with microcephaly and facial dysmorphism), both involved in DNA repair, leading to defective V(D)J recombination of the antigen receptors. Defects in DNA repair enzymes carry the risk of radiosensitivity and malignancy as well as suppression of hematopoiesis. T- and B-cell development may not be totally arrested and "leaky" forms of this subtype often result in severe erythematous rashes and autoimmune cytopenia due to oligoclonal expansion of autoreactive lymphocytes.

T⁻, B⁻, NK⁻ SCID

This subtype most commonly results from adenosine deaminase (ADA) deficiency. Reticular dysgenesis and PNP (purine nucleoside phosphorylase) deficiency also display similar lymphocyte distribution (reticular dysgenesis additionally impacts all hematopoietic lineages). ADA catabolizes the deamination of adenosine and $2'$-deoxyadenosine, converting them to inosine [45]. Lack of ADA results in the intracellular accumulation of adenosine and $2'$-deoxyadenosine, leading to the accumulation of deoxyadenosine triphosphate (deoxyATP), which has a feedback inhibition effect on ribonucleotide reductase, an enzyme required for normal DNA synthesis. Overall, DNA synthesis is impaired, and no lymphocyte cellular proliferation occurs with activation. In addition, $2'$-deoxyadenosine is a cellular toxin reported to cause chromosome breakage and ultimately severe lymphopenia resulting in absent T cells, B cells, and NK cells. Enzyme replacement therapy with polyethylene glycol (PEG) modified bovine ADA given by subcutaneous injection once weekly has resulted in clinical and immunologic improvement [45–48]. Trials of gene therapy are currently underway to treat ADA deficiency, and an ex vivo gene therapy is approved in Europe [49].

Combined Immunodeficiency (CID)

Clinical phenotypes of CIDs are generally less profound and more variable in their manifestations than SCID. However, they carry similar risk for susceptibility to opportunistic infections and autoimmune cytopenias during the newborn period. Similar to SCID, different lymphocyte populations are affected and pathogenesis is variable [38]. For example, major histocompatibility complex (MHC) class-I or class-II deficiencies are associated with low levels of the CD8⁺ or CD4⁺ subsets, respectively. ZAP-70 deficiency results in a defective T-cell receptor signaling cascade resulting in poor proliferation to mitogens with normal numbers of CD3⁺ and CD4⁺ T cells but low numbers of CD8⁺ T cells. DOCK8 deficiency is characterized by low B and NK cell numbers, lymphopenia, elevated IgE, low IgM, eosinophilia, severe atopic disease, and recurrent staphylococcal and viral infections.

Combined Immunodeficiency with Associated Syndromic Features

Conditions that affect cellular and humoral immunity but have clearly recognizable clinical phenotypes can involve single or multiple genes. The majority have multiple organ systems involved beyond the immune system, and immune dysfunction may be a minor component of the syndrome. Representative examples seen in the newborn period are listed below.

Wiskott–Aldrich Syndrome (WAS)

The triad of immunodeficiency, thrombocytopenia, and eczema characterizes WAS. It is an X-linked recessive disorder associated with mutations in the WAS gene located in Xp11.23 encoding a protein known as Wiskott–Aldrich syndrome protein (WASp). Expressed by hematopoietic cells, this gene stabilizes actin polymerization and cytoskeleton arrangement. Multiple mutations have been identified resulting in different phenotypes (as in X-linked thrombocytopenia) within the syndrome but all share features indicating abnormal WASp function [50–55]. Platelets and lymphocytes have abnormal size, shape, and function. In particular, platelets are small, aggregate poorly, and are sequestered and destroyed in the spleen. Hemorrhage is the most common complication of WAS in infancy, and a major cause of morbidity and mortality [56]. T cells are also small with abnormal cytoskeleton leading to skewing toward a Th2 cytokine profile. There is a characteristic immunoglobulin profile of elevated IgA and IgE levels, with low IgM levels.

Clinical manifestations that can be seen in early infancy include eczema, autoimmune hemolytic anemia, and thrombocytopenia. There is increased susceptibility to serious viral infections including disseminated herpes simplex, varicella-zoster, and molluscum contagiosum, as well as severe infections with encapsulated bacteria [34, 57, 58]. Infants with WAS may also experience an accelerated phase, with features of hemophagocytic lymphohistiocytosis (HLH, see the subsection on HLH later). Because of the long-term complications of immunodeficiency and malignancy, bone marrow transplantation is commonly applied to WAS and gene therapy is in development.

Ataxia–Telangiectasia

Ataxia–telangiectasia (AT) is an autosomal recessive disorder caused by biallelic mutations in DNA repair enzyme ATM (ataxia–telangiectasia mutated), a serine/threonine kinase encoded on chromosome 11q22.3, leading to DNA repair defects affecting all nucleated cells in the body [59]. Characteristic clinical features include progressive cerebellar ataxia as well as oculocutaneous telangiectasia that is rarely evident in the newborn. However, the enzyme defect also causes thymic hypoplasia which may result in abnormal TREC levels in the newborn screen due to low naive T-cell numbers [60]. Other laboratory manifestations include elevated serum α-fetoprotein and carcinoembryonic antigen, low B- and T-cell numbers, and selective IgA deficiency [61]. A subset of patients has hyper IgM phenotype with hypogammaglobulinemia and high or normal IgM levels [60]. Overall, immunodeficiency in AT is combined, remains low over time, and is not progressive [62]. Radiation sensitivity increases risk for lymphoreticular malignancies so early recognition is critical in clinical management. Treatment is based on disease manifestations. Prophylactic antibiotics may be used for recurrent sinopulmonary infections, and immune globulin replacement therapy can be considered for those with hypogammaglobulinemia or impaired specific antibody production.

The 22q11 Deletion Syndrome (DiGeorge Syndrome, DGS)

The combination of thymic defects with varying degrees of T-cell deficiency and associated congenital conotruncal cardiac defects, facial dysmorphism, cleft palate, and hypoparathyroidism are typical of DGS [63]. This syndrome is relatively common affecting up to 1 in 1,200 individuals [64, 65]. Abnormal migration of neural crest cells forming the third and fourth pharyngeal arches during early gestation is postulated to impair embryonic development of the thymus, parathyroid gland, heart, and face. Approximately 90% of patients with DGS have an underlying microdeletion within chromosomal region 22q11.2 but genetic deletions in chromosomes 10p13 and 17p13 are also associated with similar phenotypes [66, 67]. Within 22q11 deletions, T-box transcription-factor family, TBX1, has been implicated as a cause of most of the clinical manifestations [68, 69]. While most 22q11 deletions are sporadic, the deletion is inherited as an autosomal codominant condition; half of the siblings may be affected, and 10% of affected children have an affected parent. Conotruncal cardiac defects, including truncus arteriosus, tetralogy of Fallot, interrupted aortic arch type b, or aberrant right subclavian artery are the most frequent cardiac features. Dysmorphic facial features include prominent nasal root with bulbous tip, protuberant ears, cup-shaped helices, and small, carp-like mouth. Cleft lip and palate and velopharyngeal insufficiency result in speech abnormalities. Hypoparathyroidism leads to hypocalcemia, often associated with neonatal tetany and seizures. Developmental and language delay, learning disabilities, and neuropsychiatric problems including schizophrenia are common [63, 67, 70]. Other genetic syndromes associated with thymic aplasia include CHARGE syndrome most commonly associated with mutations in chromodomain helicase DNA-binding protein 7 (CHD7) gene on chromosome 8q12 or mutations in semaphorin-3E gene (SEMA3E) on chromosome 7q21 [71, 72]. Clinical manifestations of CHARGE include coloboma of the eyes, heart anomalies, choanal atresia, CNS abnormalities, developmental delay, and genital, and ear malformations [73].

Arrested T-cell development due to thymic aplasia or hypoplasia is a hallmark of the immune defects as the thymus maybe absent or reduced in size based on imaging. When T cells are completely absent (naive T cells < 50 cells/μl, termed complete DiGeorge syndrome) infection risk is extremely high and treatment requires thymic transplantation. With low $CD3^+$ T counts less than 500/μL, there can be a poor proliferation response to T-cell mitogens, elevated CD4 to

CD8 T cell ratios, and low numbers of naive T cells. Partial thymic hypoplasia is associated with antibody abnormalities such as poor response to immunizations, selective IgA deficiency, hypogammaglobulinemia, and autoimmunity (primarily autoimmune cytopenias) [74].

The treatment for individuals with DGS usually involves prophylaxis alone as most patients have the partial form and show a gradual improvement in T-cell development. Treatment for complete DGS involves intravenous immunoglobulin (IVIg) and thymus transplantation [75]. Thymic tissues obtained during elective cardiac surgery can be implanted, and this has been successfully carried out without human leukocyte antigen (HLA) matching or the risk of GVHD [75]. Otherwise, treatment is focused on correction of the cardiac and parathyroid defects and prevention of opportunistic infections with prophylactic antibiotics.

Cartilage Hair Hypoplasia (CHH)

Cartilage hair hypoplasia is characterized by short-limbed dwarfism with metaphyseal dysostosis, sparse hair, bone marrow failure, autoimmunity, and neuronal dysplasia of the intestine. Affected individuals are susceptible to developing lymphoma and other cancers [76]. It is also associated with varying degrees of thymic hypoplasia ranging from SCID to normal thymic output, thus infants with this condition may have abnormal newborn screen with low TRECs. Mutation in RMRP gene is responsible for the condition [76]. CHH presenting with SCID require HSCT. HSCT corrects immune deficiency and autoimmunity but does not improve the musculoskeletal or growth features. Careful monitoring of bowel function during the first year of life is important as Hirschsprung's disease is common.

Netherton Syndrome

Netherton syndrome is a rare autosomal recessive skin disorder caused by mutations in the serine protease inhibitor of Kazal type 5 gene (SPINK5) located on chromosome 5q32 [77, 78]. Typical presentation is characterized by the classic triad of congenital ichthyosiform erythroderma, specific hair shaft abnormality termed *trichorrhexis invaginata* ("bamboo hair"), and atopy (severe atopic dermatitis, elevated serum levels of IgE, and later development of asthma and hay fever)

[79]. Infants with this condition typically present at birth with generalized scaling erythroderma, and have life-threatening complications such as hypernatremic dehydration (from water loss through the dysfunctional skin barrier), failure to thrive, and bacterial infections. IgE and IgA are elevated and other immunoglobulins may be decreased [78]. These infants should be managed in an intensive care unit, with careful monitoring of body temperature, fluid, and electrolytes, as well as prevention and treatment of infections. Dermatitis should be managed with good skin care with liberal application of moisturizers, topical anti-inflammatory agents (corticosteroids, calcineurin inhibitors), and oral antihistamines for the management of pruritis.

Dyskeratosis Congenita (DC)

Dyskeratosis congenita is characterized by nail dystrophy, abnormal skin pigmentation (poikiloderma), and oral leukoplakia. Individuals with DC are predisposed to cancers and bone marrow failure. Some may present with palmar hyperkeratosis, pancytopenia, intrauterine growth retardation (IUGR), sparse scalp hair and eyelashes, recurrent infections, developmental delay, and in severe cases, cerebellar hypoplasia, microcephaly, and organ fibrosis (pulmonary fibrosis, esophageal stricture, liver cirrhosis) [80]. Immune phenotypes are variable, but lymphopenia, low B-cell numbers, hypogammaglobulinemia, and decreased T-cell function are frequently found. Onset of disease in infancy is associated with more severe immunologic and somatic features, especially severe enteropathy [81]. It is a condition of defective maintenance of telomeres resulting in shortened telomere length. Various inheritance patterns have been observed depending on the affected gene, including autosomal dominant, autosomal recessive, and X-linked. Treatment is based on clinical manifestations and ongoing screening is recommended for bone marrow failure, myelodysplastic syndrome, solid tumors, pulmonary fibrosis, liver disease, thyroid function, and osteopenia.

NEMO (NF-κB Essential Modulator) Deficiency Syndrome

NEMO deficiency syndrome is a rare X-linked recessive disorder characterized by anhidrotic ectodermal dysplasia with immunodeficiency (EDA-ID) caused by hypomorphic mutations in the IKBKG (inhibitor of nuclear factor kappa-B kinase regulatory subunit gamma) gene encoding NEMO protein, a key regulator of the canonical NF-κB signaling pathway. Loss-of-function mutations of IKBKG leads to X-linked incontinentia pigmenti, which is usually lethal in male fetuses. Hypomorphic IKBKG mutation leads to EDA-ID with diverse clinical manifestations [82]. Infants with NEMO deficiency present with abnormal development of ectodermal tissue including skin, hair, teeth, and sweat glands, along with severe infections. Typical EDA-ID presentation includes conical teeth, sparse scalp hair, frontal bossing, absence of sweat glands, along with early multiple and severe bacterial infections with pyogenic bacteria (*Streptococcus pneumoniae, Staphylococcus aureus, Haemophilus influenzae*) or mycobacteria (*Mycobacterium avium*) [83]. Infants may present with eczematous dermatitis soon after birth. Clinical manifestations may be evident soon after birth and their life expectancy depends on the degree of immune deficiency. Immunologic manifestations include hypogammaglobulinemia, some with hyper IgM, impaired specific antibody production, impaired T-cell receptor activation, monocyte dysfunction, poor cytotoxic NK cell activity, and variable T and B cell dysfunction (such as low naive T cells, low memory CD27 +/CD19+ B cells) [82, 84]. Treatment includes immune globulin replacement therapy and antimycobacterial prophylaxis. Chronic herpes antiviral prophylaxis may also be used in those with herpesvirus infections. HSCT is recommended for those with severe disease course.

Predominantly Antibody Deficiencies

Clinical Manifestations of Disorders in Antibody Production

Deficiencies in B-cell function are difficult to recognize during the newborn period due to passive acquisition of maternal IgG and low IgA levels throughout infancy. Defects in antibody production are characterized by bacterial sinopulmonary infections, meningitis, and sepsis as well as persistent enteroviral infections of the gastrointestinal tract or central nervous system [37]. Catabolism of passively acquired antibody occurs with a half-life of approximately 30 days, although maternal antibody can be detected throughout the first eighteen months of life [6]. As the levels of maternal antibody decline, immunoglobulin deficiency in the neonate becomes apparent and generally can be detected after age six months, or even earlier in preterm infants.

Transient Hypogammaglobulinemia of Infancy (THI)

The question remains as to whether THI is a true primary immune deficiency or an extension of the physiologic nadir that occurs as maternal antibody disappears and the infant begins its own antibody production [85]. Normal IgG nadir occurs between 3 and 6 months in term infants with significantly lower values seen in premature infants [33]. In THI, IgG levels are greater than two standard deviations below normal age-related ranges and all immunoglobulin isotypes can be affected (see Tables 5.2–5.4) [85–87]. This phenomenon should be considered in chronically ill infants who remain hospitalized for several months, as recurrent infection, malnutrition, and repeated phlebotomy accentuate antibody loss. Examination of the impact of low serum gammaglobulin (levels <4 g/ L total serum IgG) in preterm infants (24–32 weeks gestational age) revealed an increased risk for infection but not mortality compared to those with levels >4 g/L after controlling for gestational age, and the risk did not decrease with use of IVIg [88, 89]. There is evidence that infants with THI have a transient defect in $CD4^+$ T helper cell function when compared to normal infants [90]. However, B-cell numbers in these children are normal and they are able to generate specific antibody responses following immunization with T-dependent antigens such as tetanus toxoid [89].

X-Linked Agammaglobulinemia (XLA)

XLA results in profoundly diminished levels of all immunoglobulin isotypes that remain depressed for life. The defect in XLA is due to a mutation in the gene encoding B cell-specific src-associated tyrosine kinase (Bruton's tyrosine kinase or BTK). This protein plays a pivotal role in early B cell development at the pre-B-cell stage in the bone marrow leading to absent B cells in peripheral blood and lymphoid tissues [91]. Lack of circulating CD19 and CD20 B cells allows the condition to be diagnosed by flow cytometry analysis [92]. T-cell development, numbers, and function are normal. Clinical manifestations that have been observed in newborns include overwhelming enteroviral sepsis [93]. Treatment for XLA is immune globulin replacement therapy.

Hyper-IgM (HIGM) Syndrome

In the most common form of HIGM syndrome, a molecular defect in immunoglobulin class-switch results from a mutation in CD40 ligand (CD40L) which mediates class switch through cognate interaction between CD40L on the T cell and CD40 expressed on B cells. There are low or absent levels of serum IgG, IgA, and IgE with normal to elevated levels of IgM [94]. During the neonatal period, immunoglobulin profiles can appear very similar to those of normal infants or infants with an intrauterine infection. B-cell numbers are normal but infections with encapsulated organisms are common. More than half of the infants with hyper-IgM syndrome have neutropenia with associated peri-rectal abscesses and oral ulcers [95]. In addition, pneumonitis due to infection with *P. jirovecii* is frequent and cholangitis due to *Cryptosporidium* has been reported. There is an increased susceptibility to diarrhea due to *Salmonella*, *Giardia*, and *Entamoeba* [96]. The disorder has also been reported in association with congenital rubella. Nodular lymphoid hyperplasia of the intestinal tract and generalized lymphadenopathy and splenomegaly can occur in young infants [96]. HIGM is most commonly inherited as X-linked primary immune deficiency but autosomal recessive forms have also been recognized [95, 97]. The mutation in the *CD40LG* gene in the X-linked form has been mapped to Xq26 [97, 98]. Other rare molecular defects that present with hyper-IgM syndrome phenotype include CD40 deficiency (mutations in *CD40* gene, inherited AR), AID deficiency (mutations in *AIDCA* gene, AD, or AR), UNG deficiency (mutations in *UNG* gene, AR), and more recently identified mutations in *PIK3CD* and *PI3KR1* genes [95, 99, 100].

All patients with HIGM are treated with immune globulin replacement therapy. Additional therapies depend on the type of hyper-IgM and the disease manifestations of each patient. PCP prophylaxis should be considered for those with CD40L and CD40 deficiency as these defects lead to combined immunodeficiency [96]. G-CSF (granulocyte-colony stimulating factor) may be considered for those with severe chronic neutropenia [101]. HSCT is the only curative approach for patients with CD40L deficiency and early transplant may prevent liver disease [102].

Antibody Deficiency Associated with Secondary Immune Disorders

Many conditions seen in neonates accompany antibody deficiency as part of their clinical spectrum. Specifically, Turner syndrome is often associated with decreased IgG and IgM levels [103]. Immunodeficiency, centromeric heterochromatin, and facial abnormalities (ICF) syndrome results in the instability of chromosomes 1, 9, 16, and 20 with associated findings of low total immunoglobulin levels, absent isohemagglutinins, and dysgammaglobulinemia [104, 105]. Hypogammaglobulinemia is a common associated finding in Trisomy 21, Monosomy 22, Trisomy 8, and Chromosome 18q-syndrome [106]. Not surprisingly, sickle cell disease and congenital asplenia syndromes have increased susceptibility to sepsis due to encapsulated bacteria [107]. The functional asplenia observed in sickle-cell disease actually begins during the first year of life. Congenital infections with rubella, CMV, HIV, Epstein–Barr virus (EBV), and toxoplasmosis can impair both antibody production and function [6]. Antibody deficiency can occur due to protein losing enteropathies and any other conditions that result in excessive loss of protein. Low total IgG levels at birth in the term infant suggests a maternal antibody deficiency disease [108].

Diseases of Immune Dysregulation

Hemophagocytic Lymphohistiocytosis (HLH)

Hemophagocytic lymphohistiocytosis is characterized by immune dysregulation with hyperinflammatory response associated with aberrant activation of macrophages and lymphocytes leading to overwhelming cytokine release. It typically affects infants from birth to 18 months of age. Infants may present in the newborn period with a constellation of symptoms including persistent fever, splenomegaly with cytopenia, hypertriglyceridemia, and hypofibrinogenemia. Other common laboratory findings include elevated ferritin and sIL-2Rα levels, reduced NK cell function, elevated sCD163, and elevated granzyme B. B- and NK cell numbers may be decreased with normal T-cell numbers and variable immunoglobulin levels. Evidence of Hemophagocytosis in the bone marrow on liver biopsy confirms the diagnosis. The syndrome can be divided into two subtypes: primary or familial HLH and secondary HLH

[109–112]. Primary forms are most common in the newborn period.

Familial HLH (FHL)

Familial HLH is associated with inherited gene mutations, categorized into five subtypes (FHL 1–5) and identified mutations to date include mutations of *PRF1* (encoding perforin, in type 2 FHL), *UNC13D* (Munc13-4, type 3), *STX11* (syntaxin 11, type 4), and *STXBP2* (Munc18-2, type 5). In type 1 FHL, a gene mutation has not been identified. These gene mutations affect T and NK cell functions related to target cell cytolysis (target cell pore formation, membrane fusion, intracellular transport, release of cytotoxic granules) [109–111].

Management of acutely ill HLH patients with deteriorating organ function include HLH-specific treatment with dexamethasone and etoposide, with the most commonly used protocol being HLH-94 [113]. Intrathecal chemotherapy (such as methotrexate, hydrocortisone) may be used for patients with central nervous system (CNS) involvement.

There are primary immunodeficiency diseases associated with HLH, and some of these conditions may present in the neonatal period, including Wiskott–Aldrich Syndrome (described earlier), Chédiak–Higashi syndrome, Griscelli syndrome type 2, and X-linked inhibitor of apoptosis (XIAP) deficiency, described next [109, 112].

Chédiak–Higashi Syndrome (CHS)

Chédiak–Higashi syndrome is a rare autosomal recessive condition of aberrant lysosomal trafficking characterized by recurrent bacterial infections (neutrophil defects), oculocutaneous albinism (OCA, hypopigmented skin, hair, and eyes), mild coagulation defects, and progressive neurological deterioration. The diagnosis of CHS can be made by examining peripheral blood smear for pathognomonic giant cytoplasmic granules in leukocytes and platelets. A mutation in the *CHS1/LYST* gene at 1q42.1–2 is responsible for the condition [114]. In 85% of cases, affected individuals with CHS develop an accelerated phase consistent with HLH. Once individuals with CHS enter the accelerated phase, prognosis is poor. Early diagnosis and hematopoietic stem cell transplantation (HSCT) corrects the hematologic and immunologic defect, but does not prevent development of neurological deterioration in adolescence and early adulthood [115]. Treatment includes prophylactic antibiotics to prevent infections, G-CSF to correct neutropenia, and interferon gamma. HSCT corrects immunologic and hematologic manifestations, but does not prevent neurologic deterioration or oculocutaneous albinism [116].

Griscelli Syndrome Type 2 (GS2)

Griscelli syndrome type 2 is a rare autosomal recessive condition characterized by partial albinism, neutropenia, thrombocytopenia, and progressive neurologic deterioration thought to be due to cerebral lymphohistiocytic infiltration, and development of accelerated phase (HLH, only in type 2). GS2 results from a mutation in *RAB27A*, a GTP-binding protein involved in cytotoxicity and cytolytic granule exocytosis of lymphocytes [117]. Diagnosis can be made via microscopic examination of the hair shaft showing clumps of pigment. The absence of giant granules and the histologic characteristics of hypopigmentation differentiate this condition from CHS. Griscelli syndrome should be considered in infants with silvery-gray hair, hepatosplenomegaly, and immunodeficiency [118].

X-Linked Inhibitor of Apoptosis (XIAP) Deficiency

XIAP deficiency is a rare X-linked immunodeficiency that can affect boys during early infancy. Mutations in the *XIAP* gene at Xq25 leads to the condition that resembles familial HLH [119]. The most frequent clinical manifestations are HLH, recurrent splenomegaly, and to a lesser extent, IBD (often intractable) [120, 121]. EBV often triggers HLH, but HLH can also be triggered by CMV, HHV-6 infections, or even in the absence of a documented infection. Splenomegaly may be the initial clinical presentation of the disease in many cases.

Secondary HLH

Secondary HLH is usually associated with infectious diseases (most commonly with EBV), autoinflammatory and autoimmune diseases (more commonly known as macrophage activation syndrome), malignancy, HIV infection, hematopoietic stem cell or organ transplantation, immunosuppression, or metabolic diseases.

IPEX Syndrome

Immunodysregulation, polyendocrinopathy and enteropathy, X-linked (IPEX) syndrome is a primary immunodeficiency that can present in the newborn period and can even be diagnosed by fetal ultrasound [122–124]. This condition is commonly (60%–90%) associated with a mutation in the forkhead box protein 3 (*FOXP3*) gene located on the X chromosome (125, 126). FOXP3 is a DNA-binding protein that functions as a transcriptional repressor necessary for the development of T_{REG}, which in turn is responsible for regulating other immune cell functions including peripheral immunologic tolerance [127]. T_{REG} in infants with IPEX syndrome exhibit impaired suppressor function as well as decreased IL-2 and IFN-γ production by peripheral blood mononuclear cells following activation [128]. Although mutations in the *FOXP3* gene are associated with IPEX syndrome, FoxP3 *protein* expression does not appear to correlate with disease severity [123]. Clinical manifestations include autoimmune enteropathy (severe watery diarrhea and failure to thrive), eczematous dermatitis, and type I diabetes mellitus, which can all present during the neonatal period. In addition, a chronic inflammatory state is observed due to excessive cytokine production and autoantibody formation [129, 130]. The diagnosis of IPEX syndrome is primarily based on clinical signs. Laboratory findings may include elevated serum IgE, autoantibodies to pancreatic islet antigens, thyroid antigens, or small bowel mucosa, autoimmune cytopenias (anemia, thrombocytopenia, and/or neutropenia), intermittent eosinophilia, and decreased numbers of FoxP3-expressing T cells in peripheral blood [123]. Other serum immunoglobulins (IgG, IgA, IgM) and levels of complement are normal, as are circulating leukocyte counts including neutrophils, T cells, and B cells [131]. Treatment involves immune suppression with tacrolimus or sirolimus and HSCT.

Congenital Defects of Phagocytic Function

Phagocytic disorders are classified based on whether they are associated with neutropenia (Chapter 16) or defective phagocyte function (Chapter 17). Associated symptoms include bacterial and fungal infections of soft tissues, cellulitis, and chronic recurrent lymphadenitis. Recurrent abscesses in lung, liver, and bone are also frequent as well as pneumonia, sepsis, meningitis, and osteomyelitis.

Leukocyte Adhesion Deficiency (LAD)

LAD is an autosomal recessive disorder of immune trafficking, where leukocytes are unable to adhere to vascular endothelium and migrate to the sites of infection or inflammation (see Chapter 16). Infants with LAD may present with classic symptoms of delayed separation of umbilical cord, impaired wound healing, and serious/recurrent bacterial infections primarily localized to skin and mucosal surfaces with absent pus formation, accompanied by persistent leukocytosis (>25,000 cells/uL). The most common subtype LAD-I results from mutations in ITGB2 gene that encodes CD18, the β_2 subunit of the β_2 integrins, leading to decreased or absent expression [132]. Diagnosis can be made by flow cytometry showing absence of CD18 and the associated alpha subunit of the integrin molecules CD11a, CD11b, and CD11c on leukocytes. Abnormal or low amount of functional CD18 can be still expressed in some cases of LAD I, but CD11a is demonstrated to be absent in all cases [132]. Management depends on the clinical severity. Careful oral hygiene is important to control periodontitis and prevent oral infections. HSCT is the only curative treatment for the severe phenotype. The other subtypes, LAD-II and LAD-III are extremely rare.

Chronic Granulomatous Disease (CGD)

CGD is characterized by recurrent life-threatening bacterial and fungal infections along with inflammatory granuloma formation. Defects in the phagocyte nicotinamide adenine dinucleotide phosphate (NADPH) oxidase complex results in the inability of phagocytes (neutrophils, monocytes, and macrophages) to destroy catalase positive organisms [133] (see Chapter 16). Lack of functional NADPH oxidase at the cell membrane level leads to failure to generate superoxide and H_2O_2, responsible for intracellular killing of bacteria and fungi. Both neutrophils and monocytes are affected. Diagnosis is made through testing neutrophil's ability to produce superoxide, most frequently done via dihydrorhodamine (DHR) 123 flow cytometry assay. Frequent sites of infection include lung, skin, lymph nodes, liver, and soft tissues, often causing micro-abscesses and non-caseating granulomas. Many infants show signs of persistent immune activation as demonstrated by hypergammaglobulinemia and elevated C-reactive protein. Granuloma formation is common in the lungs, GI, and GU tracts. Colitis occurs in 30%–40% of all patients with CGD regardless of residual superoxide production and genotype [133]. Defects in NCF4 gene (encoding p40phox) cause a mildly impaired respiratory burst activity (DHR assay may be normal) but severe early-onset inflammatory bowel disease [134].

Treatment of CGD involves lifelong antibacterial (usually trimethoprim-sulfamethoxazole, TMP-SMX) and antifungal (usually itraconazole) prophylaxis [135, 136]. Immunomodulatory therapy with interferon-gamma are also used, mainly within the United States [137]. Combination of these drugs dramatically reduces rate of severe infections. Systemic glucocorticoids are commonly used for inflammatory manifestations of CGD usually involving GI or GU system after infection is ruled out (colitis, esophageal stricture, gastric outlet obstruction, bladder granuloma, ureteral/urethral strictures) [138]. HSCT is currently the only established curative therapy for CGD [139]. Gene therapy trials for CGD are currently underway.

Defect in Innate Immunity

Toll-Like Receptor 3 (TLR3) Deficiency

TLR3 resides within endolysosomes of myeloid dendritic cells, B cells, T cells, and NK cells. TLR3 utilizes the MYD88 (myeloid differentiation primary response protein 88) independent pathway to signal intracellularly via the molecule TIR domain-containing adapter-inducing interferon-beta (IFN-β) (TRIF), and induces production of type 1 IFN-β [140]. TLR3 binds double-stranded RNA (dsRNA), which is produced in the process of viral replication [141]. Interestingly, human TLR3 deficiency results in isolated susceptibility to HSV-1 encephalitis, while TLR3 deficient mice are susceptible to numerous viruses [142]. Additionally, mutations in the genes involved in TLR3 signaling pathway (TLR3, UNC93B1, TRIF, TRAF3, and TBK1) all pose susceptibility to HSV encephalitis, which may present in early infancy [143].

Neonatal-Onset Multisystem Inflammatory Disorder (NOMID)

NOMID is a type of autoinflammatory disorder of innate immunity in the group of cryopyrin-associated periodic syndromes (CAPS) that presents in the neonatal period, as the name implies. It is also known as chronic infantile neurologic

cutaneous and articular (CINCA) syndrome [20]. This cryopyrinopathy arises from mutations in the gene NLRP3 at chromosome 1q44 encoding protein cryopyrin (also known as nacht-domain leucine-rich repeat and pyrin domain-containing protein 3, or NALP3), which is a NOD-like receptor (NLR) [20, 144]. Cryopyrin is a part of the multiprotein NALP3 inflammasome complex and is activated by intracellular pathogens (PAMPs – pathogen-associated molecular patterns), and danger signals (DAMPS – danger-associated molecular patterns), and amplifies the activation of caspase-1, which in turn generates active form of interleukin 1β (IL-1β), and augments the inflammatory response. Mutations in the NLRP3 are thought to promote aberrant formation and overproduction of active IL-1β [145]. At or shortly after birth, infants with this condition typically present with characteristic abnormal facies including frontal bossing, protruding eyes, and saddle-shaped nose, fevers, migratory erythematous rash resembling urticaria, and impaired growth. Other clinical manifestations include chronic aseptic meningitis, sensorineural hearing loss, cerebral atrophy, uveitis, lymphadenopathy, and hepatosplenomegaly [146, 147]. Severely affected infants may die prematurely. Other milder cryopyrinopathies include Muckle–Wells syndrome and familial cold autoinflammatory syndrome (FCAS), and these present later in life. Cryopyrinopathies are generally inherited autosomal dominant, but de novo mutations have been reported [20, 144, 145]. Treatment with IL-1 receptor antagonist such as anakinra has improved signs and symptoms of inflammation in a portion of affected individuals, but not all [148]. Bone and joint abnormalities may not be as responsive to IL-1 blockade.

Complement Deficiency

Inherited disorders of the complement system are rarely recognizable during the neonatal period. The diagnosis of complement deficiencies during the neonatal period is complicated by the transient deficiencies within both the classical and alternative complement pathway that stem from immune immaturity [149]. However, inherited complement deficiencies may present early with increased susceptibility to bacterial pathogens [150]. For example, a deficiency of mannose-binding lectin (MBL), which is capable of activating the complement system via the lectin pathway, increases the risk for neonatal sepsis [151].

Acquired Immunodeficiency

Perinatal HIV-1 Infection

In spite of enormous strides in application of antiretroviral (ART) therapy to reduce maternal to child transmission (MCT) of HIV-1, perinatal HIV infection remains a significant cause of immune deficiency worldwide [152]. Identification of HIV infection during pregnancy and the implementation ART during pregnancy for the mother and post-partum for the infant reduces the risk of infection by >99%. Without antiretroviral intervention for mother and child, about one third of HIV-infected mothers transmit the virus to their infants [153]. However, uninfected infants remain at risk for acquisition through breastfeeding. All infants born to pregnant women living with HIV will have positive HIV antibody tests due to passively acquired maternal IgG antibody that persists for up to a year even if the child is not infected. As a result, HIV-1 infection in newborns and infants is diagnosed using PCR-based detection of proviral DNA within blood lymphocytes. However, only about 20% of infected infants will have a positive HIV polymerase chain reaction (PCR) at birth so repeated testing is needed over the first 6 months after birth [154]. Disease progression to AIDS in infants varies as infants infected in utero, based on positive HIV PCR at birth, show more rapid disease progression than infants infected at the time of birth or through breastfeeding. Other factors influencing progression include maternal disease stage, viral load, and HLA type. Similarly, clinical manifestations are variable during the neonatal period as some infants are totally asymptomatic while others can display mucocutaneous candidiasis, splenomegaly, lymphadenopathy, lymphopenia, or thrombocytopenia [155]. Concurrent co-infections with CMV and toxoplasmosis are common. PCP is rare in infants less than 2 months of age [156]. Laboratory findings include hypergammaglobulinemia, elevated IgA for age, and inverted CD4:CD8 T-cell ratios. Decreased numbers of T cells with a naive phenotype denotes intra-thymic infection and is a poor prognostic sign. HIV infection impacts humoral immunity as B cell dysfunction leads to dysgammaglobulinemia and increased susceptibility to sepsis and pneumonia with encapsulated bacteria. Infants born to HIV-infected mothers should not be breastfed due to the increased transmission risk. Vaginal delivery also increases the risk of transmission, particularly in women with high viral loads at the time of delivery. Guidelines for the optimal management of HIV infection and their infants is a rapidly evolving field and current recommendations can be found online at https://clinicalinfo.hiv.gov/en/guidelines/perinatal/whats-new-guidelines [157].

Diagnosis and Management of Neonatal Immunodeficiencies

General Principles

The pattern of clinical manifestations of primary and secondary immune deficiencies can be attributed to specific defects in particular components of the immune system allowing for a rationale for a stepwise diagnostic approach [158]. Once recognized, the treatment and long-term management can be implemented. Neonates, especially those in an intensive care unit setting, have multiple risk factors beyond immune immaturity that predispose them to infection. Therefore, it is far more likely that opportunistic infections in the neonate are the result of immune immaturity rather than a primary immunodeficiency. As a result, immune deficiencies may go unrecognized. The true incidence or prevalence of primary immunodeficiency that manifests during the neonatal period is unknown. Specific primary immune deficiency diseases are rare, but when evaluated as a group, may occur as often as 1 in 2,000 children [159]. It is an important, but difficult task for the neonatologist or pediatrician to be able to identify and properly investigate a neonate suspected of having a primary immunodeficiency disorder.

Diagnostic Approach to a Neonate with a Suspected Primary Immune Deficiency

Newborn Screening (NBS) for Congenital T-Cell Deficiencies

Screening for congenital T-cell abnormalities, initially implemented in 2008 as a pilot for all newborns in Wisconsin, is now recommended across the

United States [160]. Testing utilizes molecular detection of T-cell excision circles (TREC) within existing newborn screening tools (Guthrie card) of dried blood spots obtained from heel sticks obtained at birth (see Fig. 5.2a). The assay is based on TCR D-J and V-DJ gene recombination with the intervening DNA forming a circular TREC with a single copy staying within naive T cell leaving the thymus. When T cells are activated and undergo clonal expansion, number of TRECs per total T cells are diluted. This method provides a quantitative detection of T-cell development within the thymus [161]. Testing has shown to be inexpensive, in addition to being sensitive and specific in detecting cellular immune deficiencies. If TREC copies are below the threshold (generally < 25 or < 40 copies depending on the assays) then normal lymphocyte enumeration performed using flow cytometry serves as the confirmatory test. Testing of dried blood spots are done in tandem with an internal positive control to assure that the input DNA is adequate. In most states, the positive control is β actin. Quantitative reverse transcription polymerase chain reaction (RT-qPCR) of blood TREC levels identifies infants with low numbers of naive T cells such as SCID as well as other conditions that affect T-cell development, including complete DiGeorge syndrome, combined immune deficiency, and other conditions with low T-cell numbers at birth including trisomy 21, ataxia–telangiectasia (AT), cartilage hair hypoplasia (CHH), and CHARGE syndrome. Secondary T-cell impairment leading to low TREC include thymectomy associated with cardiac surgery, chylothorax, and loss of lymphocytes due to GI tract malformations [162]. Initial TREC numbers can be low in very premature infants but normalize as they approach term gestational age. In addition, heparin contamination in the specimen results in inactivation of the *Taq* polymerase used in the PCR reactions and will result in a falsely positive NBS. Preterm infants with low TREC should either have confirmatory testing by flow cytometry or repeat TREC assays (protocols vary between centers). An algorithm for NBS using the TREC assay is shown in Fig. 5.2b [162].

Among the over 5 million newborns screened, overall incidence of significant T-cell lymphopenia is 1 in 19,900. The incidence of SCID requiring hematopoietic stem cell transplant (HSCT) is approximately 1 in 60,000 and survival in these infants is >90% if transplantation occurs before 3 months of age [163]. The TREC NBS assay is highly specific as only 0.08% of newborns required repeat testing with 0.016% requiring confirmatory flow cytometry testing [162]. Most forms of SCID are not evident at birth by routine physical and laboratory exam, as infants appear normal and healthy until they encounter an infection. Therefore, it is imperative that infants with a positive TREC on NBS be evaluated quickly for implementation of early definitive therapy.

Lymphocyte Enumeration Using Flow Cytometry

Flow cytometry involves analysis of individual lymphocyte populations using a fluidics system interrogated to measure laser light deflected from cells tagged with fluorochrome-conjugated monoclonal antibodies binding to cell surface proteins, most commonly cluster of differentiation (CD) complexes [164]. Multiple monoclonal antibodies, each with its unique fluorochrome, bind surface markers of T cells, B cells, or NK cells, as well as markers identifying recent thymic emigrants or naive T cells. Measurements of the relative proportion of lymphocytes provides a valuable diagnostic tool in classifying different types of immune deficiencies. All mature T cells express CD3 on their surface, as part of T-cell receptor complex, with co-expression of either CD4 or CD8. These markers identify helper T cells or cytotoxic T cells respectively. B cells express both CD19 and CD20, either of which can be used in B-cell enumeration. Natural killer (NK) cells, which do not express CD3, are identified by co-expression of CD56 and CD16. Together, the sum of these three populations make up the *lymphosome*, consisting of 100% of the lymphocytes within a blood sample. These percentages are multiplied by the absolute lymphocyte count to quantify both as percentage and absolute numbers of lymphocyte subsets measured as cells/microliter. In newborns, CD3 T cells make up 50% to 70% of the total lymphocyte populations with term newborns having similar lymphocyte percentages but higher absolute T-cell counts when compared to those of adults. The normal ratio of CD4 to CD8 T cells is greater than 1.0 and generally approaches 2:1 to 3.5:1 in term and preterm infants. Inverted CD4/CD8 ratios are abnormal, reflecting increased CD8 T-cell activation and expansion, or declines in CD4 T cell

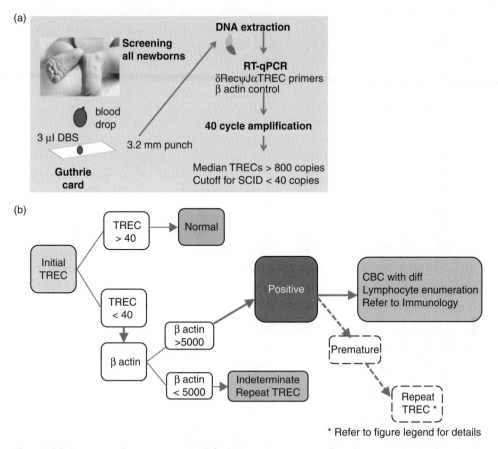

Fig. 5.2 (a) Steps in newborn screening (NBS) for SCID involve screening all newborns via a heel stick with a drop of blood (3 µl) applied to a Guthrie filter paper card. The dried blood spot (DBS) is removed from the card by a 3.2 mm punch and placed in DNA extraction buffer. The TREC (shown as a circle) are amplified by a reverse transcriptase quantitative PCR (RT-qPCR) using primers specific for δRecψJαTREC. β actin is amplified as a control to verify the integrity of the DNA. After 40 cycles of amplification the median TREC number from normal newborns is >800 copies. The cutoff for infants with suspected T cell deficiency vary from assay to assay and state to state, but in general, TREC results of <40 copies require further evaluation. Internal positive control for the assay is generally performed with β actin. (b) Algorithm for management of abnormal results with TREC newborn screen. While cutoff values vary from assay to assay, an abnormal TREC (in general <40 copies) first requires validation to confirm the quality of the DNA sample with a positive internal control, in most cases β actin. If the β actin is abnormal (<5,000 copies) then the results are considered indeterminate and the TREC assay repeated. If the β actin is normal (>5,000 copies) then the results should be considered positive for possible T-cell immune deficiency and confirmatory testing with CBC and differential and lymphocyte enumeration should be done along with referral to an Immunologist. Management of abnormal TREC results in preterm (<35 weeks) infants are not uniform across centers. *Some centers will do confirmatory testing regardless of gestational age while others will repeat the TREC assay every 2 weeks, or wait to repeat the assay until after 35 weeks gestational age.

numbers as in HIV infection. B cells (up to 20% of lymphocytes in newborns) and NK cell percentages and numbers are higher in infants compared to adults. Total CD3+ T cells can be further subdivided in naive (recent thymic emigrants) or memory T cells. Naive T cells co-express CD45RA, CD62L, CCR7, or CD31 while memory T cells express CD45RO. The normal distribution of lymphocyte subpopulations in normal newborns and children is shown in Table 5.1 [26]. Quantitative abnormalities may range from complete absence or pronounced deficiency of all or just a proportion of given lymphocyte population.

Measurements of T-Cell Function

Human lymphocytes can be stimulated in vitro by specific antigens or by mitogens, plant lectins which nonspecifically activate large numbers of lymphocytes to induce cellular proliferation that can be measured by incorporation of tritiated thymidine (^{3}H-Tdr) in cell culture system. The most commonly used T-lymphocyte mitogen are phytohemagglutinin (PHA), concanavalin A and pokeweed mitogen (PWM, activates both T and B lymphocytes). Thymidine uptake by cells activated by the mitogen is compared to proliferation of lymphocytes incubated in media alone. Results are expressed either as total ^{3}H-Tdr update or as a stimulation index that divides the maximum ^{3}H-Tdr uptake in the presence of the mitogen by the unstimulated cells without mitogen. In normal individuals, the mitogen stimulation index is 100- to 200-fold greater than the media control. Defects in T-cell signaling pathways result in mitogen responses many times lower (stimulation indexes of <10) than those of normal individuals [165]. Lymphocyte proliferation responses to mitogens are very useful in confirming the diagnosis of many of the T-cell immune disorders.

Measurements of Antibodies

Due to passively acquired maternal IgG and delay in class switch to produce IgG and IgA, occult B cell immunodeficiency exists during the neonatal period. In spite of the challenges associated with changing immunoglobulin levels during infancy, profiles of IgG, IgA, IgM, and IgE can identify distinct immune deficiencies that manifest during early infancy. Conditions with abnormal immunoglobulin profiles were described earlier in the subsection Predominantly Antibody Deficiencies. Unique immunoglobulin profiles are associated with immune dysregulation such as IPEX syndrome and WAS as well.

Testing Phagocytic Cell Function

Evaluation begins with a complete blood count with differential (see Chapter 16). Diagnosis of leukocyte adhesion deficiency is based on flow cytometry as loss of expression of CD18/11a and 11b on granulocytes and monocytes can confirm the diagnosis of LADI in patients with persistently elevated white cell counts. CGD diagnosis is based on the application of the neutrophil respiratory burst assay. Dihydrorhodamine (DHR) 123 flow cytometry assay measures the neutrophil oxidative burst by fluorescence changes in neutrophils stimulated with phorbol myristate acetate (PMA). Activation of neutrophils with PMA leads to oxidation of DHR to a fluorescent compound rhodamine 123, which can be measured by flow cytometry. The respiratory burst assay can also detect female carriers of X-linked CGD.

Diagnostic Testing Using Molecular Genetics

Over 300 genes are known to cause primary immune deficiency diseases. Confirming the genetic mutation is essential to the initiation of optimal treatments, determination of prognosis and future associated risks, identification of carriers, implementation of effective family counseling, and perhaps even gene therapy to correct the deficiency. While some primary immune deficiencies, such as 22q11.2 deletion syndrome, can be diagnosed based on chromosomal cytogenetic studies, the majority result from single gene mutations, deletions, or duplications requiring careful sequencing of targeted genetic regions that cannot be detected by karyotyping or microarray alone [166]. The advent of DNA-based techniques has allowed clinicians to accurately diagnose the majority of primary immune deficiency disorders [42]. First, the patient needs to be sufficiently characterized by laboratory-based assays, described earlier, to define the immune phenotype, followed by targeted gene sequencing to identify the precise mutations. Many patients lack a strong family history for the suspected underlying genetic mutation because as many as 40% of newly diagnosed primary immune deficiency cases represent new mutations within the family or results from compound heterozygous mutations inherited from maternal and paternal alleles. If a genetic disorder is identified, all family members at risk should be screened as the penetrance of most primary immune deficiencies varies greatly among family members [167].

The most common and straightforward way to identify single gene defects is via Sanger sequencing of genomic DNA from blood or buccal swab. For example, a single panel can probe the coding regions and splice junctions of the 26 different genes known to cause SCID. This method is accurate, inexpensive, and only takes a few weeks to determine the results. Multiple commercial DNA sequencers are currently available, and the assays have been validated by the College of American Pathologists. However, if the initial genetic screen is not informative or the patient's clinical phenotype does not conform to a known primary immune deficiency, then whole exome massive parallel (or Next Generation) sequencing can be performed using several available platforms. These assays involve paired-end reads and bidirectional sequencing [168]. Reads are assembled and aligned to reference gene sequences and analyzed for sequence variants. Next Generation sequencing (NGS) should be done as a trio including the index patient, as well as maternal and paternal samples to identify which alleles carry the pathogenic variants. There are limitations to this technology as deletions/duplications affecting exons are not detected nor can it identify mutations in introns or epigenetic modification that affect gene expression.

Diagnostic Criteria for Hemophagocytic Lymphohistiocytosis (HLH)

HLH can be diagnosed via genetic testing for known mutations of primary HLH or by meeting at least 5 of 8 diagnostic criteria. Diagnostic criteria are as follows [110, 111]:

1. Fever
2. Splenomegaly
3. Cytopenias (affecting ≥2 of 3 cell lineages):
    i. Hemoglobin <9 g/dl or <10 g/dl in infants <4 weeks of age
    ii. Platelet count <100 × 10³/mcL
    iii. neutrophils <1 × 10³/mcL
4. Hypertriglyceridemia and/or hypofibrinogenemia:
    i. fasting triglyceride level ≥265 mg/dL
    ii. fibrinogen level ≤1.5 g/L
5. Hemophagocytosis in bone marrow/spleen/lymph nodes with no evidence of malignancy
6. Low or absent natural killer cell activity,
7. Ferritin level ≥500 mcg/L
8. Soluble IL-2 receptor (CD25) level ≥2,400 U/mL

Management of Neonate with a Suspected or Known Primary Immune Deficiency Disease

Management of T-Cell Immune Deficiency

SCID and similar disorders with cellular immune deficiency should be considered as life-threatening conditions requiring immediate medical intervention [169]. Affected infants are extremely susceptible to severe, often fatal, opportunistic infections as well as at increased risk for iatrogenic conditions such as GVHD, if non-irradiated blood transfusions are given [38]. GVHD also occurs when maternal T cells cross the placenta during its separation and results in maternal-to-fetal hemorrhage. Early recognition can lead to appropriate initiation of prophylactic therapies and allows prompt initiation of definitive treatment to correct the defect [38, 170–174]. Survival for patients with SCID is vastly improved if definitive therapy such as bone marrow transplantation, enzyme replacement, or gene therapy is initiated prior to 3 months of age [38, 45, 163, 175, 176]. Enzyme replacement therapy with polyethylene glycol (PEG) modified bovine ADA, given by subcutaneous injection, is used prior to definitive gene therapy in ADA deficiency [46–48, 177]. Clinical trials of gene therapy are currently underway to treat X-linked SCID and Artemis deficiency [178–181]. Because of the high complexity and rapid changes in the management of infants with T-cell deficiency and SCID, prompt referral to a tertiary care center is recommended. Thymic transplant has been successfully utilized for patients with complete DGS but is currently only available at a couple of centers [75]. Thymic tissues obtained during elective cardiac surgery implanted into the muscles of the affected recipient results in successful T-cell reconstitution. The procedure is done without HLA matching or the risk of GVHD.

The steps in the management of the neonate with suspected disorders in cell-mediated immunity are illustrated in Fig. 5.3. These management steps include reverse isolation, blood transfusions with irradiated blood products, preferably from CMV-negative blood donors, and IVIg for immune prophylaxis initiated in conditions associated with known impairment of antibody function, even if initial IgG levels are normal. Mothers who are CMV-antibody positive or those with unknown CMV status should be cautioned against breastfeeding their infants. Infants with known or suspected immune deficiencies affecting T-cell function should receive PCP prophylaxis with TMP-SMX after the second month of life. If T cells are very low (<100 cells/μ) prophylaxis for fungal and mycobacterial infections should be added. Vaccinations with live viruses and BCG should not be given [182]. Household contacts may receive all age- and exposure-appropriate vaccines with the exception of smallpox vaccine and oral polio virus vaccine [183, 184]. The live MMR, varicella, and rotavirus vaccines may be administered to household contacts when indicated. The MMR vaccine viruses are not transmitted to contacts, and transmission of varicella-zoster virus vaccine strain is rare [184, 185]. If the varicella vaccine recipient develops a rash after vaccination, contact with the immune deficient patient should be avoided until the rash resolves, although risk of transmission is minimal unless blisters develop at the site of the vaccine administration [184, 186]. Latest recommendation from the American Academy of Pediatrics and the Centers for Disease Control for vaccinating children with immune deficiency should be followed (available online at www.aap.org and www.cdc.gov). Unnecessary radiographic imaging studies should be avoided in infants with suspected immune deficiency associated with radiosensitivity, such as Artemis deficiency, ligase IV deficiency, or ataxia–telangiectasia. Compared to B cell and other primary immune deficiency diseases, individuals with defects in cell-mediated immunity are more likely to present with initial clinical manifestations during the neonatal period [176]. The approach to the neonate with suspected T-cell immunodeficiency and the associated clinical and laboratory findings characteristic of specific T-cell deficiency diseases are summarized in Fig. 5.2 and Table 5.7, respectively.

Management of Infants with Antibody Deficiency Disorders

Management consists of administration of intravenous or subcutaneous gammaglobulin (IVIg or SCIg). Human Ig infusions contain pooled human immunoglobulin obtained from thousands of healthy adult plasma donors and therefore consists of a broad array of antibodies to multiple antigens [170]. For the most part, IgA and IgM have been removed and the solution is enriched for monomeric human IgG. Unlike other blood products, the risk of infusion-associated infections is exceedingly low because the fractionation process includes inactivation and nanofiltration steps to assure that the product is pathogen free [170]. Risks for infusion-related reactions such as fever and rigors are lower in infants compared to children or adults. IVIg is given as a slow intravenous infusion over 2 to 4 hours. It is given as a 5 or 10% solution depending on the specific product. The usual dose for replacement therapy is 500 to 800 mg/kg [170, 187–189]. Antibody replacement is given every 3 to 4 weeks in order to maintain IgG trough levels of >500 mg/dl. The use of IVIg is indicated in the treatment of XLA, Hyper IgM, and SCID, but not for selective IgA deficiency or THI of infancy [85, 189].

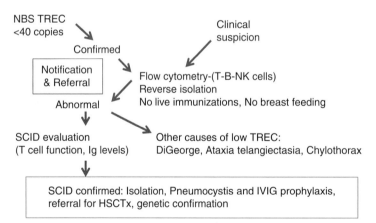

Fig. 5.3 Algorithm for management of child with suspected SCID. Clinical evaluation is warranted either based on clinical signs and symptoms suggestive of SCID or an abnormal newborn screen (NBS) TREC assay result. Infants with low TREC numbers are referred for confirmatory testing consisting with flow cytometry to enumerate T cells, B cells, and NK cells. While awaiting results, the child is placed on reverse isolation and breastfeeding is withheld. Oral trimethoprim/sulfamethoxazole prophylaxis should be initiated if over 2 months of age. All live immunizations should be delayed until test results are confirmed. If the results of flow cytometry studies are normal, then prophylaxis is discontinued and no further evaluation is needed. If the results confirm SCID or other cellular immune deficiency then further testing is carried to determine antibody levels, T-cell function, and replacement immunoglobulin is started for prophylaxis. Referral to a transplant center should be made as quickly as possible for genetic confirmation, HLA typing, and HSC transplant. If the T cells are low due to a condition that does not warrant transplant, then care is provided for that particular condition. While genetic confirmation should be obtained, results should not delay definitive therapy.

The use of IVIg for preventing infections in preterm infants is controversial as meta-analysis of multiple clinical trials only demonstrated a 3%–4% reduction in nosocomial infections without a reduction in mortality or other important clinical outcomes [187]. Thus, the use of IVIg for prophylactic use in premature infants varies across centers. IVIg may also be used for suspected or proven infection in neonates, however, a meta-analysis provided insufficient evidence to support the routine use of IVIg to prevent mortality in neonates with suspected or proven infection [190]. Prior clinical studies did demonstrate improvement in neutrophil counts with no evidence of toxicity [191, 192]. Even with the effective implementation of IVIg, patients remain susceptible to infections because of ongoing deficiency in IgA and IgM, which is not provided by IVIg infusion. IVIg does not penetrate into mucosal surfaces and does not normally cross the blood–brain barrier (in an uninflamed state).

Management of Mothers with Antibody Deficiency Conditions

Pregnant women with antibody deficiency disease, such as common variable immune deficiency (CVID), require additional antibody replacement during pregnancy to compensate for increased catabolism and enable adequate transplacental transfer of IgG to the fetus [108]. In the presence of reduced maternal serum immunoglobulin levels and absence of replacement IVIg therapy, affected mothers and their infants are at risk for life-threatening infections [108]. Gammaglobulin has been safely administered to women without adverse effects in either mother or fetus [193]. However, doses of up to 600 mg/kg every 3 weeks over the third trimester may be required to maintain adequate IgG levels for both mother and newborn child [193]. In the case of mothers with IgA deficiency, the breast milk and colostrum are deficient in IgA, compromising the mucosal immunity of their children [194].

References

1. PrabhuDas M, Adkins B, Gans H, et al. Challenges in infant immunity: Implications for responses to infection and vaccines. *Nat Immunol* 2011;**12** (3):189–94.

2. Yoshio H, Lagercrantz H, Gudmundsson GH, Agerberth B. First line of defense in early human life. *Semin Perinatol* 2004;**28**(4):304–11.

3. Martin CR, Walker WA. Probiotics: Role in pathophysiology and prevention in necrotizing enterocolitis. *Semin Perinatol* 2008;**32**(2):127–37.

4. Rakoff-Nahoum S, Paglino J, Eslami-Varzaneh F, Edberg S, Medzhitov R. Recognition of commensal microflora by toll-like receptors is required for intestinal homeostasis. *Cell* 2004;**118**(2):229–41.

5. Wynn JL, Scumpia PO, Winfield RD, et al. Defective innate immunity predisposes murine neonates to poor sepsis outcome but is reversed by TLR agonists. *Blood* 2008;**112**(5):1750–8.

6. Lewis DB, Wilson CB. Developmental immunology and role of host defenses in fetal and neonatal susceptibility to infection. In Remington JS, Klein JO, Wilson CB, Baker CJ, eds. *Infectious Diseases of the Fetus and Newborn Infant*, 6th ed. (Philadelphia, PA: Elsevier Saunders, 2006), pp. 87–210.

7. Wright JR. Host defense functions of pulmonary surfactant. *Biol Neonate* 2004;**85**(4):326–32.

8. Engle WA. Surfactant-replacement therapy for respiratory distress in the preterm and term neonate. *Pediatrics* 2008;**121**(2):419–32.

9. Pfister RH, Soll RF. New synthetic surfactants: The next generation? *Biol Neonate* 2005;**87**(4):338–44.

10. Kawai T, Akira S. The roles of TLRs, RLRs and NLRs in pathogen recognition. *Int Immunol* 2009;**21**(4):317–37.

11. Takeuchi O, Akira S. Pattern recognition receptors and inflammation. *Cell* 2010;**140**(6):805–20.

12. Kumagai Y, Takeuchi O, Akira S. Pathogen recognition by innate receptors. *J Infect Chemother* 2008;**14**(2):86–92.

13. Trinchieri G, Sher A. Cooperation of toll-like receptor signals in innate immune defence. *Nat Rev Immunol* 2007;**7**(3):179–90.

14. Krumbiegel D, Zepp F, Meyer CU. Combined toll-like receptor agonists synergistically increase production of inflammatory cytokines in human neonatal dendritic cells. *Hum Immunol* 2007;**68** (10):813–22.

15. Hotchkiss RS, Karl IE. The pathophysiology and treatment of sepsis. *N Engl J Med* 2003;**348** (2):138–50.

16. Levy O, Zarember KA, Roy RM, et al. Selective impairment of TLR-mediated innate immunity in human newborns: Neonatal blood plasma reduces monocyte TNF-alpha induction by bacterial lipopeptides, lipopolysaccharide, and imiquimod, but preserves the response to R-848. *J Immunol* 2004;**173**(7):4627–34.

17. Ng PC, Li K, Wong RP, et al. Proinflammatory and anti-inflammatory cytokine responses in preterm infants with systemic infections. *Arch Dis Child*

Fetal Neonatal Ed 2003;**88**(3): F209nousinfusionover2to4hours-13.

18. Sadeghi K, Berger A, Langgartner M, et al. Immaturity of infection control in preterm and term newborns is associated with impaired toll-like receptor signaling. *J Infect Dis* 2007;**195** (2):296–302.

19. Wen H, Miao EA, Ting JP. Mechanisms of NOD-like receptor-associated inflammasome activation. *Immunity* 2013;**39**(3):432–41.

20. Aksentijevich I, Nowak M, Mallah M, et al. De novo CIAS1 mutations, cytokine activation, and evidence for genetic heterogeneity in patients with neonatal-onset multisystem inflammatory disease (NOMID): A new member of the expanding family of pyrin-associated autoinflammatory diseases. *Arthritis Rheum* 2002;**46**(12):3340–8.

21. Rechavi E, Lev A, Lee YN, et al. Timely and spatially regulated maturation of B and T cell repertoire during human fetal development. *Sci Transl Med* 2015;**7**(276):276ra25.

22. Schroeder HW, Jr., Zhang L, Philips JB, 3rd. Slow, programmed maturation of the immunoglobulin HCDR3 repertoire during the third trimester of fetal life. *Blood* 2001;**98**(9):2745–51.

23. Zinkernagel RM. Maternal antibodies, childhood infections, and autoimmune diseases. *N Engl J Med* 2001;**345**(18):1331–5.

24. Rechavi E, Somech R. Survival of the fetus: Fetal B and T cell receptor repertoire development. *Semin Immunopathol* 2017;**39**(6):577–83.

25. Perfetto SP, Chattopadhyay PK, Roederer M. Seventeen-colour flow cytometry: Unravelling the immune system. *Nat Rev Immunol* 2004;**4** (8):648–55.

26. Shearer WT, Rosenblatt HM, Gelman RS, et al. Lymphocyte subsets in healthy children from birth through 18 years of age: The Pediatric AIDS Clinical Trials Group P1009 study. *J Allergy Clin Immunol* 2003;**112**(5):973–80.

27. Martin VG, Wu YB, Townsend CL, et al. Transitional B cells in early human B cell development: Time to revisit the paradigm? *Front Immunol* 2016;**7**:546.

28. Zhou ZH, Zhang Y, Hu YF, et al. The broad antibacterial activity of the natural antibody repertoire is due to polyreactive antibodies. *Cell Host Microbe* 2007;**1**(1):51–61.

29. Siegrist CA, Aspinall R. B-cell responses to vaccination at the extremes of age. *Nat Rev Immunol* 2009;**9**(3):185–94.

30. van Zelm MC, Szczepanski T, van der Burg M, van Dongen JJ. Replication history of B lymphocytes reveals homeostatic proliferation and extensive antigen-induced B cell expansion. *J Exp Med* 2007;**204**(3):645–55.

31. Nonoyama S, Penix LA, Edwards CP, et al. Diminished expression of CD40 ligand by activated neonatal T cells. *J Clin Invest* 1995;**95** (1):66–75.

32. Wilcox CR, Holder B, Jones CE. Factors affecting the FcRn-mediated transplacental transfer of antibodies and implications for vaccination in pregnancy. *Front Immunol* 2017;**8**:1294.

33. Ballow M, Cates KL, Rowe JC, Goetz C, Desbonnet C. Development of the immune system in very low birth weight (less than 1500 g) premature infants: Concentrations of plasma immunoglobulins and patterns of infections. *Pediatr Res* 1986;**20**(9):899–904.

34. Bousfiha A, Jeddane L, Picard C, et al. The 2017 IUIS Phenotypic Classification for Primary Immunodeficiencies. *J Clin Immunol* 2018;**38** (1):129–43.

35. Cotten CM, Taylor S, Stoll B, et al. Prolonged duration of initial empirical antibiotic treatment is associated with increased rates of necrotizing enterocolitis and death for extremely low birth weight infants. *Pediatrics* 2009;**123**(1):58–66.

36. Stoll BJ, Hansen N. Infections in VLBW infants: Studies from the NICHD Neonatal Research Network. *Semin Perinatol* 2003;**27**(4):293–301.

37. Buckley RH. Humoral immunodeficiency. *Clin Immunol Immunopathol* 1986;**40**(1):13–24.

38. Buckley RH. Primary cellular immunodeficiencies. *J Allergy Clin Immunol* 2002;**109**(5):747–57.

39. Kwan A, Church JA, Cowan MJ, et al. Newborn screening for severe combined immunodeficiency and T-cell lymphopenia in California: Results of the first 2 years. *J Allergy Clin Immunol* 2013;**132** (1):140–50.

40. Roifman CM. Hematopoietic stem cell transplantation for profound T-cell deficiency (combined immunodeficiency). *Immunol Allergy Clin North Am* 2010;**30**(2):209–19.

41. Roberts JL, Lauritsen JP, Cooney M, et al. T-B+NK+ severe combined immunodeficiency caused by complete deficiency of the CD3zeta subunit of the T-cell antigen receptor complex. *Blood* 2007;**109** (8):3198–206.

42. Notarangelo LD. Primary immunodeficiencies. *J Allergy Clin Immunol* 2010;**125**(2 Suppl 2): S182–94.

43. Sleasman JW, Harville TO, White GB, et al. Arrested rearrangement of TCR V beta genes in thymocytes from children with X-linked severe combined immunodeficiency disease. *J Immunol* 1994;**153**(1):442–8.

44. Routes J, Abinun M, Al-Herz W, et al. ICON: The early diagnosis of congenital immunodeficiencies. *J Clin Immunol* 2014;**34**(4):398–424.

45. Hershfield MS. Adenosine deaminase deficiency: Clinical expression, molecular basis, and therapy. *Semin Hematol* 1998;**35**(4):291–8.

46. Hershfield MS. PEG-ADA replacement therapy for adenosine deaminase deficiency: An update after 8.5 years. *Clin Immunol Immunopathol* 1995;**76**(3 Pt 2):S228–32.

47. Hershfield MS. PEG-ADA: An alternative to haploidentical bone marrow transplantation and an adjunct to gene therapy for adenosine deaminase deficiency. *Hum Mutat* 1995;**5**(2):107–12.

48. Hershfield MS, Buckley RH, Greenberg ML, et al. Treatment of adenosine deaminase deficiency with polyethylene glycol-modified adenosine deaminase. *N Engl J Med* 1987;**316**(10):589–96.

49. Aiuti A, Roncarolo MG, Naldini L. Gene therapy for ADA-SCID, the first marketing approval of an ex vivo gene therapy in Europe: Paving the road for the next generation of advanced therapy medicinal products. *EMBO Mol Med* 2017;**9**(6):737–40.

50. Finan PM, Soames CJ, Wilson L, et al. Identification of regions of the Wiskott–Aldrich syndrome protein responsible for association with selected Src homology 3 domains. *J Biol Chem* 1996;**271**(42):26291–5.

51. Schindelhauer D, Weiss M, Hellebrand H, et al. Wiskott–Aldrich syndrome: No strict genotype-phenotype correlations but clustering of missense mutations in the amino-terminal part of the WASP gene product. *Hum Genet* 1996;**98**(1):68–76.

52. Schwartz M, Bekassy A, Donner M, et al. Mutation spectrum in patients with Wiskott–Aldrich syndrome and X-linked thrombocytopenia: Identification of twelve different mutations in the WASP gene. *Thromb Haemost* 1996;**75**(4):546–50.

53. Schwarz K. WASPbase: A database of WAS- and XLT-causing mutations. *Immunol Today* 1996;**17**(11):496–502.

54. Thrasher AJ. WASp in immune-system organization and function. *Nat Rev Immunol* 2002;**2**(9):635–46.

55. Park JY, Kob M, Prodeus AP, et al. Early deficit of lymphocytes in Wiskott–Aldrich syndrome: Possible role of WASP in human lymphocyte maturation. *Clin Exp Immunol* 2004;**136**(1):104–10.

56. Sullivan KE. Recent advances in our understanding of Wiskott–Aldrich syndrome. *Curr Opin Hematol* 1999;**6**(1):8–14.

57. Ochs HD, Thrasher AJ. The Wiskott–Aldrich syndrome. *J Allergy Clin Immunol* 2006;**117**(4):725–38; quiz 39.

58. Buckley RH. Primary immunodeficiency diseases due to defects in lymphocytes. *N Engl J Med* 2000;**343**(18):1313–24.

59. Gatti RA, Berkel I, Boder E, et al. Localization of an ataxia-telangiectasia gene to chromosome 11q22–23. *Nature* 1988;**336**(6199):577–80.

60. van Os NJH, Jansen AFM, van Deuren M, et al. Ataxia-telangiectasia: Immunodeficiency and survival. *Clin Immunol* 2017;**178**:45–55.

61. Chopra C, Davies G, Taylor M, et al. Immune deficiency in ataxia-telangiectasia: A longitudinal study of 44 patients. *Clin Exp Immunol* 2014;**176**(2):275–82.

62. Kraus M, Lev A, Simon AJ, et al. Disturbed B and T cell homeostasis and neogenesis in patients with ataxia telangiectasia. *J Clin Immunol* 2014;**34**(5):561–72.

63. Kobrynski LJ, Sullivan KE. Velocardiofacial syndrome, DiGeorge syndrome: The chromosome 22q11.2 deletion syndromes. *Lancet* 2007;**370**(9596):1443–52.

64. Devriendt K, Fryns JP, Mortier G, van Thienen MN, Keymolen K. The annual incidence of DiGeorge/velocardiofacial syndrome. *J Med Genet* 1998;**35**(9):789–90.

65. Goodship J, Cross I, LiLing J, Wren C. A population study of chromosome 22q11 deletions in infancy. *Arch Dis Child* 1998;**79**(4):348–51.

66. Lindstrand A, Malmgren H, Verri A, et al. Molecular and clinical characterization of patients with overlapping 10p deletions. *Am J Med Genet A* 2010;**152A**(5):1233–43.

67. Sullivan KE. Chromosome 22q11.2 deletion syndrome: DiGeorge syndrome/velocardiofacial Syndrome. *Immunol Allergy Clin North Am* 2008;**28**(2):353–66.

68. Yagi H, Furutani Y, Hamada H, et al. Role of TBX1 in human del22q11.2 syndrome. *Lancet* 2003;**362**(9393):1366–73.

69. Stoller JZ, Epstein JA. Identification of a novel nuclear localization signal in Tbx1 that is deleted in DiGeorge syndrome patients harboring the 1223delC mutation. *Hum Mol Genet* 2005;**14**(7):885–92.

70. Jawad AF, McDonald-Mcginn DM, Zackai E, Sullivan KE. Immunologic features of chromosome 22q11.2 deletion syndrome (DiGeorge syndrome/velocardiofacial syndrome). *J Pediatr* 2001;**139**(5):715–23.

71. Jyonouchi S, McDonald-McGinn DM, Bale S, Zackai EH, Sullivan KE. CHARGE (coloboma, heart defect, atresia choanae, retarded growth and development, genital hypoplasia, ear anomalies/deafness) syndrome and chromosome 22q11.2 deletion syndrome: A comparison of immunologic and nonimmunologic phenotypic features. *Pediatrics* 2009;**123**(5):e871–7.

72. de Geus CM, Free RH, Verbist BM, et al. Guidelines in CHARGE syndrome and the missing link: Cranial imaging. *Am J Med Genet C Semin Med Genet* 2017;**175**(4):450–64.

73. Hale CL, Niederriter AN, Green GE, Martin DM. Atypical phenotypes associated with pathogenic CHD7 variants and a proposal for broadening CHARGE syndrome clinical diagnostic criteria. *Am J Med Genet A* 2016;**170A**(2):344–54.

74. Junker AK, Driscoll DA. Humoral immunity in DiGeorge syndrome. *J Pediatr* 1995;**127**(2):231–7.

75. Markert ML, Devlin BH, Chinn IK, McCarthy EA. Thymus transplantation in complete DiGeorge anomaly. *Immunol Res* 2009;**44**(1–3):61–70.

76. Kostjukovits S, Klemetti P, Valta H, et al. Analysis of clinical and immunologic phenotype in a large cohort of children and adults with cartilage-hair hypoplasia. *J Allergy Clin Immunol* 2017;**140**(2):612–4 e5.

77. Chavanas S, Bodemer C, Rochat A, et al. Mutations in SPINK5, encoding a serine protease inhibitor, cause Netherton syndrome. *Nat Genet* 2000;**25**(2):141–2.

78. Hovnanian A. Netherton syndrome: Skin inflammation and allergy by loss of protease inhibition. *Cell Tissue Res* 2013;**351**(2):289–300.

79. Netherton EW. A unique case of trichorrhexis nodosa; bamboo hairs. *AMA Arch Derm* 1958;**78**(4):483–7.

80. Giri N, Lee R, Faro A, et al. Lung transplantation for pulmonary fibrosis in dyskeratosis congenita: Case report and systematic literature review. *BMC Blood Disord* 2011;**11**:3.

81. Jyonouchi S, Forbes L, Ruchelli E, Sullivan KE. Dyskeratosis congenita: A combined immunodeficiency with broad clinical spectrum–a single-center pediatric experience. *Pediatr Allergy Immunol* 2011;**22**(3):313–9.

82. Fusco F, Pescatore A, Conte MI, et al. EDA-ID and IP, two faces of the same coin: How the same IKBKG/NEMO mutation affecting the NF-kappaB pathway can cause immunodeficiency and/or inflammation. *Int Rev Immunol* 2015;**34**(6):445–59.

83. Puel A, Picard C, Ku C-L, Smahi A, Casanova J-L. Inherited disorders of NF-κB-mediated immunity in man. *Curr Opin Immunol* 2004;**16**(1):34–41.

84. Miot C, Imai K, Imai C, et al. Hematopoietic stem cell transplantation in 29 patients hemizygous for hypomorphic IKBKG/NEMO mutations. *Blood* 2017;**130**(12):1456–67.

85. Tiller TL, Jr., Buckley RH. Transient hypogammaglobulinemia of infancy: Review of the literature, clinical and immunologic features of 11 new cases, and long-term follow-up. *J Pediatr* 1978;**92**(3):347–53.

86. McGeady SJ. Transient hypogammaglobulinemia of infancy: Need to reconsider name and definition. *J Pediatr* 1987;**110**(1):47–50.

87. Dressler F, Peter HH, Muller W, Rieger CH. Transient hypogammaglobulinemia of infancy: Five new cases, review of the literature and redefinition. *Acta Paediatr Scand* 1989;**78**(5):767–74.

88. Fanaroff AA, Korones SB, Wright LL, et al. A controlled trial of intravenous immune globulin to reduce nosocomial infections in very-low-birth-weight infants. National Institute of Child Health and Human Development Neonatal Research Network. *N Engl J Med* 1994;**330**(16):1107–13.

89. Sandberg K, Fasth A, Berger A, et al. Preterm infants with low immunoglobulin G levels have increased risk of neonatal sepsis but do not benefit from prophylactic immunoglobulin G. *J Pediatr* 2000;**137**(5):623–8.

90. Geha RS. Antibody deficiency syndromes and novel immunodeficiencies. *Pediatr Infect Dis J* 1988;**7**(5 Suppl):S57–60.

91. Vetrie D, Vorechovsky I, Sideras P, et al. The gene involved in X-linked agammaglobulinaemia is a member of the src family of protein-tyrosine kinases. *Nature* 1993;**361**(6409):226–33.

92. Cunningham-Rundles C, Ponda PP. Molecular defects in T- and B-cell primary immunodeficiency diseases. *Nat Rev Immunol* 2005;**5**(11):880–92.

93. Ochs HD, Smith CI. X-linked agammaglobulinemia: A clinical and molecular analysis. *Medicine* 1996;**75**(6):287–99.

94. Fuleihan RL. The hyper IgM syndrome. *Curr Allergy Asthma Rep* 2001;**1**(5):445–50.

95. Conley ME, Dobbs AK, Farmer DM, et al. Primary B cell immunodeficiencies: Comparisons and contrasts. *Annu Rev Immunol* 2009;**27**:199–227.

96. Levy J, Espanol-Boren T, Thomas C, et al. Clinical spectrum of X-linked hyper-IgM syndrome. *J Pediatr* 1997;**131**(1 Pt 1):47–54.

97. Padayachee M, Feighery C, Finn A, et al. Mapping of the X-linked form of hyper-IgM syndrome (HIGM1) to Xq26 by close linkage to HPRT. *Genomics* 1992;**14**(2):551–3.

98. Schwaber J, Rosen FS. X chromosome linked immunodeficiency. *Immunodefic Rev* 1990;**2**(3):233–51.

99. Crank MC, Grossman JK, Moir S, et al. Mutations in PIK3 CD can cause hyper IgM syndrome (HIGM) associated with increased cancer susceptibility. *J Clin Immunol* 2014;**34**(3):272–6.

100. Petrovski S, Parrott RE, Roberts JL, et al. Dominant splice site mutations in PIK3R1 cause hyper IgM syndrome, lymphadenopathy and short stature. *J Clin Immunol* 2016;**36**(5):462–71.

101. Wang WC, Cordoba J, Infante AJ, Conley ME. Successful treatment of neutropenia in the hyper-immunoglobulin M syndrome with granulocyte colony-stimulating factor. *Am J Pediatr Hematol Oncol* 1994;**16**(2):160–3.

102. de la Morena MT, Leonard D, Torgerson TR, et al. Long-term outcomes of 176 patients with X-linked hyper-IgM syndrome treated with or without hematopoietic cell transplantation. *J Allergy Clin Immunol* 2017;**139**(4):1282–92.

103. Lorini R, Ugazio AG, Cammareri V, et al. Immunoglobulin levels, T-cell markers, mitogen responsiveness and thymic hormone activity in Turner's syndrome. *Thymus* 1983;**5**(2):61–6.

104. Maraschio P, Zuffardi O, Dalla Fior T, Tiepolo L. Immunodeficiency, centromeric heterochromatin instability of chromosomes 1, 9, and 16, and facial anomalies: The ICF syndrome. *J Med Genet* 1988;**25**(3):173–80.

105. Wijmenga C, van den Heuvel LP, Strengman E, et al. Localization of the ICF syndrome to chromosome 20 by homozygosity mapping. *Am J Hum Genet* 1998;**63**(3):803–9.

106. Grimbacher B, Schaffer AA, Peter HH. The genetics of hypogammaglobulinemia. *Curr Allergy Asthma Rep* 2004;**4**(5):349–58.

107. Price VE, Dutta S, Blanchette VS, et al. The prevention and treatment of bacterial infections in children with asplenia or hyposplenia: Practice considerations at the Hospital for Sick Children, Toronto. *Pediatr Blood Cancer* 2006;**46**(5):597–603.

108. Schaffer FM, Newton JA. Intravenous gamma globulin administration to common variable immunodeficient women during pregnancy: Case report and review of the literature. *J Perinatol* 1994;**14**(2):114–7.

109. Verbsky JW, Grossman WJ. Hemophagocytic lymphohistiocytosis: Diagnosis, pathophysiology, treatment, and future perspectives. *Ann Med* 2006;**38**(1):20–31.

110. Ishii E. Hemophagocytic lymphohistiocytosis in children: Pathogenesis and treatment. *Front Pediatr* 2016;**4**:47.

111. Esteban YM, de Jong JLO, Tesher MS. An overview of hemophagocytic lymphohistiocytosis. *Pediatr Ann* 2017;**46**(8): e309–e13.

112. Mehta RS, Smith RE. Hemophagocytic lymphohistiocytosis (HLH): A review of literature. *Med Oncol* 2013;**30**(4):740.

113. Trottestam H, Horne A, Arico M, et al. Chemoimmunotherapy for hemophagocytic lymphohistiocytosis: Long-term results of the HLH-94 treatment protocol. *Blood* 2011;**118**(17):4577–84.

114. Ward DM, Shiflett SL, Kaplan J. Chediak–Higashi syndrome: A clinical and molecular view of a rare lysosomal storage disorder. *Curr Mol Med* 2002;**2**(5):469–77.

115. Kaplan J, De Domenico I, Ward DM. Chediak–Higashi syndrome. *Curr Opin Hematol* 2008;**15**(1):22–9.

116. Eapen M, DeLaat CA, Baker KS, et al. Hematopoietic cell transplantation for Chediak–Higashi syndrome. *Bone Marrow Transpl* 2007;**39**(7):411–15.

117. Menasche G, Pastural E, Feldmann J, et al. Mutations in RAB27A cause Griscelli syndrome associated with haemophagocytic syndrome. *Nat Genet* 2000;**25**(2):173–6.

118. Masri A, Bakri FG, Al-Hussaini M, et al. Griscelli syndrome type 2: A rare and lethal disorder. *J Child Neurol* 2008;**23**(8):964–7.

119. Rigaud S, Fondaneche MC, Lambert N, et al. XIAP deficiency in humans causes an X-linked lymphoproliferative syndrome. *Nature* 2006;**444**(7115):110–4.

120. Marsh RA, Madden L, Kitchen BJ, et al. XIAP deficiency: A unique primary immunodeficiency best classified as X-linked familial hemophagocytic lymphohistiocytosis and not as X-linked lymphoproliferative disease. *Blood* 2010;**116**(7):1079–82.

121. Horn PC, Belohradsky BH, Urban C, et al. Two new families with X-linked inhibitor of apoptosis deficiency and a review of all 26 published cases. *J Allergy Clin Immunol* 2011;**127**(2):544–6.

122. Powell BR, Buist NR, Stenzel P. An X-linked syndrome of diarrhea, polyendocrinopathy, and fatal infection in infancy. *J Pediatr* 1982;**100**(5):731–7.

123. Gambineri E, Perroni L, Passerini L, et al. Clinical and molecular profile of a new series of patients with immune dysregulation, polyendocrinopathy, enteropathy, X-linked syndrome: Inconsistent correlation between forkhead box protein 3 expression and disease

severity. *J Allergy Clin Immunol* 2008;**122**(6):1105–12.e1.

124. Louie RJ, Tan QK, Gilner JB, et al. Novel pathogenic variants in FOXP3 in fetuses with echogenic bowel and skin desquamation identified by ultrasound. *Am J Med Genet A* 2017;**173**(5):1219–25.

125. Bennett CL, Brunkow ME, Ramsdell F, et al. A rare polyadenylation signal mutation of the FOXP3 gene (AAUAAA–>AAUGAA) leads to the IPEX syndrome. *Immunogenetics* 2001;**53**(6):435–9.

126. Bennett CL, Christie J, Ramsdell F, et al. The immune dysregulation, polyendocrinopathy, enteropathy, X-linked syndrome (IPEX) is caused by mutations of FOXP3. *Nat Genet* 2001;**27**(1):20–1.

127. Mills KH. Regulatory T cells: Friend or foe in immunity to infection? *Nat Rev Immunol* 2004;**4**(11):841–55.

128. Bacchetta R, Passerini L, Gambineri E, et al. Defective regulatory and effector T cell functions in patients with FOXP3 mutations. *J Clin Invest* 2006;**116**(6):1713–22.

129. Torgerson TR, Ochs HD. Immune dysregulation, polyendocrinopathy, enteropathy, X-linked: Forkhead box protein 3 mutations and lack of regulatory T cells. *J Allergy Clin Immunol* 2007;**120**(4):744–50; quiz 51–2.

130. Halabi-Tawil M, Ruemmele FM, Fraitag S, et al. Cutaneous manifestations of immune dysregulation, polyendocrinopathy, enteropathy, X-linked (IPEX) syndrome. *Br J Dermatol* 2009;**160**(3):645–51.

131. Tan QK, Louie RJ, Sleasman J. IPEX Syndrome. In Adam MP, Ardinger HH, Pagon RA, et al., eds. *GeneReviews®* [Internet] (Seattle, WA: University of Washington, 2004/2018). Available online at www.ncbi.nlm.nih.gov/books/NBK1118/.

132. Cabanillas D, Regairaz L, Deswarte C, et al. Leukocyte adhesion deficiency Type 1 (LAD1) with expressed but nonfunctional CD11/CD18. *J Clin Immunol* 2016;**36**(7):627–30.

133. Holland SM. Chronic granulomatous disease. *Hematol Oncol Clin North Am* 2013;**27**(1):89–99, viii.

134. van de Geer A, Nieto-Patlan A, Kuhns DB, et al. Inherited p40phox deficiency differs from classic chronic granulomatous disease. *J Clin Invest* 2018;**128**(9):3957–75.

135. Margolis DM, Melnick DA, Alling DW, Gallin JI. Trimethoprim-sulfamethoxazole prophylaxis in the management of chronic granulomatous disease. *J Infect Dis* 1990;**162**(3):723–6.

136. Gallin JI, Alling DW, Malech HL, et al. Itraconazole to prevent fungal infections in chronic granulomatous disease. *N Engl J Med* 2003;**348**(24):2416–22.

137. A controlled trial of interferon gamma to prevent infection in chronic granulomatous disease. The International Chronic Granulomatous Disease Cooperative Study Group. *N Engl J Med* 1991;**324**(8):509–16.

138. Chin TW, Stiehm ER, Falloon J, Gallin JI. Corticosteroids in treatment of obstructive lesions of chronic granulomatous disease. *J Pediatr* 1987;**111**(3):349–52.

139. Güngör T, Teira P, Slatter M, et al. Reduced-intensity conditioning and HLA-matched haemopoietic stem-cell transplantation in patients with chronic granulomatous disease: A prospective multicentre study. *Lancet* 2014;**383**(9915):436–48.

140. Pisegna S, Pirozzi G, Piccoli M, et al. p38 MAPK activation controls the TLR3-mediated up-regulation of cytotoxicity and cytokine production in human NK cells. *Blood* 2004;**104**(13):4157–64.

141. Schroder M, Bowie AG. TLR3 in antiviral immunity: Key player or bystander? *Trends Immunol* 2005;**26**(9):462–8.

142. Zhang SY, Jouanguy E, Ugolini S, et al. TLR3 deficiency in patients with herpes simplex encephalitis. *Science* 2007;**317**(5844):1522–7.

143. Lim HK, Seppanen M, Hautala T, et al. TLR3 deficiency in herpes simplex encephalitis: High allelic heterogeneity and recurrence risk. *Neurology* 2014;**83**(21):1888–97.

144. Aksentijevich I, Putnam CD, Remmers EF, et al. The clinical continuum of cryopyrinopathies: Novel CIAS1 mutations in North American patients and a new cryopyrin model. *Arthritis Rheum* 2007;**56**(4):1273–85.

145. Baroja-Mazo A, Martin-Sanchez F, Gomez AI, et al. The NLRP3 inflammasome is released as a particulate danger signal that amplifies the inflammatory response. *Nat Immunol* 2014;**15**(8):738–48.

146. Hull KM, Shoham N, Chae JJ, Aksentijevich I, Kastner DL. The expanding spectrum of systemic autoinflammatory disorders and their rheumatic manifestations. *Curr Opin Rheumatol* 2003;**15**(1):61–9.

147. Ahmadi N, Brewer CC, Zalewski C, et al. Cryopyrin-associated periodic syndromes: Otolaryngologic and audiologic manifestations. *Otolaryngol Head Neck Surg* 2011;**145**(2):295–302.

148. Goldbach-Mansky R, Dailey NJ, Canna SW, et al. Neonatal-onset multisystem inflammatory disease responsive to interleukin-1beta inhibition. *N Engl J Med* 2006;**355**(6):581–92.

149. Berger M. Complement deficiency and neutrophil dysfunction as risk factors for bacterial infection in newborns and the role of granulocyte transfusion in therapy. *Rev Infect Dis* 1990;**12** Suppl 4:S401–9.

150. Frank MM. Complement deficiencies. *Pediatr Clin North Am* 2000;**47**(6):1339–54.

151. Dzwonek AB, Neth OW, Thiebaut R, et al. The role of mannose-binding lectin in susceptibility to infection in preterm neonates. *Pediatr Res* 2008;**63**(6):680–5.

152. UNAIDS. Global report: UNAIDS report on the global AIDS epidemic. Available online at https://www.unaids.org/en/resources/publications/all

153. Mofenson LM. Mother–child HIV-1 transmission: Timing and determinants. *Obstet Gynecol Clin North Am.* 1997;**24**(4):759–84.

154. Shearer WT, Quinn TC, LaRussa P, et al. Viral load and disease progression in infants infected with human immunodeficiency virus type 1. Women and Infants Transmission Study Group. *N Engl J Med* 1997;**336**(19):1337–42.

155. Havens PL, Mofenson LM. Evaluation and management of the infant exposed to HIV-1 in the United States. *Pediatrics* 2009;**123**(1):175–87.

156. 1993 revised classification system for HIV infection and expanded surveillance case definition for AIDS among adolescents and adults. *MMWR Recomm Rep* 1992;**41**(Rr-17):1–19.

157. Panel on Antiretroviral Therapy and Medical Management of Children Living with HIV. Recommendations for the Use of Antiretroviral Drugs in Pregnant Women with HIV Infection and Interventions to Reduce Perinatal HIV Transmission in the United States. 2020. Available online at https://clinicalinfo.hiv.gov/guidelines/perinatal/introduction

158. Bonilla FA, Bernstein IL, Khan DA, et al. Practice parameter for the diagnosis and management of primary immunodeficiency. *Ann Allergy Asthma Immunol* 2005;**94**(5 Suppl 1):S1–63.

159. Boyle JM, Buckley RH. Population prevalence of diagnosed primary immunodeficiency diseases in the United States. *J Clin Immunol* 2007;**27**(5):497–502.

160. Chase NM, Verbsky JW, Routes JM. Newborn screening for T-cell deficiency. *Curr Opin Allergy Clin Immunol* 2010;**10**(6):521–5.

161. Baker MW, Grossman WJ, Laessig RH, et al. Development of a routine newborn screening protocol for severe combined immunodeficiency. *J Allergy Clin Immunol* 2009;**124**(3):522–7.

162. Kwan A, Abraham RS, Currier R, et al. Newborn screening for severe combined immunodeficiency in 11 screening programs in the United States. *JAMA* 2014;**312**(7):729–38.

163. Pai SY, Logan BR, Griffith LM, et al. Transplantation outcomes for severe combined immunodeficiency, 2000–2009. *N Engl J Med* 2014;**371**(5):434–46.

164. Brown M, Wittwer C. Flow cytometry: Principles and clinical applications in hematology. *Clin Chem* 2000; **46**(8 Pt 2):1221–9.

165. Shearer WT, Dunn E, Notarangelo LD, et al. Establishing diagnostic criteria for severe combined immunodeficiency disease (SCID), leaky SCID, and Omenn syndrome: The Primary Immune Deficiency Treatment Consortium experience. *J Allergy Clin Immunol* 2014;**133**(4):1092–8.

166. Pena LDM, Jiang YH, Schoch K, et al. Looking beyond the exome: A phenotype-first approach to molecular diagnostic resolution in rare and undiagnosed diseases. *Genet Med* 2018;**20**(4):464–9.

167. Shashi V, McConkie-Rosell A, Schoch K, et al. Practical considerations in the clinical application of whole-exome sequencing. *Clin Genet* 2016;**89**(2):173–81.

168. Green RC, Berg JS, Grody WW, et al. ACMG recommendations for reporting of incidental findings in clinical exome and genome sequencing. *Genet Med* 2013;**15**(7):565–74.

169. Buckley RH. Transplantation of hematopoietic stem cells in human severe combined immunodeficiency: Longterm outcomes. *Immunol Res* 2011;**49**(1–3):25–43.

170. Buckley RH. Breakthroughs in the understanding and therapy of primary immunodeficiency. *Pediatr Clin North Am* 1994;**41**(4):665–90.

171. Fischer A. Primary T-cell immunodeficiencies. *Curr Opin Immunol* 1993;**5**(4):569–78.

172. Dorsey MJ, Petrovic A, Morrow MR, Dishaw LJ, Sleasman JW. FOXP3 expression following bone marrow transplantation for IPEX syndrome after reduced-intensity conditioning. *Immunol Res* 2009;**44**(1–3):179–84.

173. Seidel MG, Fritsch G, Lion T, et al. Selective engraftment of donor CD4+25high FOXP3-positive T cells in IPEX syndrome after nonmyeloablative hematopoietic stem cell transplantation. *Blood* 2009;**113**(22):5689–91.

174. Zhan H, Sinclair J, Adams S, et al. Immune reconstitution and recovery of FOXP3 (forkhead

box P3)-expressing T cells after transplantation for IPEX (immune dysregulation, polyendocrinopathy, enteropathy, X-linked) syndrome. *Pediatrics* 2008;**121**(4):e998–1002.

175. Fischer A. Severe combined immunodeficiencies. *Immunodefic Rev* 1992;**3**(2):83–100.

176. Rosen FS. Severe combined immunodeficiency: A pediatric emergency. *J Pediatr* 1997;**130**(3):345–6.

177. Ferrua F, Aiuti A. Twenty-five years of gene therapy for ADA-SCID: From bubble babies to an approved drug. *Hum Gene Ther* 2017;**28** (11):972–81.

178. Cavazzana M, Six E, Lagresle-Peyrou C, Andre-Schmutz I, Hacein-Bey-Abina S. Gene therapy for X-Linked severe combined Immunodeficiency: Where do we stand? *Hum Gene Ther* 2016;**27**(2):108–16.

179. Cavazzana-Calvo M, Hacein-Bey S, de Saint Basile G, et al. Gene therapy of human severe combined immunodeficiency (SCID)-X1 disease. *Science* 2000;**288**(5466):669–72.

180. Hacein-Bey-Abina S, Le Deist F, Carlier F, et al. Sustained correction of X-linked severe combined immunodeficiency by ex vivo gene therapy. *N Engl J Med* 2002;**346**(16):1185–93.

181. Punwani D, Kawahara M, Yu J, et al. Lentivirus mediated correction of Artemis-deficient severe combined immunodeficiency. *Hum Gene Ther* 2017;**28**(1):112–24.

182. Succi RC, Farhat CK. Vaccination in special situations. *J Pediatr (Rio J)* 2006;**82**(3 Suppl):S91–100.

183. Petersen BW, Harms TJ, Reynolds MG, Harrison LH. Use of vaccinia virus smallpox vaccine in laboratory and health care personnel at risk for occupational exposure to orthopoxviruses: Recommendations of the Advisory Committee on Immunization Practices (ACIP), 2015. *Morb Mortal Wkly Rep* 2016;**65**(10):257–62.

184. Medical Advisory Committee of the Immune Deficiency F, Shearer WT, Fleisher TA, Buckley RH, et al. Recommendations for live viral and bacterial vaccines in immunodeficient patients and their close contacts. *J Allergy Clin Immunol* 2014;**133**(4):961–6.

185. Marin M, Guris D, Chaves SS, Schmid S, Seward JF. Prevention of varicella: Recommendations of the Advisory Committee on Immunization Practices (ACIP). *MMWR Recomm Rep* 2007;**56**(RR-4):1–40.

186. Grossberg R, Harpaz R, Rubtcova E, et al. Secondary transmission of varicella vaccine virus in a chronic care facility for children. *J Pediatr* 2006;**148**(6):842–4.

187. Ohlsson A, Lacy JB. Intravenous immunoglobulin for preventing infection in preterm and/or low birth weight infants. *Cochrane Database Syst Rev* 2013(7):CD000361.

188. Skull S, Kemp A. Treatment of hypogammaglobulinaemia with intravenous immunoglobulin, 1973–93. *Arch Dis Child* 1996;**74**(6):527–30.

189. Berger M. Principles of and advances in immunoglobulin replacement therapy for primary immunodeficiency. *Immunol Allergy Clin North Am* 2008;**28**(2):413–37, x.

190. Ohlsson A, Lacy JB. Intravenous immunoglobulin for suspected or subsequently proven infection in neonates. *Cochrane Database Syst Rev* 2004(1):Cd001239.

191. Christensen RD, Brown MS, Hall DC, Lassiter HA, Hill HR. Effect on neutrophil kinetics and serum opsonic capacity of intravenous administration of immune globulin to neonates with clinical signs of early-onset sepsis. *J Pediatr* 1991; **118** (4 Pt 1):606–14.

192. Weisman LE, Stoll BJ, Kueser TJ, et al. Intravenous immune globulin therapy for early-onset sepsis in premature neonates. *J Pediatr* 1992;**121**(3):434–43.

193. Madsen DL, Catanzarite VA, Varela-Gittings F. Common variable hypogammaglobulinemia in pregnancy: Treatment with high-dose immunoglobulin infusions. *Am J Hematol* 1986;**21**(3):327–9.

194. Barros MD, Porto MH, Leser PG, Grumach AS, Carneiro-Sampaio MM. Study of colostrum of a patient with selective IgA deficiency. *Allergol Immunopathol (Madr)* 1985;**13**(4):331–4.

195. Buckley M, Dees SC, O'Fallon WM. Serum immunoglobulins. I. Levels in normal children and in uncomplicated childhood allergy. *Pediatrics* 1968;**41**:600–11.

Chapter

6

Newborn Genetic Screening for Blood Disorders

Parul Rai, Ewelina K. Mamcarz, and Jane S. Hankins

Introduction

The newborn screening (NBS) program is a well-established comprehensive public health initiative with the main goal of identifying newborns affected by genetic disorders, for whom early interventions may prevent disease morbidity and mortality. The early-in-life screening for genetic conditions not only permits early institution of specific therapeutic measures for those affected, but also creates the opportunity for genetic counselling for carriers (e.g., parents). Several hematologic conditions have benefited from NBS, most notably hemoglobinopathies, particularly sickle cell disease (SCD), for which early diagnosis with preemptive penicillin initiation has substantively reduced pediatric mortality [1, 2]. The inclusion of severe combined immune deficiency (SCID) in the panel of screened genetic disorders has allowed for early referral to hematopoietic stem cell transplantation and the soon-to-be scaled up, gene therapy [3, 4].

Principles of a NBS program should include informed consent, use of accurate laboratory methods, provision of relevant education and counseling, procurement and immediate care institution, preferably within the comprehensive care programs. In addition, NBS should be voluntary, every effort made to protect patient and family confidentiality, and avoid labeling and stigmatization.

In the United States (US), the number of genetic conditions screened at birth varies by state, however all 50 states screen for hemoglobinopathies. Severe combined immunodeficiency (SCID), although not a primary hematologic genetic condition, may present with hematologic symptoms at birth (e.g., lymphopenia), and has been part of the recommended universal newborn screening panel (RUSP) since 2010. Currently, all states in the US include SCID in their NBS panel. On the other hand, only the NBS programs of Pennsylvania and District of Columbia screen for glucose-6 phosphate dehydrogenase (G6PD) deficiency. The next subsections will discuss the NBS efforts for quantitative and qualitative hemoglobinopathies, and for G6PD deficiency which is the most common red blood cell (RBC) enzymopathy. In addition, the efforts to screen and treat different forms of SCID have also been described.

NBS Implementation for Blood Disorders in the United States and Worldwide

The first legislatively mandated state NBS program in the US was established in 1963, when Massachusetts began testing dried blood specimens (DBS) obtained from newborns heel prick for phenylketonuria (PKU), using the Guthrie test [5]. PKU testing was eventually implemented nationwide by 1969–1970. By the mid 1970s many states had expanded their screening panel to include other metabolic (maple syrup disease, homocystinuria), and endocrine (congenital hypothyroidism) disorders [6, 7]. New York was the first to include testing for SCD on its NBS panel in 1975. The solubility tube test to screen for hemoglobin S (HbS) has been known since 1949 [8]. However, despite the refinement (by using a more stable reducing agent than dithionite) and automation of this technique, it was limited because it was unable to distinguish among homozygous (HbSS), trait (HbAS), and compound heterozygous (e.g., HbSC) HbS mutations [9–11]. The development of cellulose acetate

Neonatal Hematology, Pathogenesis, Diagnosis, and Management of Hematologic Problems, 3rd edition, ed. Pedro A. de Alarcón, Eric J. Werner, Robert D. Christensen, and Martha C. Sola-Visner. Published by Cambridge University Press. © Cambridge University Press 2021.

electrophoresis technique in 1969 to separate Hb variants, and its eventual adaptation to test elutes from DBS in 1973, enabled large-scale screening for SCD in conjunction with PKU testing using the same specimen [12, 13]. Since then, techniques such as isoelectric focusing (IEF) and high performance liquid chromatography (HPLC) have increasingly been utilized by NBS state programs [14]. Introduction of tandem mass spectrometry (MS/MS) technology in the 1990s revolutionized the field as it enabled rapid, cost effective, and highly sensitive testing for multiple simultaneous metabolic disorders using a single assay [15]. Its application has recently been extended to screen for clinically relevant Hb variants [16]. In 1972, a centralized Hemoglobinopathy Reference Laboratory was established at the Centers for Disease Control and Prevention (CDC) to formulate protocols, standardize laboratory techniques, and perform regular evaluation to ensure regulated quality controlled testing for hemoglobinopathies nationwide [17, 18]. After its closure in 1993, this role was transitioned to the Newborn Screening Quality Assurance Program at the CDC, to ensure the continued quality and accuracy of testing provided by NBS laboratories nationwide [19, 20].

Two NHLBI-sponsored studies, in 1977 and 1983, namely the Co-operative Study of Sickle Cell Disease (CSSD) and Prophylactic Penicillin Study, respectively, demonstrated that penicillin prophylaxis started in infancy significantly decreased invasive pneumococcal infection and associated mortality [1, 21]. Based on these findings, the NIH consensus conference in 1987 emphasized the importance of early identification of SCD by universal NBS so as to prevent fatal complications during infancy [22]. Despite this recommendation, it was only in 2007 that screening for SCD was adopted by all 50 states [23]. In 2005, the American College of Medical Genetics (ACMG) was commissioned to give recommendations for a universal screening panel (RUSP) [24]. This panel identified 29 disorders (20 metabolic and 9 non-metabolic), including SCD, that comprised the core screening panel for NBS programs in the US. These disorders were selected based on the following criteria: (1) they could be identified in pre-symptomatic newborns 24–48 hours after birth, (2) their natural history was well understood, (3) validated screening tests with appropriate sensitivity and specificity existed, and (4) effective treatment to mitigate

the disease-associated adverse outcomes were available. G6PD screening was excluded from this panel due to insufficient knowledge of the natural history of the G6PD mutations [25]. An additional 25 disorders that did not fulfil the above criteria, but could be incidentally detected during the screening for the core panel conditions, were considered secondary/target conditions, and the state programs were then required to report their findings. Since then, the ACMG has continued to expand the RUSP. In November 2016, the RUSP included 34 core and 26 secondary conditions, however, its implementation into state NBS programs has not been uniform. This is due to the rarity of these conditions, heterogeneity in their clinical presentation and disease course, and the lack of established infrastructure required to provide high-quality medical services for afflicted children, raising questions regarding the cost-effectiveness and benefit of their early screening [26–27].

Since the implementation of NBS for hemoglobinopathies in the US, other countries have adopted it. In low and middle income countries (LMICs), NBS coverage depends on federal financing and prioritization. Other sources of funding include private laboratories, which offer screening on a fee-for-service basis, and collaboration among local non-government agencies and the World Health Organization regional offices. Except for Brazil, Panama, Costa Rica, and Cuba [28], the NBS coverage for hemoglobinopathies in LMICs is variable [29]. In Brazil, the NBS program was introduced in stages, and it has been universal (available in all states) since 2013 [30–32]. The Caribbean islands of Guadeloupe and Martinique both have universal NBS for SCD, however, administratively, they are considered territories of France. Jamaica achieved universal status in 2018, but only in the public sector. India, with an estimated 15% of the global SCD births, currently has not implemented nationwide NBS for SCD [33], despite recommendations by government driven programs, and multiple pilot studies showing the feasibility of establishing such programs in rural settings [34–38]. Sub-Saharan Africa accounts for 79% of new SCD cases in the world, and this proportion is projected to increase to 88% by the year 2050 [33]. In this region, while there are a few regional screening programs (Angola, Ghana, Uganda) [39–41], the coverage remains incomplete [42]. Due to global migration and the resulting increasing prevalence of hemoglobinopathies in Europe, some European countries have initiated screening for hemoglobinopathies and G6PD [29, 43]. Of the Western European countries, Spain, France, the Netherlands, Monaco, and the United Kingdom are the only ones with universal coverage.

The screening for SCID was piloted in 2008 in Wisconsin [44], and as of December 2018, it is fully implemented by all US states. Universal screening is also available in Israel, and several pilot programs are ongoing in Europe, the Middle East and Asia [45–48]. In addition to early detection of SCID, implementation of SCID NBS has allowed for an accurate measurement of its incidence. With 1:58,000 births, its incidence has almost doubled from what was previously estimated (1:100,000 births), highlighting that SCID was previously underdiagnosed in the absence of unbiased population screening [49].

Blood Disorders Screened via NBS

In the US, approximately 100,000 people are affected with SCD (~1/360 African American births) [50]. Of the 300,000–400,000 annual new hemoglobinopathy cases worldwide, approximately 80% have SCD and 20% have thalassemia (13% with β-thalassemia and 7% with α-thalassemia) [51]. The prevalence varies by region of the world and it is estimated that 80% of these affected births occur in malaria-endemic LMICs [52]. While sickle variants are predominantly seen in sub-Saharan Africa, thalassemia mutations have high prevalence in the Southeast Asian region. The overlap in the geographical distribution of malaria and hemoglobinopathies is attributed to the malarial-protective effects of both sickle cell trait (HbAS) [53], and α-thalassemia trait [54]. The malarial protection conferred by HbAS appears to be due to increased clearance of infected erythrocyte and reduced parasite growth, rather than decreased infectivity [55]. This protection is, however, lost when the sickle trait mutation is co-inherited with α-thalassemia trait [56].

Sickle Cell Disease

Sickle cell disease (SCD) is an autosomal recessive condition in which an abnormal sickle hemoglobin (HbS) is inherited either as homozygous (HbSS) or as double heterozygous with other Hb variants (e.g., HbSC, HbSD, HbSE, HbSO) or β-thalassemia (HbS/β-thalassemia). SCD is considered a qualitative

hemoglobinopathy, as abnormal sickle globin chains are produced in normal numbers, but how they behave in the RBCs leads to the pathophysiology of the disease. Polymerization of HbS in certain conditions (e.g., hypoxia, acidosis, dehydration), results in sickling of RBCs. Sickle erythrocytes have abnormal rheology and are not very pliable, causing vascular obstruction, or microvascular vaso-occlusion. This vaso-occlusion causes both acute and chronic complications. Acute complications from the disease include recurrent episodes of pain, acute chest syndrome, priapism, acute splenic sequestration, and overt stroke. Endothelial dysfunction mediated by hemolysis of sickle RBCs and ischemia-reperfusion injury secondary to microvasculature occlusion, causes ongoing end-organ damage, constituting the chronic complications of the disease [57]. Among the chronic organ damage observed, the brain (cognitive dysfunction, silent cerebral infarcts), spleen (asplenia), kidneys (sickle nephropathy), lungs (obstructive and restrictive disease, pulmonary hypertension), heart (sickle cardiomyopathy), bones (low mineral density, osteonecrosis), and eyes (sickle retinopathy), are particularly affected. The amount of fetal hemoglobin (HbF, $\alpha_2\gamma_2$) present is of prognostic significance and ameliorates disease severity, forming the basis for therapies which can induce its production, such as hydroxyurea [58]. While HbSS and HbS/β° thalassemia genotypes have a severe phenotype, the compound heterozygous states (HbSC, HbSE) may have a less severe course which might correlate with the proportion of sickle versus non-sickle hemoglobin.

Thalassemia

Thalassemia is a quantitative hemoglobinopathy where there is either decreased globin production ($\alpha°$, α^+, $\beta°$, β^+ deletional mutations) or globin structural instability ($\alpha^{Constant\ Spring}$, β^{Lepore} nondeletional mutations). Decreased synthesis of α globin chain affects production of stable heterotetramers (HbA = α2β2, HbA2 = α2δ2, HbF = α2γ2) and an excess of unbound γ and β globin chains, which polymerize to form homotetramers β4 (HbH) and γ4 (Hb Bart, also called fast band). These homotetramers have high oxygen affinity resulting in tissue hypoxia. In addition, owing to their decreased stability, they precipitate in erythroid precursors and circulating erythrocytes, resulting in ineffective erythropoiesis and peripheral hemolysis.

The clinically significant α-thalassemias include hydrops fetalis (four-gene deletion, $-/-$) where fetal/newborn demise from severe anemia occurs if not rescued by intra-uterine or post-delivery transfusions [59]. Deletional HbH occurs when three α genes are deleted ($\alpha-/--$). This form of HbH tends to have a milder clinical course than the one resulting from homozygous ($\alpha^{Tsaudi}\alpha/\alpha^{Tsaudi}\alpha$) or compound heterozygous ($\alpha^{Tsaudi}\alpha/\alpha^{Agrinio}\alpha$), ($-/\alpha^{Constant\ Spring}\alpha$) non-deletional α mutations. In non-deletional HbH, growth deficits, splenomegaly, and transfusion requirements begin in infancy compared to deletional HbH mutations, where they occur after the first decade of life [60, 61]. Non-clinically significant forms of α-thalassemia include α-thalassemia trait (two-gene deletion, either in cis, $\alpha\alpha/--$ or in trans, $\alpha-/\alpha-$), or the silent carrier (one-gene deletion, $\alpha-/\alpha\alpha$). Alpha-thalassemia trait is common in African Americans, who primarily have the trans deletion, as opposed to Southeast Asians who have the α deletion in cis. In β-thalassemia, the α:β globin chain imbalance diminishes production of HbA, causing it to either be absent (thalassemia major: $\beta^0\beta^0$) or decreased (thalassemia intermedia $\beta^0\beta^+$, $\beta^+\beta^+$, and thalassemia trait $\beta\beta^0$, $\beta\beta^+$). Additionally, elevated HbA$_2$ levels from increased δ-globin synthesis is an important parameter for identifying β-thalassemia trait, but may be falsely low in the presence of iron deficiency anemia [62]. Beta-thalassemia major usually becomes symptomatic (severe anemia requiring transfusions) in the first 6 months of life, when the switch from fetal (γ) to adult (β, δ) globin expression occurs [63]. Beta-thalassemia intermedia, hemoglobin Lepore (homozygous and compound heterozygous with β-thalassemia), and dominant β-thalassemia mutations can have a variable phenotype and may occasionally require blood transfusions later in life for worsening anemia [64–66]. The co-inheritance of α-thalassemia silent carrier and trait can act as genetic modifiers of β hemoglobinopathies, mitigating clinical severity [67]. While, co-inheritance of α gene triplication mutations might increase their disease severity by worsening the globin chain imbalance [68].

Glucose-6 Phosphate Dehydrogenase Deficiency

Glucose-6 phosphate dehydrogenase (G6PD) deficiency is an X-linked disorder, where mutations in the G6PD gene (~200 mutations) result in many allelic variants with different levels of erythrocyte enzyme activity and clinical severity. G6PD enzyme is crucial for erythrocyte antioxidant defense, as it catalyzes the first step in the pentose phosphate pathway, the only NADPH-producing pathway in erythrocytes. The NADPH generated maintains a reducing environment in the cell by restoring the level of reduced glutathione. G6PD-deficient erythrocytes have increased susceptibility to oxidative stress from certain drugs, infections, naphthalene balls, and fava beans, resulting in acute intravascular hemolysis. This hemolysis is usually self-limiting, as the hemolyzed older red cells are replaced with younger red cells with higher enzyme activity [69]. The more serious consequences of G6PD deficiency can occur in the neonatal period (particularly in the premature born), where failure to promptly manage the resulting hyperbilirubinemia can cause permanent neurological damage (bilirubin encephalopathy or kernicterus). Concomitant mutation in the uridine-diphosphate-glucuronosyl transferase-I promoter gene (Gilbert's syndrome) can further increase the risk of developing hyperbilirubinemia [70]. The G6PD A-variant (10%–60% enzyme activity) is commonly seen in individuals of African ancestry and is present in approximately 10% of black males in the United States [71]. Despite being considered less severe than the Mediterranean variant (enzyme activity <10%), G6PD A-variant has the potential to cause hazardous hyperbilirubinemia as highlighted in studies in Nigerian neonates in whom this variant is widely encountered [72, 73].

Immunologic Disorders with Hematologic Abnormalities Screened via NBS

Primary immunodeficiency disorders are a group of more than 300 rare, mostly inherited, diseases resulting from defects of the development and/or function of the adaptive or innate immune system [74]. Most patients are diagnosed within the first year of life due to failure to thrive and/or recurrent and persistent infections such as sinusitis, otitis media, pneumonia, thrush, or skin abscesses. Following diagnosis, supportive treatment with prophylactic antimicrobials and intravenous immunoglobulin infusions is started immediately to prevent occurrence of infections before definitive therapy is performed.

Table 6.1 The most common genetic defects in SCID

T−B+NK−	T−B+NK+	T−B−NK−	T−B−NK+
IL-2R common gamma chain (IL2RG)	IL-7Ra chain (IL7RA)	Adenosine deaminase (ADA)	Recombinase-activating genes 1 and 2 (RAG1/RAG2)
Janus kinase 3 (JAK3)	CD3 subunits: delta, epsilon, and zeta (CD3D, CD3E, CD3Z)		DNA cross-link repair enzyme 1C (Artemis)
	CD45: protein tyrosine phosphatase, receptor type, C (PTPRC)		DNA ligase IV (LIG4)
			DNA-dependent protein kinase (PRKDC)

Patients affected with SCID, a form of primary immunodeficiency, present with profound defects in cellular and humoral immunity at 4–6 months of life, coinciding with weaning of protective maternal antibodies. Laboratory studies demonstrate a combination of usually absent or nonfunctional T, B, NK cells, and lack of responses to vaccine antigens [75]. SCID is genetically heterogeneous and in the past, was classified based on the presence or absence of T, B, and NK cells. Currently, mutations in approximately 20 genes controlling maturation of the immune system have been identified in various types of SCID [76]. The list of common gene defects is listed in Table 6.1. Diagnosis can be determined by whole-exome or whole-genome sequencing. Typical patients with SCID have absent or very low number of T cells (<300 autologous T cells/microliter) or T cells of maternal origin and none or very low T-cell function (<10% of lower limit of normal) as measured by response to phytohemagglutinin. The number of B and NK cells can vary in different types of SCID (Table 6.1) [77].

SCID is inherited in an autosomal recessive pattern in most patients, and adenosine deaminase (ADA) deficiency is the best-known form of autosomal recessive SCID in which infants lack the ADA enzyme necessary for T-cell survival. However, the most common type of SCID is X-linked, which is caused by mutations in the interleukin 2 receptor gamma gene (IL2RG) gene, encoding the common gamma chain (γ_c). The γ_c is shared by multiple cytokine receptors necessary for lymphocyte development and function. Despite a wide variety of genotypes, all patients are susceptible to severe infections, and often develop chronic diarrhea and failure to thrive. Persistent mucocutaneous candidiasis is a usual early finding as well as infections with viral pathogens, such as adenovirus, cytomegalovirus, Epstein–Barr virus, norovirus, respiratory syncytial virus, influenza, and parainfluenza. These, along with some opportunistic infection such as *Pneumocystis jirovecii*, can frequently be fatal [78]. In countries where NBS is not available, patients succumb to infections following live-attenuated vaccines such as rotavirus, varicella, and Bacillus Calmette–Guerin [79]. Hence, early diagnosis is crucial making this disease a target for NBS programs.

NBS Procedures for Hemoglobinopathies

Screening Methods for Hemoglobinopathies

The majority of the hemoglobinopathy screening programs currently use IEF or HPLC as the primary biochemical screening methods, replacing the dual electrophoresis (cellulose acetate/citrate agar electrophoresis) technique. Although more expensive than electrophoresis, IEF, and HPLC are more suitable for NBS programs as they can provisionally identify and precisely quantify a larger number of Hb variants, require small-volume blood samples and are less labor intensive [14]. However, despite their high sensitivity and specificity, they might be unable to identify variants with similar mobility or retention time, and which co-migrate or co-elute. Hence a two-tiered approach is used by NBS programs wherein the initial test is followed by a complementary secondary technique (dual electrophoresis technique, IEF, HPLC, or DNA based assays). Definitive diagnosis can be obtained with molecular techniques such as Multiplex gap PCR assays (for detecting α gene duplications and α deletional thalassemia mutations), reverse dot blot genotyping (to detect β globin variants and β thalassemia mutations), and DNA sequencing [80–82]. While DNA-based testing is part of the screening protocol in a few states (New York, Texas, Washington, California, Mississippi), its application is limited by high cost, complex instrumentation, and longer time required for analysis.

Utilization of these biochemical screening techniques in low-resource countries (sub-Saharan African countries, India) is difficult, due to the lack of laboratory infrastructure, funding and system of care required for standardized sample testing. Point of care (POC) diagnostics, which are easy to operate and interpret, allow for rapid testing at a low cost. However, depending on the test methodology, they may have limitations. Sickledex (based on decreased solubility of sickle hemoglobin) is unable to distinguish between HbAS and HbSS [83], while Aqueous Multiphase System (based on the high density of sickle RBC) [84], and Paper based SCD assay (paper-based solubility assay) [85], are limited in their ability to differentiate between HbSS and compound heterozygote state such as HbSC. On the other hand, Sickle Scan (lateral flow immunoassay using polyclonal antibodies) [86, 87], and HemoTypeSC (immunoassay using monoclonal antibodies) can identify various variants (HbS, HbC) and distinguish between HbSS and HbSC [88]. The recently introduced HemeChip (micro electrophoresis assay) can identify and even quantitate them [89]. These POC diagnostics are still being investigated and their implementation being evaluated.

Interpretation of NBS Results for Hemoglobinopathies

The expression of β-globin gene cluster (ε, γ, β, δ) is developmentally regulated [90]. HbF is the major hemoglobin for most of intrauterine life and is predominant at birth (60%–95%). The transcriptional switch to predominant adult hemoglobin (HbA = $\alpha_2\beta_2$) occurs soon after birth [63]. While the steepest changes in the Hb fractions occur in the first year of life, it may continue beyond infancy at a slower rate [91]. This decrease might be slower with SCD, with mean HbF levels as high as 20% at 1 year of age [92]. The Hb fraction at birth and later during the adult period determines the hemoglobinopathy diagnosis (Table 6.2).

Limitations of Non-Genetic NBS Testing for Hemoglobinopathies

Although hemoglobinopathy screening methodologies are highly sensitive, they are limited in their ability to detect certain mutations in the β globin gene cluster until the adult Hb pattern has developed. Hereditary persistence of fetal hemoglobin (HPFH) disorder can be identified only beyond the neonatal period, as HbF (>80%) is physiologically high at birth. Additionally, neonatal screening is unable to distinguish between certain mild and severe disease states where the hemoglobin pattern is similar at birth (Table 6.3). Furthermore, the HbA level at birth is highly gestational-age dependent, hence HbA fraction estimation is not a reliable method to distinguish the asymptomatic β thalassemia trait ($\beta^0\beta$, $\beta^+\beta$) and silent β thalassemia mutations from the symptomatic β thalassemia intermedia ($\beta^+\beta^0$, $\beta^+\beta^+$) and dominant β thalassemia (clinically symptomatic heterozygous β-thalassemia mutations) mutations, as they all present with the same hemoglobin pattern on NBS (FA). However, follow-up screening outside of the neonatal period, when the hematological parameters and Hb fractions are expected to have reached adult levels, might help differentiate between these disorders. As the switch from hemoglobin F to A is determined by gestational age, premature infants (gestational age <28 weeks) even without a hemoglobinopathy mutation, have only HbF on their NBS. Additionally, heterozygous sickle cell trait might be confused for a homozygous mutation on the NBS in preterm newborns, especially if the abnormal hemoglobin (HbS or HbC) level is higher than that of HbA [93]. Hence, it is essential to repeat the testing in preterm newborns by age 2 months. Parent testing and DNA-based testing are warranted in some cases. Confirmatory testing with HPLC or IEF during infancy might not be able to differentiate certain thalassemia genotypes ($\beta^0\beta^0$ vs. HPFH vs δβ^0 thalassemia or $\beta^E\beta^E$ vs. $\beta^E\beta^0$ thalassemia). Hence a definitive diagnosis for at-risk infants <12 months of age, with a suggestive NBS results can be made by confirmatory testing with DNA-based methods [94]. Alpha locus mutations or deletions resulting in α globin deficiency, is reflected by presence of Hb Bart on the NBS. Although highly sensitive, absence of Hb Bart cannot exclude silent thalassemia carrier (1 α gene deletion). This is specially seen with

Table 6.2 Newborn and adult hemoglobin fractionation patterns of sickle and non-sickle hemoglobinopathies

Diagnosis	Birth Hb fractionation	Hb pattern	Adulthood Hb fractionation	Hb genotype	Blood count	Parent genotype
Normal	HbF 80%–90%, HbA 10%–20%,* HbA$_2$ 0	FA	HbA 96%–97%, HbA$_2$ <3.5%, HbF 1%–2%	AA	Normal for age and sex	Not applicable
Sickling hemoglobinopathies						
Sickle cell trait	HbF 80%–90%, HbA ~6%, HbS ~4%, HbA$_2$ 0	FAS	HbA 55–60%, HbS 35%–40%, HbA$_2$ < 3.5%, HbF 1–2%	AS	Normal for age and sex	At least one parent with one or more β^s gene (e.g., HbAS, HbSS)
Sickle cell trait with alpha thalassemia trait**	HbF 80–90%, HbA ~7%, HbS ~3%, HbA$_2$ 0, Hb Bart 5–10%	FAS + Fast Band	HbA 60%–70%, HbS 20%–30%, HbA2 <3.5%, HbF 1%–2%	AS	Mild anemia (Hb 10–12 g/dL and microcytosis (MCV 70–75fL). Target cells seen on the peripheral blood smear	At least one parent with one or more β^s gene (e.g., HbAS, HbSS) and both parents with at least one α gene deletion each (e.g., −α/αα, −−/αα, −α/−α) or one parent with at least two α gene cis- deletion (−−/αα, −−/−α)
Sickle cell anemia (homozygous β^s)	HbF 80%–90%, HbS 10%–20%, HbA 0, HbA$_2$ 0	FS	HbS 80%–90%, HbF 1%–30%, *** HbA$_2$ <3.5%, HbA 0	SS	Mild to severe anemia (Hb 6–10 g/dL) and normal MCV (80–90 fL).	Both parents with one or more β^s gene (e.g., HbAS, HbSS)
Sickle cell anemia (homozygous β^s) with alpha thalassemia trait**	HbF 80%–90%, HbS 10%–20%, HbA 0, HbA$_2$ 0, Hb Barts 5%–10%	FS + Fast Band	HbS 80%–90%, HbF 5%–10%, *** HbA$_2$ <3.5% (but may be higher), HbA 0	SS	Mild to moderate anemia (Hb 8–11g/dL) and microcytosis (MCV 70–75 fL). Target cells seen on the peripheral blood smear	Both parents with one or more β^s gene each (e.g., HbAS, HbSS) and both parents with at least one α gene deletion each (e.g., −α/αα, −−/αα, −α/−α) or one parent with at least two α gene cis- deletion (−−/αα, −−/−α)
Sickle beta zero thalassemia	HbF 80%–90%, HbS 10%–20%, HbA 0, HbA$_2$ 0	FS	HbS 80%–95%, HbF 5%–10%, *** HbA$_2$ 4%–6%, HbA 0	Sβ^0 thalassemia	Mild to severe anemia (Hb 7– 9g/dL) and microcytosis (MCV 60–80 fL). Target cells seen on the peripheral blood smear	One parent with one or more β^s gene (e.g., HbAS, HbSS) and the other with at least one β^0 gene (e.g., β^{0}β^0 or β^{A}β^0)
Sickle beta plus thalassemia	HbF 80%–90%, HbS ~7%, HbA ~3%, HbA2 0	FSA	HbS 50–80%, HbA 5%–30% (occasionally higher, but always lower than HbS), HbF 1%–20%,*** HbA$_2$ 4%–6%	Sβ$^+$ thalassemia	Moderate anemia (Hb 9–12g/dL) and microcytosis (MCV 60–80 fL). Target cells seen on the peripheral blood smear	One parent with one or more β^s gene (e.g., HbAS, HbSS) and the other with at least one β$^+$ gene (e.g., β^{A}β$^+$, β$^+$β$^+$, or β$^+$β^0)
Sickle hemoglobin C disease	HbF 80%–90%, HbS ~4.5%, HbC ~4.5%, HbA 0, HbA$_2$ 0	FSC	HbS 45%–50%, HbC 45%–50%, HbF 1%–6%,*** HbA$_2$ <3.5%, HbA 0	HbSC	Mild anemia (Hb 9–14g/dL) and microcytosis (MCV 70–75). Target cells seen on the peripheral blood smear	One parent with one or more β^s gene (e.g., HbAS, HbSS) and the other with one or more β^c gene (e.g., β^{c}β^c, β^{A}β^c)

Table 6.2 (cont.)

Diagnosis	Birth		Adulthood		Blood count	Parent genotype
Sickle hemoglobin E disease	HbF 80%–90%, HbS 6%, HbE 4%,**** HbA 0	FSE	HbS 55%–60% HbE ~30%–35%,***** HbF 1-5%,*** HbA 0	HbSE	Mild anemia (Hb 8–14 g/dL) and microcytosis (MCV 71–97 fL). Target cells seen on the peripheral blood smear	One parent with one or more β^S gene (e.g., HbAS, HbSS) and the other with one or more β^E gene (e.g., $\beta^E\beta^E$, $\beta^A\beta^E$)
Sickle cell with $\delta\beta^0$ thalassemia	HF 80%–90%, HbS 10%–20%, HbA 0, HbA_2 0	FS	HbS 60–80%, HbF 15%–20% ***(heterocellular pattern), HbA_2 <3.5, HbA 0	HbS/$\delta\beta^0$ thalassemia	Mild anemia (Hb 10–12 g/dL) and microcytosis (MCV 76–85 fL)	One parent with one or more β^S gene (e.g., HbAS, HbSS) and the other with at least one $\delta\beta^0$ gene
Sickle cell with hereditary persistence of fetal hemoglobin (HPFH)	HbF 80%–90%, HbS 10%–20%, HbA 0, HbA_2 0	FS	HbS 60%–70%, HbF 25%–35% ***(pancellular pattern), HbA_2 <3.5, HbA 0 (deletion-HPFH)	Hb S/HPFH	Mild or no anemia (Hb 10–15 g/dL) and microcytosis (MCV 68–88 fL)	One parent with one or more β^S gene (e.g., HbAS, HbSS) and the other with homozygous or heterozygous non-deletional HPFH mutation

Non-sickling hemoglobinopathies

Diagnosis	Birth		Adulthood		Blood count	Parent genotype
Beta thalassemia trait (minor)	HbF 80%–90%, HbA 10%–20%, HbA_2 0	FA	HbA 85%–90%, HbA_2 5%–7%,**** HbF 2–7%	Hb$\beta\beta^0$ or Hb$\beta\beta^+$	Microcytic (MCV 60–80 fL) and mild anemia 12–14 g/dL. Target cells seen on the peripheral blood smear	At least one parent with one or more β^+ or β^0 gene
Beta thalassemia intermedia	HbF 80%–90%, HbA 3%–10%, HbA_2 0	FA	HbA 70%–90%, HbF 10–35%, HbA_2 5%–7%****	Hb$\beta^+\beta^+$ or Hb$\beta^0\beta^+$	Moderate to severe anemia (Hb 7–10 g/dL), microcytosis (MCV 50–80 fL) and hypochromia (MCH 16–24 pg). Target cells, basophilic stippling, anisocytosis, poikilocytosis, and polychromasia seen on the peripheral blood smear	Both parents with one or more β^+ or β^0 gene each
Beta thalassemia major (Cooley's anemia)	HbF 100%, HbA 0, HbA_2 0	F only	$\beta^0\beta^0$: HbF 90%–95%, HbA_2 <3.5%, HbA 0 $\beta^0\beta^+$: HbF 70%–90%, HbA ~30%, HbA_2 >5%	Hb$\beta^0\beta^0$ or Hb$\beta^0\beta^+$	Severe anemia (Hb 3–7 g/dL), microcytosis (MCV 50–60 fL) and hypochromia (MCH 12–18 pg). Marked anisocytosis, poikilocytosis, polychromasia, and nucleated red blood cells seen on the peripheral blood smear	One parent has one or more β^0 gene, and the other with one or more β^+ and/or β^0 gene
Hemoglobin E with beta zero thalassemia	HbF 80%–90%, HbE ~10%,**** HbA 0	FE	HbE 30%–70%,***** HbF 10–60%, HbA 0	HbE/β^0 thalassemia	Anemia (Hb <8 g/dL) and microcytosis (MCV 60–70 fL) Peripheral blood similar to Cooley's anemia	One parent with at least one β^E gene, and the other with at least one β^0 gene
Hemoglobin E with beta plus thalassemia	HbF ~90%, HbE ~6%,**** HbA 4%	FEA	HbE 30%–60%,***** HbA 10%–30%, HbF 4–30%	HbE/β^+ thalassemia	Anemia (Hb ~9.5 g/dL) and microcytosis (MCV 70–80 fL)	One parent with at least one β^E gene and the other with at least one β^+ gene

Condition	Newborn Hb quantification	Band pattern	Older child/adult Hb quantification	Genotype	CBC/clinical findings	Inheritance
Alpha thalassemia silent carrier	HbF 80%–90%, HbA 10%–20%, HbA$_2$ 0, Hb Bart ~1%–2%	FA	HbA 96%–97%, HbA$_2$ <3.5%, HbF 1%–2%	αα/α−	Normal for age and sex	At least one parent with at least one missing a globin gene (e.g., αα/α− or α−/α−)
Alpha thalassemia trait **	HbF 90%, HbA 10%, HbA$_2$ 0, Hb Bart 5%–10%	FA + Fast bands	HbA 96%–97%, HbA$_2$ <3.5%, HbF 1–2%	α−/α− or αα/−−	Mild anemia (Hb 11–13 g/dL) and microcytosis (MCV 65–80 fL)	Both parents with at least one missing a globin gene each (e.g., αα/α− or α−/α−) or one parent with at least two α gene cis- deletion (−−/αα, −−/α−)
Hemoglobin H disease	HbF 60%–80%, HbA ~5%, HbA$_2$ 0, Hb Bart 20%–50% (>25%)	FA + Fast bands	Hb A 80%–90%, HbA$_2$ <3.5, HbF 1%–3%, HbH 1%–40%	α−/−−	Anemia (Hb 7–10 g/dL), microcytosis (MCV 50–65 fL) and hypochromia (MCHC 25–30 g/dL). Basophilic stippling, anisocytosis, poikilocytosis and polychromasia seen on the peripheral blood smear******	One parent with −−/αα (cis deletion) and the other with at least one missing a globin gene (e.g., αα/α− or α−/α−)
Hydrops fetalis	Hb Bart 70%–100%, Hb Portland 10%–15%, HbA 0, HbA2 0	Fast bands	Not applicable	−−/−−	Can be normocytic with severe hypochromic anemia (Hb 3–8 g/dL)	Both parents have −−/αα (cis deletion)

Notes: Hemoglobin quantification results as measured by high performance liquid chromatography (HPLC). Hb denotes hemoglobin. β^s denotes the sickle mutation in the beta globin gene. β^C denotes the C mutation in the beta globin gene. β^E denotes the E mutation in the beta globin gene. β^0 denotes absence of beta globin gene function. β$^+$ denotes decreased beta globin production.

*HbA is lower is premature babies.

** Alpha thalassemia trait can be a deletion either in cis (−−/αα) or in trans (α−/α−).

*** HbF varies by β^s haplotype (e.g., higher in Arab–Indian haplotype) and variants in other locus (e.g., BCL11a) and may be as high as 30% even in the absence of exposure to hydroxyurea.

**** In some cases, HbA$_2$ can be between 3.5% and 5%. It can be even <3.5% in presence of iron deficiency or concomitant δ-gene deletional mutation.

*****HbE co-elutes with HbA2 on HPLC, hence not distinguishable from each other.

****** β precipitate inclusions ("golf-ball inclusions") can be seen in 35%–90% of red blood cells on HbH preparation.

Table 6.3 Phenotype differences in similar NBS pattern results

Hemoglobin pattern on the NBS	Mild disease phenotype	Moderate or severe disease phenotype
FS	HbS/HPFH	HbSS, HbS/β^0 thalassemia, HbS/β^+ thalassemia*
F only	Hbβ^0/HPFH, homozygous Hb HPFH	Hb $\beta^0\beta^0$ thalassemia, Hb β^0/$\delta\beta$ thalassemia, homozygous Hb $\delta\beta^0$ thalassemia
FE	HbEE	HbE/β^0 thalassemia
FA + Hb Barts	α thalassemia trait**	HbH***

Notes: NBS denotes newborn screening.

* Although rare, HbA fraction might be low or undetectable at birth in certain β thalassemia mutations, causing HbS/β^+ thalassemia to be misclassified as HbS/β^0 thalassemia.

** 2 α genes deleted or mutated.

*** When Hb H is caused by non-deletional α thalassemia, hemoglobin H is not always detectable.

heterozygous $\alpha^{3.7Kb}$ mutation (affecting the α_1 gene), where the Hb Bart level might be too low to be measured reliably. The amount of Hb Bart cannot distinguish between the trans and cis thalassemia trait genotypes.

Technical errors might also result in failing to diagnose an underlying hemoglobinopathy on initial testing. This can occur if there is contamination of sample with maternal blood or transfused donor blood. Testing needs to be done on a pre-transfusion sample, and if not available, repeated 3–4 months post-transfusion. Alternatively, DNA-based methods testing can be done [95]. Delay in transporting and analyzing samples can result in denaturation/precipitation of the unstable Hb variant and, therefore, failure to detect it [96]. Degradation of the extracted dried blood sample can lead to less accurate quantification of Hb Barts, and may result in misdiagnosis [97]. Alternatively, cord blood sample can be used for Hb Barts screening, however these samples are not easily transported and there is a risk of maternal blood contamination.

Follow-Up Strategies for Newly Diagnosed Sickling Hemoglobinopathies

In the US, initial screening for SCD is usually performed on DBS collected 24–72 hours after birth or prior to hospital discharge. Some US states require repeat testing with a second sample collected at 1–2 weeks of age. As the structure of the NBS programs varies by state, there are some differences regarding the follow-up algorithms of presumptive positive/abnormal screening results.

In general, for all initial screening results showing presence of HbS fraction, the state department refers all new cases to the PCP or the SCD treatment center. Following referral, a fresh sample is performed for confirmatory testing (~6–8 weeks of age). Neonates with confirmatory results concerning for a clinically significant sickle hemoglobinopathy including FS (HbF >HbS), FSA (Hb F> HbS> HbA), FSC (HbF> HbS = HbC), and FSV (HbF> HbS> HbV, where HbV is referred to as the unknown hemoglobin variant other than S or C) patterns, should have care established with a SCD treatment center and prophylactic penicillin initiated by age 2 months. Repeat testing at 6–12 months of age may be performed if the sickle genotype is still unclear or in the absence of parent studies (Fig. 6.1). The impact of newborn screening in reducing early mortality in SCD was largely due to the integration of newborn screening with comprehensive follow-up care [2, 98]. This integration ensures that the affected newborns have access to ongoing routine health maintenance (routine immunization, parental education, monitoring of growth and development, and disease-modifying therapies) and special healthcare services (stroke risk screening, access to blood bank services, and screening for organ damage) required to improve their quality of life and decrease disease morbidity and mortality [99].

Follow-Up Strategy for newly Diagnosed Non-Sickling Hemoglobinopathies

Screening for non-sickle hemoglobinopathies is not mandated by all the NBS state programs in

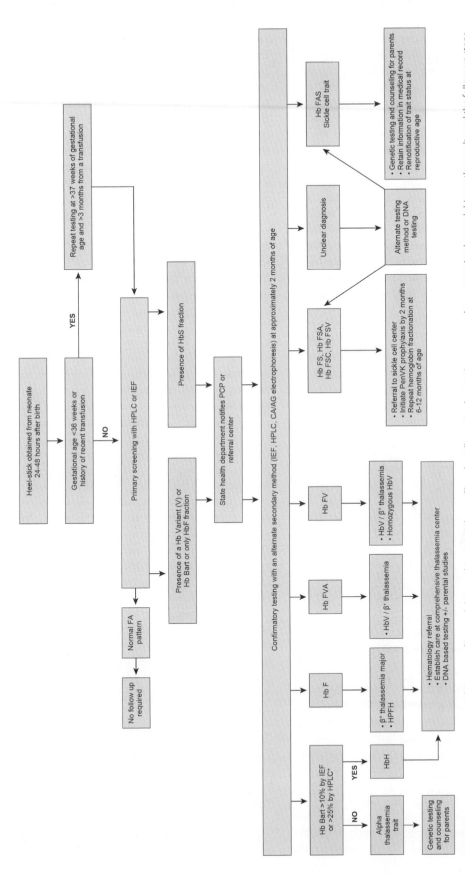

Fig. 6.1 Approach to screening and follow up of hemoglobinopathies in newborns. Flowchart illustrating how to interpret newborn screening hemoglobinopathy results and the follow-up steps to confirm diagnosis and establish early care. HPLC: high performance liquid chromatography, IEF: isoelectric focusing, Hb F: fetal hemoglobin, Hb A: adult hemoglobin A, Hb V: variant hemoglobin, Hb S: sickle hemoglobin, CA/AG electrophoresis: cellulose acetate/agarose gel electrophoresis, PCP: primary care provider, HPFH: hereditary persistence of fetal hemoglobin, *Confirmatory DNA alpha globin gene analysis can also be done to diagnose Hb H disease and alpha thalassemia trait.

the US. Hence, while incidental findings (Hb variants, Hb Bart, or absence of HbA) suggestive of a clinically significant non-sickle hemoglobinopathy are reported by most states to the PCP and family, the confirmatory testing of these abnormal screening results is directed by the PCP and/or pediatric hematology referral center and not the state. The lack of standard guidelines also has resulted in wide variability in the state based recommendations regarding follow up of abnormal initial screening results (Fig. 6.1). While 7 out of 50 states in the US do not report low levels of Hb Barts, 12 out of 50 states have no follow-up recommendations. The remaining states provide recommendations ranging from complete blood count to alpha globin gene analysis (Wisconsin) [100]. California's NBS does diagnostic DNA-based second tier testing on samples with clinically significant level of Hb Bart (>25%), for a definitive diagnosis of HbH [101]. Expansion of NBS core panel to include non-sickle hemoglobinopathies would ensure early identification for the clinically significant thalassemia mutations ($\beta^0\beta^0$, $\beta^E\beta^0$, hydrops fetalis, non-deletional HbH) in infancy, and where early intervention (blood transfusion) can improve survival. Integration of this screening with comprehensive follow-up care is also beneficial for the clinically significant thalassemia mutations with varied phenotypic expression where close surveillance, parental education, and long-term follow up ensures decreased disease morbidity and improved quality of life [101]. Early identification of milder mutations (trait and carrier) would help avoid unnecessary iron supplementation for microcytosis in the absence of iron deficiency and aid in identifying couples who are carriers.

NBS Procedures for G6PD Deficiency

The American Academy of Pediatrics (AAP) recognizes G6PD deficiency as a major risk factor for development of hyperbilirubinemia and kernicterus in the newborn, therefore, it recommends pre-discharge bilirubin screening in conjunction with investigation of hyperbilirubinemia risk factors. The AAP recommends that G6PD screening is only done on jaundiced neonates who are at risk of having G6PD based on their family history, ethnicity, and geographic origin or if they are responding poorly to phototherapy [102]. The World Health Organization

recommends universal screening for G6PD using fluorescent spot test in areas with a male G6PD prevalence of 3%–5% or more [103]. Reports from working groups have concluded that screening for G6PD using point-of-care biochemical assays during birth hospitalization and timely result notification (<48 hrs) is clinically feasible [104], however, there is no consensus yet regarding how to screen and whether knowledge of G6PD status in the immediate newborn period will prevent neonatal kernicterus [102].

A subset of female neonates who are heterozygous for G6PD-deficient mutation may have a severe presentation with hemolysis, hyperbilirubinemia, and kernicterus [105–107]. In female heterozygotes with random X-inactivation, two erythrocyte populations (~1:1 ratio) are seen, where one population has normal G6PD activity while the other is G6PD deficient and susceptible to hemolysis. Variation in X-inactivation with skewing towards the erythrocyte deficient population may lead to a more severe G6PD-deficient phenotype [108]. Biochemical assays, including the widely recommended semi-quantitative fluorescent spot test, can assess the G6PD enzyme activity by detecting NADPH level [109]. Due to their low cutoff value, they are sensitive in identifying hemizygous males and homozygous females with complete deficiency of G6PD. However, when used to screen female heterozygotes, the result representing the average enzyme activity of both erythrocyte populations (enzyme deficient and sufficient) might be falsely normal, despite the presence of a sizable enzyme-deficient erythrocyte population [110]. Additionally, this assay can be falsely negative when screening G6PD deficient individuals undergoing or recovering from an acute hemolytic event due to the high number of young erythrocytes (with higher G6PD level), necessitating repeat testing in a few weeks [111]. Alternatively, DNA-based analysis can reliably identify female heterozygotes and is also unaffected by a recent hemolytic event. A DNA-based newborn screening assay capable of detecting the five most common G6PD mutations in the USA and estimated to identify approximately 90% of all G6PD-deficient neonates, is currently used by the NBS programs of Pennsylvania and the District of Columbia [112].

DNA technology, though highly sensitive and specific, especially when using DBS elutes, might be limited in their clinical usefulness if the results are not obtained within the typical hyperbilirubinemia risk period [113]. This testing is expensive and can miss new mutations, unless whole exome sequencing is done, and requires technical expertise and infrastructure (a centralized core laboratory) to be scalable. Newer point-of-care screening tools, such as tandem mass spectrometry and digital microfluidics, might help by providing rapid diagnosis at a lower cost and perhaps, enable large scale screening [114, 115].

NBS Procedures for Severe Combined Immune Deficiency

Although all typical infants with SCID have low or absent production of T cells from the thymus, and most cases can be identified by low absolute lymphocyte counts (ALC), this test alone is not sufficient for screening. In patients with maternally engrafted T cells, or high or normal B cells, ALC may be normal to high, causing false negative results. To capture all the cases, ALC cutoff would have to be at a level leading to an unacceptable number of false positive results. Therefore, ALC is not considered an adequate population-based screening test for SCID. Because SCID is characterized by severe deficiency of T cells, the screening test currently available for infants is an indicator of thymic production of de novo (naive) T cells. This screening test is a real-time polymerase chain reaction (PCR) assay that amplifies DNA extracted from DBS to detect T-cell receptor excision circles (TRECs). TRECs are circular DNA fragments that are byproducts of the T-cell receptor rearrangement that physiologically occurs in the thymus, and thus a direct measure of thymic output of naive T cells.

The use of NBS by TREC quantification has shortened time to diagnosis, making treatment possible at a very early age and therefore improving patients' outcomes [4, 116]. Given heterogeneity of SCID, there is no standard treatment regimen that can be applied to all infants. Patients can be successfully treated by hematopoietic stem cell transplantation (HCT), particularly if they have a human leukocyte antigen-matched sibling donor (MSD) as long-term survival rates in these patients are as high as 97% [78]. In most cases, however, a MSD is not available and patients receive grafts from their parents (haploidentical), matched unrelated donors (MUD) [117–119], or from a matched umbilical cord blood (UCB) unit. This cohort has a significantly worse outcome with an overall survival rate of 60%–85%, which is due to post-transplant complications such as graft versus host disease, autoimmunity, incomplete immune reconstitution or even graft rejection [120]. Based on these studies, it is currently unclear what the best alternative donor source and conditioning regimen is for SCID patients who do not have a MSD. These studies are being conducted by individual centers and/or through the pediatric immune deficiency treatment consortium to determine the best approach for newly diagnosed SCID patients.

Unlike other SCID forms, newly diagnosed patients with ADA deficiency can receive enzyme replacement therapy (ERT) with intramuscular injections of exogenous polyethylene-glycol-conjugated bovine ADA (PEG-ADA). Although ERT is effective and can be continued for life, it is particularly useful as a bridging therapy prior to HCT to stabilize patients, however it provides inadequate long-term reconstitution and its effect tends to decrease over time with survival rates of 78% at 20 years [121, 122]. Patients treated with ERT require close monitoring and weekly or twice-weekly injections of PEG-ADA to maintain high ADA activity. In addition, wide application of ERT is limited due to its cost and lack of availability in some countries.

Due to limitations of transplantation and limited availability of ERT, gene therapy has also been explored as a potentially curative treatment for ADA-deficiency and X-linked SCID [123, 124]. Gene therapy is an experimental technique inserting a normal copy of a patient's mutated gene into the genome of his/her own hematopoietic stem cell. This approach has some potential advantages over existing therapies for patients without a suitable MSD. It may be immediately available with no delay due to donor search and eliminates the risk of GVHD and graft rejection. Furthermore, immunosuppressive prophylaxis or high dose conditioning regimens are not required, decreasing treatment-related organ toxicity, prolonged immunosuppression, and the risk of infection, compared with traditional HCT. However, this kind of therapy has complications. Early gene therapy trials for X-linked SCID utilizing retroviral vectors without conditioning restored only T-cell immunity and were complicated by leukemia in 25% of cases [125]. Leukemogenesis was due to the expression of genes, which were located in close proximity to the integrated retroviral vector. Since then, lentiviral vectors have been developed that eliminate this risk; in addition, non-myeloablative conditioning regimens have been explored to improve the engraftment of gene-corrected HSCs. This progress is highlighted by early phase clinical studies for X-linked SCID, in which the infusion of lentiviral-gene corrected HSCs post non-myeloablative busulfan conditioning restored full immunity of T, B, and NK cells without complications [126, 127]. Gene therapy for ADA deficiency has also been successful without complications and gene therapy for other forms of SCID such as Artemis deficiency are in progress [128, 129]. While gene therapy for SCID has been mainly spearheaded by academic centers, based of its success thus far, several centers have now partnered with biotech companies to obtain FDA approval for its widespread administration. Thus, gene therapy may become a viable alternative to transplantations and/or ERT, following the NBS diagnosis.

Carrier Testing

Carrier screening programs for autosomal recessive genetic disorders help identify clinically asymptomatic individuals who carry a variant allele of the gene (heterozygous mutation or trait) associated with that disorder. Autosomal recessive disorder couples have a 25% risk (1 in 4) of having a child affected with the disease (homozygous mutation) with each pregnancy. Hence it is important to identify and educate these individuals of their carrier status and its genetic implications, as it may affect their reproductive decisions. Additionally, they should also be informed if their carrier state can increase their risk for certain medical complications or might influence their treatment and management in certain clinical settings (pre-operative management of patients with sickle cell trait) [130–132]. Communities with increased prevalence of a genetic disorder (due to genetic drift or founder effect) have been shown to have higher familiarity and awareness of that disorder, perceived benefit of carrier testing, acceptance of reproductive options and community support, compared to the general population, hence may support the successful implementation of ancestry-based heterozygote screening programs [133, 134].

Screening can be offered to individuals at any life stage (school age or premarital/preconception or prenatal). Premarital and preconception screening and counseling not only allows individuals and prospective parents who are carriers, to maximize on their available reproductive options (partner selection, adoption, preimplantation genetic diagnosis, donor gametes) but is also associated with less emotional distress compared to testing during pregnancy (prenatal counseling) [135–137]. School-based carrier screening programs have also shown to be successful in decreasing incidence of affected births in the targeted communities [138–140]. Nevertheless, the ethical and social implications associated with this type of prospective screening (genotypic prevention) should not be ignored [141–143]. The advancement in genetic technology, has now led to the increased availability of expanded screening panels that can screen for multiple genes and sequence variants, and is offered to individuals and couples irrespective of their ethnicity-based risk status [144]. Furthermore, this universal screening approach reduces the risk of stigmatization, allows for equitable access to relevant and valuable genetic information to couples and individuals who do not belong to the identified high-risk groups and facilitates reproductive autonomy [145, 146]. However, the impact of this improved technological capacity and expanded screening panels on newborn screening programs, is still unclear. Additionally, there is also little evidence suggesting that knowledge of their newborn's carrier state affected the future reproductive decisions of the parents [147–149].

Future Directions

The advent of economic progress in LMICs results in improvement in healthcare services and an epidemiological transition towards reduced infant and childhood mortality. Consequently, newborns with an underlying hemoglobin disorder, who would have previously died undiagnosed, now survive and tend to present for diagnosis and treatment, thus increasing the disease population [150, 151]. The high birth rate in LMIC regions impacts the proportion of SCD-affected births, which is estimated to increase by approximately 11% in sub-Saharan Africa [33]. Whereas based on United Nations demographic projections, the proportion of affected births in other HbS regions, such as North America, Eurasia, and Arab–India, is expected to decrease by 2050 [33]. These projections underline the importance of close surveillance of new hemoglobinopathy cases. Greater effort in creating NBS programs and ongoing cohort studies that have the ability to follow children into adulthood will facilitate the understanding of the beneficial impact of early interventions on the long-term clinical, social, and economic Effectiveness of NBS programs. Finally, the recent addition of SCID to the genetic NBS panel poses both a challenge and an opportunity. To avoid inequity, greater emphasis will be needed to create specialized centers with the capacity to receive and treat these complex cases, even using the most recent technology (e.g., gene therapy) for newly found cases.

References

1. Gaston MH, Verter JI, Woods G, et al. Prophylaxis with oral penicillin in children with sickle cell anemia. A randomized trial. *N Engl J Med* 1986;**314** (25):1593–9.

2. Vichinsky E, Hurst D, Earles A, Kleman K, Lubin B. Newborn screening for sickle cell disease: Effect on mortality. *Pediatrics* 1988;**81**(6):749–55.

3. Cowan MJ, Neven B, Cavazanna-Calvo M, Fischer A, Puck J. Hematopoietic stem cell transplantation for severe combined immunodeficiency diseases. *Biol Blood Marrow Transplant* 2008;**14**(1 Suppl 1):73–5.

4. Myers LA, Patel DD, Puck JM, Buckley RH. Hematopoietic stem cell transplantation for severe combined immunodeficiency in the neonatal period leads to superior thymic output and improved survival. *Blood* 2002;**99**(3):872–8.

5. Guthrie R, Susi A. A simple phenylalanine method for detecting phenylketonuria in large populations of newborn infants. *Pediatrics* 1963;**32**:338–43.

6. Levy HL. Genetic screening. *Adv Hum Genet* 1973;**4**:1–104.

7. Dussault JH, Coulombe P, Laberge C, et al. Preliminary report on a mass screening program for neonatal hypothyroidism. *J Pediatr* 1975;**86** (5):670–4.

8. Itano HA, Pauling L. A rapid diagnostic test for sickle cell anemia. *Blood* 1949;**4**(1):66–8.

9. Nalbandian RM, Nichols BM, Camp FR, Jr., et al. Dithionite tube test – a rapid, inexpensive technique for the detection of hemoglobin S and non-S sickling hemoglobin. *Clin Chem* 1971;**17** (10):1028–32.

10. Nichols BM, Nalbandian RM, Henry RL, Wolf PL, Camp FR, Jr. Murayama test for hemoglobin S: Simplification in technique. *Clin Chem* 1971;**17** (10):1059–60.

11. Hicksg EJ, Griep JA, Nordschow CD. Comparison of results for three method of hemoglobin S identification. *Clin Chem* 1973;**19**(5):533–5.

12. Garrick MD, Dembure P, Guthrie R. Sickle-cell anemia and other hemoglobinopathies: Procedures and strategy for screening employing spots of blood on filter paper as specimens. *N Engl J Med* 1973;**288**(24):1265–8.

13. Kohn J. Separation of haemoglobins on cellulose acetate. *J Clin Pathol* 1969;**22**(1):109–11.

14. Benson JM, Therrell BL, Jr. History and current status of newborn screening for hemoglobinopathies. *Semin Perinatol* 2010;**34** (2):134–44.

15. Rashed MS, Ozand PT, Bucknall MP, Little D. Diagnosis of inborn errors of metabolism from blood spots by acylcarnitines and amino acids profiling using automated electrospray tandem mass spectrometry. *Pediatr Res* 1995;**38** (3):324–31.

16. Moat SJ, Rees D, King L, et al. Newborn blood spot screening for sickle cell disease by using tandem mass spectrometry: Implementation of a protocol to identify only the disease states of sickle cell disease. *Clin Chem* 2014;**60**(2):373–80.

17. Schmidt RM, Holland S. Standardization in abnormal hemoglobin detection. An evaluation of hemoglobin electrophoresis kits. *Clin Chem* 1974;**20**(5):591–4.

18. Schmidt RM, Brosious EM. Evaluation of proficiency in the performance of tests for abnormal hemoglobins. *Am J Clin Pathol* 1974;**62** (5):664–9.

19. De Jesus VR, Mei JV, Bell CJ, Hannon WH. Improving and assuring newborn screening laboratory quality worldwide: 30-year experience at the Centers for Disease Control and Prevention. *Semin Perinatol* 2010;**34** (2):125–33.

20. De Jesus VR, Mei JV, Cordovado SK, Cuthbert CD. The Newborn Screening Quality Assurance Program at the Centers for Disease Control and Prevention: Thirty-five year experience assuring newborn screening laboratory quality. *Int J Neonatal Screen* 2015;**1** (1):13–26.

21. Gaston M, Rosse WF. The cooperative study of sickle cell disease: Review of study design and objectives. *Am J Pediatr Hematol Oncol* 1982;**4** (2):197–201.

22. Consensus conference. Newborn screening for sickle cell disease and other hemoglobinopathies. *JAMA* 1987;**258**(9):1205–9.

23. Therrell BL, Jr., Lloyd-Puryear MA, Eckman JR, Mann MY. Newborn screening for sickle cell diseases in the United States: A review of data spanning 2 decades. *Semin Perinatol* 2015;**39**(3):238–51.

24. Watson MS, Mann MY, Lloyd-Puryear MA, et al., American College of Medical Genetics Newborn Screening Expert Group. Newborn screening: Toward a uniform screening panel and system: Executive summary. *Pediatrics* 2006; **117** (5 Pt 2): S296–307.

25. Koopmans J, Hiraki S, Ross LF. Attitudes and beliefs of pediatricians and genetic counselors regarding testing and screening for CF and G6PD: Implications for policy. *Am J Med Genet A* 2006;**140**(21):2305–11.

26. Natowicz M. Newborn screening: Setting evidence-based policy for protection. *N Engl J Med* 2005;**353**(9):867–70.

27. Botkin JR, Clayton EW, Fost NC, et al. Newborn screening technology: Proceed with caution. *Pediatrics* 2006;**117**(5):1793–9.

28. Heredero-Baute L. Community-based program for the diagnosis and prevention of genetic disorders in Cuba: Twenty years of experience. *Community Genet* 2004;**7**(2–3):130–6.

29. Therrell BL, Padilla CD, Loeber JG, et al. Current status of newborn screening worldwide: 2015. *Semin Perinatol* 2015;**39**(3):171–87.

30. Fernandes AP, Januario JN, Cangussu CB, Macedo DL, Viana MB. Mortality of children with sickle cell disease: A population study. *J Pediatr* 2010;**86**(4):279–84.

31. Sabarense AP, Lima GO, Silva LM, Viana MB. Survival of children with sickle cell disease in the comprehensive newborn screening programme in Minas Gerais, Brazil. *Paediatr Int Child Health* 2015;**35**(4):329–32.

32. Silva-Pinto AC, Alencar de Queiroz MC, Antoniazzo Zamaro PJ, Arruda M, Pimentel dos Santos H. The neonatal screening program in Brazil, focus on sickle cell disease (SCD). *Int J Neonatal Screen* 2019;**5**(1):11.

33. Piel FB, Hay SI, Gupta S, Weatherall DJ, Williams TN. Global burden of sickle cell anaemia in children under five, 2010–2050: Modelling based on demographics, excess mortality, and interventions. *PLoS Med* 2013;**10**(7):e1001484.

34. Upadhye DS, Jain DL, Trivedi YL, et al. Neonatal screening and the clinical outcome in children with sickle cell disease in central India. *PLoS One* 2016;**11**(1):e0147081.

35. Dixit S, Sahu P, Kar SK, Negi S. Identification of the hot-spot areas for sickle cell disease using cord blood screening at a district hospital: An Indian perspective. *J Community Genet* 2015;**6**(4):383–7.

36. Upadhye D, Das RS, Ray J, et al. Newborn screening for hemoglobinopathies and red cell enzymopathies in Tripura State: A malaria-endemic state in northeast India. *Hemoglobin* 2018;**42**(1):43–6.

37. Panigrahi S, Patra PK, Khodiar PK. Neonatal screening of sickle cell anemia: A preliminary report. *Indian J Pediatr* 2012;**79**(6):747–50.

38. Howson CP, Cedergren B, Giugliani R, et al. Universal newborn screening: A roadmap for action. *Mol Genet Metab* 2018;**124**(3):177–83.

39. McGann PT, Ferris MG, Ramamurthy U, et al. A prospective newborn screening and treatment program for sickle cell anemia in Luanda, Angola. *Am J Hematol* 2013;**88**(12):984–9.

40. McGann PT, Grosse SD, Santos B, et al. A cost-effectiveness analysis of a pilot neonatal screening program for sickle cell anemia in the Republic of Angola. *J Pediatr* 2015;**167**(6):1314–9.

41. Ndeezi G, Kiyaga C, Hernandez AG, et al. Burden of sickle cell trait and disease in the Uganda Sickle Surveillance Study (US3): A cross-sectional study. *Lancet Glob Health* 2016;**4**(3):e195–200.

42. McGann PT, Hernandez AG, Ware RE. Sickle cell anemia in sub-Saharan Africa: Advancing the clinical paradigm through partnerships and research. *Blood* 2017;**129**(2):155–61.

43. Streetly A, Sisodia R, Dick M, et al. Evaluation of newborn sickle cell screening programme in England: 2010–2016. *Arch Dis Child* 2018;**103**(7):648–53.

44. Holtzman NA. Newborn screening for severe combined immunodeficiency: Progress and challenges. *JAMA* 2014;**312**(7):701–2.

45. Adams SP, Rashid S, Premachandra T, et al. Screening of neonatal UK dried blood spots using a duplex TREC screening assay. *J Clin Immunol* 2014;**34**(3):323–30.

46. Audrain M, Thomas C, Mirallie S, et al. Evaluation of the T-cell receptor excision circle assay performances for severe combined immunodeficiency neonatal screening on Guthrie cards in a French single centre study. *Clin Immunol* 2014;**150**(2):137–9.

47. Somech R, Lev A, Simon AJ, et al. Newborn screening for severe T and B cell immunodeficiency in Israel: A pilot study. *Isr Med Assoc J* 2013;**15**(8):404–9.

48. Chien YH, Chiang SC, Chang KL, et al. Incidence of severe combined immunodeficiency through

newborn screening in a Chinese population. *J Formos Med Assoc* 2015;**114**(1):12–6.

49. Kwan A, Church JA, Cowan MJ, et al. Newborn screening for severe combined immunodeficiency and T-cell lymphopenia in California: Results of the first 2 years. *J Allergy Clin Immunol* 2013;**132** (1):140–50.

50. Hassell KL. Population estimates of sickle cell disease in the US. *Am J Prev Med* 2010;**38**(4 Suppl): S512–21.

51. Modell B, Darlison M. Global epidemiology of haemoglobin disorders and derived service indicators. *Bull World Health Organ* 2008;**86** (6):480–7.

52. Weatherall DJ. The inherited diseases of hemoglobin are an emerging global health burden. *Blood* 2010;**115**(22):4331–6.

53. Pasvol G, Weatherall DJ, Wilson RJ. Cellular mechanism for the protective effect of haemoglobin S against *P. falciparum malaria. Nature* 1978;**274**(5672):701–3.

54. Allen SJ, O'Donnell A, Alexander ND, et al. Alpha +–thalassemia protects children against disease caused by other infections as well as malaria. *Proc Natl Acad Sci USA* 1997;**94**(26):14736–41.

55. Taylor SM, Parobek CM, Fairhurst RM. Haemoglobinopathies and the clinical epidemiology of malaria: A systematic review and meta-analysis. *Lancet Infect Dis* 2012;**12** (6):457–68.

56. Williams TN, Mwangi TW, Wambua S, et al. Negative epistasis between the malaria-protective effects of alpha+–thalassemia and the sickle cell trait. *Nat Genet* 2005;**37**(11):1253–7.

57. Sundd P, Gladwin MT, Novelli EM. Pathophysiology of sickle cell disease. *Annu Rev Pathol* 2019;**14**:263–92.

58. Serjeant GR. Natural history and determinants of clinical severity of sickle cell disease. *Curr Opin Hematol* 1995;**2**(2):103–8.

59. Chui DH, Waye JS. Hydrops fetalis caused by alpha-thalassemia: An emerging health care problem. *Blood* 1998;**91**(7):2213–22.

60. Fucharoen S, Viprakasit V. Hb H disease: Clinical course and disease modifiers. *Hematology Am Soc Hematol Educ Program* 2009;**2009**(1):26–34.

61. Lal A, Goldrich ML, Haines DA, et al. Heterogeneity of hemoglobin H disease in childhood. *N Engl J Med* 2011;**364**(8):710–18.

62. Menzel S, Garner C, Rooks H, Spector TD, Thein SL. HbA2 levels in normal adults are influenced by two distinct genetic mechanisms. *Br J Haematol* 2013;**160**(1):101–5.

63. Olivieri NF. The beta-thalassemias. *New Engl J Med* 1999;**341**(2):99–109.

64. Ho PJ, Hall GW, Luo LY, Weatherall DJ, Thein SL. Beta-thalassaemia intermedia: Is it possible consistently to predict phenotype from genotype? *Br J Haematol* 1998;**100**(1):70–8.

65. Ho PJ, Wickramasinghe SN, Rees DC, et al. Erythroblastic inclusions in dominantly inherited beta thalassemias. *Blood* 1997;**89**(1):322–8.

66. Efremov DG, Efremov GD, Zisovski N, et al. Variation in clinical severity among patients with Hb Lepore-Boston-beta-thalassaemia is related to the type of beta-thalassaemia. *Br J Haematol* 1988;**68**(3):351–5.

67. Thein SL. Genetic modifiers of beta-thalassemia. *Haematologica* 2005;**90**(5):649–60.

68. Higgs DR, Clegg JB, Weatherall DJ, Serjeant BE, Serjeant GR. Interaction of the alpha alpha alpha globin gene haplotype and sickle haemoglobin. *Br J Haematol* 1984;**57**(4):671–8.

69. Cappellini MD, Fiorelli G. Glucose-6-phosphate dehydrogenase deficiency. *Lancet* 2008;**371** (9606):64–74.

70. Kaplan M, Renbaum P, Levy-Lahad E, et al. Gilbert syndrome and glucose-6-phosphate dehydrogenase deficiency: A dose-dependent genetic interaction crucial to neonatal hyperbilirubinemia. *Proc Natl Acad Sci USA* 1997;**94**(22):12128–32.

71. Frank JE. Diagnosis and management of G6PD deficiency. *Am Fam Physician* 2005;**72** (7):1277–82.

72. Kaplan M, Hammerman C. Glucose-6-phosphate dehydrogenase deficiency: A hidden risk for kernicterus. *Semin Perinatol* 2004;**28**(5):356–64.

73. Slusher TM, Vreman HJ, McLaren DW, et al. Glucose-6-phosphate dehydrogenase deficiency and carboxyhemoglobin concentrations associated with bilirubin-related morbidity and death in Nigerian infants. *J Pediatr* 1995;**126** (1):102–8.

74. Al-Mousa H, Al-Saud B. Primary immunodeficiency diseases in highly consanguineous populations from Middle East and North Africa: Epidemiology, diagnosis, and care. *Front Immunol* 2017;**8**:678.

75. Griffith LM, Cowan MJ, Notarangelo LD, et al. Improving cellular therapy for primary immune deficiency diseases: Recognition, diagnosis, and management. *J Allergy Clin Immunol* 2009;**124** (6):1152–60 e12.

76. Cossu F. Genetics of SCID. *Ital J Pediatr* 2010;**36**:76.

77. Shearer WT, Dunn E, Notarangelo LD, et al. Establishing diagnostic criteria for severe combined immunodeficiency disease (SCID), leaky SCID, and Omenn syndrome: The Primary Immune Deficiency Treatment Consortium experience. *J Allergy Clin Immunol* 2014;**133**(4):1092–8.

78. Pai SY, Logan BR, Griffith LM, et al. Transplantation outcomes for severe combined immunodeficiency, 2000–2009. *N Engl J Med* 2014;**371**(5):434–46.

79. Sarmiento JD, Villada F, Orrego JC, Franco JL, Trujillo-Vargas CM. Adverse events following immunization in patients with primary immunodeficiencies. *Vaccine* 2016;**34**(13):1611–6.

80. Chong SS, Boehm CD, Higgs DR, Cutting GR. Single-tube multiplex-PCR screen for common deletional determinants of alpha-thalassemia. *Blood* 2000;**95**(1):360–2.

81. Harteveld CL, Refaldi C, Cassinerio E, Cappellini MD, Giordano PC. Segmental duplications involving the alpha-globin gene cluster are causing beta-thalassemia intermedia phenotypes in beta-thalassemia heterozygous patients. *Blood Cells Mol Dis* 2008;**40**(3):312–16.

82. Old JM. Screening and genetic diagnosis of haemoglobinopathies. *Scand J Clin Lab Invest* 2007;**67**(1):71–86.

83. Bond M, Hunt B, Flynn B, et al. Towards a point-of-care strip test to diagnose sickle cell anemia. *PLoS One* 2017;**12**(5):e0177732.

84. Kumar AA, Chunda-Liyoka C, Hennek JW, et al. Evaluation of a density-based rapid diagnostic test for sickle cell disease in a clinical setting in Zambia. *PLoS One* 2014;**9**(12):e114540.

85. Yang X, Kanter J, Piety NZ, et al. A simple, rapid, low-cost diagnostic test for sickle cell disease. *Lab Chip* 2013;**13**(8):1464–7.

86. Kanter J, Telen MJ, Hoppe C, et al. Validation of a novel point of care testing device for sickle cell disease. *BMC Med* 2015;**13**:225.

87. McGann PT, Schaefer BA, Paniagua M, Howard TA, Ware RE. Characteristics of a rapid, point-of-care lateral flow immunoassay for the diagnosis of sickle cell disease. *Am J Hematol* 2016;**91**(2):205–10.

88. Quinn CT, Paniagua MC, DiNello RK, Panchal A, Geisberg M. A rapid, inexpensive and disposable point-of-care blood test for sickle cell disease using novel, highly specific monoclonal antibodies. *Br J Haematol* 2016;**175**(4):724–32.

89. Ung R, Alapan Y, Hasan MN, et al. Point-of-care screening for sickle cell disease by a mobile micro-electrophoresis platform. *Blood* 2015;**126**(23).

90. Grosveld F, Antoniou M, Berry M, et al. The regulation of human globin gene switching. *Philos Trans R Soc Lond B Biol Sci* 1993;**339**(1288):183–91.

91. Colombo B, Kim B, Atencio RP, Molina C, Terrenato L. The pattern of fetal haemoglobin disappearance after birth. *Br J Haematol* 1976;**32**(1):79–87.

92. Davis LR. Changing blood picture in sickle-cell anaemia from shortly after birth to adolescence. *J Clin Pathol* 1976;**29**(10):898–901.

93. Hustace T, Fleisher JM, Sanchez Varela AM, Podda A, Alvarez O. Increased prevalence of false positive hemoglobinopathy newborn screening in premature infants. *Pediatr Blood Cancer* 2011;**57**(6):1039–43.

94. Hoppe CC. Newborn screening for non-sickling hemoglobinopathies. *Hematology Am Soc Hematol Educ Program* 2009; **2009**:19–25.

95. Reed W, Lane PA, Lorey F, et al. Sickle-cell disease not identified by newborn screening because of prior transfusion. *J Pediatr* 2000;**136**(2):248–50.

96. Yates AM, Mortier NA, Hyde KS, Hankins JS, Ware RE. The diagnostic dilemma of congenital unstable hemoglobinopathies. *Pediatr Blood Cancer* 2010;**55**(7):1393–5.

97. Alauddin H, Langa M, Mohd Yusoff M, et al. Detection of alpha-thalassaemia in neonates on cord blood and dried blood spot samples by capillary electrophoresis. *Malays J Pathol* 2017;**39**(1):17–23.

98. Frempong T, Pearson HA. Newborn screening coupled with comprehensive follow-up reduced early mortality of sickle cell disease in Connecticut. *Conn Med* 2007;**71**(1):9–12.

99. Okpala I, Thomas V, Westerdale N, et al. The comprehensiveness care of sickle cell disease. *Eur J Haematol* 2002;**68**(3):157–62.

100. Fogel BN, Nguyen HLT, Smink G, Sekhar DL. Variability in state-based recommendations for management of alpha thalassemia trait and silent carrier detected on the newborn screen. *J Pediatr* 2018;**195**:283–7.

101. Michlitsch J, Azimi M, Hoppe C, et al. Newborn screening for hemoglobinopathies in California. *Pediatr Blood Cancer* 2009;**52**(4):486–90.

102. Watchko JF, Kaplan M, Stark AR, Stevenson DK, Bhutani VK. Should we screen newborns for glucose-6-phosphate dehydrogenase deficiency in the United States? *J Perinatol* 2013;**33**(7):499–504.

103. WHO Working Group. Glucose-6-phosphate dehydrogenase deficiency. *Bull World Health Organ* 1989;**67**(6):601–11.

104. Nock ML, Johnson EM, Krugman RR, et al. Implementation and analysis of a pilot in-hospital newborn screening program for glucose-6-phosphate dehydrogenase deficiency in the United States. *J Perinatol* 2011;**31**(2):112–17.

105. Watchko JF. Hyperbilirubinemia in African American neonates: Clinical issues and current challenges. *Semin Fetal Neonatal Med* 2010;**15**(3):176–82.

106. Kaplan M, Hammerman C, Vreman HJ, Stevenson DK, Beutler E. Acute hemolysis and severe neonatal hyperbilirubinemia in glucose-6-phosphate dehydrogenase-deficient heterozygotes. *J Pediatr* 2001;**139**(1):137–40.

107. Herschel M, Ryan M, Gelbart T, Kaplan M. Hemolysis and hyperbilirubinemia in an African American neonate heterozygous for glucose-6-phosphate dehydrogenase deficiency. *J Perinatol* 2002;**22**(7):577–9.

108. Beutler E, Baluda MC. The separation of glucose-6-phosphate-dehydrogenase-deficient erythrocytes from the blood of heterozygotes for glucose-6-phosphate-dehydrogenase deficiency. *Lancet* 1964;**1**(7326):189–92.

109. Beutler E, Blume KG, Kaplan JC, et al. International Committee for Standardization in Haematology: Recommended screening test for glucose-6-phosphate dehydrogenase (G-6-PD) deficiency. *Br J Haematol* 1979;**43**(3):465–7.

110. Luzzatto L. Glucose 6-phosphate dehydrogenase deficiency: From genotype to phenotype. *Haematologica* 2006;**91**(10):1303–6.

111. Beutler E. G6PD deficiency. *Blood* 1994;**84**(11):3613–36.

112. Lin Z, Fontaine JM, Freer DE, Naylor EW. Alternative DNA-based newborn screening for glucose-6-phosphate dehydrogenase deficiency. *Mol Genet Metab* 2005;**86**(1–2):212–19.

113. Kaplan M, Hammerman C. Neonatal screening for glucose-6-phosphate dehydrogenase deficiency: Biochemical versus genetic technologies. *Semin Perinatol* 2011;**35**(3):155–61.

114. Carpenter KH, Wiley V. Application of tandem mass spectrometry to biochemical genetics and newborn screening. *Clin Chim Acta* 2002;**322**(1–2):1–10.

115. Millington DS, Sista R, Eckhardt A, et al. Digital microfluidics: A future technology in the newborn screening laboratory? *Semin Perinatol* 2010;**34**(2):163–9.

116. Heimall J, Logan BR, Cowan MJ, et al. Immune reconstitution and survival of 100 SCID patients post-hematopoietic cell transplant: A PIDTC natural history study. *Blood* 2017;**130**(25):2718–27.

117. Griffith LM, Cowan MJ, Kohn DB, et al. Allogeneic hematopoietic cell transplantation for primary immune deficiency diseases: Current status and critical needs. *J Allergy Clin Immunol* 2008;**122**(6):1087–96.

118. Gaspar HB, Qasim W, Davies EG, et al. How I treat severe combined immunodeficiency. *Blood* 2013;**122**(23):3749–58.

119. Dvorak CC, Cowan MJ. Hematopoietic stem cell transplantation for primary immunodeficiency disease. *Bone Marrow Transplant* 2008;**41**(2):119–26.

120. Wahlstrom JT, Dvorak CC, Cowan MJ. Hematopoietic stem cell transplantation for severe combined immunodeficiency. *Curr Pediatr Rep* 2015;**3**(1):1–10.

121. Malacarne F, Benicchi T, Notarangelo LD, et al. Reduced thymic output, increased spontaneous apoptosis and oligoclonal B cells in polyethylene glycol-adenosine deaminase-treated patients. *Eur J Immunol* 2005;**35**(11):3376–86.

122. Gaspar HB, Aiuti A, Porta F, et al. How I treat ADA deficiency. *Blood* 2009;**114**(17):3524–32.

123. Ferrua F, Aiuti A. Twenty-five years of gene therapy for ADA-SCID: From bubble babies to an approved drug. *Hum Gene Ther* 2017;**28**(11):972–81.

124. Cavazzana M, Six E, Lagresle-Peyrou C, Andre-Schmutz I, Hacein-Bey-Abina S. Gene therapy for X-linked severe combined immunodeficiency: Where do we stand? *Hum Gene Ther* 2016;**27**(2):108–16.

125. Hacein-Bey-Abina S, Pai SY, Gaspar HB, et al. A modified gamma-retrovirus vector for X-linked severe combined immunodeficiency. *N Engl J Med* 2014;**371**(15):1407–17.

126. De Ravin SS, Wu X, Moir S, et al. Lentiviral hematopoietic stem cell gene therapy for X-linked severe combined immunodeficiency. *Sci Transl Med* 2016;**8**(335):335ra57.

127. Mamcarz E, Zhou S, Lockey T, et al. Lentiviral gene therapy with low dose busulfan for infants with SCID-X1 (revised). *N Engl J Med* 2019;**380**:1525–34.

128. Aiuti A, Roncarolo MG, Naldini L. Gene therapy for ADA-SCID, the first marketing approval of an ex vivo gene therapy in Europe: Paving the road for the next generation of advanced therapy medicinal products. *EMBO Mol Med* 2017;**9**(6):737–40.

129. Punwani D, Kawahara M, Yu J, et al. Lentivirus mediated correction of Artemis-deficient severe

combined immunodeficiency. *Hum Gene Ther* 2017;**28**(1):112–24.

130. Atlas SA. The sickle cell trait and surgical complications: A matched-pair patient analysis. *JAMA* 1974;**229**(8):1078–80.

131. Metras D, Coulibaly AO, Ouattara K, et al. Open-heart surgery in sickle-cell haemoglobinopathies: Report of 15 cases. *Thorax* 1982;**37**(7):486–91.

132. Naik RP, Haywood C, Jr. Sickle cell trait diagnosis: Clinical and social implications. *Hematol Am Soc Hematol Educ Prog* 2015;**2015**:160–7.

133. Holtkamp KCA, Mathijssen IB, Lakeman P, et al. Factors for successful implementation of population-based expanded carrier screening: Learning from existing initiatives. *Eur J Public Health* 2017;**27**(2):372–7.

134. Kaback MM. Population-based genetic screening for reproductive counseling: The Tay–Sachs disease model. *Eur J Pediatr* 2000;**159** Suppl 3: S192–5.

135. De Wert GM, Dondorp WJ, Knoppers BM. Preconception care and genetic risk: Ethical issues. *J Community Genet* 2012;**3**(3):221–8.

136. Henneman L, Borry P, Chokoshvili D, et al. Responsible implementation of expanded carrier screening. *Eur J Hum Genet* 2016;**24**(6):e1–e12.

137. Bombard Y, Miller FA, Hayeems RZ, Avard D, Knoppers BM. Reconsidering reproductive benefit through newborn screening: A systematic review of guidelines on preconception, prenatal and newborn screening. *Eur J Hum Genet* 2010;**18**(7):751–60.

138. Mitchell JJ, Capua A, Clow C, Scriver CR. Twenty-year outcome analysis of genetic screening programs for Tay–Sachs and beta-thalassemia disease carriers in high schools. *Am J Hum Genet* 1996;**59**(4):793–8.

139. Lena-Russo D, Badens C, Aubinaud M, et al. Outcome of a school screening programme for carriers of haemoglobin disease. *J Med Screen* 2002;**9**(2):67–9.

140. Amato A, Cappabianca MP, Lerone M, et al. Carrier screening for inherited haemoglobin disorders among secondary school students and young adults in Latium, Italy. *J Community Genet* 2014;**5**(3):265–8.

141. van Elderen T, Mutlu D, Karstanje J, et al. Turkish female immigrants' intentions to participate in preconception carrier screening for hemoglobinopathies in the Netherlands: An empirical study. *Public Health Genomics* 2010;**13** (7–8):415–23.

142. Saffi M, Howard N. Exploring the effectiveness of mandatory premarital screening and genetic counselling programmes for beta-thalassaemia in the Middle East: A scoping review. *Public Health Genomics* 2015;**18**(4):193–203.

143. Kihlbom U. Ethical issues in preconception genetic carrier screening. *Ups J Med Sci* 2016:1–4.

144. Langlois S, Benn P, Wilkins-Haug L. Current controversies in prenatal diagnosis 4: Pre-conception expanded carrier screening should replace all current prenatal screening for specific single gene disorders. *Prenat Diagn* 2015;**35**(1):23–8.

145. Nazareth SB, Lazarin GA, Goldberg JD. Changing trends in carrier screening for genetic disease in the United States. *Prenat Diagn* 2015;**35**(10):931–5.

146. Lazarin GA, Haque IS. Expanded carrier screening: A review of early implementation and literature. *Semin Perinatol* 2016;**40**(1):29–34.

147. Ciske DJ, Haavisto A, Laxova A, Rock LZ, Farrell PM. Genetic counseling and neonatal screening for cystic fibrosis: An assessment of the communication process. *Pediatrics* 2001;**107** (4):699–705.

148. Lewis S, Curnow L, Ross M, Massie J. Parental attitudes to the identification of their infants as carriers of cystic fibrosis by newborn screening. *J Paediatr Child Health* 2006;**42** (9):533–7.

149. Hayeems RZ, Bytautas JP, Miller FA. A systematic review of the effects of disclosing carrier results generated through newborn screening. *J Genet Couns* 2008;**17**(6):538–49.

150. Omran AR. The epidemiologic transition. A theory of the epidemiology of population change. *Milbank Mem Fund Q* 1971;**49** (4):509–38.

151. Darlison MW, Modell B. Sickle-cell disorders: Limits of descriptive epidemiology. *Lancet* 2013;**381**(9861):98–9.

A Guide to Identifying the Cause of Anemia in a Neonate

Robert D. Christensen

Diagnosing anemia in a neonate is only a first step in a process that includes: clarifying the pathology responsible for the anemia, instituting the best-known therapy (if indeed a treatment is warranted), and then evaluating whether the therapy administered was effective in alleviating the anemia. Chapters 4, 6–10, and 20 focus on the principal varieties of anemia that occur in the neonatal period. The purpose of this chapter is not to repeat material detailed there, but to provide a method for navigating the somewhat unique process of diagnosing neonatal anemia and then discovering its cause. To accomplish this purpose, the chapter is organized into two parts: (1) making the diagnosis of anemia in neonates using reference intervals appropriate for gestational and postnatal age, and (2) following an evaluative algorithm to identify the underlying *cause* of the anemia in a neonatal patient.

Making the Diagnosis of Anemia

Simply stated, anemia is a pathological decrease, below normal, in the quantity of red blood cells [1]. In neonatal hematology, anemia is typically defined by a hemoglobin concentration, or a hematocrit, below the 5th percentile of the appropriate reference interval [2]. Comparison with an "appropriate reference interval" is essential for diagnosing anemia in neonates. This is because the hemoglobin and hematocrit normally increase steadily in a fetus during gestation, and then decrease in a characteristic pattern for several weeks after birth [2]. These physiological perinatal changes in what the hemoglobin and hematocrit "should be" necessitate that to properly label a neonate as "anemic," the patient's hemoglobin and hematocrit must be compared with

appropriate normative figures or tables, such as those provided in Chapter 24.

For adult patients, the diagnosis of anemia involves comparing the patient's hemoglobin/hematocrit with normative values of healthy volunteers of the same *sex*. This is because mature males tend to have somewhat higher hemoglobin/hematocrit values than do mature females [3]. However, this female–male difference is not observed in neonates at birth or during the neonatal period [4]. Therefore, separate sex-specific figures/tables are not needed to diagnose anemia in neonates. Moreover, for adult patients, the diagnosis of anemia requires comparing the patient's hemoglobin/hematocrit with values obtained at a grossly similar altitude above sea level. This is because patients living at high altitude develop somewhat higher hemoglobin/hematocrit values than do those living at sea level [5]. This altitude difference does not appear to apply to neonates at birth, at least not at altitudes up to 5,000 ft (1,524 m) or so above sea level [4]. It is not clear whether neonates born at extremely high altitudes (such as La Rinconada, Peru at 16,830 ft [5,130 m]) have significantly higher hemoglobin/hematocrit values at birth than those in the reference intervals of Chapter 24. Thus, it is not known whether new reference interval figures/tables are needed to assist in diagnosing anemia of babies born in very high altitude settlements such as certain communities in Peru, China, Nepal, Argentina, and Bolivia.

Not every neonate with anemia (as defined by a hemoglobin/hematocrit below the 5th percentile of the appropriate reference interval) requires a diagnostic evaluation to determine the cause of the anemia. If they did, 5% of all neonates would

Neonatal Hematology, Pathogenesis, Diagnosis, and Management of Hematologic Problems, 3rd edition, ed. Pedro A. de Alarcón, Eric J. Werner, Robert D. Christensen, and Martha C. Sola-Visner. Published by Cambridge University Press. © Cambridge University Press 2021.

need to undergo such an evaluation. With four million births annually in the USA, this would mean 200,000 neonates/year would be classified as anemic, and in need of a diagnostic evaluation. Rather, some neonates will have a hemoglobin/hematocrit only slightly below the 5th percentile cutoff limit. If such a neonate is well appearing, with normal vital signs, and with a normal physical examination, one can forego a detailed diagnostic evaluation to seek the cause of the anemia; perhaps simply repeating the hemoglobin/hematocrit after a few days or weeks. Contrariwise, neonates with hematocrit/hemoglobin levels far below the 5th percentile level, or with signs of anemia, such as pallor, tachycardia, and or tachypnea, should undergo a diagnostic evaluation to identify the underlying cause of the anemia and to assist in selecting the best treatment and follow-up plans.

An algorithm that can be followed to confirm a diagnosis of anemia in a neonate is shown as Fig. 7.1. It involves applying the proper reference intervals (found in Chapter 24), and considering whether the anemia might be too mild, trivial, or asymptomatic to warrant commencing a larger and more definitive evaluation of causation.

The algorithm in Fig. 7.1 begins by applying the appropriate reference intervals for hemoglobin and hematocrit. These ranges gradually increase during the period in utero. In applying these reference intervals, it should be remembered that in newborn infants the anatomic site of the blood drawn to measure the hemoglobin and hematocrit influences the test result [6]. Perfusion of small vessels in the extremities can be relatively poor, particularly in the hours immediately after birth or during hypotension or skin cooling, and this can result in increased transudation of fluid and capillary hemoconcentration. Consequently, the hemoglobin and hematocrit of capillary blood can be 5% to 10% higher than from venous blood [7]. The difference between capillary and venous values is greatest on the day of birth and typically disappears by about 3 months of age. The discrepancy is greatest in preterm infants and in those with hypotension, hypovolemia, and acidosis. Differences can be minimized, but not fully resolved, by warming the extremity before sampling, obtaining freely flowing blood, and discarding the first few drops [7]. The interpretation of serial observations necessitates the consistent use of one anatomic site of blood sampling (i.e., all vascular or all capillary).

Hemoglobin concentrations should increase during the first hours after birth, attributable in part to a shift of fluid from the intravascular

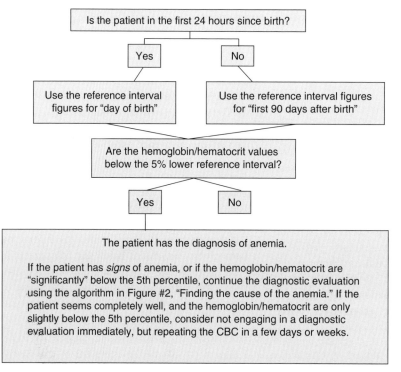

Fig. 7.1 Using the reference interval charts (see Chapter 24) to diagnose anemia in a neonate.

compartment, but also to the transfusion of fetal red cells from the placenta at the time of birth [6, 7]. After the first day, the reference intervals for hemoglobin and hematocrit gradually decrease, as shown in Fig. 24.2 (term and late preterm neonate) and Fig. 24.3 (preterm neonates). Once anemia has been diagnosed in a neonate, and it has been decided that this is not a minimal or trivial condition, attention should next be turned to discovering its *cause*.

Finding the Underlying Cause of the Anemia

An initial impression of the *cause* of the anemia often derives from: (1) the history, (2) the physical examination, and (3) the CBC on which the diagnosis of anemia was made. These three elements

can be termed "first-line" evidence for discovering the cause of the neonatal anemia, because they are generally readily available at the time the diagnosis of anemia is made. The initial putative cause of the anemia, derived from first-line evidence, can almost always be categorized into one of three groups: (1) hemorrhage, (2) hemolysis, or (3) hyporegenerative (see the algorithm in Fig. 7.2).

Very rarely, neonatal anemia has a mixed causative mechanism. For instance, hemorrhage and hemolysis can co-exist in an anemic neonate with disseminated intravascular coagulation (DIC), where internal and external bleeding is significant and brisk hemolysis accompanies microangiopathic schistocytosis [8]. However, generally a neonatal anemia has a single cause and is not due to a complicated combination of nutritional,

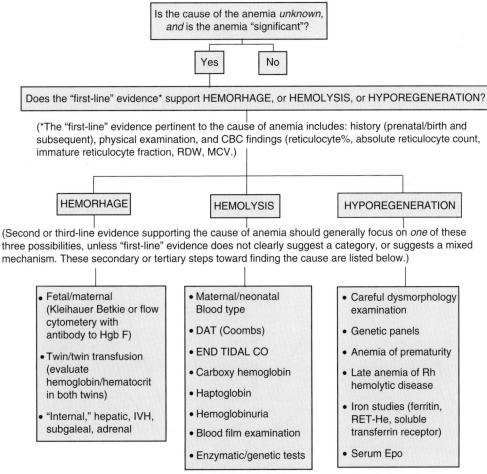

Fig. 7.2 Finding the cause of the anemia.

inflammatory, inherited, and/or neoplastic disorders, as can occur in anemic adult patients. Therefore, after gaining an initial impression of causation from first-line evidence, it can be wise to focus on the *one* most likely cause (hemorrhage, hemolysis, hyporegenerative). Identifying the most likely one will suggest second-line testing to give confirmation and will lead to specific diagnostic testing where such is appropriate. Focusing the secondary tests on *one* of the three causative categories will diminish unnecessary testing, thus reducing costs, lowering phlebotomy losses, and saving time. The following sections review second-line tests to consider when focusing on one of the three groups as the cause of the anemia.

Hemorrhage

A reticulocyte count is sometimes an instructive second-line test in seeking the cause of anemia in a neonate. This is because reticulocytosis is expected when anemia is the result of hemorrhage *or* hemolysis, but not when anemia is due to erythrocyte hyporegeneration. Likewise, following a significant hemorrhage in a neonate, nucleated red blood cells (NRBC) can emerge into the circulation, thereby increasing the NRBC count. However, a caveat should be appreciated if using an elevated reticulocyte count, and an elevated NRBC count, to identify hemorrhage or hemolysis as the cause of anemia. Namely, an elevation in reticulocytes and NRBC is a physiologic response to significant anemia, but this response does not occur *immediately* after

a hemorrhage or a sudden brisk hemolytic episode. Rather, a period of at least 12 to 24 hours is typically required between hemorrhage or hemolysis and reticulocytosis, and a period of 24 to 36 hours is typically required between hemorrhage or hemolysis and a NRBC elevation [9, 10].

Figure 7.3 illustrates the time required for an elevation in reticulocyte count and NRBC count after administering a single dose of long-acting erythropoietin (darbepoetin). Such administration serves as a model of the time required for elevation in reticulocytes and NRBC after hemorrhage, based on the assumption that hemorrhage produces tissue hypoxia, which in turn results in generation of erythropoietin, which in turn stimulates erythropoiesis to replace the erythrocytes lost by hemorrhage. Since reticulocytosis and an elevation in NRBC occur only 12–36 hours after a severe hemorrhage, one should anticipate a *normal* reticulocyte count and NRBC count if these tests are obtained very early after an acute hemorrhage or abrupt hemolysis. Thus, if a large fetal/maternal hemorrhage occurs within minutes to a few hours preceding birth, the principal pathology in the neonate will be related to hypovolemia, and the requirement for intravenous fluid. The fall in hemoglobin and hematocrit may not occur for an hour or more, once fluid has moved into the circulation and perhaps intravenous fluids have been administered. An increase in reticulocyte count and NRBC count, characteristic of severe hemorrhage, might not be evident for many hours.

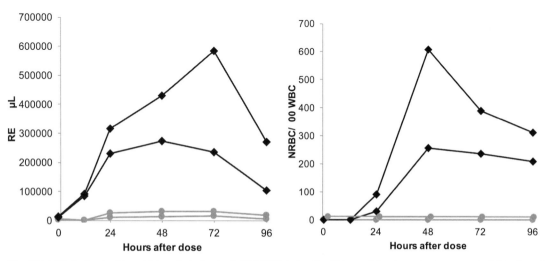

Fig. 7.3 (a) Reticulocytes/µL and (b) nucleated red cells/100 WBC during the 96 hours following subcutaneous administration of darbepoetin 10 µg/mL subcutaneous (black symbols and lines) or vehicle control (gray symbols and lines) to four newborn sheep. (From [10].)

If hemorrhage is thought to be the cause of neonatal anemia, and the site of the blood loss is not obvious, another second-level test could include a search for fetal cells in the mother's circulation, using either the Kleihaur–Betke acid elution test or flow cytometery of mother's blood using antibody against hemoglobin-F [11]. Either test, if positive, identifies and somewhat quantifies a fetal to maternal hemorrhage. More in-depth discussion of this problem is found in Chapter 23. One important caveat should be recalled when interpreting the tests that seek fetal erythrocytes in the mother's blood; namely, one should expect false negative results when the mother has antibody against her fetus' blood group antigens. As an example, if a mother is a recipient of a fetal hemorrhage, and mother is blood group O, and her fetus is group A (or B or AB), she will very likely rapidly lyse the fetal cells in her circulation. Therefore testing the mother's blood for fetal cells will reveal none, but this will be a false negative result. In such cases, although the usual testing is negative, mothers will often recall chills and or fever and malaise at a time the fetal to maternal hemorrhage occurred, somewhat reminiscent of a transfusion reaction.

Hemolysis

Hemolysis is a pathological shortening of the red blood cell life span. Hemolysis is a different process than the natural physiologic removal of red cells at the end of their normal life span by a process termed senescence [12]. Hemolysis can be the result of either inherited mutations in genes involved in erythrocyte structure or function, or the result of acquired disorders that disrupt erythrocytes by immune-mediated mechanisms or mechanical disruption [13].

Second-line tests to consider, when hemolysis is considered the likely cause of neonatal anemia, include the non-invasive measurement of end tidal carbon monoxide (CO) [14–16], or if a blood gas is needed, measuring the carboxyhemoglobin percentage [17]. Elevation in either measurement of CO can confirm hemolysis and can at the same time give a general impression of its severity, based on the degree of CO elevation. Figure 7.4 illustrates non-invasive assessment of the hemolytic rate using end tidal CO quantification. Figure 7.5 shows the expected reference interval for ETCOc (end tidal carbon monoxide concentration) in neonates and older children. An ETCOc above the upper reference interval can be taken as evidence of hemolysis.

If these tests of CO are not available, other markers of hemolysis can be used, including absent serum haptoglobin (note - haptoglobin levels can be lower in neonates than in adults, but should not be absent, unless hemolysis is brisk), marked hemoglobinuria, and rapidly rising

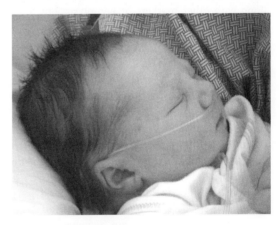

Fig. 7.4 ETCOc measurement on term neonate, using a single-nare cannula. (CoSense, shown with permission, Capnia Inc., Redwood Shores, California.)

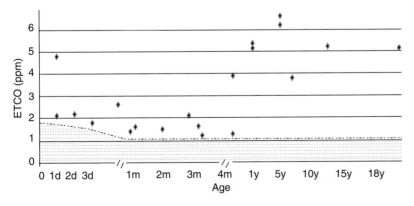

Fig. 7.5 ETCOc normative values. The hatched zone, below the dashed line, represent the reference interval for ETCO of healthy subjects from 1 hour to over 18 years of age. The diamonds show ETCO values of neonates and children with proven hemolytic disorders. (From [15].)

indirect bilirubin. The other important second-line testing needed if hemolysis is considered as the cause of anemia is blood typing of mother and neonate and direct antiglobin test (DAT; Coombs) testing.

Examination of a stained blood film specifically focusing on erythrocyte morphology can also give relevant information about hemolysis [18]. Once hemolytic disease has been identified as the cause of the neonatal anemia, the specific reason for the hemolysis can be sought, and the problems of hyperbilirubinemia and worsening anemia can be anticipated and managed expectantly. Details of this process are found in Chapter 10.

Hemolytic anemia in a neonate is usually accompanied by indirect hyperbilirubinemia. However, this is not invariant; some neonates conjugate and excrete bilirubin much more rapidly than do others. Consequently, rarely a neonate with anemia is found to have a hemolytic disorder but does not have significant hyperbilirubinemia. These unusual cases will have an elevated ETCOc along with other markers of hemolysis, but their jaundice will be only mild to moderate.

Hyporegenerative

Second-line testing to consider when hyporegenerative anemia is considered includes a careful physical examination to look for minor dysmorphic features as detailed in Chapter 4. When a genetic cause is suspected for the hyporegenerative neonatal anemia, sequencing panels can be selected, as indicated in Chapter 4.

Iron deficiency anemia is a rare cause of hyporegenerative anemia in the neonatal period [19]. Neonates at high risk for iron deficiency include extremely preterm neonates, small for gestational age infants, and infants of diabetic mothers. Particularly when mothers of babies in these three groups are obese [20]. Iron deficiency as a cause of neonatal anemia can be sought by typical iron studies including reticulocyte hemoglobin content, ferritin, serum iron, and transferrin saturation, and soluble transferrin receptor [19, 20]. However the amount of blood needed for a complete battery of iron tests is generally in excess of what should reasonable be withdrawn from an anemic neonate.

Hyporegenerative anemia in a neonate can occur for reasons other than genetic mutations and iron deficiency. Treatments administered in a neonatal intensive care unit (NICU) can reduce

erythropoietin production and lead to anemia with a low reticulocyte count. Specifically, neonates treated with supplemental oxygen in amounts greatly exceeding that needed can reduce erythropoiesis. The responsible mechanism involves hypoxia-inducible factors (HIFs), which are transcription factors that respond to oxygen at the cellular level. HIF-2α regulates erythropoietin (EPO) production in the fetal liver [21]. Inadequate delivery of oxygen results in a rapid inhibition of a prolyl-hydroxylase, which uses oxygen as a co-substrate. This leads to translocation of HIF-2α to the nucleus where the alpha units heterodimerize and bind to the hypoxia responsive elements in the regulatory portion of the *EPO* gene. This binding induces a >1,000-fold increase in EPO production, significantly raising circulating EPO levels [21, 22]. Contrariwise, delivery of very high physiologically abnormal quantities of oxygen to a neonate results in the reverse, with a reduction of EPO production, a subsequently low circulating EPO level, followed by a very low reticulocyte count, followed by a hyporegenerative anemia. Thus, if a neonate who is receiving supplemental O_2 has intermittent or persistent hyperoxia, endogenous EPO production can be significantly reduced, leading to at least a mild or moderate hyporegenerative anemia.

References

1. Beutler E, Waalen J. The definition of anemia: What is the lower limit of normal of the blood hemoglobin concentration? *Blood* 2006;**107**:1747–50.

2. Henry E, Christensen RD. Reference intervals in neonatal hematology. *Clin Perinatol* 2015;**42**:483–97.

3. Wintrobe MM. Blood of normal men and women. *Bull John Hopkins Hosp* 1933;**53**:118–40.

4. Jopling J, Henry E, Wiedmeier SE, Christensen RD. Reference ranges for hematocrit and blood hemoglobin concentration during the neonatal period: Data from a multihospital health care system. *Pediatrics* 2009;**123**:e333–7.

5. Ruíz-Argüelles GJ, Sanchez-Medal L, Loria A, et al. Red cell indices in normal adults residing at altitude from sea level to 2670 meters. *Am J Hematol* 1980;**8**:265–71.

6. Oh W, Lind J. Venous and capillary hematocrit in newborn infants and placental transfusion. *Acta Paediatr Scand* 1966;**55**:38–42.

7. Linderkamp O, Versmold HT, Strohhacker I, et al. Capillary–venous hematocrit differences in

newborn infants. 1. Relationship to blood volume, peripheral blood flow, and acid-base parameters. *Eur J Pediatr* 1977:**127**;9–14.

8. Judkins AJ, MacQueen BC, Christensen RD, et al. Automated quantification of fragmented red blood cells: Neonatal reference intervals and clinical disorders of neonatal intensive care unit patients with high values. *Neonatology.* 2018;**115**:5–12.

9. Christensen RD, Lambert DK, Richards DS. Estimating the nucleated red blood cell 'emergence time' in neonates. *J Perinatol* 2014;**34**:116–19.

10. Christensen RD, Albertine KH, Dahl MJ, et al. Nucleated red blood cell counts in term neonates following fetal hypoxia. *Neonatology* (in press).

11. Kim YA, Makar RS. Detection of fetomaternal hemorrhage. *Am J Hematol* 2012;**87**:417–23.

12. Badior KE, Casey JR. Molecular mechanism for the red blood cell senescence clock. *IUBMB Life* 2018;**70**:32–40.

13. Christensen RD, Yaish HM. Hemolytic disorders causing severe neonatal hyperbilirubinemia. *Clin Perinatol* 2015;**42**:515–27.

14. Christensen RD, Lambert DK, Henry E, et al. End-tidal carbon monoxide as an indicator of the hemolytic rate. *Blood Cells Mol Dis* 2015;**54**:292–6.

15. Christensen RD, Malleske DT, Lambert DK, Baer VL, et al. Measuring end-tidal carbon monoxide of jaundiced neonates in the birth hospital to identify those with hemolysis. *Neonatology* 2016;**109**:1–5.

16. Bhutani VK, Maisels MJ, Schutzman DL, Castillo Cuadrado ME, et al. Identification of risk for neonatal haemolysis. *Acta Paediatr* 2018;**107**:1350–6.

17. Tidmarsh GF, Wong RJ, Stevenson DK. End-tidal carbon monoxide and hemolysis. *J Perinatol* 2014;**34**:577–81.

18. Christensen RD, Yaish HM, Lemons RS. Neonatal hemolytic jaundice: Morphologic features of erythrocytes that will help you diagnose the underlying condition. *Neonatology* 2014;**105**:243–9.

19. MacQueen BC, Christensen RD, Ward DM, et al. The iron status at birth of neonates with risk factors for developing iron deficiency: A pilot study. *J Perinatol* 2017;**37**:436–40.

20. MacQueen BC, Robert D. Christensen RD, Baer VL, Ward DM, Snow GL. Screening umbilical cord blood for congenital iron deficiency. *Blood Cells Mol Dis* 2019;**77**:95–100.

21. Yoon D, Ponka P, Prchal JT. Hypoxia 5. Hypoxia and hematopoiesis. *Am J Physiol Cell Physiol* 2011;**300**:C1215–C1222.

22. Shih HM, Wu CJ, Lin SL. Physiology and pathophysiology of renal erythropoietin-producing cells. *J Formos Med Assoc* 2018;**117**:955–63.

Anemia of Prematurity and Indications for Erythropoietin Therapy

Pamela J. Kling

Introduction

Anemia of prematurity is a multifactorial anemia, characterized by relatively low plasma erythropoietin (EPO) levels, iatrogenic blood loss, low circulating blood volumes, and insufficient erythropoiesis. This anemia has been long characterized as nutritionally insensitive, but nutrition may influence its clinical course. Anemia of prematurity is treated with erythrocyte transfusions. However, delaying umbilical cord clamping may increase initial hematocrit percentages, improve infant iron status, prevent erythrocyte transfusions, decrease necrotizing enterocolitis (NEC), and decrease intraventricular hemorrhage (IVH). Many published studies have examined the potential of therapy with recombinant human EPO or other erythropoietic stimulating agent (ESA). Although EPO therapy is associated with statistically lower number of total erythrocyte transfusions, most early transfusions are not eliminated. However, early erythropoietic EPO dosing may also decrease NEC and IVH as well as improve neurocognitive outcomes. A recent systematic review refuted previous concerns that early administration of EPO was associated with increased retinopathy of prematurity (ROP). Early high dose EPO regimens are currently being studied for neuroprotection in premature infants. Iron deficiency in EPO treatment is also of potential concern, but long-term iron status of EPO treated premature infants is similar to controls.

Physiology of Anemia of Prematurity

Erythropoietin (EPO), the primary hormone regulating erythropoiesis, is measurable throughout fetal gestation [1]. In the fetus and newborn, EPO is produced primarily by the liver, which may be relatively insensitive to hypoxia, compared to kidney [1, 2]. After term birth, erythropoiesis is suppressed by markedly improved postnatal oxygen delivery, a relatively depressed plasma EPO, and a fall in hemoglobin (Hb) occurs that reaches "physiologic nadir" in the first months postpartum [3]. This response is exaggerated in premature infants [4]. The anemia of prematurity reflects not only insufficient EPO production [4], but also small circulating blood volume, hemorrhage, hemolysis, shortened red blood cell (RBC) survival, and perhaps most important is the iatrogenic blood loss, coined the "anemia of phlebotomy" (summarized by Ohls) [5]. Anemia of prematurity is traditionally described as nutritionally "insensitive" in that it does not improve with addition of iron, although iron contributes to the recovery of Hb [6, 7]. Iron status is critical, in that insufficient iron supplementation may inhibit the efficacy of EPO in prematurity [7, 8].

Therapy for Anemia of Prematurity

Minimizing Blood Loss

Blood loss impacts the clinical course of the anemia of prematurity. In a typical 800 gram birth weight premature infant, with red cell mass at birth of 27 mL, avoidance of erythrocyte transfusions depends on avoidance of blood loss [9]. Lower initial Hb and acuity are major factors in determining erythrocyte transfusion [10, 11]. In the absence or presence of EPO therapy, phlebotomy clearly correlates to erythrocyte volumes

Neonatal Hematology, Pathogenesis, Diagnosis, and Management of Hematologic Problems, 3rd edition, ed. Pedro A. de Alarcón, Eric J. Werner, Robert D. Christensen, and Martha C. Sola-Visner. Published by Cambridge University Press. © Cambridge University Press 2021.

transfused [9, 10, 12–19]. This is most evident when precise transfusion criteria are employed [14]. Some centers report relatively lower phlebotomy loss on even the smallest infants [20, 21]. Inline and microsampling point of care testing minimizes blood loss in unstable infants [17, 22, 23]. Advances in perinatal care that decrease patient acuity would logically decrease blood administration [13], but erythrocyte transfusion practices vary widely [14–16]. In the neonatal intensive care unit (NICU), blood volume drawn is related to volume transfused, with phlebotomist overdraw in the blood tubes becoming significant [9, 24, 25].

Delayed Umbilical Cord Clamping

At premature delivery, administering an autologous placental transfusion by delaying umbilical cord clamping decreases number of erythrocyte transfusions [26–30]. Delayed clamping may sufficiently augment the initial red blood cell volume by 10%–15% [31, 32]. In a Cochrane Systematic Review, delayed clamping for up to 180 seconds was associated with higher hematocrit values after birth, fewer erythrocyte transfusions for anemia, fewer cases of intraventricular hemorrhage (IVH; all grades), and fewer cases of necrotizing enterocolitis (NEC) [29]. Recent review of delayed clamping in extremely preterm infants confirmed fewer transfusions and less IVH, with both blood pressure and survival higher [33]. It is not known whether delayed clamping either works as well as EPO in preventing erythrocyte transfusions or whether delayed clamping augments the efficacy of EPO in premature infants. Additionally, iron [34] contained in the red blood cell mass may improve long-term iron status and decrease iron deficiency anemia [35], but red cell breakdown results in higher peak bilirubin levels after delayed clamping [29]. Nonetheless, the American College of Obstetricians and Gynecologists and American Academy of Pediatrics recommend delaying cord clamping for premature infants when feasible [30].

Erythrocyte Transfusions

Although covered in another chapter in more detail (see Chapter 20), any review of EPO therapy should cover erythrocyte transfusions and transfusion triggers [25, 36]. Conservative erythrocyte transfusion criteria were developed as part of the clinical trials of EPO in prematurity, and these were recognized as safe and effective tools in limiting transfusions [12, 14, 37]. The desire of clinicians to limit blood donor exposure, with or without EPO therapy, has led to lower numbers of erythrocyte transfusions per infant [10, 13, 38, 39]. Recently, randomized studies examined the safety of lower Hb or hematocrit triggers [17, 40], showing no consistent adverse sequelae at hospital discharge of restrictive triggers for erythrocyte transfusion [41, 42], with conflicting findings in the two large studies [17, 40]. In follow up, one study found lower white matter volumes in toddlers with liberal transfusions [43] that adversely impacted function [43], and white matter correlated with function in females at school age [44], while the larger study found no differences in death, cerebral palsy, cognitive delay, or hearing loss in toddlers with restrictive or liberal transfusion criteria, but higher mental development index (MDI) with in post hoc analysis in liberal transfusions [41, 45].

EPO Therapy for Anemia of Prematurity

Since 1990, over 65 studies have been published reporting use of EPO or erythropoietic stimulating agents (ESAs) to prevent transfusions in prematurity. ESAs are new drugs either structurally altering EPO in order to increase half-life or are EPO mimetic by binding to EPO receptor, with only limited number of newborns studied [46]. See Table 8.1 for a summary of EPO trials in prematurity. These EPO studies have undergone meta-analyses and Cochrane Systematic Reviews evaluating early or late EPO, or comparing early vs. late EPO [47–50]. Early EPO was defined as beginning therapy at <8 days and late EPO beginning at ≥ 8 days [48–50]. Primary or secondary endpoints to these studies include avoidance of transfusion, number of transfusions, transfusion volume, rise in reticulocytes, or rise in hematocrit. The studies are diverse with respect to degree of stability and birth weight of infants. These studies vary according to timing of initiation, EPO dose, dosing interval, duration of therapy, and route of administration. Initial data supported that EPO might be more efficacious if initiated earlier (before 4 days postnatal age) [36, 51, 52]. However, the Cochrane review did not support this finding [50]. Compared to older individuals, premature infants need a greater per kilogram dosage of subcutaneous (SQ) or intravenous (IV) EPO, secondary to greater plasma clearance, greater distribution volume and shorter mean residence time in premature neonates (see Table 8.1) [53, 54]. Various subcutaneous dosing intervals and continuous intravenous infusion have been examined, with comparable dosing showing no difference in plasma EPO levels, clearance and

Table 8.1 EPO trials in prematurity

Timing of initiation of therapy:	Day of life (DOL) 2 to DOL 28 (≥ DOL 8)
rhEPO dose:	150 to 1,500 U/kg per wk (750 U/kg per wk)
Dosing interval:	Twice weekly to daily (3 times/wk)
Duration of therapy:	DOL 10 until 6 weeks, or until hospital D/C (stop before 34 weeks' gestation)
Route of administration:	IV bolus, IV continuous drip, SQ
Nutritional supplementation:	
Oral iron	2 mg/kg daily to 36 mg/kg daily (≥4 mg/kg per day optimal, but monitor iron status)
Parenteral iron	None to 3 mg/kg daily or 20 mg/kg weekly
Folate	40 μg daily to 1,000 μg daily
Vitamin E	5–25 IU daily (25 IU)
B12	None to 21 μg/kg/wk SQ

Source: From Refs. [12, 21, 36, 57, 58, 61, 62, 66, 67, 70, 73, 78, 90, 111, 112, 115, 147–154].

reticulocyte counts as daily [55]. However, more frequent subcutaneous dosing may be more efficacious [56].

Data also support that optimal nutritional supplementation impacts EPO efficacy, Table 8.1. Optimal caloric and protein intake may optimize the effect of EPO [57–59]. Optimal vitamin B12, folate, and iron supplementation may also increase EPO efficacy [60, 61]. In published studies, oral iron supplementation during EPO therapy ranges from 2 mg/kg daily to 36 mg/kg daily; and parenteral iron administration ranges from 1–3 mg/kg daily or 6–20 mg/kg as a weekly injection [36, 52, 55, 62–65]. Optimal nutritional supplementation during EPO therapy remains under investigation.

Meta-analyses from controlled and randomized EPO studies have been performed. Meta-analysis conclusions are limited due to heterogeneity of the studies, including differences in erythrocyte transfusion criteria [47–50]. In Vamvakas and Strauss [47], only 20% met optimal design criteria [12, 36, 66–68]. Table 8.2 summarizes the studies as analyzed by the Cochrane review, early (<8 postnatal days) vs. late (≥8 postnatal days) dosing [48–50]. The meta-analyses of early and late EPO dosing concluded that EPO decreases erythrocyte transfusion number, with the average number of children needed to treat in order to prevent an erythrocyte transfusion being 6–7 [48–50]. Early dosing is not more effective than late and high dosing (>500 IU/kg per week) is not more effective than low (≤500 IU/kg per week) [48–50]. Eliminating early erythrocyte transfusions should be the focus of additional work.

Table 8.2 EPO findings from Cochrane Systematic Reviews

	# Infants (EPO/control)	# Studies	Prevent all Tx	Decreased % Tx (% Tx)	Decreased Tx# (#)	Mortality	Morbidity
Early	907/843	19	No	Yes (52 vs. 69%)	Yes (2.0 vs. 3.0)	Same (10.0 vs. 9.2%)	None
Late	605/537	20	No	Yes (42 vs 60%)	Yes (1.5 vs 2.2)	Same (5.0 vs. 6.3%)	None

	# Infants (early/late)	# Studies	Prevent all Tx	Decreased % Tx (% Tx)	Decreased Tx# (#)	Mortality	Morbidity
Early/Late	131/131	2	No/No	Same (68 vs. 75%)	Yes (2.1 vs. 2.4)	Same (10 vs. 13%)	Early ROP ≥ late

Notes: Early <8 days of age, Late >8 days of age. All dosages are included.

Transfusion (Tx). Percent of infants transfused (% Tx). Mean number of transfusions/infant (#).

Retinopathy of prematurity (ROP).

Other morbidities examined: IVH, PVL, Sepsis, BPD, NEC, SIDS, hospital stay, neurodevelopment.

Source: From [48–50].

Typical side effects of EPO therapy are relatively uncommon in premature neonates. Those seen in adults, including hypertension, thrombosis, bone pain, rash, and seizures are generally not seen. Pure red cell aplasia, which has been reported in adults on chronic therapy, has not been reported in infants [69]. Some studies show decreased absolute neutrophil counts, but no increase in infections [67, 70–72]. Some studies show increased platelet numbers, but no thromboses [71–73]. Some studies cite poor weight gain [69], but this is not a consistent finding. The most concerning potential risk was first seen in retrospective analyses and unique to premature infants, that is, an association between EPO and retinopathy of prematurity (ROP) [74]. Risk factors included >20 cumulative doses of EPO, or later introduction of EPO dosing [74]. A previous Cochrane Systematic Review teased out a greater incidence of ROP in early ESA/EPO group, but a recent update did not find this outcome [48–50]. The physiologic basis for this concern is that EPO serves as a vascular growth factor [75]. However, early ESA/EPO administration occurs during phase I vaso-obliterative stage, characterized by cessation of retinal vascular growth due to hyperoxia, while later EPO dosing coincides with phase II vaso-proliferative stage, which theoretically would be responsive to EPO. Another theoretical EPO complication is iron deficiency, a situation more worrisome in premature infants than other populations due to irreversible learning deficits found in infants with severe iron deficiency [76]. Monitoring iron status is somewhat cumbersome in premature infants and is discussed in more detail later in the chapter.

Potential protective effects of erythropoietic ESA/EPO treatment were decreased incidences of NEC [77] and decreased patent ductus arteriosis [78]. Early erythropoietic EPO dosing may also decrease NEC (number needed to benefit of 33) and IVH (number needed to benefit of 25), [48, 49]. In the Cochrane Systematic Reviews, neurodevelopmental outcome was improved in early ESA/EPO vs. control (number needed to benefit of 13) [48], but was not found in later EPO treatment, although late EPO treatment is due for an update [49]. Exogenous EPO exerts neuroprotective effects in animals. Premature infants given lower, erythropoietic dosages of ESA/EPO were reported to have better neurocognitive outcome and improved as toddlers or preschoolers [79, 80], with improved outcome is potentially related to higher peak EPO levels [79]. One group extended findings to teenage years, finding overall development and IQ scores improved in EPO vs. not, finding that the differences were attributed to those without vs. with intraventricular hemorrhage [81].

EPO for Neuroprotection

The impact of very high dose EPO given immediately after birth for neuroprotection is currently under study in two populations. High dose EPO is under study in term newborns to improve neurocognitive and motor outcomes in those with neonatal encephalopathy [82–84]. High dose neurocognitive prophylaxis using EPO is also under study in premature infants [85–88]. Although optimal dosing and timing of high dose neuroprotective EPO in premature infants still unclear, a recent meta-analysis supported that therapy improved the mental developmental index at 18–24 months, with the number needed to treat of 14 [85]. Long-term outcome assessments from multicenter trials are underway, including the Swiss study [87, 88] and the PENUT study [86]. The PENUT study underway combines high neuroprotective EPO dosing, followed by erythropoietic EPO dosing, a regimen that also may prevent some early erythrocyte transfusions.

Cost

Several studies show that EPO therapy to prevent erythrocyte transfusions in neonates is probably not cost effective [78, 89–91], but many centers dose multiple infants with aliquots from the same drug vial, decreasing cost [92]. In light of worldwide blood shortage and safety issues, cost effectiveness may be less important, but studies in countries with limited resources found that EPO treatment did not decrease erythrocyte transfusions [93, 94].

Summary of rhEpo in Prematurity 2018

In premature infants, advances to improve stability of, minimize phlebotomy, and delaying umbilical cord clamping may decrease the early erythrocyte transfusions in premature infants not normally prevented by erythropoietic dosing of EPO alone. It is also feasible that EPO may be more effective when combined with delayed umbilical cord clamping.

EPO is indicated in some premature infants, especially in those born to families of Jehovah's Witnesses or to parents who object to blood transfusions [47]. EPO at both erythropoietic and high doses may be neuroprotective, making EPO, although moderately effective in prevent erythrocyte transfusions, a better option than multiple transfusions in treating anemia of prematurity.

Iron Status of Premature Infants

Perinatal Iron Acquisition

Iron stores in premature infants increase in proportion to gestational age and birth weight. The healthy term infant's total body iron content is 75 mg/kg body weight [95, 96]. Normally, fetal iron is accrued at 1.6–2.0 mg/kg daily, even with poor maternal iron status [97, 98]. As much as 80% of body iron is contained in Hb [96]. Thus, premature infants, before their late preterm growth spurt, are born with relatively poor iron status [99, 100]. However, certain groups are endowed with poorer iron at birth, up to 17% of premature infants have biochemical iron deficiency, and thus are at risk for developing iron deficiency anemia [99–104]. These risk factors include cesarean delivery, immediate cord clamping, maternal obesity, maternal diabetes, maternal smoking, being small for gestation, and/or placental insufficiency [99–104]. Although utilized in all body tissues, the greatest demand for iron in the premature infant is erythropoiesis. As neonatal blood volume expands with rapid growth, premature infants produce massive amounts of Hb. For each gram of Hb synthesized, 3.47 mg of elemental iron is required. Erythrocyte expansion needs are more rapid for premature than for term infants, secondary to the relatively faster growth rate. Postnatal iron status for infants (and older individuals) is sensed by iron regulators and controlled through enteral iron transporters. Stable isotope studies show that infants are very efficient at intestinal iron absorption [105–108]. The implications of maintaining adequate iron status during early postnatal life include better neurocognitive outcomes [109].

Measuring Iron Status in Premature Infants

In early postnatal life, interpreting values for the battery of tests used to measure iron status in older individuals is challenging. These tests poorly reflect iron stores in early development, but investigators examining rhEPO in prematurity must try to measure iron status. Although an imprecise index of iron stores in the first months of life [6, 105, 110], plasma ferritin levels are reported in many EPO in prematurity trials [12, 63, 90, 111–115]. Plasma ferritin levels generally fall with increasing postnatal age in all infants, with prematurity no exception [6]. The lower cutoff value for normal plasma ferritin in premature infants is unknown, but is likely much higher than textbook normals of 12 µg/L [96]. In children and adults with EPO-stimulated erythropoiesis, clinicians use cutoff values of plasma ferritin as high as 60–100 µg/L [116, 117]. As with older patients, Maier, et al. recommend <100 µg/L as cutoff [90], while Meyer, et al. recommend <65 µg/L as cutoff to increase oral iron supplementation [115]. In support of these recommendations, an exclusively breastfed cohort of late preterm infants without any supplemental iron, a ferritin value of 70 µg/L at 6 weeks of age predicted developing iron deficiency anemia at 6 months of age [118].

Erythroid maturation and proliferation rely on the transferrin receptor (TfR) pathway for iron delivery [119]. Soluble TfR (sTfR) levels are reported in premature infants receiving rhEPO [64, 120, 121]. In adults, the sTFR is shed from reticulocytes entering the circulation and measures either erythropoiesis or iron status [122, 123]. An early rise in sTfR has been shown to predict erythropoietic response in adults treated with rhEPO [124]. Although sTfR levels have been reported to reflect iron status in newborns [125] and premature infants [120], we found that sTfR levels also correlated to stimulation of erythropoiesis in both term and premature infants [126, 127]. The ferritin index, the sTfR level divided by log plasma ferritin, may overcome this limitation. As in older individuals, the ferritin index could be used during EPO therapy in prematurity [128]. The newer, automated hematology counters report reticulocyte hemoglobin content (CHr), a more sensitive measure of iron-deficient erythropoiesis [117]. Combining the ferritin index with CHr may be of utility [129].

Other studies utilized different markers of iron status during rhEPO treatment in prematurity. Bechensteen, et al. recommend a cutoff value of serum iron <90 µg/100 mL to indicate iron deficiency [57]. In adults receiving rhEPO, hypochromic erythrocytes >6% are abnormal [130], and levels >8% may also be abnormal in neonates, triggering an increase in iron therapy [63, 65, 115, 121].

Zinc protoporphyrin/heme (ZnPP/H) ratios measure incomplete erythrocyte iron incorporation accompanying iron deficiency [131]. ZnPP/H ratios greater than 100 µM/M in rhEPO-treated adults measure incomplete iron incorporation into erythrocytes [132, 133]. ZnPP/H ratio correlates inversely to gestational age, suggesting that rate of erythropoiesis may impact the ratio [134]. However, ZnPP/H ratios also decrease in response to iron therapy or erythrocyte transfusion, supporting the importance of iron supply to the erythrocyte in determining the ratio [135, 136]. As with reticulocyte CHr, examining reticulocyte-enriched ZnPP/H may also be useful for monitoring iron therapy [137].

Postnatal Iron Sources

The anemia of prematurity was traditionally treated with frequent erythrocyte transfusions, but the effects of modern conservative transfusion practices on the long-term iron status of premature infants is poorly studied. Because of the high hematocrit of packed erythrocytes, up to 1 mg of iron is given per mL transfused. This iron "administration" may be clinically significant, as iron stores and plasma ferritin levels rise with erythrocyte transfusions in prematurity [138–140]. EPO treatment does not alter this the association between erythrocyte transfusions and plasma ferritin [8, 21, 59, 66, 67, 73, 111, 112, 115, 128, 141]. As clinical practice increasingly limits number of erythrocyte transfusions given premature infants, the iron allotment from transfusions will decrease. If choosing to treat premature infants with EPO, the potential for tissue iron deficiency is great and requires meticulous monitoring for iron deficiency.

Enteral Iron Supplementation

Data in adults support that iron supplementation is necessary for EPO efficacy. EPO studies in prematurity administered between 2 mg/kg to 6 mg/kg daily oral iron. Several studies found at least one indication for iron deficient erythropoiesis in EPO-treated, oral iron-supplemented infants, compared to oral iron-supplemented controls [55, 63, 64]. High dose oral iron fumarate (18–36 mg/kg daily) is used routinely in Norway

and may be associated with less severe anemia of prematurity overall [57, 59].

Parenteral Iron Supplementation

Erythropoietin studies in adults show that parenteral iron increases effectiveness and decreases functional iron deficiency [117]. In prematurity, several neonatal studies examined EPO, combined with parenteral iron [36, 52, 55, 62]. Three studies compared EPO/parenteral with EPO/enteral iron [63–65]. All found similar hematocrit in EPO/parenteral vs. EPO/enteral iron [63–65], but Pollak, et al. found higher reticulocytes and higher plasma ferritin in the EPO/parenteral vs. EPO/enteral iron [65]. Meyer, et al. observed higher hypochromic reticulocytes with EPO/enteral iron [63], while Pollak, et al. found higher hypochromic erythrocytes in both iron groups, compared to controls [65].

Parenteral iron therapy may have toxicity. Deficient antioxidant status of prematurity may contribute to iron-induced free radical diseases of prematurity, such as bronchopulmonary dysplasia, ROP and necrotizing enterocolitis [142–144]. No clinical evidence of iron toxicity was seen in the EPO/parenteral iron studies above, but only one study investigated measures of lipid peroxidation. Immediately after a 2-hour IV infusion of 2 mg iron sucrose, Pollak, et al. found a transient rise in plasma malondialdehyde levels [65]. Because significant hemolysis is observed after erythrocyte transfusion [145], we studied and found elevated plasma malondialdehyde levels in premature infants after erythrocyte transfusion [146]. Caution should be exerted when administering parenteral iron in conjunction with erythrocyte transfusions, at least until further evidence supports that EPO, parenteral iron, and simultaneous erythrocyte transfusions are safe.

Long-Term Iron Status of Premature Infants

Long-term iron status is of major concern in rapidly growing premature infants. Only three studies followed iron status of EPO/enteral iron-treated infants after hospital discharge. Although lower plasma ferritin levels are seen in EPO/enteral iron vs. control infants, it is reassuring that both EPO and control infants have similar plasma ferritin levels at 4–12 months of age [111, 128, 141]. Less reassuring are the extremely low ferritin levels seen (mean levels 21–40 µg/L), with several individual plasma ferritin levels below the 12 µg/L cutoff for iron deficiency in adults [111, 128, 141]. It is possible that avoiding erythrocyte transfusions could endanger the long-term iron stores of rapidly growing premature infants. One recent study determined that human milk is an inadequate iron source for the growing number of late preterm infants, a population unlikely to be transfused and thus to benefit from the iron within erythrocyte transfusions, so must be supplemented early [118].

Conclusion

The anemia of prematurity is multifactorial, but recovers more quickly if blood loss is minimized. EPO is effective, but does not completely eliminate early erythrocyte transfusions in most premature infants. However, delayed cord clamping or enacting restrictive erythrocyte transfusion criteria are also effective as well. Many unanswered, but testable questions include: Which group of premature infants would benefit the most from EPO? How does nutritional supplementation optimize EPO efficacy? Does EPO impair long-term iron status? How are EPO and ROP related? Clinicians should be judicious with its implementation and duration, as it is not yet standard of care. For now, efforts should be focused on measures to prevent early erythrocyte transfusions in premature infants.

References

1. Zanjani ED, Ascensao JL, McGlave PB, Banisadre M, Ash RC. Studies in the liver to kidney switch of erythropoietin production. *J Clin Invest* 1981;**67**:1183–8.

2. Eckardt K-U, Ratcliffe PJ, Tan CC, Bauer C, Kurtz A. Age-dependent expression of the erythropoietin gene in rat liver and kidneys. *J. Clin. Invest* 1992;**89**:753–60.

3. Kling PJ, Schmidt RL, Roberts RA, Widness JA. Serum erythropoietin levels during infancy: Associations with erythropoiesis. *J Pediatr* 1996;**128**:791–6.

4. Stockman JA, III, Garcia JF, Oski FA. The anemia of prematurity: Factors governing the erythropoietin response. *N Engl J Med* 1977;**296**:647–50.

5. Ohls RK. Evaluation and treatment of anemia in the neonate. In Christensen RD, ed. *Hematologic Problems of the Neonate* (Philadelphia, PA: WB Saunders, 2000). pp. 137–69.

6. Lundstrom U, Siimes MA. At what age does iron supplementation become necessary in low-birth weight infants? *J Pediatr* 1977;**91**:878–83.

7. Ohls RK. Erythropoietin to prevent and treat the anemia of prematurity. *Curr Opin Pediatr* 1999;**11**:108–14.

8. Maier RF, Obladen M, Messinger D, Wardrop CAJ. Factors related to transfusion in very low birthweight infants treated with erythropoietin. *Arch Dis Child* 1996;**74**:F182–F186.

9. Ohls RK. Erythropoietin treatment in extremely low birth weight infants: Blood in versus blood out. *J Pediatr* 2002;**141**:3–6.

10. Kling PJ, Sullivan TM, Leftwich ME, Roe DJ. Score for neonatal acute physiology predicts erythrocyte transfusions in premature infants. *Arch Dis Pediatr Adolesc Med* 1997;**151**:27–31.

11. Ekhaguere OA, Morriss FH, Jr., Bell EF, Prakash N, Widness JA. Predictive factors and practice trends in red blood cell transfusions for very-low-birth-weight infants. *Pediatr Res* 2016;**79**:736–41.

12. Shannon KM, Keith JM, Mentzer WC, et al. Recombinant human erythropoietin stimulates erythropoiesis and reduces erythrocyte transfusions in very low birth weight preterm infants. *Pediatrics* 1995;**95**:1–10.

13. Widness JA, Seward VJ, Kromer IJ, et al. Changing patterns of red blood cell transfusion in very low birth weight infants. *J Pediatr* 1996;**129**:680–7.

14. Hume H. Red blood cell transfusions for preterm infants: The role of evidence-based medicine. *Sem Perinatol* 1997;**21**:8–19.

15. Bednarek FJ, Weisberger S, Richardson DK, et al. Variations in blood transfusions among newborn intensive care units. *J Pediatr* 1998;**133**:601–7.

16. Ringer SA, Richardson DK, Sacher RA, Keszler M, Churchill WH. Variations in transfusion practice in neonatal intensive care. *Pediatrics* 1998;**101**:194–200.

17. Bell EF, Strauss RG, Widness JA, et al. Randomized trial of liberal versus restrictive guidelines for red blood cell transfusion in preterm infants. *Pediatrics* 2005;**115**:1685–91.

18. Luban NL. Management of anemia in the newborn. *Early Hum Dev* 2008;**84**:493–8.

19. Becquet O, Guyot D, Kuo P, et al. Respective effects of phlebotomy losses and erythropoietin treatment on the need for blood transfusion in very premature infants. *BMC Pediatr* 2013;**13**:176.

20. Maier RF, Sonntag J, Walka MM, et al. Changing practices of red blood cell transfusions in infants with birth weights less than 1000 g. *J Pediatr* 2000;**136**:220–4.

21. Donato H, Vain N, Rendo P, et al. Effect of early versus late administration of human recombinant erythropoietin on transfusion requirements in premature infants: Results of a randomized, placebo-controlled, multicenter trial. *Pediatrics* 2000;**105**:1066–1072.

22. Widness JA, Kulhavy JC, Johnson KJ, et al. Clinical performance of an in-line point-of-care monitor in neonates. *Pediatrics* 2000;**106**:497–504.

23. Moya MP, Clark RH, Nicks J, Tanaka DT. The effects of bedside blood gas monitoring on blood loss and ventilator management. *Biol Neonate* 2001;**80**:257–61.

24. Lin JC, Strauss RG, Kulhavy JC, et al. Phlebotomy overdraw in the neonatal intensive care nursery. *Pediatrics*.2000;**106**:e19.

25. Bishara N, Ohls RK. Current controversies in the management of the anemia of prematurity. *Semin Perinatol* 2009;**33**:29–34.

26. Kinmond S, Aitchison TC, Holland BM, et al. Umbilical cord clamping and preterm infants: A randomised trial. *Brit Med J* 1993;**306**:172–5.

27. Wardrop CAJ, Holland BM. The roles and vital importance of placental blood to the newborn infant. *J Perinat Med* 1995;**23**:139–43.

28. Ibrahim HM, Krouskop RW, Lewis DF, Dhanireddy R. Placental transfusion: Umbilical cord clamping and preterm infants. *J Perinatol*.2000;**20**:351–4.

29. Rabe H, Diaz-Rossello JL, Duley L, Dowswell T. Effect of timing of umbilical cord clamping and other strategies to influence placental transfusion at preterm birth on maternal and infant outcomes. *Cochrane Database Syst Rev* 2012;**8**: CD003248.

30. Committee on Obstetric Practice. Committee opinion no. 684: Delayed umbilical cord clamping after birth. *Obstet Gynecol* 2017;**129**:e5–e10.

31. Strauss RG. How I transfuse red blood cells and platelets to infants with the anemia and thrombocytopenia of prematurity. *Transfusion* 2008;**48**:209–17.

32. Aladangady N, Aitchison TC, Beckett C, et al. Is it possible to predict the blood volume of a sick preterm infant? *Arch Dis Child Fetal Neonatal Ed* 2004;**89**:F344–7.

33. Backes CH, Rivera BK, Haque U, et al. Placental transfusion strategies in very preterm neonates: A systematic review and meta-analysis. *Obstet Gynecol* 2014;**124**:47–56.

34. Hutton EK, Hassan ES. Late vs early clamping of the umbilical cord in full-term neonates: Systematic review and meta-analysis of controlled trials. *JAMA* 2007;**297**:1241–52.

35. Chaparro CM, Neufeld LM, Alvarez GT, Cedillo RE-L, Dewey KG. Effect of timing of umbilical cord clamping on iron status in Mexican infants: A randomised controlled trial. *Lancet* 2006;**367**:1997–2004.

36. Ohls RK, Ehrenkranz RA, Wright LL, et al. The effects of early erythropoietin therapy on the transfusion requirements of preterm infants below 1250 grams birthweight: A multicenter, randomized controlled trial. *Pediatrics* 2001;**108**:934–42.

37. Roseff SD, Luban NL, Manno CS. Guidelines for assessing appropriateness of pediatric transfusion. *Transfusion* 2002;**42**:1398–413.

38. Strauss RG. Practical issues in neonatal transfusion practice. *Am J Clin Path* 1997;**107**: S57–S63.

39. Simon TL, Alverson DC, AuBuchon J, et al. Practice parameter for the use of red blood cell transfusions. *Arch Pathol Lab Med* 1998;**122**:130–8.

40. Kirpalani H, Whyte RK, Andersen C, et al. The Premature Infants in Need of Transfusion (PINT) study: A randomized, controlled trial of a restrictive (low) versus liberal (high) transfusion threshold for extremely low birth weight infants. *J Pediatr* 2006;**149**:301–7.

41. Whyte R, Kirpalani H. Low versus high haemoglobin concentration threshold for blood transfusion for preventing morbidity and mortality in very low birth weight infants. *Cochrane Database Syst Rev* 2011;**11**:CD000512.

42. Ibrahim M, Ho SK, Yeo CL. Restrictive versus liberal red blood cell transfusion thresholds in very low birth weight infants: A systematic review and meta-analysis. *J Paediatr Child Health* 2014;**50**:122–30.

43. McCoy TE, Conrad AL, Richman LC, et al. Neurocognitive profiles of preterm infants randomly assigned to lower or higher hematocrit thresholds for transfusion. *Child Neuropsychol* 2011;**17**:347–67.

44. McCoy TE, Conrad AL, Richman LC, et al. The relationship between brain structure and cognition in transfused preterm children at school age. *Dev Neuropsychol* 2014;**39**:226–32.

45. Whyte RK, Kirpalani H, Asztalos EV, et al. Neurodevelopmental outcome of extremely low birth weight infants randomly assigned to restrictive or liberal hemoglobin thresholds for blood transfusion. *Pediatrics* 2009;**123**:207–13.

46. Warwood TL, Ohls RK, Lambert DK, et al. Intravenous administration of darbepoetin to NICU patients. *J Perinatol* 2006;**26**:296–300.

47. Vamvakas EC, Strauss RG. Meta-analysis of controlled clinical trials studying the efficacy of rHuEPO in reducing blood transfusions in the anemia of prematurity. *Transfusion* 2001;**41**:406–15.

48. Ohlsson A, Aher SM. Early erythropoiesis-stimulating agents in preterm or low birth weight infants. *Cochrane Database Syst Rev* 2017;**11**:CD004863.

49. Aher SM, Ohlsson A. Late erythropoietin for preventing red blood cell transfusion in preterm and/or low birth weight infants. *Cochrane Database Syst Rev* 2014;**4**:CD004868.

50. Aher SM, Ohlsson A. Early versus late erythropoietin for preventing red blood cell transfusion in preterm and/or low birth weight infants. *Cochrane Database Syst Rev* 2012;**10**: CD004865.

51. Maier RF, Obladen M, Kattner E, et al. High- versus low-dose erythropoietin in extremely low birth weight infants. *J Pediatr* 1998;**132**:866–70.

52. Carnielli VP, D Riol R, Montini G. Iron supplementation enhances response to high doses of recombinant human erythropoietin in preterm infants. *Arch Dis Child* 1998;**79**:F44–F48.

53. Brown MS, Jones MA, Ohls RK, Christensen RD. Single-dose pharmacokinetics of recombinant human erythropoietin in preterm infants after intravenous and subcutaneous administration. *J Pediatr* 1993;**122**:655–7.

54. Widness JA, Veng-Pedersen P, Peters C, et al. Erythropoietin pharmacokinetics in premature infants: Developmental, non-linearity, and treatment effects. *J Appl Physiol* 1996;**80**:140–8.

55. Ohls RK, Veerman MW, Christensen RD. Pharmacokinetics and effectiveness of recombinant erythropoietin administered to preterm infants by continuous infusion in total parenteral nutrition solution. *J Pediatr* 1996;**128**:518–23.

56. Brown MS, Keith JF. Comparison between two and five doses a week of recombinant human erythropoietin for anemia of prematurity: A randomized trial. *Pediatrics* 1999;**104**:210–15.

57. Bechensteen AG, Håga P, Halvorsen S, et al. Erythropoietin, protein, and iron supplementation and the prevention of anaemia of prematurity. *Arch Dis Child* 1993;**69**:19–23.

58. Messer J, Haddad J, Donato L, Astruc D, Matis J. Early treatment of premature infants with recombinant human erythropoietin. *Pediatrics* 1993;**92**:519–23.

59. Bechensteen AG, Halvorsen S, Haga P, PM C, Liestøl K. Erythropoietin (EPO), protein and iron supplementation and the prevention of anaemia of prematurity: Effects on serum immunoreactive Epo, growth and protein and iron metabolism. *Acta Paediatr* 1996;**85**:490–5.

60. Worthington-White D, Behnke M, Gross S. Premature infants require additional folate and vitamin B-12 to reduce the severity of the anemia of prematurity. *Am J Clin Nutr* 1994;**60**:930–5.

61. Haiden N, Schwindt J, Cardona F, et al. Effects of a combined therapy of erythropoietin, iron, folate, and vitamin B12 on the transfusion requirements of extremely low birth weight infants. *Pediatrics* 2006;**118**:2004–13.

62. Carnielli VP, Montini G, Da Riol R, Dall'Amico R, Cantarutti F. Effect of high doses of human recombinant erythropoietin on the need for blood transfusions in preterm infants. *J Pediatr* 1992;**121**:98–102.

63. Meyer MP, Haworth C, Meyer JH, Commerford A. A comparison of oral and intravenous iron supplementation in preterm infants receiving recombinant erythropoietin. *J Pediatr* 1996;**129**:258–63.

64. Kivivuori SM, Virtanen M, Raivio KO, Viinikka L, Siimes MA. Oral iron is sufficient for erythropoietin treatment of very low birth-weight infants. *Eur J Pediatr* 1999;**158**:147–51.

65. Pollak A, Hayde M, Hayn M, et al. Effect of intravenous iron supplementation on erythropoiesis in erythropoietin-treated premature infants. *Pediatrics* 2001;**107**:78–85.

66. Ohls RK, Harcum J, Schibler KR, Christensen RD. The effect of erythropoietin on the transfusion requirements of preterm infants weighing 750 grams or less: A randomized, double-blind, placebo-controlled study. *J Pediatr* 1997;**131**:661–5.

67. Kumar P, Shankaran S, Krishnan RG. Recombinant human erythropoietin therapy for treatment of anemia of prematurity in very low birth weight infants: A randomized, double-blind, placebo-controlled trial. *J Perinatol* 1998;**18**:173–7.

68. Ohls RK, Ehrenkranz RA, Lemons JA, et al. A multicenter randomized double-masked placebo-controlled trial of early erythropoietin and iron administration to preterm infants. *Pediatr Res* 1999;**45**:216A.

69. Zipursky A. The risk of hematopoietic growth factor therapy in newborn infants. *Pediatr Res* 2002;**51**:549.

70. Ohls RK, Christensen RD. Recombinant erythropoietin compared with erythrocyte transfusion in the treatment of anemia of prematurity. *J Pediatr* 1991;**119**:781–8.

71. Beck D, Masserey E, Meyer M, Calame A. Weekly intravenous administration of recombinant human erythropoietin in infants with the anaemia of prematurity. *Eur J Pediatr* 1991;**150**:767–72.

72. Halperin DS, Wacker P, Lacourt G, et al. Effects of recombinant human erythropoietin in infants with anemia of prematurity: A pilot study. *J Pediatr* 1990;**116**:779–86.

73. Emmerson A. Double blind trial of recombinant human erythropoietin in preterm infants: Comment. *Archives Dis Child* 1993;**69**:542.

74. Brown MS, Baron AE, France EK, Hamman RF. Association between higher cumulative doses of recombinant erythropoietin and risk for retinopathy of prematurity. *J AAPOS* 2006;**10**:143–9.

75. Ashley RA, Dubuque SH, Dvorak B, et al. Erythropoietin stimulates vasculogenesis in neonatal rat mesenteric microvascular endothelial cells. *Pediatr Res* 2002;**51**:472–8.

76. Rao R, Georgieff MK. Iron in fetal and neonatal nutrition. *Semin Fetal Neonatal Med* 2007;**12**:54–63.

77. Ledbetter DJ, Juul SE. Erthropoietin and the incidence of necrotizing enterocolitis in infants with very low birth weight. *J Pediatr Surg* 2000;**35**:178–82.

78. Ohls RK, Osborne KA, Chrstensen RD. Efficacy and cost analysis of treating very low birth weight infants with erythropoietin during their first two weeks of life: A randomized, placebo-controlled trial. *J Pediatr* 1995;**126**:421–6.

79. Bierer R, Peceny MC, Hartenberger CH, Ohls RK. Erythropoietin concentrations and neurodevelopmental outcome in preterm infants. *Pediatrics.* 2006;**118**:e635-640.

80. Ohls RK, Cannon DC, Phillips J, et al. Preschool assessment of preterm infants treated with darbepoetin and erythropoietin. *Pediatrics* 2016;**137**:e20153859.

81. Neubauer AP, Voss W, Wachtendorf M, Jungmann T. Erythropoietin improves neurodevelopmental outcome of extremely preterm infants. *Ann Neurol* 2010;**67**:657–66.

82. Massaro AN, Wu YW, Bammler TK, et al. Plasma biomarkers of brain injury in neonatal hypoxic-ischemic encephalopathy. *J Pediatr* 2018;**194**:67–75.

83. Juul SE, Comstock BA, Heagerty PJ, et al. High-dose erythropoietin for asphyxia and encephalopathy (HEAL): A randomized controlled trial – background, aims, and study protocol. *Neonatology* 2018;**113**:331–8.

84. Garg B, Sharma D, Bansal A. Systematic review seeking erythropoietin role for neuroprotection in neonates with hypoxic ischemic encephalopathy: Presently where do we stand. *J Matern Fetal Neonatal Med* 2018;**31**:3214–24.

85. Fischer HS, Reibel NJ, Buhrer C, Dame C. Prophylactic early erythropoietin for neuroprotection in preterm infants: A meta-analysis. *Pediatrics* 2017;**139**:e20164317.

86. Juul SE, Mayock DE, Comstock BA, Heagerty PJ. Neuroprotective potential of erythropoietin in neonates; design of a randomized trial. *Matern Health Neonatol Perinatol* 2015;**1**:27.

87. Fauchere JC, Koller BM, Tschopp A, et al. Swiss erythropoietin neuroprotection trial g. safety of early high-dose recombinant erythropoietin for neuroprotection in very preterm infants. *J Pediatr* 2015;**167**:52–7 e53.

88. Natalucci G, Latal B, Koller B, et al. Swiss EPONTG. Effect of early prophylactic high-dose recombinant human erythropoietin in very preterm infants on neurodevelopmental outcome at 2 years: A randomized clinical trial. *JAMA* 2016;**315**:2079–85.

89. Shireman TI, Hilsenrath PE, Strauss RG, Widness JA, Mutnick AH. Recombinant human erythropoietin vs transfusions in the treatment of anemia of prematurity. *Arch Pediatr Adolesc Med* 1994;**148**:582–8.

90. Maier RF, Obladen M, Scigalla P, et al. The effect of epoetin beta (recombinant human erythropoietin) on the need for transfusion in very-low-birth-weight infants. *N Engl J Med* 1994;**330**:1173–8.

91. Fain J, Hilsenrath P, Widness JA, Strauss RG, Mutnick AH. A cost analysis comparing erythropoietin and red cell transfusions in the treatment of anemia of prematurity. *Transfusion* 1995;**35**:936–43.

92. Yeo CL, Choo S, Ho LY. Effect of recombinant human erythropoietin on transfusion needs in preterm infants. *J Paediatr Child Health* 2001;**37**:352–8.

93. Atasay B, Gunlemez A, Akar N, Arsan S. Does early erythropoietin therapy decrease transfusions in anemia of prematurity. *Indian J Pediatr* 2002;**69**:389–91.

94. Avent M, Cory BJ, Galpin J, et al. A comparison of high versus low dose recombinant human erythropoietin versus blood transfusion in the management of anaemia of prematurity in a developing country. *J Tropical Pediatr* 2002;**48**:227–33.

95. Oski FA. Iron deficiency in infancy and childhood. *New Engl J Med* 1993;**329**:190–3.

96. Oski FA. Differential diagnosis of anemia. In Nathan DG, Oski FA, eds. 4th ed. *Hematology of Infancy and Childhood* (Philadelphia, PA: W.B. Saunders, 1993). pp. 346–53.

97. Dallman PR. Iron deficiency in the weanling: A nutritional problem on the way to resolution. *Acta Paediatr Scand Suppl* 1986;**323**:59–67.

98. Harthoorn-Lasthuizen EJ, Lindemans J, Langenhuijsen MM. Does iron-deficient erythropoiesis in pregnancy influence fetal iron supply? *Acta Obstet Gynecol Scand* 2001;**80**:392–6.

99. McCarthy PJ, Zundel HR, Johnson KR, Blohowiak SE, Kling PJ. Impact of growth restriction and other prenatal risk factors on cord blood iron status in prematurity. *J Pediatr Hematol Oncol* 2016;**38**(3):210–15.

100. Mukhopadhyay K, Yadav RK, Kishore SS, et al. Iron status at birth and at 4 weeks in preterm-SGA infants in comparison with preterm and term-AGA infants. *J Matern Fetal Neonatal Med* 2012;**25**:1474–8.

101. McLimore HM, Phillips AK, Blohowiak SE, et al. Impact of multiple prenatal risk factors on newborn iron status at delivery. *J Pediatr Hematol Oncol* 2013;**35**:473–77.

102. Jones AD, Zhao G, Jiang YP, et al. Maternal obesity during pregnancy is negatively associated with maternal and neonatal iron status. *Eur J Clin Nutr* 2016;**70**(8):918–24.

103. MacQueen BC, Christensen RD, Ward DM, et al. The iron status at birth of neonates with risk factors for developing iron deficiency: A pilot study. *J Perinatol* 2017;**37**:436–40.

104. McCarthy EK, Kenny LC, Hourihane JOB, et al. Impact of maternal, antenatal and birth-associated factors on iron stores at birth: Data from a prospective maternal-infant birth cohort. *Eur J Clin Nutr* 2017;**71**:782–7.

105. Fomon SJ. Iron. In Fomon S, ed. *Nutrition of Normal Infants* (St. Louis, MO: Mosby, 1993). pp. 239–60.

106. Ehrenkranz RA. Iron requirements of preterm infants. *Nutrition* 1994;**10**:77–8.

107. Fomon SJ, Ziegler EE, Nelson SE, Serfass RE, Frantz JA. Erythrocyte incorporation of iron by 56-day-old infants fed a 58Fe-labeled supplement. *Pediatr Res* 1995;**38**:373–8.

108. Widness JA, Lombard KA, Ziegler EE, et al. Erythroctye incorporation and absorption of 58Fe in premature infants treated with erythropoietin. *Pediatr Res* 1997;**41**:416–23.

109. Georgieff MK. Long-term brain and behavioral consequences of early iron deficiency. *Nutr Rev* 2011;**69** Suppl 1:S43–48.

110. Saarinen UM, Siimes MA. Serum ferritin in assessment of iron nutrition in healthy infants. *Acta Paediatr Scand* 1978;**67**:745–51.

111. Al-Kharfy T, Smyth JA, Wadsworth L, et al. Erythropoietin therapy in neonates at risk of having bronchopulmonary dysplasia and requiring multiple transfusions. *J Pediatr* 1996;**129**:89–96.

112. Bader D, Blondheim O, Jonas R, et al. Decreased ferritin levels, despite iron supplementation, during erythropoietin therapy in anaemia of prematurity. *Acta Paediatr* 1996;**85**:496–501.

113. Bechensteen AG, Halvorsen S, Haga P, Cotes PM, Liestol K. Erythropoietin, protein and iron supplementation and the prevention of anaemia of prematurity: Effects on serum immunoreactive Epo, growth and protein and iron metabolism. *Acta Paediatr.* 1996;**85**:490–5.

114. Emmerson A. Role of erythropoietin in the newborn. *Archives Dis Child* 1993;**69**:273–5.

115. Meyer MP, Meyer JH, Commerford A, et al. Recombinant human erythropoietin in the treatment of the anemia of prematurity: Results of a double-blind, placebo-controlled study. *Pediatrics* 1994;**93**:918–23.

116. Morris KP, Watson S, Reid MM, Hamilton PJ, Coulthard MG. Assessing iron status in children with chronic renal failure on erythropoietin: Which measurements should we use? *Pediatr Nephrol* 1994;**8**:51–6.

117. Goodnough LT, Skikne B, Brugnara C. Erythropoietin, iron and erythropoiesis. *Blood* 2000;**96**:823–33.

118. Akkermans MD, Uijterschout L, Abbink M, et al. Predictive factors of iron depletion in late preterm infants at the postnatal age of 6 weeks. *Eur J Clin Nutr* 2016;**70**:941–6.

119. Taetle R. The role of transferrin receptors in hemopoietic cell growth. *Exp Hematol* 1990;**18**:360–5.

120. Kivivuori SM, Heikinheimo M, Teppo A-M, Siimes MA. Early rise in serum concentration of transferrin receptor induced by recombinant human erythropoietin in very-low-birth-weight infants *Pediatr Res.* 1994;**36**:85–9.

121. Bechensteen AG, Haga P, Halvorsen S, et al. Effect of low and moderate doses of recombinant human erythropoietin on the haematological response in premature infants on a high protein and iron intake. *Eur J Pediatr* 1997;**156**:56–61.

122. Kohgo Y, Niitsu Y, Kondo H, et al. Serum transferrin receptor as a new index of erythropoiesis. *Blood* 1987;**70**:1955–8.

123. Beguin Y, Clemons GK, Pootrakul P, Fillet G. Quantitative assessment of erythropoiesis and functional classification of anemia based on measurements of serum transferrin receptor and erythropoietin. *Blood* 1993;**81**:1067–76.

124. Beguin Y, Loo M, S. RZ, et al. Early prediction of response to recombinant human erythropoietin in patients with the anemia of renal failure by serum transferrin receptor and fibrinogen. *Blood* 1993;**82**:2010–16.

125. Rusia U, Flowers C, Madan N, Agarwal N, Sood SK. Serum transferrin receptor levels in the evaluation of iron deficiency in the neonate. *Acta Paediatr Japon* 1995;**38**:455–9.

126. Kling PJ, Widness JA. Transfusions, (RBC Tx) and erythropoiesis indicators influence serum transferrin receptors (TfR) levels in premature infants. *Pediatr Res* 1995;**37**:282A.

127. Kling PJ, Roberts RA, Widness JA. Plasma transferrin receptor levels and indices of erythropoiesis and iron status in healthy term infants. *Am J Pediatr Hem/Onc* 1997;**20**:309–14.

128. Krallis N, Cholevas V, Mavridis A, et al. Effect of recombinant human erythropoietin in preterm infants. *Eur J Haematol* 1999;**63**:71–6.

129. Kasper DC, Widness JA, Haiden N, Berger A, et al. Characterization and differentiation of iron status in anemic very low birth weight infants using a diagnostic nomogram. *Neonatology* 2009;**95**:164–71.

130. Braun J, Lindner K, Schreiber M, Heidler RA, Horl WH. Percentage of hypochromic red blood cells as predictor of erythropoietic and iron response after i.v. iron supplementation in maintenance haemodialysis patients. *Nephrol Dial Transplan* 1997;**12**:1173–81.

131. Rettmer RL, Carlson TH, Origenes ML, Jack RM, Labbe RF. Zinc protoporphyrin/heme ratio for diagnosis of preanemic iron deficiency. *Pediatrics* 1999;**104**:e37.

132. Kaltwasser JP, Gottschalk R. Erythropoietin and iron. *Kidney Int* 1999;**55**:S49–S56.

133. National Kidney Foundation. *Clinical Practice Guidelines for the Treatment of Anemia of Chronic Renal Failure* (New York: National Kidney Foundation; 1999), available online at https://bit .ly/33S1B23.

134. Lott DG, Zimmerman MB, Labbe' RF, Kling PJ, Widness JA. Erythrocyte zinc protoporphyrin ratios are elevated with prematurity and with fetal hypoxia. *Pediatrics* 2005;**116**:414–22.

135. Miller SM, McPherson RJ, Juul SE. Iron sulfate supplementation decreases zinc protoporphyrin to heme ratio in premature infants. *J Pediatr* 2006;**148**:44–8.

136. Winzerling JJ, Kling PJ. Iron deficient erythropoiesis in premature infants measured by blood zinc protoporphyrin/heme. *J Pediatr* 2001;**139**:134–6.

137. Blohowiak SE, Chen ME, Repyak KS, et al. Reticulocyte enrichment of zinc protoporphyrin/ heme discriminates impaired iron supply during early development. *Pediatr Res* 2008;**64**:63–7.

138. Shaw JCL. Iron absorption by the premature infant: The effect of transfusion and iron supplements on the serum ferritin levels. *Acta Paediatr Scand Suppl* 1982;**299**:83–9.

139. Arad I, Konijn AM, Linder N, Goldstein MDM, Kaufmann NA. Serum ferritin levels in preterm infants after multiple blood transfusions. *Am J Perinatol* 1988;**5**:40–3.

140. Brown MS. Effect of transfusion and phlebotomy on serum ferritin levels in low birth weight infants. *J Perinatol* 1996;**16**:39–42.

141. Soubasi V, Kremenopoulos G, Diamanti E, et al. Follow-up of very low birth weight infants after erythrpoietin treatment to prevent anemia of prematurity. *J Pediatr* 1995;**127**:291–7.

142. Sullivan JL. Iron, plasma antioxidants and the 'oxygen radical disease of prematurity'. *Am J Dis Child* 1988;**142**:1341–4.

143. Evans PJ, Evans R, Kovar IZ, Holton AF, Halliwell B. Bleomycin-detectable iron in the plasma of premature and full-term neonates. *FEBS Letters* 1992;**303**:210–12.

144. Miller NJ, Rice-Evans C, Davies MJ, Gopinathan V, Milner A. A novel method for measuring antioxidant capacity and its application to monitoring the antioxidant status in premature neonates. *Clin Sci* 1993;**84**:407–12.

145. Humphrey MJ, Harrell-Bean HA, Eskelson C, Corrigan JJ. Blood transfusion in the neonate: Effects of dilution and age of blood on hemolysis. *J Pediatr* 1982;**101**:605–7.

146. Kling PJ, Reichard RD, Roberts RA, Winzerling JJ, Woodward SS. The effects of transfusions on oxidative stress and plasma erythropoietin levels in premature infants. *Ann Hematol* 2000;**79**:B13.

147. Obladen M, Maier R, Grauel L, et al. Recombinant human erythropoietin (rhEPO) for prevention of anaemia of prematurity: A randomized multicentre trial. *Pediatr Res* 1990;**28**:287A(Abstr).

148. Shannon KM, Mentzer WC, Abels RI, et al. Recombinant human erythropoietin in anemia of prematurity: Preliminary results of a double-blind placebo controlled pilot study. *J Pediatr* 1991;**118**:949–55.

149. Shannon KM, Mentzer WC, Abels RI, et al. Enhancement of erythropoiesis by recombinant human erythropoietin in low birth weight infants: A pilot study. *J Pediatr* 1992;**120**:586–92.

150. Soubasi V, Kremenpoulos G, Diamandi E, Tsantali C, Tsakiris D. In which neonates does early recombinant human erythropoietin treatment prevent anemia of prematurity? Results of a randomized, controlled study. *Pediatr Res* 1993;**34**:675–9.

151. Ronnestad A, Moe PJ, Breivik N. Enhancement of erythropoiesis by erythropoietin, bovine protein and energy fortified mother's milk during anaemia of prematurity. *Acta Paediatrica* 1995;**84**:809–11.

152. Samanci N, Ovali F, Dagoglu T. Effects of recombinant human erythropoietin in infants with very low birth weights. *J Int Med Res* 1996;**24**:190–8.

153. Giannakopoulou C, Bolonaki I, Stiakaki E, et al. Erythropoietin (rHuEPO) administration to premature infants for the treatment of their anemia. *Pediatr Hematol Oncol* 1998;**15**:37–43.

154. Maier RF, Obladen M, Mueller-Hansen I, et al. Early treatment with erythropoietin beta ameliorates anemia and reduces transfusion requirements in infants with birth weights below 1000 g. *J Pediatr* 2002;**141**:8–15.

Chapter

9

Hemolytic Disease of the Fetus and Newborn
Maternal Antibody Mediated Hemolysis

Mary Elizabeth Ross, Stephen P. Emery, Pedro A. de Alarcón, and Jon F. Watchko

Introduction

Hemolytic disease of the fetus and newborn (HDFN) is the immune mediated destruction of fetal and neonatal red blood cells by maternal antibody. HDFN occurs when the fetal red blood cells express a paternally inherited antigen not present on maternal red blood cells. The spectrum of illness ranges from clinically insignificant to that of a critically ill, anemic, hydropic, and jaundiced infant at risk for bilirubin-induced brain damage (kernicterus).

It was the pivotal paper by Dr. Louis K. Diamond in 1932 that clearly identified the development of the maternal antibody in response to the incompatibility of the fetal red cells with maternal red cells even though the Rhesus red cell antigen had not yet been identified [1]. Parallel to the understanding of HDFN, Landsteiner began the process of identification of the red cell antigens at the start of the twentieth century, first with the identification of the ABO system and then with the identification of the Rh system [2]. He described the development of antibodies against rhesus monkeys red cells in rabbits. He suggested that this was a new antigen distinct from the ABO system and called it the Rhesus antigen. This name is now well established in spite of the early controversy, since the antigen identified was a simian antigen which is related but is not the same as the human antigen. Current International Society of Blood Transfusion terminology for this blood group is Rh and the symbol is RH.

The term HDFN replaced the original term, erythroblastosis fetalis, when the immunological mechanisms responsible for fetal anemia and jaundice were confirmed [3]. The D antigen of the Rh blood group, designated RHD, continues to be the most commonly identified antigenic stimulus for HDFN. RHD negative mothers give birth to RHD positive fetuses in about 9% of European-ancestry pregnancies. In a first pregnancy, without prophylaxis, 15%–17% of these at-risk mothers would become immunized against RHD and more than 20% of the babies had HDFN requiring treatment [4]. Subsequent pregnancies with the same maternal fetal antigen mismatch have a higher frequency of affected infants. Overall, among women with *established* anti-D antibodies, 50% of RHD babies with HDFN will have minimal disease requiring no intervention, 25% will have disease requiring intervention after birth to prevent brain injury by bilirubin and the effects of significant anemia, and 25% will require in utero intervention to prevent severe morbidity or mortality [4]. The case fatality rate for RHD HDFN in 1986 in the USA was 2.6% [5]. In 1998 the death rate attributed to HDFN in USA was reported to be nine infants per million live newborns [6]. During the period from 1970 through the late 1990s the use of prophylactic anti-D antibody increased, and the frequency of both maternal alloimmunization and RHD HDFN decreased dramatically [7]. At the same time there has been a gradual increase in the frequency in HDFN due to other antigens [8]. A review of antibodies recognizing red cell antigens that have been detected either in maternal serum during pregnancy or described to cause HDFN are listed in Table 9.1. This chapter will review maternal anti-erythrocyte antibody development, the red cell antigens involved, the diagnosis of HDFN in neonates, and management of the affected neonate and fetus.

Neonatal Hematology, Pathogenesis, Diagnosis, and Management of Hematologic Problems, 3rd edition, ed. Pedro A. de Alarcón, Eric J. Werner, Robert D. Christensen, and Martha C. Sola-Visner. Published by Cambridge University Press. © Cambridge University Press 2021.

Development of Maternal Anti-Erythrocyte Antibodies

There are essentially three mechanisms for the development of maternal anti-erythrocyte antibodies: (1) innate production, (2) sensitization via fetomaternal hemorrhage, and (3) iatrogenic exposure in the form of prior RBC transfusion. The major blood group system, ABO, is characterized by innate antibody production. Individuals with blood type O innately produce anti-A and anti-B antibodies. No prior maternal blood exposure is necessary for formation of these antibodies.

The second mechanism, fetomaternal hemorrhage (FMH) is infrequent prior to the start of the third trimester [9–11]. Less than 15% of all new anti-RHD antibodies identified prior to term in primigravida women are detected before 28 weeks'

gestation [9]. FMH occurs most frequently around the time of delivery. The association between the week of gestation and increasing frequency of FMH is likely a direct effect of the growing fetus exerting greater force on placental tissue with normal maternal movement. Additionally, the fetal blood volume increases with increasing fetal age. Events during pregnancy associated with an increased risk of FMH are detailed in Table 9.2 [12]. Knowledge of the association of FMH with these events drives the recommendation for additional doses of anti-RHD to prevent maternal isoimmunization.

The third mechanism is iatrogenic exposure through maternal transfusion which may be required for obstetric complications. Additionally, with the increasing medical success, children with complex medical problems are living into young adulthood. Some of these young adults will have

Table 9.1 Maternal antibodies recognizing blood group antigens. Blood group antigens involved in HDFN

System name[i]	Symbol[ii]	ISBT number[iii]	Antigens[iv]	Frequency HDFN[v]	Severity[vi]	References (population)[vii]
ABO	ABO	001	ABO	Common	Mild–moderate	[23, 158–159]
Rh	RH	004	D, c, C, E, e	Common	Severe	[53–54, 57–58, 60–61, 63, 160–161]
			C^w, C^x	Described	Severe	[162–163] (Pakistan)
			E^w, G, Rh17	Described		[164–166]
Kell	KEL	006	K, k, Ku	Common	Severe	[65–66, 69–70, 167–168, 169–170, 171]
			Js^b		Moderate–severe	[74–75]
			Kp^a, Kp^b		Mild–moderate	[73]
			Js^a, Ula		Mild–moderate	
Duffy	FY	008	Fy^a	Described	Severe	[87–89, 172]
			Fy^b	Uncommon		[86]
			Fy3	Described	Mild–moderate	[91]
Kidd	JK	009	Jk^a, Jk^b, Jk3		Mild–moderate	[95–96, 98, 97, 172, 173]
MNS	MNS	002	M	Described	Mild–severe delayed	[103–105, 172, 174–175] (Japan)
			N	Described		[176]
			S, U, Vw	Moderate	Severe	[106, 172, 107–108, 177]
			s			
			Mta	Described	Mild–moderate	[178–179]
			Hil, Mur			[175, 180] (Taiwan)
Langereis	LAN	033	Lan	Described	Severe	[181]
Landsteiner–Wiener	LW	016	LW	Described		[182]
P	P1PK	003	P1	Not described	Maternal antibody	[172]
Lutheran	LU	005	Lu^a	Described	Mild	[183–184]
			Lu^b	Not described	Maternal antibody	[185]

Table 9.1 (cont.)

System name[i]	Symbol[ii]	ISBT number[iii]	Antigens[iv]	Frequency HDFN[v]	Severity[vi]	References (population)[vii]
Lewis	LE	007	Le^a	Described	Mild	[186, 187]
			Le^b	Not described	Possible	[188–189]
Diego	DI	010	Di	Described	Mild to severe	[64]
Colton	CO	015	Coa, Co3	Described	Mild	[190]
Gerbich	GE	020	Ge2, Ge3	Described	Mild–severe	[191, 149, 192] (Hispanic)
Scianna	SC	013	Sc2, Rd	Described	Mild–severe or delayed	[193–194]
JR	JR	032	Jr^a	Described	Mild–severe	[195–198] (Japan)
Dombrock	DO	014		Not described	Maternal antibody	[199]
Yt	YT	011		Not described	Maternal antibody	[200]
Chido/ Rodgers	CH/RG	017		Not described	Maternal antibody	[201]
JMH	JMH	026		Not described	Maternal antibody	[201]
Knops	KN	022		Not described	Maternal antibody	[201]
Cromer	CROM	021		Not described	Maternal antibody	[61–64]

Gill, GIL (029); Globoside, GLOB (028); I (027); Kx, XK (019); OK (024); RAPH (025); XG (012) no reports of maternal AB or HDFN

Notes:

i Common blood group system by common name.

ii International Society of Blood Transfusion (ISBT) blood group symbol.

iii ISBT blood group system number.

iv Specific antigens within the blood group system.

v Indicates whether HDFN has been described. In the situation of maternal antibody detected without apparent HDFN, the designation "Not described" is used.

vi This gives the reader a brief overall sense of severity of HDFN described in the literature for the particular red blood cell group system.

vii Citations regarding HDFN or maternal antibody detection. Parentheses indicate any specific ethnic populations described with HDFN from the anti-RBC antibodies.

received blood transfusions as part of their medical care. Although transfused mothers represent only a small percentage of patients at risk for HDFN, they represent 50% of the pregnancies affected by Kell HDFN [13]. Now that RHD HDFN is largely preventable, preventing iatrogenic cases of HDFN should be a priority [14–15].

The expanded utilization of reproductive technology has led to unexpected risk for development of HDFN. Frequent changes in health-care providers creates the opportunity for both intentional and unintentional omission of details of medical history. The use of donor oocytes, donor sperm, or adopted embryos may go unshared with a subsequent obstetrics provider or pediatrician. Reproductive technologies can lead to a fetus or neonate with HDFN presenting with fetomaternal red cell antigen mismatches that appear biologically impossible based on known maternal and paternal red cell phenotypes [16–17]. For example, the AB+ adopted embryo born to an O– mother and O– father.

Red Blood Cell Antigen Systems

The International Society of Blood Transfusion (ISBT) currently recognizes 36 red blood cell systems, each consisting of one or more red cell surface antigens controlled at a single gene locus or

Table 9.2 Risk factors associated with HDN

Known previous transfusions

Medical history with potential for unappreciated history of transfusions
Prolonged hospital stay as a newborn
Survivor of childhood cancer
Return to operating room within seven days after prior pregnancy
Major surgical procedure
  Repair of craniosynostosis
  Correction congenital heart defect
  Abdominal surgery
  Splenectomy for unclear indication could suggest maternal red cell defect

Risk for unappreciated fetal maternal hemorrhage
Ectopic pregnancy
Spontaneous abortion
Induced abortion
Abnormal placental insertion
Amniocentesis
Chorionic villus sampling
Cordocentesis
Fetal version maneuvers
Maternal abdominal trauma
Placental abruption
Fetal surgery
Prenatal fetal demise
Delivery of infant

Prior pregnancy history
In utero transfusion
Early delivery for HDN
Maternal interventions including IVIg, plasma exchange
Prior infant requiring an exchange transfusion or phototherapy

two very closely linked homologous genes that have little or no observable recombination. Each system has a name, a 2–3 letter symbol, and a 3-digit number (mainly used in computer logging). Within each system are a variable number of antigens. Tables linking system names, gene designations, chromosomal locations, cluster of differentiation (CD) numbers, and the numeric designations are available on the ISBT website page "Red Cell Immunogenetics and Blood Group Terminology" (available at http://www.isbtweb.org/working-parties/red-cell-immunogenetics-and-blood-group-terminology). We have included the current ISBT terminology in Table 9.1 which outlines the blood groups antigens that have been described to result in a spectrum of symptoms from simply detectable maternal antibody to red cell antigen up to severe HDFN requiring a high level intervention.

Immunoglobulin is transported across the placenta by an energy dependent process that uses an Fc receptor, FcRn [18]. IgA and IgM are not

transported since they are not bound by FcRn, and there is no other transfer mechanism. Maternal IgG transfer appears to begin in the 15th week, but it is minimal up to the 22nd week of gestation in normal pregnancies. After the 22nd week IgG transport rapidly accelerates, such that the IgG concentration in term neonates equals or exceeds the maternal level [19]. In addition to the amount and avidity of antibody produced, the IgG subclass that is produced can also affect transport across the placenta and hemolysis [20, 21].

ABO

ABO was the first red blood cell antigen system identified. There are two antigens (A, B) resulting in four blood types (A, B, AB, O). The A and B antigens are glycotransferases that differ by four amino acids. The O allele contains a single nucleotide deletion resulting in a frame-shift mutation and coding for a protein without enzymatic activity [22]. Every immune competent person who does not express the A or B protein, will innately produce antibody to that antigen. Symptomatic HDFN due to ABO mismatch occurs almost exclusively in infants whose mothers are blood type O [23]. Some A or B infants born to blood type O mothers will develop more severe hemolytic disease than others. HDFN from ABO mismatch is characterized predominantly by hyperbilirubinemia and less anemia compare to HDFN as a result of anti-RHD. A blood type B infant of a blood type O mother is associated with greater hyperbilirubinemia risk than a blood type A infant of an O mother [24–25]. The greater risk for hyperbilirubinemia appears to be particularly in neonates with mothers of African origin [26–29]. One recent report highlights several such neonates who experienced progressive hyperbilirubinemia despite phototherapy and required an exchange transfusion [30].

Routine cord blood screening of infants born to type O mothers has been recommended in the past and remains common practice in many nurseries. The literature, however, suggests that such screening is not warranted given the cost and low yield [23, 24, 31]. Recommendations by the American Association of Blood Banks, and the American Academy of Pediatrics state cord blood testing for infant's blood type and direct antiglobin test (direct Coombs test, DAT) is not required provided there is appropriate birth hospitalization bilirubin surveillance and risk assessment before discharge [32–33]. A blood type, DAT, and measurement of total serum bilirubin is indicated in the evaluation of any newborn with jaundice developing in the first 24 hours of life and/or clinically significant hyperbilirubinemia including those treated with phototherapy.

Rh System

The RH antigens are coded for by two closely related genes on chromosome 1, RHD and RHCE. The genes are codominant which results in protein product of the gene inherited from each parent. The RHCE gene codes for C, c, E, and e polypeptides [34, 35]. The RH proteins are only expressed in erythroid cells [35–36]. In fetal development the RHD antigen can be detected on red blood cells (RBC) as early as the 7th week of gestation. The highest density of red cell antigens is on mature red blood cells.

The RHD gene codes for the D protein. Unlike small c and e, small d only indicates the absence of D protein expression (in this chapter designated as RHD negative). In Caucasian populations the lack of RHD expression is due to gene deletion, and occurs in 11%–35% of Caucasian ethnic groups [37]. Among the 0.5%–7% eastern Asian and southern Africans who are serologically RHD negative, as many as 66% have a grossly intact RHD gene [38–42]. RHD negative status in Africans can be due to a 37 bp insertion which encodes a premature stop codon [35].

RHD is the most immunogenic of the RBC antigens [43]. The sensitivity of the immune system to RHD is illustrated by the fact that multiple 0.01 ml doses of whole blood can be sufficient for immunization [44]. Untreated, 1%–2% of RHD negative mothers of RHD positive, ABO compatible fetuses will have anti-RHD detectable at the end of a first pregnancy [45–46]. At 3 to 6 months postpartum a total of 9% of this group of mothers will have a positive IAT, with the increase attributable to immunization by FMH at delivery. During a second RHD positive, ABO compatible pregnancy an additional 8% of RHD negative mothers will have anti-RHD detected, consistent with secondary immunization following undetected primary immunization during the first pregnancy. Thus, 15%–17% of mothers will be immunized following a first ABO compatible, RHD incompatible pregnancy without immunoprophylaxis.

Type O RHD negative mothers carrying type A or B RHD fetuses have a lower frequency of anti-RHD immunization [47–50]. This is due to the removal of fetal red blood cells from maternal circulation by the agglutinating IgM anti-A or anti-B antibody preventing sensitization to the RHD antigen [15].

Anti-E antibodies are the most frequently found anti-Rh system antibodies found in pregnancy but are less immunogenic than anti-D antibodies [51, 52, 53]. However, significant HDFN may occur in up to 20% of infants of sensitized mothers and severe disease including hydrops may occur. Anti-e is less frequent and significant HDFN is less frequent but may occur [54].

The rare RH null phenotype results from deletion of RHAG which must be present for RH antigens to be present on the surface of the red blood cell. Rh null appears serologically the same as RHcde but is characterized hematologically by normochromic, hemolytic anemia, and complete lack of the RH antigens in the RBC membrane [55].

Anti-RHc, "little c" occurs less frequently than anti-RHE, at an incidence of about 0.7 per 1,000 pregnancies, but 20%–30% of affected neonates will require postnatal intervention [56–58]. Therefore anti-RHc is second only to RHD as a cause of HDFN. Importantly, one report described a frequency of 13% of anti-c positive pregnancies resulting in severe anemia or hydrops [59]. Others have reported the same with anti-c, but at a lower rate [60–61]. RHC, "big C" is reported to be the target of maternal hemolytic antibodies in 0.1 to 0.2 per 1,000 pregnancies. Of those with anti-C antibodies, one-third of affected babies showed some sign of being affected, but less than 10% required any treatment.

RHC^w, an antigen associated with HDFN, is a mutated form of RHC and differs from RHC by a single amino acid [62]. Each of the RH antigens (D, C, c, E, e), the RH variants C^w, C^x, E^w, Ce^s, and G, have been implicated as causes of significant HDFN (see Table 9.1). Anti-e antibody, as the least immunogenic of the Rh group antigens, is uncommon and has been reported to cause by comparison more mild HDFN [43, 63].

Kell

The Kell antigen system (KEL) was named for the woman in whom the antibody was first identified

[64]. Many of the KEL variants differ only by a single amino acid. Although the majority of these antigens are without clinical relevance to newborns, antibody to K, k, Ku, and Js[b] are significant causes of moderate to severe HDFN [65–66].

The KEL glycoprotein is the first erythroid specific antigen known to be expressed during erythroid development [67]. Thus, antibody targeted against this antigen can profoundly affect red blood cell production. This observation helps to explain the manifestations of HDFN caused by antibodies to KEL in which anemia and reticulocytopenia may be more severe, and hyperbilirubinemia less severe, than when other antigens are involved [68–70].

Anti-K antibody is found in about 0.1% of pregnant women [71]. However, most of these women have developed antibodies due to transfusion exposure [13]. Since only 9% of people of European ancestry and 2% of people of African ancestry are antigen positive for K, and almost all are heterozygous, the likelihood that a fetus will express K is small [72]. Antibody to KEL has been associated with a lower critical titer, 8, than for RH antigens [65]. When an antibody to K is detected in initial prenatal screens, there is great importance in determination of paternal antigen status. With paternal heterozygosity and a titer of 1:8 or greater, fetal antigen determination is indicated to guide future monitoring. Of those infants born to mothers with anti-K and known to express the K antigen, 40% in one series were severely affected, 24% required phototherapy, and the remainder received no intervention [13]. In another series 73% of antigen positive infants were severely affected [68]. The other KEL associated antigens: k, Kp[b] [73], and Js[b] [67, 74–75] have been associated with HDFN that in the case of Js[b] was severe.

Duffy

The Duffy (FY) antigen is a red cell membrane glycoprotein which functions as an attachment site for the malaria agent, *Plasmodium vivax*, and as a receptor for multiple chemokines [76–79]. There are two principal forms, Fy[a] and Fy[b], which are codominant and differ by a single amino acid [80]. The null variant genotype *FY/FY* and phenotype Fy(a−b−) is a single base pair change in the promoter region at the binding site

for the hematopoietic transcription factor GATA-1 [81–82]. The null variant Fy(a−b−) is found in 95% of West Africans and 68% of African Americans [77]. The lack of erythroid expression of Fy[a] and Fy[b] in the *FY/FY* individuals is considered to be among the many RBC adaptations to the environmental pressure of malaria [83]. The molecular basis for the null variant is an example of tissue-specific gene regulation, as the Duffy antigen is expressed in nonerythroid tissues, including those with the *FY/FY* genotype, apparently under control of other transcription factors [84].

Although Western African ancestry individuals have a high frequency of lacking the Fy[a] and Fy[b] antigens on red blood cells, a population based study in the United States did not find an increased frequency of antibody to Fy[a] among individuals self-classified as black compared to those self-classified as white [85]. In this series in which 45 patients had developed antibody to Fy[a], none had developed antibody to Fy[b]. Fy[b] is calculated to have an immunogenic potency one-eighth that of Fy[a] [85]. It has not been implicated as a cause of HDFN requiring treatment except in a single case [8, 86]. In two case series that included pregnant women with anti-Fy[a], two-thirds of mothers had a history of blood transfusion [56, 87]. Antibody to Fy[a] has been implicated in significant HDFN [88–89]. The anti-Fy[a] titer has been a poor predictor of severity of neonatal disease [89]. Two case series described 40 Fy[a] positive infants born to mothers with anti-Fy[a]. Of these 40, 2 received intrauterine transfusions, 3 received exchange transfusions, and 3 were treated with phototherapy alone [57, 89]. Fetal genotype determination of Fy[a] is described [89–90].

Another distinct antigenic site, Fy3, is absent on those who are Fy(a−b−), but detectable on those who are Fy(a+b−) and those who are Fy(a−b+). Anti-Fy3 has been associated with alloimmunization and very rarely with moderate HDFN [91].

Kidd

Kidd (JK) antigen is a glycoprotein, which functions as a constitutive urea transporter in red blood cells and kidney [92]. Jk[a] and Jk[b], differ by a single base pair and amino acid [93]. The Kidd glycoprotein carries an additional antigen, Jk3, which appears to generate an antibody response only in Kidd null Jk(a−b−) subjects. Anti-Jk3 will react with all Jk^a or Jk^b positive cells. Jk(a−b−) is uncommon except among people of Polynesian ancestry [94].

Each of these three epitopes has been associated with HDFN requiring intervention in a small number of cases [95–98]. Antibody to the Jk^a and Jk^b antigens has been associated with positive direct antiglobulin test and hyperbilirubinemia requiring phototherapy [95–96].

MNS

Antigens of the MN reside on GYPA and Ss resides on GYPB. GYPA and GYPB are heavily glycosylated and are considered sialomucins. Cells lacking GYPA have altered ion transport capabilities. GYPA may interact with the red cell protein band 3, an anion exchange protein altering membrane flexibility [99, 100]. Glycophorin A (GYPA) is one of the most abundant red cell proteins. During erythroid maturation GYPA is detectable shortly after the KEL antigenic group [67]. Anti-M is usually an IgM antibody. In one series, antibodies to MNS accounted for less than 5% of the HDFN [101]. While more recent series report 10% HDFN due to anti-M/N [102–103]. Intervention required ranged from no intervention to exchange transfusion [104–105]. In a review of Japanese cases, severe HDFN occurred despite low maternal titers. Additionally, some of these infants developed late onset anemia suggesting anti-M may be able to suppress hematopoiesis analogous to Kell [103]. The frequency of detected anti-S is about 5% that of anti-RHD in the post immunoprophylaxis era. A strong association with transfusion history is reported, but the antibody is too weak to titrate in two-thirds of the cases. Moderately severe HDFN has occurred and there is one case report of IUT for HDFN due to anti-S [106]. The glycophorin B molecule carries the U antigen as well as S/s. Rarely anti-U has been implicated in HDFN, but among the 15 reported cases all affected infants had an DAT titer of greater than 1:256 [107]. Another infant had low titers and required only phototherapy for mild HDFN [108].

Clinical Management

With the advent of prevention strategies, prenatal screening, management of affected pregnancies, and effective in-utero treatment, HDFN has become a relatively rare and, usually, manageable disease. It is important, however, to not underestimate its ability to cause significant harm in the form of perinatal loss, prematurity, and neonatal morbidity when it does occur.

Prenatal Prevention

Women who are RH negative lack the RHD antigen on their red cells. If the fetus inherits the RHD gene from the father, RH positive fetal cells can, through the course of normal pregnancy, access the maternal intravascular compartment and elicit a maternal immune response in the form of IgG antibodies against the RHD antigen. The antibody can cross the placenta and attack fetal red cells, resulting in HDFN.

In the absence of prevention strategies, 14% of affected pregnancies result in stillbirth and half result in neonatal death or severe morbidity [109]. In the United States, the strategy of postnatal injection of anti-RHD immune globulin resulted in a steady decline in the frequency of anti-D in pregnant women and a concomitant decrease in the frequency of perinatal death due to anti-D HDFN [5, 110]. During the period from its introduction in 1968 to its widespread use by 1983, the reduction in maternal immunization and perinatal death were each about 90%. After 10 to 15 years of routine administration of postnatal IM anti-D immune globulin to RHD negative, and anti-RHD antibody negative mothers, the immunization rate of at-risk mothers had decreased from 16% to 2%, and deaths due to HDFN were decreased from 22–45 per 100,000 live births to 3.9–7.5 per 100,000 live births [46, 110–111]. This decrease was primarily attained by the application of postnatal anti-RHD prophylaxis, but it was aided during that time by the birth pattern of a smaller number of second and subsequent pregnancies with the accompanying risk for repeat antigen exposure [112].

The addition of a dose of anti-RHD immune globulin at 28 weeks further decreased the frequency of immunization ten-fold from approximately 2% with postnatal prophylaxis alone to 0.2% with pre- and postnatal anti-RHD immune globulin [45–46, 113]. In addition, specific antepartum events including spontaneous or induced abortion [114–115], amniocentesis [116–117], cordocentesis [118–119], chorionic villus sampling [120–121], antepartum hemorrhage, blunt abdominal trauma [122], external cephalic version [123], and others were identified as increasing the risk of immunization to RHD. (See Table 9.2.) Subsequent studies showed a decrease in immunization when anti-D immune globulin was given following amniocentesis and pregnancy termination [124–125]. Policies were developed for additional immune prophylaxis to prevent immunization following the above specific high-risk events for FMH [126].

The American College of Obstetricians and Gynecologists has published evidence-based clinical practice guidelines for the prevention of RHD alloimmunization that simplify and standardize prenatal care [127]. These recommendations include maternal ABO blood type and antibody screen at the first prenatal visit. RHD negative, antibody negative women are rescreened at 24–28 weeks and, if still antibody screen negative, are given a 300 microgram intramuscular injection of anti-D immune globulin. After delivery of an RHD positive infant, RH negative women who remain antibody negative are given a repeat 300 microgram dose of anti-D immune globulin within 72 hours of delivery.

This antepartum strategy is predicated on the fetal antigen status being an unknown. Paternal blood typing may be helpful if the father is RH negative. If paternity is certain, then the fetus is also negative, and no further intervention is warranted. Alternatively, cell-free fetal DNA in the maternal circulation, even in the first trimester, is highly sensitive (99%) and specific (95%) for fetal RHD genotype [128–130]. Knowing the fetal genotype can eliminate the need for further intervention. Although this strategy may not be cost-effective or pragmatic currently, it is likely to become so as the price and availability of the technology improve and could eventually change the management algorithm.

According to the American Association of Blood Banks, pregnant patients who are blood grouped as weak D (formerly Du) have historically been categorized as D antigen negative with recommendations to utilize RHD immune globulin. The College of American Pathologists now recommends RHD genotype. This would allow weak D phenotypes 1, 2, and 3 to be treated as RH positive. Such a shift could potentially save 24,700 injections of RHD IgG [131].

If the maternal antibody screen is positive at pregnancy registration or becomes positive for anti-D or other red cell antigen antibodies known to cause fetal immune-mediated hemolysis, the fetus is at risk for HDFN, and additional surveillance is warranted. Available diagnostic and surveillance options for determining the presence and severity of HDFN include serial testing of maternal antibody titer by indirect antiglobin test (IAT). Other techniques include: determination of fetal genotype by DNA-based techniques on maternal blood or amniotic fluid, middle cerebral artery Doppler velocity studies by ultrasound, amniocentesis using optical density change of the amniotic fluid as an indicator of hemolytic activity in the fetus, and direct determination of fetal hemoglobin level and red cell antigen type by percutaneous umbilical cord blood sampling. The best option to employ is determined by the antigen involved, the mother's obstetric history, the father's genotype, and the gestational age at which the antibody is first detected. An algorithm for the monitoring of pregnancies at risk for RHD alloimmunization is demonstrated in Table 9.3. Much of the algorithm applies to pregnancies at risk for HDFN from alloimmunization against any red cell antigen.

A notable exception to this surveillance strategy is Kell alloimmunization. The Kell antibody has the ability to not only attack mature red cells in the fetal circulation, but it can also attack progenitor cells in the fetal bone marrow resulting in decreased red cell production. This two-pronged attack of decreased red cell production and increased destruction can result in rapid and severe anemia irrespective of maternal antibody concentration. MCA Doppler surveillance is initiated at 18 weeks [65].

For a pregnant woman who is newly identified to be at risk for HDFN based on an antibody screen result, the IAT titer continues to be the measure that is most widely used to determine whether invasive testing should be done. Serial antibody titers are performed at regular intervals, usually every 2 to 4 weeks in the second trimester and every 1 to 2 weeks in the last trimester. Each lab that performs serial measurement of maternal anti-blood group antibodies determines a critical titer defined as the lowest titer that has been associated with fetal compromise at their institution. The critical titer is specific for a given antigen since it varies with the antigen. An additional criterion that may be employed is the sequential increase in titer greater than 2 dilutions, for example, 2 increasing to 16. Given the limited frequency of HDFN, many labs do not have the volume of patients

Table 9.3 Interpreting maternal antibody status of RHD negative women

Maternal antibody status at beginning of pregnancy	Maternal antibody status (prior to Rhogam) 24–28 weeks	Rhogam given?	Maternal antibody status at delivery	Maternal antibody	Diagnosis	Infant risk for HDFN
Negative	Negative	Yes	Positive	Anti-D	Passive anti-D; Rhogam effect	Unlikely*
Negative	Negative	No	Positive	Anti-D	**Late** RHD sensitization	Yes
Negative	Positive	No	Positive	Anti-D	**Early** RHD sensitization	Yes
Positive	Positive	No	Positive	Anti-D	Sensitized pregnancy to RHD	Yes
Negative	Negative	Yes	Positive	Non-D antibody	**Late** sensitization to non-D antigen	Yes

Notes: * At times, the infant will also have a positive direct Coombs test secondary to maternal RhIg administration. This finding is generally not thought to indicate a hemolytic risk [32, 45, 202]. There are rare reports of HDFN [203].
Based on [30, 143].

to determine their own critical titers. Therefore, any titer between 16 and 32 is generally used.

Historically, an IAT anti-D titer of 32 or greater triggered the need for close follow up and the use of more invasive procedures. Amniocentesis could then begin as early as 14 weeks in antigen-sensitized mothers. The fluid was evaluated for bilirubin pigment concentration, by measuring the optical density of the amniotic fluid specimen at 450 nm, the spectral peak for bilirubin, and subtracting the value for the control fluid at 450 nm producing the OD450. The results were then plotted on Liley's original graph that used data from samples taken from 27 weeks' gestation to term and was divided into three regions by two curves [132]. Later, Queenan et al. collected data for fetuses from 14 weeks to term and constructed a graph with four regions [133].

Noninvasive ultrasound monitoring using the middle cerebral artery (MCA) peak systolic velocity (PSV) has almost entirely replaced invasive monitoring. Using current MCA velocity criteria to identify significant anemia the false negative rate is 0%, and the false positive rate is 12%. Importantly, the ability to identify fetuses with significant anemia is independent of ultrasound changes associated with hydrops [134]. This technology has now become the standard for monitoring pregnancies at risk of HDFN, avoiding invasive procedures such as amniocentesis and cordocentesis that carry an inherent risk and can accelerate the disease via additional FMH.

In women with an obstetric history of a prior affected fetus/neonate who carry an RH-positive fetus in the current pregnancy, HDFN can be expected to be more severe. MCA PSV monitoring should begin earlier and applied more frequently in this instance.

In Utero Therapy

The mainstay of treatment for severe HDFN is intrauterine transfusion (IUT). IUT corrects fetal anemia and decreases the volume of circulating fetal RBCs carrying the antigen responsible for HDFN. After several IUTs, the percent of fetal RBCs is negligible. The pregnancy can, therefore, continue to term with periodic transfusions. In experienced hands, the fetal risk of IUT is remarkably low [135]. Long-term outcome studies suggest low levels of neurodevelopment impairment of survivors [136].

Intrauterine transfusion can be accomplished by two approaches: intraperitoneal and intravascular transfusion. Historically, intraperitoneal transfusion preceded intravascular for technical reasons. With the advent of high-resolution, real-time ultrasound, which allowed for fetal intravascular access, intravascular transfusion replaced intraperitoneal except in unusual circumstances. Intraperitoneal transfusion relies on packed red blood cells (PRBCs) to be gradually absorbed from the intraperitoneal compartment. It is still employed when intravascular access is technically impossible, such as in maternal obesity and early gestation, or as an adjunct to intravascular transfusion to potentially extend the interval between transfusions. Intraperitoneal IUT is less effective, however, in the presence of ascites. Importantly, it does not provide direct information about the effectiveness of the treatment. Intravascular access, however, holds multiple advantages over intraperitoneal. Not only does it quickly correct the anemia, but it also allows for accurate and direct assessment of anemia and monitoring of the treatment's success. It allows for the sampling of fetal blood, which can be used for a myriad of informative laboratory tests such as blood type, hemoglobin level, platelet count, reticulocyte count, and Kleihauer–Betke. These laboratory values allow for an accurate assessment of the degree of anemia as well as the fetal response to treatment and can be used to guide management.

Donor blood must be negative for the RBC antigen(s) involved in HDFN and cross-matched with the mother to avoid sensitization to a new antigen. They should be as fresh as possible, spun to a high concentration (hematocrit of 75%), CMV negative, irradiated, and leukodepleted (see Chapter 20, Table 20.4). Considerable time may be required for the blood bank to match and prepare donor blood, especially if multiple antibodies are involved. Close communication with the blood bank and transfusion medicine is helpful in procedure planning. Maternal blood may be the best source of PRBCs in cases of multiple maternal alloantibodies, but pregnant women are often excluded from blood donation for various reasons [137]. See Chapter 20 on Transfusion Practices for more information.

The procedure consists of two distinct components: percutaneous umbilical blood sampling (PUBS) and IUT. Sampling involves achieving intravascular access and collecting a sample of fetal blood. If fetal anemia (2 standard deviations below the gestational age mean) is confirmed, transfusion is initiated immediately [138]. Given the challenge and inherent risks of obtaining intravascular access, all equipment, supplies, and personnel must be in place and prepared to perform an IUT. The major risk of IUT is fetal bradycardia, most often secondary to a large bolus of viscous blood. Bradycardia typically, but not always, resolves with temporary interruption of IUT. Contingency planning must include the ability to perform an emergency cesarean section after a gestational age when neonatal survival would be anticipated. This planning must include the informed consent of the patient and advanced notification of anesthesia, nursing, and neonatology teams. Antenatal corticosteroids should be administered in proximity to the next planned IUT after viability is achieved.

Intrauterine transfusion is initiated when convincing evidence for severe fetal anemia exists, usually by middle cerebral artery Doppler assessment 1.5 multiples of the median [134]. Once transfusion is initiated, it is generally repeated at progressively elongated intervals of 2, 3, and then 4 weeks. This strategy takes into account the volume of fetal cells within the intravascular compartment. Repeated IUTs increase the volume of donor RBCs and decreases the percent of fetal RBCs, which can be monitored by the fetal reticulocyte count and Kleihauer–Betke on subsequent samplings. Donor blood cells have a longer half-life than fetal cells, allowing for extension of the interval between IUTs. An alternative strategy is to follow MCA Doppler studies after the first IUT to determine the timing of the next. The efficiency of this strategy diminishes after the second IUT as donor RBCs have different flow properties than fetal cells [139]. Typically, the last IUT is performed at 35 weeks with delivery at 38 weeks. Cesarean section may be reserved for routine indications.

In the rare circumstance of severe disease at very early gestation, both plasmapheresis and intravenous immunoglobulin (IVIg) have been used to mitigate the disease until intrauterine transfusion is technically achievable. Both interventions are associated with maternal side effects, high cost, and short duration of effect [139–140].

Pregnancies complicated by HDFN managed by IUT evidence an overall survival of approximately 90%. Long-term neurologic outcomes are generally favorable, matching the baseline incidence for neurologic impairment in the general population, except in the case of severe hydrops fetalis [136]. The presence of hydrops fetalis decreases survival, highlighting the importance of efforts to prevent its occurrence [141–142].

Perinatal Communication: A Critical Handoff

To assure timely and effective neonatal care, all medical providers attending the mother *and newborn* must know the status of the maternal anti-erythrocyte antibody screen and *if positive* recognize its potential to herald significant hyperbilirubinemia in the neonate [143]. If known prenatally, obstetric providers should communicate the finding of the positive maternal anti-erythrocyte antibody screen to labor and delivery, the newborn nursery and neonatal care takers well prior to delivery. Prenatal neonatology consultation for pregnancies complicated by maternal alloimmunization should be solicited to provide parental counsel on the postnatal evaluation and management of the newborn and to coordinate neonatal care.

Similarly, if first identified during the delivery hospitalization, newborn caretakers should be notified of a positive maternal anti-erythrocyte antibody screen in a timely fashion, prior to and no later than the time of delivery. This is necessary to secure cord blood typing and direct antiglobulin testing to determine whether the maternal anti-erythrocyte antibody or antibodies pose a risk for neonatal hemolysis and ensure there are no delays in identifying significant early hyperbilirubinemia or in initiating treatment.

Immune mediated hemolysis is often quite robust and resultant early hyperbilirubinemia can be rapidly progressive. It is therefore essential that the critical information of a positive maternal anti-erythrocyte antibody screen be clearly communicated across the perinatal continuum between obstetric and newborn caretakers to ensure newborn safety.

Additionally, post-natal diagnosis of HDFN should be transmitted *back* to the obstetrics provider in preparation for future pregnancies.

Interpreting a Positive Maternal Antibody Screen at the Time of Delivery

Accurate interpretation of a positive maternal anti-erythrocyte antibody screen at the time of delivery is necessary to ensure proper newborn care. This will include the determination of what red blood cell antigen the maternal antibody is directed toward and when the mother became antibody positive. This may require a call to the blood bank to clarify or confirm the antibody screen results. Then it is necessary to determine if the infant carries the antigen to which the antibody is directed. This requires a blood type and DAT on the infant, ideally from cord blood to ensure a timely evaluation.

If the mother is RHD positive and has a positive anti-erythrocyte antibody screen, then she is sensitized, and the blood bank will tell you which non-RHD antigen the antibody is directed toward. Alternatively, if the mother is RHD negative and has a positive anti-erythrocyte antibody screen then it is necessary to determine whether she was antibody negative at the beginning of the pregnancy, antibody negative at 24–28 weeks' gestation prior to RH immunoglobulin administration, determine whether she received RH immunoglobulin, and whether the antibody is anti-D. Table 9.3 shows how to interpret the maternal antibody status in RHD negative woman at the time of delivery [30]. Figure 9.1 is an algorithm to help newborn care takers determine how best to evaluate and manage the neonate in the context of a positive maternal anti-erythrocyte antibody screen [143].

It is also important to recognize that a RHD positive infant delivered to a RHD-negative woman during the *first* isoimmunized pregnancy (antibody screen negative at the beginning of the pregnancy but then turns positive) is at risk for HDFN. In fact, at least 20% of such infants are affected and require treatment in terms of either phototherapy or exchange transfusion [144]. The same holds true for RHD positive women during the first alloimmunized pregnancy.

Diagnosis in the Neonate

The diagnosis of non-ABO HDFN is predicated on the finding of a positive maternal anti-erythrocyte antibody screen coupled with a positive DAT in the neonate. ABO immune mediated hemolytic disease on the other hand is diagnosed in a heterospecific mother infant pair where mother is type O and the infant type A or B, coupled with a positive DAT in the infant. Given the pivotal role of the DAT in the diagnosis of immune mediated hemolytic disease, it is usually straightforward to differentiate HDFN from other causes of hemolysis in newborns including red cell membrane defects (e.g., hereditary spherocytosis) and red cell enzymopathies (e.g., glucose-6-phosphate dehydrogenase deficiency). In fact, infants born of ABO incompatible mother–infant pairs who have a negative DAT appear to be at no greater risk for developing hyperbilirubinemia than their ABO compatible counterparts [23]. The development of significant hyperbilirubinemia in such neonates should prompt evaluation

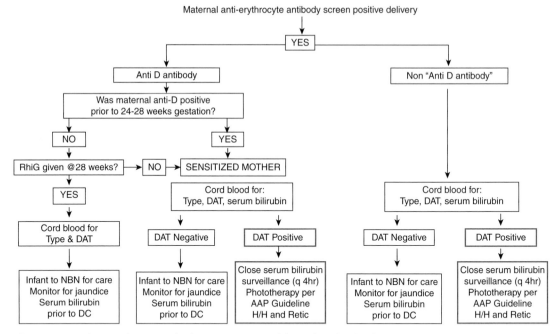

Fig. 9.1 Maternal anti-erythrocyte antibody screen positive at delivery algorithm. [143]

for a cause other than isoimmunization [145]. Hemolysis, regardless of etiology, should be suspected with early onset or rapidly progressive hyperbilirubinemia as well as hyperbilirubinemia that is not responsive to intensive phototherapy.

Other findings of HDFN may include: a maternal past pregnancy history of an infant with severe anemia, hydrops, or marked hyperbilirubinemia; a history of maternal transfusion; severe intrauterine anemia; hydrops fetalis; prolonged neonatal hyperbilirubinemia; hemolysis on review of neonatal red blood cell smear; history of in vitro fertilization involving donor sperm, donor ovum, or adopted embryo; and known red cell antigen mismatch between mother and infant.

Postnatal Management

Delivery Room

As an antibody-sensitized pregnancy passes the age of fetal viability, delivery should be scheduled in a perinatal level three center with interdisciplinary fetomaternal medicine and neonatology services. Relative to the unaffected fetus matched for gestational age, the fetus with severe HDFN appears to be at increased risk of neonatal respiratory distress syndrome. This is probably secondary to intrauterine

fetal compromise and possibly related to fetal hyperinsulinemia, which may down regulate fetal surfactant production. If the infant is delivered before term, the combination of anemia, hyperbilirubinemia, and respiratory distress may require neonatal resuscitation and intensive care.

The timing and mode of delivery can be planned according to fetal condition and obstetrical considerations. If delivery appears necessary before 34 weeks of gestation, lung maturation can be accelerated by a 48-hour course of antenatally administered glucocorticoids. Unless antenatal evaluation shows evidence of severe fetal compromise already present, most patients with HDFN will tolerate delivery by induction of labor, with close electronic and bedside monitoring. Mild to moderately anemic fetuses generally tolerate labor well, although severely anemic fetuses or those with incipient high output cardiac failure may not. Cesarean section should be immediately available in case of fetal intolerance to labor or the development of untoward obstetrical complications, and cesarean section may be the preferred route of delivery for severe fetal compromise or for other high-risk obstetrical indications. A neonatology team should attend the delivery.

In the current era of close fetal surveillance during sensitized pregnancies and management using intrauterine transfusion it is unusual for infants to be born with severe anemia, high output cardiac failure, signs of hydrops fetalis, or shock. However, should such signs be evident, the neonate requires timely treatment. Transfusion with O negative, appropriate red cell antigen negative, irradiated packed RBC, cross-matched against the mother, can be given to profoundly anemic infants as a partial exchange transfusion of 25–50 ml/kg, removed and infused in 5 ml/kg aliquots per 3–4 minute "cycle." Anemic but more stable infants can be transfused slowly at 10 ml/kg over 2–3 hours [146] (see also Chapter 20). The mortality of hydrops fetalis remains substantial despite advances in obstetrical care and neonatal intensive management.

Infants without evidence of profound anemia or cardiovascular compromise can be stabilized and observed without emergency transfusion until the postnatal course of their anemia and hyperbilirubinemia is further evaluated. After initial neonatal stabilization and assessment including cord blood assessments of total serum bilirubin (TSB), and hemoglobin, hemoglobin and bilirubin concentrations should be determined again within 4 hours, and serially thereafter as a guide to further management. Even if hyperbilirubinemia is controlled, supplemental transfusions of 10–15 ml/kg for anemia may be needed one or more times before birth hospitalization discharge.

Clinical Management Beyond the Delivery Room

Hemolytic conditions, including HDFN, are noted in many cases of kernicterus with recent evidence suggesting hemolysis is *the* "unifying feature" of bilirubin-induced neurotoxicity risk [147]. These findings reflect the important role hemolysis plays both in excessive bilirubin production with resultant hyperbilirubinemia *and* in potentiating the risk of brain damage in an infant with severe hyperbilirubinemia. Although the mechanism(s) of the neurotoxicity intensifying effect is unclear, the augmented risk for bilirubin-induced neurotoxicity is the basis for lower bilirubin treatment threshold when a hemolytic condition is present.

Phototherapy

High intensity phototherapy should be initiated at birth if severe HDFN is diagnosed prenatally or upon determination of early hyperbilirubinemia.

Phototherapy in the blue light spectrum should be used in combination with a fiberoptic/LED blanket or mattress to optimize the surface area exposed. Irradiance should be at least 30 microwatts/cm^2. Hyperbilirubinemia in symptomatic neonatal ABO hemolytic disease is generally milder but may also require timely treatment, if severe, or early onset in nature, for example, 10–15 mg/dL or higher before 24 hours of age. The American Academy of Pediatrics clinical practice guideline on the management of hyperbilirubinemia in the newborn 35 or more weeks' gestation provides hour specific bilirubin phototherapy thresholds based on gestational age and neurotoxicity risk [33].

Intravenous Immune Globulin (IVIg)

Controlled trials have confirmed that the administration of IVIg to infants with RH and ABO hemolytic disease will significantly reduce the need for exchange transfusion [148]. The AAP recommends IVIg in immune mediated hemolytic disease if the TSB is rising despite intensive phototherapy or the TSB level is within 2–3 mg/dL of the exchange level [148]. Two Cochrane reviews (in 2002 and 2018) have raised concerns regarding the quality of the IVIg clinical trials and recommend additional, large randomized controlled trials [149, 150].

Exchange Transfusion

Advances in phototherapy effectiveness coupled with aggressive early determination of bilirubin levels, has reduced the need for exchange transfusion to prevent kernicterus. Exchange transfusion is now performed infrequently and reserved for those few infants in whom intensive phototherapy and IVIg do not control hyperbilirubinemia, or those neonates who show signs of intermediate to advanced stages of acute bilirubin encephalopathy (hypertonia, arching, retrocollis, opisthotonus, fever, high-pitched cry) even if the TSB is falling. The readers are referred to the 2004 AAP hyperbilirubinemia guideline for operative TSB exchange thresholds based on gestational age and neurotoxicity risk factors [33].

To secure blood for exchange transfusion as quickly as possible a type and cross should be sent to the blood bank immediately upon determination that an exchange transfusion is merited. At the same time blood bank and transfusion medicine should be contacted to review the planned exchange transfusion and shepherd the preparation of reconstituted blood for as timely delivery to the NICU as circumstances permit. Reconstituted blood, that is, washed PRBC mixed with adult fresh frozen plasma (FFP) thawed to a hematocrit approximating 40%, is the preferred exchange replacement product [151]. In HDFN the blood bank must locate compatible PRBC units, a process that may take several hours depending on the nature of the maternal antibody or antibodies present. In total, it usually takes the blood bank a minimum of 3–4 hours to prepare cross-matched reconstituted blood for exchange transfusion; often longer in HDFN. All blood products for infants should be irradiated to prevent transfusion associated graft vs. host disease and are cytomegalovirus (CMV) safe.

Delayed Anemia

HDFN due to RH can be complicated by prolonged and progressive postnatal anemia with an extended need for neonatal transfusion. Proposed mechanisms have included marrow suppression by intrauterine or postnatal transfusion, erythropoietin deficiency, ongoing hemolysis or destruction of erythroid progenitors. A report of HDFN due to anti-Ge3 suggests both ongoing hemolysis and inhibition of early hematopoietic progenitors [152]. Another case of HDFN resulting from high titers of anti-D resulted in anemia through week 15 of life. In this case erythropoietin levels were normal, a bone marrow aspirate demonstrated increased erythropoiesis up through the stage of terminal differentiated red cell but without reticulocytes. In this study the authors were unable to demonstrate any direct cytotoxic effect of anti-D serum on erythroid progenitors [153]. Prolonged transfusion requirements are more frequent when HDFN is due to Kell antigen than RH [154].

Around the World

As discussed above, in high income countries, the introduction of anti-D immunoglobulin initially postpartum, at 28 weeks of gestation, after miscarriages and early termination of pregnancies in unsensitized women at risk for developing anti-RHD is an effective preventive measure. This is not the case in middle-income and low-income countries where there is no preventive strategy or it is inconsistently applied. Bhutani and collaborators, utilizing birth rate statistics, market distribution of anti-D immunoglobulin, infant mortality rate and

prevalence of RHD negativity estimated that a global incidence of RH disease is 276/100,000 live births with estimated rates of 57, 252, 278, 385, and 386 for Southeast Asia/Pacific countries, Latin America, North Africa/the Middle East, South Asia, sub-Saharan Africa and eastern Europe respectively compared to 2.5 for countries that have a well-established preventive strategy [155]. The incidence of RHD negativity varies within ethnicity [156–154], but even with a low prevalence rate the estimate of burden is high in sub-Saharan Africa [155–156].

Future Direction

The severity of disease can be highly variable for many of the antigens. Antibody titer alone is not sufficient to determine severity of HDFN. Some antibodies produce severe disease at low titers while other antibodies produce very little hemolysis at high titers. Further research is needed to determine what other factors can be utilized to predict the severity of HDFN.

More work is needed to develop effective prevention strategies in low resource environments.

References

1. Diamond LK, Blackfan KD, Baty JM. Erythroblastosis fetalis and its association with universal edema of the fetus, icterus gravis neonatorum and anemia of the newborn. *J Pediatr* 1932;**1**:269–309.

2. Landsteiner K, Weiner A. An agglutinable factor in human blood recognized by immune sera for Rhesus blood. *Pro Soc Exp Biol Med* 1940;**43**:223.

3. Mollison PL. Methods of determining the posttransfusion survival of stored red cells. *Transfusion* 1984;**24**:93–6.

4. Bowman JM. Treatment options for the fetus with alloimmune hemolytic disease. *Transfus Med Rev* 1990;**4**:191–207.

5. Chavez GF, Mulinare J, Edmonds LD. Epidemiology of Rh hemolytic disease of the newborn in the United States. *JAMA* 1991;**265**:3270–4.

6. Murphy SL. Deaths: Final data for 1998. *Natl Vital Stat Rep* 2000;**48**:1–105.

7. Liumbruno GM, D'Alessandro A, Rea F, et al. The role of antenatal immunoprophylaxis in the prevention of maternal-foetal anti-Rh(D) alloimmunisation. *Blood Transfus* 2010;**8**:8–16.

8. Moise KJ, Jr. Non-anti-D antibodies in red-cell alloimmunization. *Eur J Obstet Gynecol Reprod Biol* 2000;**92**:75–81.

9. Bowman JM, Pollock JM, Penston LE. Fetomaternal transplacental hemorrhage during pregnancy and after delivery. *Vox Sang* 1986;**51**:117–21.

10. Cohen F, Zuelzer WW. Mechanisms of isoimmunization. II. Transplacental passage and postnatal survival of fetal erythrocytes in heterospecific pregnancies. *Blood* 1967;**30**:796–804.

11. Huchet J, Defossez Y, Brossard Y. Detection of transplacental hemorrhage during the last trimester of pregnancy. *Transfusion* 1988;**28**:506.

12. Feldman N, Skoll A, Sibai B. The incidence of significant fetomaternal hemorrhage in patients undergoing cesarean section. *Am J Obstet Gynecol* 1990;**163**:855–8.

13. McKenna DS, Nagaraja HN, O'Shaughnessy R. Management of pregnancies complicated by anti-Kell isoimmunization. *Obstet Gynecol* 1999;**93**:667–73.

14. Howard H, Martlew V, McFadyen I, et al. Consequences for fetus and neonate of maternal red cell allo-immunisation. *Arch Dis Child Fetal Neonatal Ed* 1998;**78**:F62–6.

15. Clarke CA. Preventing rhesus babies: The Liverpool research and follow up. *Arch Dis Child* 1989;**64**:1734–40.

16. Doyle B, Quigley J, Allen C, Fitzgerald J. Homozygous expression of fetal red cell antigen in donor oocyte pregnancy complicated by allo-immunisation: Are current antibody thresholds to trigger increased monitoring relevant? *Transfus Med* 2014;**24**:182–3.

17. Alsaati G, Sandler SG. Assisted reproductive technology: An uncommon, but increasing, cause of parent–child ABO discrepancy. *Transfusion* 2015;**55**:2048–9.

18. Simister NE, Story CM. Human placental Fc receptors and the transmission of antibodies from mother to fetus. *J Reprod Immunol* 1997;**37**:1–23.

19. Palfi M, Selbing A. Placental transport of maternal immunoglobulin G. *Am J Reprod Immunol.* 1998;**39**:24–6.

20. Devey ME, Voak D. A critical study of the IgG subclasses of Rh anti-D antibodies formed in pregnancy and in immunized volunteers. *Immunology* 1974;**27**:1073–9.

21. Palfi M, Hilden JO, Gottvall T, Selbing A. Placental transport of maternal immunoglobulin G in pregnancies at risk of Rh (D) hemolytic disease of the newborn. *Am J Reprod Immunol* 1998;**39**:323–8.

22. Yamamoto F, Clausen H, White T, Marken J, Hakomori S. Molecular genetic basis of the histo-blood group ABO system. *Nature* 1990;**345**:229–33.

23. Ozolek JA, Watchko JF, Mimouni F. Prevalence and lack of clinical significance of blood group incompatibility in mothers with blood type A or B. *J Pediatr* 1994;**125**:87–91.

24. Maisels MJ, Stevenson DK, Watchko JF. *Care of the Jaundiced Neonate* (New York: McGraw Hill, 2012).

25. Kaplan M, Hammerman C, Vreman HJ, Wong RJ, Stevenson DK. Hemolysis and hyperbilirubinemia in antiglobulin positive, direct ABO blood group heterospecific neonates. *J Pediatr* 2010;**157**:772–7.

26. Naiman JL. *Erythroblastosis Fetalis* (Philadelphia: W.B. Saunders, 1982).

27. Adewuyi JO, Gwanzura C, Mvere D. Characteristics of anti-A and anti-B in black Zimbabweans. *Vox Sang* 1994;**67**:307–9.

28. Adewuyi JO, Gwanzura C. Racial difference between white and black Zimbabweans in the haemolytic activity of A, B, O antibodies. *Afr J Med Med Sci* 2001;**30**:71–4.

29. Murray NA, Roberts IA. Haemolytic disease of the newborn. *Arch Dis Child Fetal Neonatal Ed* 2007;**92**:F83-88.

30. Watchko JF. Common hematologic problems in the newborn nursery. *Pediatr Clin North Am* 2015;**62**:509–24.

31. Maisels MJ, Watchko JF. Routine blood typing and DAT in infants of group O mothers. *J Perinatol* 2013;**33**:579.

32. Judd WJ. Practice guidelines for prenatal and perinatal immunohematology, revisited. *Transfusion* 2001;**41**:1445–52.

33. AAP Subcommittee on Hyperbilirubinemia. Management of hyperbilirubinemia in the newborn infant 35 or more weeks of gestation. *Pediatrics* 2004;**114**:297–316.

34. Avent ND, Reid ME. The Rh blood group system: A review. *Blood*. 2000;**95**:375–87.

35. Westhoff CM. The Rh blood group system in review: A new face for the next decade. *Transfusion* 2004;**44**:1663–73.

36. Avent ND. New insight into the Rh system: Structure and function. *ISBT Science Series* 2007;**2**:35–43.

37. Colin Y, Cherif-Zahar B, Le Van Kim C, et al. Genetic basis of the RhD-positive and RhD-negative blood group polymorphism as determined by Southern analysis. *Blood* 1991;**78**:2747–52.

38. Avent ND, Martin PG, Armstrong-Fisher SS, et al. Evidence of genetic diversity underlying Rh D-,

weak D (Du), and partial D phenotypes as determined by multiplex polymerase chain reaction analysis of the RHD gene. *Blood* 1997;**89**:2568–77.

39. Daniels G, Green C, Smart E. Differences between RhD-negative Africans and RhD-negative Europeans. *Lancet* 1997;**350**:862–3.

40. Okuda H, Kawano M, Iwamoto S, et al. The RHD gene is highly detectable in RhD-negative Japanese donors. *J Clin Invest* 1997;**100**:373–9.

41. Singleton BK, Green CA, Avent ND, et al. The presence of an RHD pseudogene containing a 37 base pair duplication and a nonsense mutation in Africans with the Rh D-negative blood group phenotype. *Blood* 2000;**95**:12–18.

42. Sun CF, Chou CS, Lai NC, Wang WT. RHD gene polymorphisms among RhD-negative Chinese in Taiwan. *Vox Sang* 1998;**75**:52–7.

43. Winters JL, Pineda AA, Gorden LD, et al. RBC alloantibody specificity and antigen potency in Olmsted County, Minnesota. *Transfusion* 2001;**41**:1413–20.

44. Jakobowicz R, Williams L, Silberman F. Immunization of Rh-negative volunteers by repeated injections of very small amounts of Rh-positive blood. *Vox Sang* 1972;**23**:376–81.

45. Bowman JM, Chown B, Lewis M, Pollock JM. Rh isoimmunization during pregnancy: Antenatal prophylaxis. *Can Med Assoc J* 1978;**118**:623–7.

46. Tovey LA, Townley A, Stevenson BJ, Taverner J. The Yorkshire antenatal anti-D immunoglobulin trial in primigravidae. *Lancet* 1983;**2**:244–6.

47. Nevanlinna HR, Anttinen EE, Vainio T. Hemolytic disease of newborn due to Rh isoimmunization: Considerations on therapy and prognosis. *Duodecim* 1956;**72**:354–69.

48. Clarke C, Finn R, McConnell R, Sheppard P. The protection afforded by ABO incompatibility against erythroblastosis due to rhesus anti-D. *Int Arch Allergy Immunol* 1958;**13**:377–81.

49. Ascari WQ, Levine P, Pollack W. Incidence of maternal Rh immunization by ABO compatible and incompatible pregnancies. *Br Med J* 1969;**1**:399–401.

50. Murray S, Knox EG, Walker W. Rhesus haemolytic disease of the newborn and the ABO groups. *Vox Sang* 1965;**10**:6–31.

51. Bollason G, Hjartardottir H, Jonsson T, et al. Red blood cell alloimmunization in pregnancy during the years 1996–2015 in Iceland: A nationwide population study. *Transfusion* 2017;**57**:2578–85.

52. Awowole I, Cohen K, Rock J, Sparey C. Prevalence and obstetric outcome of women with red cell antibodies in pregnancy at the Leeds Teaching Hospitals NHS Trust, West Yorkshire, England. *Eur J Obstet Gynecol Reprod Biol* 2019;**237**:89–92.

53. Moran P, Robson SC, Reid MM. Anti-E in pregnancy. *BJOG* 2000;**107**:1436–8.

54. McAdams RM, Dotzler SA, Winter LW, Kerecman JD. Severe hemolytic disease of the newborn from anti-e. *J Perinatol* 2008;**28**:230–2.

55. Sturgeon P. Hematological observations on the anemia associated with blood type Rhnull. *Blood* 1970;**36**:310–20.

56. Bowell PJ, Allen DL, Entwistle CC. Blood group antibody screening tests during pregnancy. *Br J Obstet Gynaecol* 1986;**93**:1038–43.

57. Filbey D, Hanson U, Wesstrom G. The prevalence of red cell antibodies in pregnancy correlated to the outcome of the newborn: A 12 year study in central Sweden. *Acta Obstet Gynecol Scand* 1995;**74**:687–92.

58. Kozlowski CL, Lee D, Shwe KH, Love EM. Quantification of anti-c in haemolytic disease of the newborn. *Transfus Med* 1995;**5**:37–42.

59. Wenk RE, Goldstein P, Felix JK. Alloimmunization by hr'(c), hemolytic disease of newborns, and perinatal management. *Obstet Gynecol* 1986;**67**:623–6.

60. Bowell PJ, Brown SE, Dike AE, Inskip MJ. The significance of anti-c alloimmunization in pregnancy. *Br J Obstet Gynaecol* 1986;**93**:1044–8.

61. Babinszki A, Berkowitz RL. Haemolytic disease of the newborn caused by anti-c, anti-E and anti-Fya antibodies: Report of five cases. *Prenat Diagn* 1999;**19**:533–6.

62. Mouro I, Colin Y, Cherif-Zahar B, Cartron JP, Le Van Kim C. Molecular genetic basis of the human Rhesus blood group system. *Nat Genet* 1993;**5**:62–5.

63. Moncharmont P, Juron-Dupraz F, Rigal D, Vignal M, Meyer F. Haemolytic disease of two newborns in a Rhesus anti-e alloimmunized woman. Review of literature. *Haematologia (Budap)* 1990;**23**:97–100.

64. Coombs RR, Mourant AE, Race RR. A new test for the detection of weak and incomplete Rh agglutinins. *Br J Exp Pathol* 1945;**26**:255–66.

65. Bowman JM, Pollock JM, Manning FA, Harman CR, Menticoglou S. Maternal Kell blood group alloimmunization. *Obstet Gynecol* 1992;**79**:239–44.

66. Babinszki A, Lapinski RH, Berkowitz RL. Prognostic factors and management in pregnancies complicated with severe Kell alloimmunization: Experiences of the last 13 years. *Am J Perinatol* 1998;**15**:695–701.

67. Southcott MJ, Tanner MJ, Anstee DJ. The expression of human blood group antigens during erythropoiesis in a cell culture system. *Blood*. 1999;**93**:4425–35.

68. Weiner CP, Widness JA. Decreased fetal erythropoiesis and hemolysis in Kell hemolytic anemia. *Am J Obstet Gynecol* 1996;**174**:547–51.

69. Vaughan JI, Manning M, Warwick RM, et al. Inhibition of erythroid progenitor cells by anti-Kell antibodies in fetal alloimmune anemia. *N Engl J Med* 1998;**338**:798–803.

70. Vaughan JI, Warwick R, Letsky E, et al. Erythropoietic suppression in fetal anemia because of Kell alloimmunization. *Am J Obstet Gynecol* 1994;**171**:247–52.

71. Mayne KM, Bowell PJ, Pratt GA. The significance of anti-Kell sensitization in pregnancy. *Clin Lab Haematol* 1990;**12**:379–85.

72. Redman CM, Marsh WL. The Kell blood group system and the McLeod phenotype. *Semin Hematol* 1993;**30**:209–18.

73. Gorlin JB, Kelly L. Alloimmunisation via previous transfusion places female Kpb-negative recipients at risk for having children with clinically significant hemolytic disease of the newborn. *Vox Sang* 1994;**66**:46–8.

74. Lowe RF, Musengezi AT, Moores P. Severe hemolytic disease of the newborn associated with anti-JSb. *Transfusion* 1978;**18**:466–8.

75. Gordon MC, Kennedy MS, O'Shaughnessy RW, Waheed A. Severe hemolytic disease of the newborn due to anti-Js(b). *Vox Sang* 1995;**69**:140–1.

76. Miller LH, Mason SJ, Clyde DF, McGinniss MH. The resistance factor to *Plasmodium vivax* in blacks. The Duffy-blood-group genotype, FyFy. *N Engl J Med* 1976;**295**:302–4.

77. Hadley TJ, Peiper SC. From malaria to chemokine receptor: The emerging physiologic role of the Duffy blood group antigen. *Blood* 1997;**89**:3077–91.

78. Horuk R, Chitnis CE, Darbonne WC, et al. A receptor for the malarial parasite Plasmodium vivax: The erythrocyte chemokine receptor. *Science* 1993;**261**:1182–4.

79. Sim BK, Chitnis CE, Wasniowska K, Hadley TJ, Miller LH. Receptor and ligand domains for invasion of erythrocytes by *Plasmodium falciparum*. *Science* 1994;**264**:1941–4.

80. Tournamille C, Le Van Kim C, Gane P, Cartron JP, Colin Y. Molecular basis and PCR-DNA typing of the Fya/fyb blood group polymorphism. *Hum Genet* 1995;**95**:407–10.

81. Tournamille C, Colin Y, Cartron JP, Le Van Kim C. Disruption of a GATA motif in the Duffy gene promoter abolishes erythroid gene expression in Duffy-negative individuals. *Nat Genet* 1995;**10**:224–8.

82. Chaudhuri A, Polyakova J, Zbrzezna V, Pogo AO. The coding sequence of Duffy blood group gene in humans and simians: Restriction fragment length polymorphism, antibody and malarial parasite specificities, and expression in nonerythroid tissues in Duffy-negative individuals. *Blood* 1995;**85**:615–21.

83. Weatherall DJ. Host genetics and infectious disease. *Parasitology* 1996;**112** Suppl:S23–29.

84. Peiper SC, Wang ZX, Neote K, et al. The Duffy antigen/receptor for chemokines (DARC) is expressed in endothelial cells of Duffy negative individuals who lack the erythrocyte receptor. *J Exp Med* 1995;**181**:1311–17.

85. Sosler SD, Perkins JT, Fong K, Saporito C. The prevalence of immunization to Duffy antigens in a population of known racial distribution. *Transfusion* 1989;**29**:505–7.

86. Vescio LA, Farina D, Rogido M, Sola A. Hemolytic disease of the newborn caused by anti-Fyb. *Transfusion* 1987;**27**:366.

87. Shah VP, Gilja BK. Hemolytic disease of newborn due to anti-Duffy (Fya). *NY State J Med* 1983;**83**:244–5.

88. Weinstein L, Taylor ES. Hemolytic disease of the neonate secondary to anti-Fya. *Am J Obstet Gynecol* 1975;**121**:643–5.

89. Goodrick MJ, Hadley AG, Poole G. Haemolytic disease of the fetus and newborn due to anti-Fy(a) and the potential clinical value of Duffy genotyping in pregnancies at risk. *Transfus Med* 1997;**7**:301–4.

90. Mallinson G, Soo KS, Schall TJ, Pisacka M, Anstee DJ. Mutations in the erythrocyte chemokine receptor (Duffy) gene: The molecular basis of the Fya/Fyb antigens and identification of a deletion in the Duffy gene of an apparently healthy individual with the Fy(a-b-) phenotype. *Br J Haematol* 1995;**90**:823–9.

91. Buchanan DI, Sinclair M, Sanger R, Gavin J, Teesdale P. An Alberta Cree Indian with a rare Duffy antibody, anti-Fy 3. *Vox Sang* 1976;**30**:114–21.

92. Lawicki S, Covin RB, Powers AA. The Kidd (JK) Blood Group System. *Transfus Med Rev* 2017;**31**:165–72.

93. Olives B, Merriman M, Bailly P, et al. The molecular basis of the Kidd blood group polymorphism and its lack of association with type

1 diabetes susceptibility. *Hum Mol Genet* 1997;**6**:1017–20.

94. Woodfield DG, Douglas R, Smith J, Simpson A, Pinder L, Staveley JM. The Jk(a-b-) phenotype in New Zealand Polynesians. *Transfusion* 1982;**22**:276–8.

95. Dorner I, Moore JA, Chaplin H, Jr. Combined maternal erythrocyte autosensitization and materno-fetal Jk incompatibility. *Transfusion* 1974;**14**:212–19.

96. Merlob P, Litwin A, Reisner SH, Cohen IJ, Zaizov R. Hemolytic disease of the newborn caused by anti-Jkb. *Pediatr Hematol Oncol* 1987;**4**:357–60.

97. Thakral B, Malhotra S, Saluja K, Kumar P, Marwaha N. Hemolytic disease of newborn due to anti-Jk b in a woman with high risk pregnancy. *Transfus Apher Sci* 2010;**43**:41–3.

98. Pierce SR, Hardman JT, Steele S, Beck ML. Hemolytic disease of the newborn associated with anti-Jk3. *Transfusion* 1980;**20**:189–91.

99. Bruce LJ, Pan RJ, Cope DL, et al. Altered structure and anion transport properties of band 3 (AE1, SLC4A1) in human red cells lacking glycophorin A. *J Biol Chem* 2004;**279**:2414–40.

100. Tomita M, Furthmayr H, Marchesi VT. Primary structure of human erythrocyte glycophorin A. Isolation and characterization of peptides and complete amino acid sequence. *Biochemistry* 1978;**17**:4756–70.

101. Geifman-Holtzman O, Wojtowycz M, Kosmas E, Artal R. Female alloimmunization with antibodies known to cause hemolytic disease. *Obstet Gynecol* 1997;**89**:272–5.

102. Pal M, Williams B. Prevalence of maternal red cell alloimmunisation: A population study from Queensland, Australia. *Pathology* 2015;**47**:151–5.

103. Yasuda H, Ohto H, Nollet KE, et al. Hemolytic disease of the fetus and newborn with late-onset anemia due to anti-M: A case report and review of the Japanese literature. *Transfus Med Rev* 2014;**28**:1–6.

104. De Young-Owens A, Kennedy M, Rose RL, Boyle J, O'Shaughnessy R. Anti-M isoimmunization: Management and outcome at the Ohio State University from 1969 to 1995. *Obstet Gynecol* 1997;**90**:962–6.

105. Duguid JK, Bromilow IM, Entwistle GD, Wilkinson R. Haemolytic disease of the newborn due to anti-M. *Vox Sang* 1995;**68**:195–6.

106. Mayne KM, Bowell PJ, Green SJ, Entwistle CC. The significance of anti-S sensitization in pregnancy. *Clin Lab Haematol* 1990;**12**:105–7.

107. Smith G, Knott P, Rissik J, de la Fuente J, Win N. Anti-U and haemolytic disease of the fetus and newborn. *Br J Obstet Gynaecol* 1998;**105**:1318–21.

108. Novaretti MC, Jens E, Pagliarini T, et al. Hemolytic disease of the newborn due to anti-U. *Rev Hosp Clin Fac Med Sao Paulo* 2003;**58**:320–3.

109. Zipursky A, Paul VK. The global burden of Rh disease. *Arch Dis Child Fetal Neonatal Ed* 2011;**96**:F84–85.

110. Clarke CA, Mollison PL. Deaths from Rh haemolytic disease of the fetus and newborn, 1977–87. *J R Coll Physicians Lond* 1989;**23**:181–4.

111. McMaster Conference on Prevention of Rh Immunization 28–30 September, 1977. *Vox Sang* 1979;**36**:50–64.

112. Joseph KS, Kramer MS. The decline in Rh hemolytic disease: Should Rh prophylaxis get all the credit? *Am J Public Health* 1998;**88**:209–15.

113. Trolle B. Prenatal Rh-immune prophylaxis with 300 micrograms immune globulin anti-D in the 28th week of pregnancy. *Acta Obstet Gynecol Scand* 1989;**68**:45–7.

114. Queenan JT, Gadow EC, Lopes AC. Role of spontaneous abortion in Rh immunization. *Am J Obstet Gynecol* 1971;**110**:128–30.

115. Queenan JT, Kubarych SF, Shah S, Holland B. Role of induced abortion in rhesus immunisation. *Lancet* 1971;**1**:815–17.

116. Tabsh KM, Lebherz TB, Crandall BF. Risks of prophylactic anti-D immunoglobulin after second-trimester amniocentesis. *Am J Obstet Gynecol* 1984;**149**:225–6.

117. Brandenburg H, Jahoda MG, Pijpers L, Wladimiroff JW. Rhesus sensitization after midtrimester genetic amniocentesis. *Am J Med Genet* 1989;**32**:225–6.

118. Daffos F, Capella-Pavlovsky M, Forestier F. Fetal blood sampling during pregnancy with use of a needle guided by ultrasound: A study of 606 consecutive cases. *Am J Obstet Gynecol* 1985;**153**:655–60.

119. Bowman JM, Pollock JM, Peterson LE, et al. Fetomaternal hemorrhage following funipuncture: Increase in severity of maternal red-cell alloimmunization. *Obstet Gynecol* 1994;**84**:839–43.

120. Blakemore KJ, Baumgarten A, Schoenfeld-Dimaio M, et al. Rise in maternal serum alpha-fetoprotein concentration after chorionic villus sampling and the possibility of isoimmunization. *Am J Obstet Gynecol* 1986;**155**:988–93.

121. Jansen MW, Brandenburg H, Wildschut HI, et al. The effect of chorionic villus sampling on the

number of fetal cells isolated from maternal blood and on maternal serum alpha-fetoprotein levels. *Prenat Diagn* 1997;**17**:953–9.

122. Rose PG, Strohm PL, Zuspan FP. Fetomaternal hemorrhage following trauma. *Am J Obstet Gynecol* 1985;**153**:844–7.

123. Boucher M, Marquette GP, Varin J, Champagne J, Bujold E. Fetomaternal hemorrhage during external cephalic version. *Obstet Gynecol* 2008;**112**:79–84.

124. An assessment of the hazards of amniocentesis. Report to the Medical Research Council by their Working Party on Amniocentesis. *Br J Obstet Gynaecol* 1978;**85** Suppl **2**:1–41.

125. Simonovits I, Timar I, Bajtai G. Rate of Rh immunization after induced abortion. *Vox Sang* 1980;**38**:161–4.

126. USPST Task Force. Screening for D (Rh) Incompatibility. In USPST Task Force *Guide to Clinical Preventive Services* 2nd ed. (Washington, DC: Office of Disease Prevention and Health Promotion, 1996).

127. Committee on Practice Bulletins-Obstetrics. Practice Bulletin No. 181: Prevention of Rh D alloimmunization. *Obstet Gynecol* 2017;**130**:e57–e70.

128. Moise KJ,Jr. , GandhiM, Boring NH, et al. Circulating cell-free DNA to determine the fetal RHD status in all three trimesters of pregnancy. *Obstet Gynecol* 2016;**128**:1340–6.

129. Vivanti A, Benachi A, Huchet FX, et al. Diagnostic accuracy of fetal rhesus D genotyping using cell-free fetal DNA during the first trimester of pregnancy. *Am J Obstet Gynecol* 2016;**215**:606e601–606 e605.

130. de Haas M, Thurik FF, van der Ploeg CP, et al. Sensitivity of fetal RHD screening for safe guidance of targeted anti-D immunoglobulin prophylaxis: Prospective cohort study of a nationwide programme in the Netherlands. *BMJ* 2016;**355**:i5789.

131. Sandler SG, Flegel WA, Westhoff CM, et al. It's time to phase in RHD genotyping for patients with a serologic weak D phenotype. College of American Pathologists Transfusion Medicine Resource Committee Work Group.*Transfusion* 2015;**55**:680–9.

132. Liley AW. Liquor amnil analysis in the management of the pregnancy complicated by resus sensitization. *Am J Obstet Gynecol* 1961;**82**:1359–70.

133. Queenan JT, Tomai TP, Ural SH, King JC. Deviation in amniotic fluid optical density at a wavelength of 450 nm in Rh-immunized pregnancies from 14 to 40 weeks' gestation: A proposal for clinical management. *Am J Obstet Gynecol* 1993;**168**:1370–6.

134. Mari G, Deter RL, Carpenter RL, et al. Noninvasive diagnosis by Doppler ultrasonography of fetal anemia due to maternal red-cell alloimmunization. Collaborative Group for Doppler Assessment of the Blood Velocity in Anemic Fetuses. *N Engl J Med* 2000;**342**:9–14.

135. Zwiers C, van Kamp I, Oepkes D, Lopriore E. Intrauterine transfusion and non-invasive treatment options for hemolytic disease of the fetus and newborn: Review on current management and outcome. *Expert Rev Hematol* 2017;**10**:337–44.

136. Lindenburg IT, Smits-Wintjens VE, van Klink JM, et al. Long-term neurodevelopmental outcome after intrauterine transfusion for hemolytic disease of the fetus/newborn: The LOTUS study. *Am J Obstet Gynecol* 2012;**206**:141 e141-148.

137. Watson WJ, Wax JR, Miller RC, Brost BC. Prevalence of new maternal alloantibodies after intrauterine transfusion for severe Rhesus disease. *Am J Perinatol* 2006;**23**:189–92.

138. Nicolaides KH, Soothill PW, Clewell WH, et al. Fetal haemoglobin measurement in the assessment of red cell isoimmunisation. *Lancet* 1988;**1**:1073–5.

139. Scheier M, Hernandez-Andrade E, Fonseca EB, Nicolaides KH. Prediction of severe fetal anemia in red blood cell alloimmunization after previous intrauterine transfusions. *Am J Obstet Gynecol* 2006;**195**:1550–6.

140. Papantoniou N, Sifakis S, Antsaklis A. Therapeutic management of fetal anemia: Review of standard practice and alternative treatment options. *J Perinat Med* 2013;**41**:71–82.

141. Schumacher B, Moise KJ, Jr. Fetal transfusion for red blood cell alloimmunization in pregnancy. *Obstet Gynecol* 1996;**88**:137–50.

142. Lindenburg IT, van Kamp IL, van Zwet EW, et al. Increased perinatal loss after intrauterine transfusion for alloimmune anaemia before 20 weeks of gestation. *BJOG* 2013;**120**:847–52.

143. Vats K, Watchko JF. Coordinating care across the perinatal continuum in hemolytic disease of the fetus and newborn: The timely handoff of a positive maternal anti-erythrocyte antibody Screen. *J Pediatr* 2019;**214**:212–16.

144. Goplerud CP, White CA, Bradbury JT, Briggs TL. The first Rh-isoimmunized pregnancy. *Am J Obstet Gynecol* 1973;**115**:632–8.

145. Herschel M, Karrison T, Wen M, Caldarelli L, Baron B. Isoimmunization is unlikely to be the cause of hemolysis in ABO-incompatible but direct antiglobulin test-negative neonates. *Pediatrics* 2002;**110**:127–30.

146. Cashore WJ. Neonatal hyperbilirubinemia. In McMillan JA, Feigin RD, DeAngelis CD, Jones MDJ, eds. *Oski's Pediatrics* 4th ed. (Philadelphia, PA: Lippincott, Williams & Wilkins; 2006), pp. 235–45.

147. Christensen RD, Agarwal AM, George TI, Bhutani VK, Yaish HM. Acute neonatal bilirubin encephalopathy in the State of Utah 2009–2018. *Blood Cells Mol Dis* 2018;**72**:10–13.

148. American Academy of Pediatrics Subcommittee on Hyperbilirubinemia. Management of hyperbilirubinemia in the newborn infant 35 or more weeks of gestation [published correction appears in *Pediatrics* 2004;114(4):1138]. *Pediatrics* 2004;**114**(1):297–316.

149. Alcock GS, Liley H. Immunoglobulin infusion for isoimmune haemolytic jaundice in neonates. *Cochrane Database of Systematic Reviews* 2002;**3**: CD003313.

150. Zwiers C, Scheffer-Rath MEA, Lopriore E, de Haas M, Liley HG. Immunoglobulin for alloimmune hemolytic disease in neonates. *Cochrane Database of Systematic Reviews* 2018;**3**: CD003313.

151. Watchko JF. Emergency release uncross-matched packed red blood cells for immediate double volume exchange transfusion in neonates with intermediate to advanced acute bilirubin encephalopathy: Timely but insufficient? *J Perinatol* 2018;**38**:947–53.

152. Blackall DP, Pesek GD, Montgomery MM, et al. Hemolytic disease of the fetus and newborn due to anti-Ge3: Combined antibody-dependent hemolysis and erythroid precursor cell growth inhibition. *Am J Perinatol* 2008;**25**:541–5.

153. Dorn I, Schlenke P, Hartel C. Prolonged anemia in an intrauterine-transfused neonate with Rh-hemolytic disease: No evidence for anti-D-related suppression of erythropoiesis in vitro. *Transfusion* 2010;**50**:1064–70.

154. Rath ME, Smits-Wintjens VE, Lindenburg IT, et al. Exchange transfusions and top-up transfusions in neonates with Kell haemolytic disease compared to Rh D haemolytic disease. *Vox Sang* 2011;**100**:312–16.

155. Bhutani VK, Zipursky A, Blencowe H, et al. Neonatal hyperbilirubinemia and Rhesus disease of the newborn: Incidence and impairment estimates for 2010 at regional and global levels. *Pediatr Res* 2013;**74** Suppl 1:86–100.

156. Osaro E, Charles AT. Rh isoimmunization in sub-Saharan Africa indicates need for universal access to anti-RhD immunoglobulin and effective management of D-negative pregnancies. *Int J Womens Health* 2010;**2**:429–37.

157. Kancherla V, Oakley GP, Jr., Brent RL. Urgent global opportunities to prevent birth defects. *Semin Fetal Neonatal Med* 2014;**19**:153–60.

158. Waldron P, de Alarcón P. ABO hemolytic disease of the newborn: A unique constellation of findings in siblings and review of protective mechanisms in the fetal-maternal system. *Am J Perinatol* 1999;**16**:391–8.

159. Sherer DM, Abramowicz JS, Ryan RM, et al. Severe fetal hydrops resulting from ABO incompatibility. *Obstet Gynecol* 1991;**78**:897–9.

160. Lacey PA, Caskey CR, Werner DJ, Moulds JJ. Fatal hemolytic disease of a newborn due to anti-D in an Rh-positive Du variant mother. *Transfusion* 1983;**23**:91–4.

161. Bowman JM, Pollock JM, Manning FA, Harman CR. Severe anti-C hemolytic disease of the newborn. *Am J Obstet Gynecol* 1992;**166**:1239–43.

162. Macher S, Wagner T, Rosskopf K, et al. Severe case of fetal hemolytic disease caused by anti-C(w) requiring serial intrauterine transfusions complicated by pancytopenia and cholestasis. *Transfusion* 2016;**56**:80–3.

163. Malik S, Moiz B. Clinical significance of maternal anti-Cw antibodies: A review of three cases and literature. *J Pak Med Assoc* 2012;**62**:620–1.

164. Grobel RK, Cardy JD. Hemolytic disease of the newborn due to anti-EW. A fourth example of the Rh antigen, EW. *Transfusion* 1971;**11**:77–8.

165. Jakobowicz R, Whittingham S, Barrie JU, Simmons RT. A further investigation on polyvalent anti-C (rh') and anti-G (rhg) antibodies produced by iso-immunization in pregnancy. *Med J Aust* 1962;**49**(1):896–7.

166. Li BJ, Jiang YJ, Yuan F, Ye HX. Exchange transfusion of least incompatible blood for severe hemolytic disease of the newborn due to anti-Rh17. *Transfus Med* 2010;**20**:66–9.

167. Vaughan JI, Warwick R, Welch CR, Letsky EA. Anti-Kell in pregnancy. *Br J Obstet Gynaecol* 1991;**98**:944–5.

168. Moncharmont P, Juron-Dupraz F, Doillon M, Vignal M, Debeaux P. A case of hemolytic disease of the newborn infant due to anti-K (Cellano). *Acta Haematol* 1991;**85**:45–6.

169. Bowman JM, Harman FA, Manning CR, Pollock JM. Erythroblastosis fetalis produced by anti-k. *Vox Sang* 1989;**56**:187–9.

170. Duguid JKM, Bromilow IM. Haemolytic disease of the newborn due to anti-k. *Vox Sang* 1990;**58**:69–72.

171. Moulds JM, Persa R, Rierson D, et al. Three novel alleles in the Kell blood group system resulting in the Knull phenotype and the first in a Native American. *Transfusion* 2013;**53**:2867–71.

172. Jovanovic-Srzentic S, Djokic M, Tijanic N, et al. Antibodies detected in samples from 21,730 pregnant women. *Immunohematology* 2003;**19**:89–92.

173. Mittal K, Sood T, Bansal N, et al. Clinical significance of rare maternal anti Jk(a) antibody. *Indian J Hematol Blood Transfus.* 2016;**32**:497–9.

174. Ishida A, Ohto H, Yasuda H, et al. Anti-M antibody induced prolonged anemia following hemolytic disease of the newborn due to erythropoietic suppression in 2 siblings. *J Pediatr Hematol Oncol* 2015;**37**:e375–377.

175. Wu KH, Chu SL, Chang JG, Shih MC, Peng CT. Haemolytic disease of the newborn due to maternal irregular antibodies in the Chinese population in Taiwan. *Transfus Med* 2003;**13**:311–14.

176. Telischi M, Behzad O, Issitt PD, Pavone BG. Hemolytic disease of the newborn due to anti-N. *Vox Sang* 1976;**31**:109–16.

177. Moncharmont P, Buclet D, Trouilloud C, Peyrard T, Rigal D. Severe hemolytic disease of the fetus and the newborn associated with anti-Vw (Vw). *J Matern Fetal Neonatal Med* 2010;**23**:1066–8.

178. Field TE, Wilson TE, Dawes BJ, Giles CM. Haemolytic disease of the newborn due to anti-Mt a. *Vox Sang* 1972;**22**:432–7.

179. Cheung CC, Challis D, Fisher G, et al. Anti-Mta associated with three cases of hemolytic disease of the newborn. *Immunohematology* 2002;**18**:37–9.

180. Wu KH, Chang JG, Lin M, et al. Hydrops foetalis caused by anti-Mur in first pregnancy–a case report. *Transfus Med* 2002;**12**:325–7.

181. Brooks S, Squires JE. Hemolytic disease of the fetus and newborn caused by anti-Lan. *Transfusion.* 2014;**54**:1317–20.

182. Davies J, Day S, Milne A, Roy A, Simpson S. Haemolytic disease of the foetus and newborn caused by auto anti-LW. *Transfus Med* 2009;**19**:218–19.

183. Francis BJ, Hatcher DE. Hemolytic disease of the newborn apparently caused by anti-Lu-a. *Transfusion* 1961;**1**:248–50.

184. Scheffer H, Tamaki HT. Anti-Lu-b and mild hemolytic disease of the newborn: A case report. *Transfusion* 1966;**6**:497–8.

185. Dube VE, Zoes CS. Subclinical hemolytic disease of the newborn associated with IgG anti-Lub. *Transfusion* 1982;**22**:251–3.

186. Abhyankar S, Silfen S, Rao SP, Vinciguerra C, Dimiaio TM. Positive cord blood "DAT" due to anti-Le(a): Absence of hemolytic disease of the newborn. *Am J Pediatr Hematol Oncol* 1989;**11**:184–5.

187. Carreras Vescio LA, Torres OW, Virgilio OS, Pizzolato M. Mild hemolytic disease of the newborn due to anti-Lewis(a). *Vox Sang* 1993;**64**:194–5.

188. Bharucha ZS, Joshi SR, Bhatia HM. Hemolytic disease of the newborn due to anti-Le. *Vox Sang* 1981;**41**:36–9.

189. Reid ME, Ellisor SS. Hemolytic disease of newborn due to anti-Leb. *Vox Sang* 1982;**42**:278.

190. Joshi SR, Wagner FF, Vasantha K, Panjwani SR, Flegel WA. An AQP1 null allele in an Indian woman with Co(a-b-) phenotype and high-titer anti-Co3 associated with mild HDN. *Transfusion* 2001;**41**:1273–8.

191. Sacks DA, Johnson CS, Platt LD. Isoimmunization in pregnancy to Gerbich antigen. *Am J Perinatol* 1985;**2**:208–10.

192. Pate LL, Myers JC, Palma JP, et al. Anti-Ge3 causes late-onset hemolytic disease of the newborn: The fourth case in three Hispanic families. *Transfusion* 2013;**53**:2152–7.

193. DeMarco M, Uhl L, Fields L, et al. Hemolytic disease of the newborn due to the Scianna antibody, anti-Sc2. *Transfusion* 1995;**35**:58–60.

194. Rauch S, Ritgen J, Wisskirchen M, et al. A case of anti-Rd causing fetal anemia. *Transfusion* 2017;**57**:1485–7.

195. Nakajima H, Ito K. An example of anti-Jra causing hemolytic disease of the newborn and frequency of Jra antigen in the Japanese population. *Vox Sang* 1978;**35**:265–7.

196. Masumoto A, Masuyama H, Sumida Y, Segawa T, Hiramatsu Y. Successful management of anti-Jra alloimmunization in pregnancy: A case report. *Gynecol Obstet Invest* 2010;**69**:81–3.

197. Takabayashi T, Murakami M, Yajima H, et al. Influence of maternal antibody anti-Jra on the baby: A case report and pedigree chart. *Tohoku J Exp Med* 1985;**145**:97–101.

198. Ishihara Y, Miyata S, Chiba Y, Kawai T. Successful treatment of extremely severe fetal anemia due to anti-Jra alloimmunization. *Fetal Diagn Ther* 2006;**21**:269–71.

199. Braschler T, Vokt CA, Hustinx H, et al. Management of a pregnant woman with

anti-holley alloantibody. *Transfus Med Hemother* 2015;**42**:129–30.

200. Ferguson SJ, Boyce F, Blajchman MA. Anti-Ytb in pregnancy. *Transfusion* 1979;**19**:581–2.

201. Moulds MK. Serological investigation and clinical significance of high-titer, low-avidity (HTLA) antibodies. *Am J Med Technol* 1981;**47**:789–95.

202. Maayan-Metzger A, Schwartz T, Sulkes J, Merlob P. Maternal anti-D prophylaxis during pregnancy does not cause neonatal haemolysis. *Arch Dis Child Fetal Neonatal Ed* 2001;**84**:F60–62.

203. Cohen DN, Johnson MS, Liang WH, McDaniel HL, Young PP. Clinically significant hemolytic disease of the newborn secondary to passive transfer of anti-D from maternal RhIG. *Transfusion* 2014;**54**:2863–6.

Neonatal Hemolysis

Bertil Glader and Aditi Kamdar

This chapter focuses on the recognition and management of hemolysis in newborn infants (Table 10.1). Some of the common hemolytic anemias of childhood first appear in the newborn period, while others do not present until several months of age, and a few rare hemolytic disorders occur only in the neonatal period. These variations in the age that hemolytic anemia first presents reflect differences in neonatal erythropoiesis, hemoglobin synthesis, and the metabolism of newborn erythrocytes. When approaching an infant with a potential hemolytic disorder, the first issue to be addressed is whether there is evidence of increased red-cell destruction and accelerated production. If yes, then the next question to consider is whether the cause of neonatal hemolysis is due to extracellular (acquired) factors or an intrinsic (genetic) red-cell defect. Acquired disorders are those that are immune mediated, associated with infection, or accompany some other underlying pathology. Inherited red-cell disorders are due to defects in the cell membrane, abnormalities in red

blood cell (RBC) metabolism, or a consequence of a hemoglobin defect.

Evaluation of a neonate for hemolysis must be considered in the context of normal newborn physiology. The RBC lifespan in term neonates (80–100 days) and in premature infants (60–80 days) is shorter than in older children and adults (100–120 days) [1]. The reason for the reduced RBC survival observed in newborns is not known, but it has been thought to be due to the many biochemical differences between adult and neonatal RBCs [2–4]. Increased oxidant sensitivity of newborn red cells and relative instability of fetal hemoglobin have been considered as possible causes for this shortened lifespan [5]. Of interest, however, are recent studies using biotin labelled adult and neonatal RBC demonstrated that red cell survival in neonates was not that different: neonatal RBC survival (54.2+/−11.2 days) versus adult RBC survival (70.1+/−19.1 days) [6, 7]. Moreover, the survival of labeled adult RBC in neonates was much shorter than the 120-day lifespan seen when infused into

Table 10.1 Causes of hemolytic anemia during the newborn period

Acquired RBC Disorders
Alloimmune hemolysis (Rh and ABO incompatibility)
Immune hemolytic anemia due to maternal disease (SLE) or drugs Congenital infections (CMV, toxoplasmosis, syphilis)
Bacterial sepsis
They are separate causes of hemolysis:

1) Disseminate and localized intravascular coagulation
2) Vitamine E deficiency
3) Infantile pyknocytosis

Hereditary RBC Disorders
Membrane defects (hereditary spherocytosis, hereditary elliptocytosis)
Enzyme deficiencies (glucose-6-phosphate dehydrogenase, pyruvate kinase) Hemoglobinopathies (alpha-thalassemia syndromes, gamma-beta-thalassemia)
Unstable hemoglobins

Notes: CMV, cytomegalovirus; RBC, red blood cell; SLE, systemic lupus erythematosus

Neonatal Hematology, Pathogenesis, Diagnosis, and Management of Hematologic Problems, 3rd edition, ed. Pedro A. de Alarcón, Eric J. Werner, Robert D. Christensen, and Martha C. Sola-Visner. Published by Cambridge University Press. © Cambridge University Press 2021.

healthy adults. These studies provide evidence that the circulatory environment of infants may be an important determinant of RBC survival rather than just factors intrinsic to the neonatal RBC.

Laboratory Features of Neonatal Hemolysis

A common clinical presentation of hemolytic anemia in older children is anemia, reticulocytosis, and hyperbilirubinemia. In the newborn infant, however, because of the normal hematologic adaptations to extrauterine life, the degree of hyperbilirubinemia and reticulocytosis must be interpreted in terms of the values appropriate for gestational and postgestational age. Also, some tests used to assess RBC production and destruction in older children have limited usefulness in the newborn.

Evidence for Anemia and Increased Red Blood Cell Production

The normal hemoglobin (Hb) concentration at birth is 14–20 g/dl (mean approximately 17 g/dl), decreasing to a level of 11 g/dl over 3 to 4 months [2, 8]. This hemoglobin decrement, referred to as the physiologic anemia of infancy, occurs as part of the normal adaptation to extrauterine life. It is a transition from a hypoxic milieu with an elevated RBC mass to a well-oxygenated environment with excess oxygen-carrying capacity. In the presence of mild hemolysis (commonly seen with ABO incompatibility), the magnitude of anemia may be minimal and obscured by the physiologic anemia of infancy. In infants with more significant hemolysis, the extent of anemia also is a reflection of the infant's capacity for increasing RBC production. In many congenital hemolytic disorders, it is not uncommon to observe worse anemia in infancy compared with later in childhood, presumably a reflection of less available marrow capacity in neonates.

As fetal erythropoiesis diminishes, the mean corpuscular volume (MCV) decreases from birth (100–130 fl) to one year of age (70–85 fl). The elevated MCV at birth has implications on how we define neonatal microcytosis and thereby recognize certain disorders, such as alpha-thalassemia, in newborns [2, 9].

The normal reticulocyte count of children and older infants is 1%–2%. The reticulocyte count in term infants ranges between 3% and 7% at birth, but this decreases to 1% to 3% by 4 days and to less than 1% by 7 days of age [2]. In premature infants, reticulocyte values at birth are higher (6%–10%) and may remain elevated for a longer period of time. With significant hemolysis, neonates usually demonstrate increased reticulocytosis. However, as noted above, because the physiologic anemia of infancy is a response to excess oxygen-carrying capacity, mild hemolysis might not be sensed as an oxygen deficit and, hence, no increased erythropoiesis or reticulocytosis may be observed. Nucleated RBCs are seen in newborn infants, but they generally disappear by the third day of life in term infants and in 7 to 10 days in premature infants. The persistence of reticulocytosis or nucleated RBCs suggests the possibility of hemolysis. Hypoxia, in the absence of anemia, also can be associated with increased release of reticulocytes and nucleated RBCs. In the presence of hemolysis, the bone marrow manifests erythroid hyperplasia, but examination of the bone marrow rarely is utilized to diagnose hemolysis in neonates.

The peripheral blood smear in many hemolytic disorders reveals abnormal red-cell morphology. In newborn infants, however, the peripheral blood smear can be misleading unless "normal" RBC morphology for this age group is appreciated. Morphological characteristics of RBCs are consistent with the normal state of relative hyposplenism in newborn infants [9]. Howell–Jolly bodies, target cells, siderocytes, and other bizarre forms can be seen in normal neonates [10], and this is even more marked in premature infants. Just as with many other characteristics of the neonatal RBC, the red-cell morphologic changes found in the newborn period disappear by 3 to 4 months of age.

Evidence for Increased Red Blood Cell Destruction

Elevated serum unconjugated (indirect) bilirubin concentration with normal liver function is a useful marker of accelerated red-cell destruction in children and adults. In neonates, however, the normal increase in serum bilirubin concentration must be considered when evaluating for hemolysis. Bilirubin production in neonates is greater than in adults because of the increased circulating red-cell mass at birth, the decreased survival of neonatal red cells, and the increased enterohepatic circulation of bilirubin [11]. In addition, there is transiently reduced glucuronyl transferase activity, which impairs hepatic bilirubin conjugation

[12]. As a consequence of these phenomena, physiological hyperbilirubinemia normally occurs in newborn infants, and bilirubin concentrations as high as 12 mg/dl (peak at 4 days) are seen in term neonates, and levels up to 15 mg/dl (peak at 7 days) are observed in premature infants. However, in association with hemolysis, serum bilirubin concentrations exceed these physiological levels and clinical jaundice may appear before 36 hours of age. Moreover, since mild hemolysis can occur without anemia or significant reticulocytosis, excessive hyperbilirubinemia often is the only manifestation of neonatal hemolytic disease. The decision to monitor bilirubin levels and to evaluate for underlying hemolysis is based on the Bhutani risk curves of total bilirubin concentration as a function of age [13] . Beyond the first few days of life, other metabolic problems and breast feeding can cause hyperbilirubinemia and further confound the recognition of increased red-cell destruction.

Carbon monoxide generation in humans is from the breakdown of heme, and is transported in the blood as carboxyhemoglobin. Measurement of blood carboxyhemoglobin levels can be used as a marker of accelerated red-cell destruction [14]. Also, exhaled carbon monoxide from the lungs can be measured directly to document increased RBC destruction [15, 16]. A noninvasive instrument to measure exhaled carbon monoxide is commercially available and appears to be a reliable marker of increased breakdown of hemoglobin to bilirubin [17, 18]. A neonate with hyperbilirubinemia and increased carbon monoxide production needs close monitoring because the cause of the elevated bilirubin is due to ongoing destruction of RBCs. This infant needs further evaluation to determine the cause of hemolysis.

Elevated serum lactic dehydrogenase (LDH) also is a marker of accelerated erythrocyte destruction; however, it is usually hyperbilirubinemia that initiates a work-up for neonatal hemolysis.

Other tests are available to assess for hemolysis, but most have limited utility in newborns. Serum haptoglobin is an alpha-2 glycoprotein that reacts with free hemoglobin to form a complex that is removed by the reticuloendothelial system. Since synthesis of this protein is not stimulated by hemolysis or clearance of the hemoglobin–haptoglobin complexes, reduced levels of serum haptoglobin are a reasonable marker of intravascular hemolysis. In neonates, however, haptoglobin levels are low and normal child or adult values may not be achieved until several months of age [19]. Thus, the serum haptoglobin concentration is not a reliable parameter of hemolysis in newborns.

Acquired Hemolytic Anemias in the Newborn

Alloimmune Hemolysis

Maternal sensitization to fetal RBC antigens inherited from the father and the ensuing placental transfer of maternal antibodies directed against fetal RBC antigens is the most common cause of neonatal hemolysis (see Chapter 9). The spectrum of clinical problems ranges from minimal anemia and hyperbilirubinemia to severe anemia with hydrops. At one time, before prevention of Rh sensitization was possible, hemolytic disease of the newborn was responsible for more than 10,000 deaths annually in the USA [20], but now the overall incidence of alloimmune hemolysis has decreased dramatically. Nevertheless, hemolysis due to Rh D incompatibility does still exist worldwide in areas where immunoprophylaxis is not readily available. At our institution in California, we have observed hemolysis in several neonates whose mothers had resided in Mexico and did not receive immunoprophylaxis with previous pregnancies. Today, the majority of alloimmune hemolysis cases in neonates are due to ABO incompatibility and, to a lesser extent, due to sensitization to Kell, Duffy, Kidd, and other Rh antigens. Since alloimmune hemolysis is the most common cause of neonatal hemolytic anemia, testing for antibody on neonatal RBCs is a necessary initial step in the evaluation of any newborn with hemolysis. This is accomplished with the direct antiglobulin test (DAT), also known as the direct Coombs' test, which detects the presence of antibody on RBC. Only after alloimmune hemolysis is ruled out should one consider the work-up for other causes of neonatal hemolytic anemia. The specific tests used to diagnose other causes of hemolysis are discussed later in this chapter.

Immune Hemolytic Anemia Due to Maternal Disease

Maternal autoimmune hemolytic anemia or lupus erythematosus during pregnancy may be associated with passive transfer of immunoglobulin G (IgG) antibody to the fetus [21]. The diagnosis is suggested by the presence of neonatal hemolytic disease, a positive DAT, absence of Rh, or ABO incompatibility, and antiglobulin-positive hemolysis in the mother.

Hemolytic Anemia Due to Maternal Drug Intake

Maternal drug intake can lead to hemolysis in the fetus and neonate. One such example is seen with dapsone (diaminodiphenylsulfone), which is used for the prevention and treatment of *Pneumocystis carinii* infection, leprosy, and a variety of dermatologic disorders. A dose-related hemolytic anemia is recognized as a complication of this drug therapy in normal adults and children. Neonatal hemolysis has occurred when mothers were taking dapsone during pregnancy [22].

Infection

Congenital infections due to cytomegalovirus (CMV), toxoplasmosis, or syphilis, as well as bacterial sepsis, can be associated with hemolytic anemia, and frequently some degree of thrombocytopenia also exists. In association with congenital infections, often there is hepatosplenomegaly and other stigmata such as cataracts and microcephaly. In cases of bacterial sepsis, both the direct and indirect bilirubin may be elevated. The mechanism of hemolysis is not defined clearly, but it is thought to be related in part to RBC sequestration and macrophage activation associated with infection. In addition, certain bacteria may produce enzymes (phospholipases, neuraminidase) that affect membrane lipids or alter the normal RBC glycoprotein surface structure. Neuraminidase cleavage of sialic acid residues from membrane sialoglycoproteins results in a decreased surface charge and shortened red cell survival [23].

Microangiopathic (Schistocytic) Anemia

The presence of many fragmented RBC or schistocytes in the peripheral blood suggests that hemolysis is due to altered erythrocyte–blood-vessel wall interactions. Abnormalities of the placental microcirculation or macrovascular anomalies such as an umbilical-vein varix are rare causes of congenital schistocytic anemia [24]. Also, schistocytic hemolytic anemia occurs as a component of disseminated intravascular coagulation (DIC) and this is secondary to the deposition of fibrin within the vascular walls. When erythrocytes interact with fibrin, fragments of RBCs are broken off, producing fragile schistocytes that are removed by macrophages in the reticuloendothelial tissues.

Vitamin E Deficiency

Premature infants are endowed at birth with significantly less vitamin E than term infants. Unless supplemental vitamin E is provided, this deficiency state persists for 2 to 3 months. Vitamin E is an antioxidant compound vital to the integrity of erythrocytes; in its absence, these cells are susceptible to lipid peroxidation and membrane injury. One clinical consequence of vitamin E deficiency is that hemolytic anemia can occur in small premature infants (weighing less than 1,500 g) at 6 to 10 weeks of age [25, 26]. This hemolytic anemia, which is characterized by reduced vitamin E levels and increased RBC peroxide hemolysis, disappears rapidly following vitamin E administration. At one time, it was thought that vitamin E deficiency might contribute to the anemia of prematurity in a more general sense. In fact, in one study performed several years ago, premature infants given daily vitamin E (15 IU per day) had higher hemoglobin levels and lower reticulocyte levels than a control group not given the vitamin [25]. However, these vitamin E supplemented babies still had lower hemoglobin concentrations than term newborns, indicating that anemia of prematurity is caused largely by other factors, such as erythropoietin deficiency. Although it has become standard practice to administer vitamin E to all premature infants, some still may develop hemolytic anemia. Those with anemia, reticulocytosis and an oxygen requirement may benefit from additional vitamin E [27].

Infantile Pyknocytosis

Pyknocytes are abnormal, densely staining erythrocytes with a distorted, irregularly contracted appearance with few, irregular, short projections. Pyknocytes account for up to 2% of the erythrocytes in a term infant's peripheral blood smear and up to 6% of the erythrocytes in a preterm infant's peripheral blood smear [28]. Infantile pyknocytosis is an infrequently observed hemolytic anemia of variable severity. It was initially described by Tuffy and colleagues [29] and has been noted by several investigators since that time [30–38]. Clinical manifestations include hemolysis, pallor, jaundice, and, occasionally, hepatosplenomegaly. Laboratory features

Table 10.2 Classification of erythrocyte membrane disorders

Disorder	Gene	Protein	Inheritance
Hereditary spherocytosis	ANK1	Ankyrin-1	AD
	SPTB	Spectrin β chain	AD
	SPTA1	Spectrin α chain	AR
	SLC4A1	Band 3 anion transport protein	AD
	EPB42	Erythrocyte membrane protein band 4.2	AR
Hereditary elliptocytosis	EPB41	Protein band 4.1	AD
	SPTA1	Spectrin α chain	AD
	SPTB	Spectrin β chain	AD
Hereditary pyropoikilocytosis	SPTA1	Spectrin a chain	AR
Ovalocytosis Southeast Asian type	SLC4A1	Band 3 anion transport protein	AD
Overhydrated hereditary stomatocytosis	RHAG	Ammonium transporter Rh type A	AD
Dehydrated hereditary stomatocytosis	PIEZO1	Piezo-type mechanosensitive ion channel	AD
Familial pseudohyperkalemia	ABCB6	ATP-binding cassette sub-family B member 6	AD
Cryohydrocytosis	SLC4A1	Band 3 anion transport protein	AD

include anemia, reticulocytosis, and an elevation in aspartate aminotransferase (AST). Increased numbers of pyknocytes, blister cells and polychromatophilia are apparent on the peripheral blood smear. Infantile pyknocytosis is largely a diagnosis of exclusion. Similar morphology may be observed with other hemolytic disorders, G-6-PD deficiency [30], pyruvate kinase deficiency, and vitamin E deficiency [25]. Hereditary elliptocytosis and microangiopathic hemolytic disorders also may produce similar-appearing RBCs. These causes of hemolytic anemia should be ruled out in the evaluation of any infant with proposed infantile pyknocytosis.

Hemolysis Due to Hereditary Red Blood Cell Membrane Disorders

The RBC membrane structure has three major components: (1) a bilayer of phospholipids intercalated with molecules of unesterified cholesterol and glycolipids; (2) integral membrane proteins (antigens, receptors) that penetrate or span the lipid bilayer, interact with the hydrophobic lipid core, and are bound tightly to the membrane; and (3) a separate protein network that forms the membrane cytoskeleton (spectrin, ankyrin, and several other proteins) interacting with both the integral membrane proteins and the lipid bilayer. Abnormalities in the quantity and/or quality of these proteins and their interaction with each other are the cause of the two most common inherited RBC membrane disorders

hereditary spherocytosis and hereditary elliptocytosis (Table 10.2). Numerous DNA mutations have been identified, and several excellent reviews of the advances in these diseases are available [39, 40]. Both hereditary spherocytosis (HS) and hereditary elliptocytosis (HE) are associated with neonatal hemolysis.

Hereditary Spherocytosis

Hereditary **spherocytosis** (HS) is the most common hereditary hemolytic anemia among people of northern European background. In the USA, the incidence of the disorder is approximately 1 in 5,000 [41, 42]. In most affected families, HS is transmitted as an autosomal dominant trait, and identification of the disorder in multiple generations of affected families is the rule. Nearly one-quarter of all newly diagnosed patients do not demonstrate a dominant inheritance pattern, and the parents of these patients are clinically and hematologically normal. New mutations have been implicated to explain some of these sporadic cases. Also, autosomal recessive mode of inheritance accounts for some cases of HS and is clinically manifested only in homozygous or compound heterozygous individuals, often associated with severe hemolytic anemia [43, 44].

The hallmark of the disorder is the presence of spherocytes, RBCs that have become spheroid because of a loss of membrane surface (Fig. 10.1a).

159

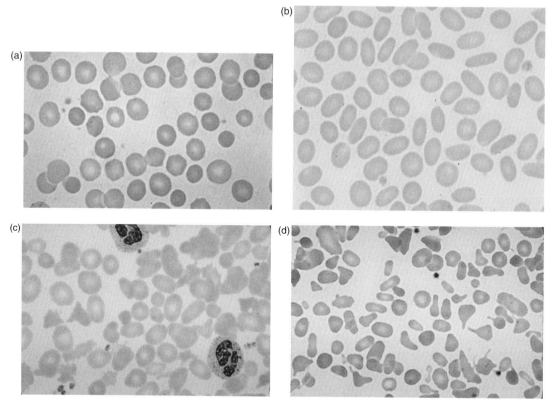

Fig. 10.1 Photomicrographs of blood smears from patients with different hereditary red blood cell (RBC) membrane disorders. (a) Hereditary spherocytosis; (b) mild, asymptomatic common hereditary elliptocytosis characterized by numerous elliptocytic cells; (c) hereditary elliptocytosis with chronic hemolysis with the presence of elliptocytes and rod-shaped cells and poikilocytes; (d) hereditary pyropoikilocytosis with a large number of microspherocytes and micropoikilocytes and relative paucity of elliptocytes. (See plate section for color version.)

This is a result of inherited mutations in genes for membrane cytoskeleton proteins (α-spectrin, β-spectrin, ankyrin, band 3, protein 4.2). These genetic mutations lead to protein abnormalities that weaken the stability of the interactions between the cytoskeleton and membrane lipid bilayer, resulting in a loss of vertical integrity of the cell membrane. As a consequence, there is vesiculation, with loss of bits of the bilayer and, thereby, progressive loss of membrane surface area. As RBCs become more spherical, there is decreased flexibility and increased vulnerability to entrapment in the spleen, and this is where metabolic depletion and macrophage interactions lead to hemolysis (Fig. 10.2). Removal of the spleen allows spherocytes to have a near-normal lifespan, although the cytoskeletal defects and abnormal RBC shape persist.

The clinical features of HS encountered most commonly are anemia, jaundice, and splenomegaly. However, signs and symptoms are highly variable, with respect to both age of onset and severity. At one extreme, some mild cases may escape recognition for many years into adulthood, while, at the other extreme, hydrops with fetal death has been reported [40]. About 30%–50% of adults with the disorder have a history of jaundice during the first week of life [46, 47]. The magnitude of hyperbilirubinemia occasionally requires exchange transfusion [48]. In contrast to the frequency of hyperbilirubinemia, most newborns with hereditary spherocytosis are not anemic at birth [46]. However, in many infants hemolytic anemia does occur in the first month of life and can require one or more RBC transfusions. It is thought that this change reflects maturation of the splenic filtering function and development of the splenic circulation, coupled with an inadequate erythropoietic response. Within a few months, erythropoiesis increases, anemia improves, and the need for red-cell transfusions disappears in all but the most

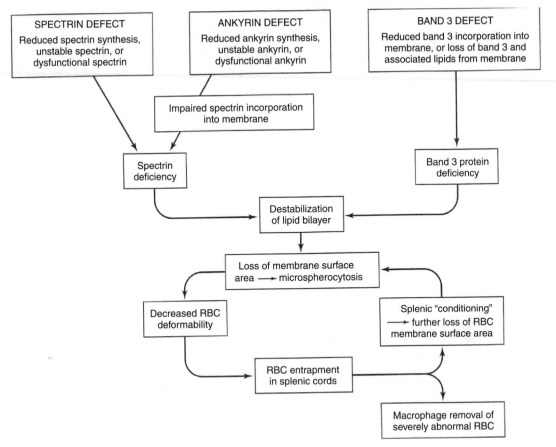

Fig. 10.2 The pathophysiology of hereditary spherocytosis is a consequence of spectrin, ankyrin, or band 3 abnormalities, which lead to membrane instability, loss of lipid microvesicles, decreased red cell surface area, reduced cellular deformability, and stagnation of red blood cells in the splenic cords. Schema modified from Palek and Jarolim [45].

severely affected infants. Beyond the neonatal period, jaundice is rarely intense. However, even when patients have no detectable jaundice, there usually is laboratory evidence of ongoing hemolysis. Splenomegaly is common in older children, and, in large family studies, palpable spleens have been detected in over 75% of affected members. No apparent correlation exists between spleen size and disease severity.

The diagnosis of HS in older children is suggested by the complete blood count (CBC), which typically reveals decreased to normal haemoglobin concentration, increased mean corpuscular hemoglobin concentration (MCHC), increased reticulocytes, spherocytes on the blood smear (see Fig. 10.1a) and laboratory evidence of increased RBC destruction (increased bilirubin). In such an individual with a family history of documented HS, no further diagnostic investigation is warranted. In the

newborn infant, morphologic assessment of the RBCs sometimes is difficult because even normal neonates may possess a minor population of spherocytes and, conversely, infants with hereditary spherocytosis may have fewer spherocytes than will be the case later in life. The possibility of HS in newborns is suggested by an increased MCHC (>36.5) and a low MCV. From the Intermountain Healthcare database, a neonatal HS ratio (MCHC/ MCV), that is >0.36, indicates the presence of HS with a 97% sensitivity, >99% specificity, and >99% negative predictive value [49].

Historically, the incubated RBC osmotic fragility (OF) test was used to confirm the diagnosis of HS. However, this test lacks both sensitivity and specificity for HS and other conditions such as red cell glycolytic enzyme deficiencies can manifest increased fragility. In neonates, alloimmune hemolysis due to ABO incompatibility must always be ruled out since the peripheral blood spherocytosis and OF are similar to that seen in HS. Blood typing and a direct antiglobulin test (DAT) usually confirm a diagnosis of ABO incompatibility, although the DAT occasionally is negative and thus misleading. In the past, a practical approach in these cases was to repeat the OF testing in 3 to 4 months when the confounding effects of maternal antibody were no longer present.

The EMA (eosin-5-maleimide) binding assay is a flow cytometry test that provides a relatively rapid and automated screening tool for HS. EMA is a fluorescent dye which covalently binds to the extracellular portion of band 3 on erythrocytes. The underlying structural protein defects in HS RBCs result in decreased EMA binding which can readily be measured with flow cytometry [50]. This is a highly specific assay for HS and has become the diagnostic test of choice for many haematologists [51].

Molecular testing is indicated for patients without a classic family history and in those cases where the diagnosis is equivocal and might represent some other RBC membrane disorder [52]. This is important because splenectomy, which is appropriate for some older children with severe HS, may be contraindicated in other RBC membrane disorders which can look like HS [53].

Treatment during the newborn period is directed toward management of hyperbilirubinemia which usually requires phototherapy and/or exchange transfusion in severe cases. In affected infants who also are homozygous for the mutation responsible for Gilbert syndrome, hyperbilirubinemia almost always requires phototherapy [54]. Occasionally, RBC transfusions may be required at birth for management of symptomatic anemia [55]. A more common occurrence is the appearance of a transient but severe anemia during the first 20 days of life due to underproduction of erythropoietin in the face of continuing hemolysis [56]. These infants should be monitored closely following discharge from the nursery. Folic acid is required to sustain erythropoiesis: 0.5–1.0 mg per day is used for older children. With young infants we teach parents how to make an oral folate solution containing 50 μg folate/ml with 1 ml of a freshly prepared vitamin solution made each day. Splenectomy is the definitive treatment for severe hereditary spherocytosis. However, surgery is deferred until the child is at least 5 years old because of the increased risk of overwhelming

sepsis with encapsulated organisms such as *Haemophilus influenzae* or *Streptococcus pneumoniae* that occurs in infants and young children following splenectomy [57]. It has been suggested that partial splenectomy may reduce the rate of hemolysis without increasing the risk of overwhelming infection, and this is a possible option in very young children with severe hemolysis [58].

Hereditary Elliptocytosis

Hereditary elliptocytosis is an autosomal dominant clinically heterogeneous group of disorders caused by mutations of RBC membrane cytoskeletal genes (usually spectrin or protein 4.1; see Table 10.2). These resultant protein abnormalities weaken skeletal protein interactions, disrupt the horizontal integrity of the membrane, and thereby increase RBC mechanical fragility [39, 40]. The hereditary elliptocytosis variants occur with an estimated frequency of 1 in 5,000, occurring in all racial and ethnic groups. Most individuals with common hereditary elliptocytosis have no clinical abnormalities or anemia, although the peripheral blood smear can be striking, with 15%–100% elliptocytes (see Figure 10.1b). In a small fraction (5%–20%) of common cases, there is some degree of hemolysis, usually compensated but occasionally leading to anemia (Hb 9–12 g/dl, reticulocytes 20%–25%). The peripheral blood smear in these hemolytic cases reveals poikilocytes in addition to elliptocytes. It is of interest that in families with common hereditary elliptocytosis, some individuals have a chronic hemolytic disorder while others do not, thus indicating that other genetic factors modify disease expression [59]. Both homozygous and compound heterozygous forms of the disease also occur and these cases are associated with clinically significant hemolytic anemia. Morphological characteristics include marked poikilocytosis, microelliptocytosis, and red-cell fragmentation (see Figure 10.1c). In some cases, both parents have nonhemolytic common hereditary elliptocytosis. Hereditary pyropoikilocytosis (HPP) is a recessively inherited severe hemolytic anemia characterized by RBC membrane budding, red-cell fragments, microspherocytes, and poikilocytes seen on the peripheral smear (see Figure 10.1d). The MCV may be extremely low (30–50 fl), while the MCHC is normal. From a clinical perspective, it is difficult to distinguish HPP from homozygous or doubly heterozygous common hereditary elliptocytosis. Once regarded as a separate condition, HPP is biochemically related to common hereditary elliptocytosis, occurs in families where other members have common hereditary elliptocytosis, and now is considered to be a variant of this disorder. During childhood, affected individuals manifest moderately severe hemolytic anemia (hemoglobin concentration 5–9 g/dl; reticulocyte count 13%–35%). Most but not all patients are of African heritage. The osmotic fragility test usually is normal in non-hemolytic forms of common hereditary elliptocytosis but is increased in those hemolytic variants with poikilocytosis and fragmentation. Molecular testing often is useful in these HE cases. No treatment is needed for most patients, although splenectomy later in childhood is beneficial for those with significant hemolysis.

Infantile poikilocytosis is a particularly interesting variant of hereditary elliptocytosis that occurs in the newborn period. Affected young infants have moderately severe hemolytic anemia and hyperbilirubinemia in the newborn period, the latter often necessitating exchange transfusion [60, 61]. The blood smear is characterized by marked red-cell fragmentation and poikilocytosis in addition to elliptocytosis. These morphologic changes are indistinguishable from those noted in patients with HPP. However, in contrast to HPP, hemolysis lessens gradually, and the clinical and hematologic features convert to those of mild hereditary elliptocytosis by 6–12 months of age [60]. In these infants, RBC membrane mechanical fragility is strikingly abnormal, probably a consequence of the destabilizing influence of large amounts of free intraerythrocytic 2,3-diphosphoglycerate (2,3-DPG) a byproduct of the presence of fetal hemoglobin [62]. As fetal hemoglobin levels decline in affected infants, membrane mechanical fragility improves, hemolysis disappears, and RBC morphology undergoes a transition from poikilocytosis to elliptocytosis. At birth, it is difficult to predict which patients will have transient poikilocytosis with ultimate recovery into common hereditary elliptocytosis and which are destined to have lifelong HPP with hemolysis. Close observation is necessary.

In addition to HS and HE variants, there are other rare RBC membrane defects than can present with neonatal hemolysis such as hereditary xerocytosis and the variable hereditary stomatocytic disorders (see Table 10.2). These are not discussed here but there are several excellent reviews of these

conditions [39, 40, 53]. Nowadays, the diagnosis of these conditions is made by molecular testing panels after the more common RBC disorders are excluded [52].

Hemolysis Due to Hereditary Enzyme Abnormalities

Glucose is the main metabolic substrate for RBCs. It is metabolized by the glycolytic or "energy-producing" pathway and, to a much lesser extent, by the hexosemonophosphate (HMP) shunt or "protective" pathway (Fig. 10.3). The initial and most important reaction of the HMP shunt is catalyzed by glucose-6-phosphate dehydrogenase (G6PD). The HMP shunt represents the sole source of NADPH in erythrocytes, providing the reducing power necessary to protect RBCs from oxidant injury. The major products of glycolysis are adenosine triphosphate (ATP), a source of energy for numerous RBC membrane and metabolic reactions, and 2,3-DPG, an important intermediate that modulates hemoglobin–oxygen affinity. A critical enzyme for the generation of ATP is pyruvate kinase (PK). Hemolytic anemia due to G6PD deficiency is very common, while glycolytic enzymopathies are rare. Abnormalities in several glycolytic enzymes have been described, although over 90% of cases associated with hemolysis are due to pyruvate kinase deficiency. Hyperbilirubinemia, anemia, and even hydrops fetalis can be seen with inherited RBC enzymopathies. Overviews of this group of disorders are available elsewhere [63–65].

Glucose-6-Phosphate Dehydrogenase Deficiency

Glucose-6-phosphate dehydrogenase (G6PD) deficiency is an X-linked disorder that affects approximately 400 million people throughout the world, particularly in Mediterranean countries, Africa, and China. In the majority of G6PD-deficient individuals, there are no symptoms or laboratory signs of anemia in the steady state. Hemolysis occurs only with oxidant stresses during infections, after exposure to certain chemicals and medications, or associated with the ingestion of fava beans. Also, being an X-linked condition hemolysis occurs primarily in males and to a much lesser extent in carrier females.

Normal RBCs contain abundant amounts of reduced glutathione (GSH), a sulfhydryl-containing

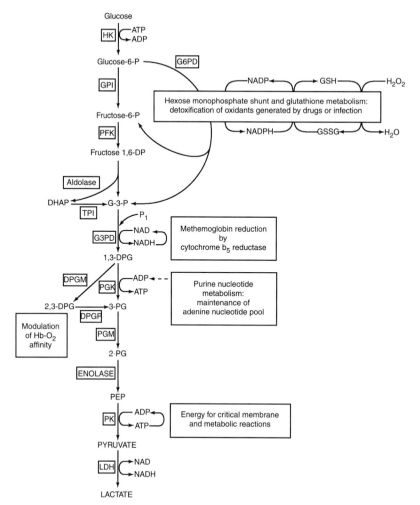

Fig.10.3 Overall red cell metabolism and function. Substrate abbreviations: (GSH) reduced glutathione; (GSSG) oxidized glutathione; (G-3-P) glyceraldehyde-3-phosphate; (DHAP) dihydroxyacetone phosphate; (1,3-DPG) 1,3-diphosphoglycerate; (2,3-DPG) 2,3-diphosphoglycerate; (3-PG) 3-phosphoglycerate; (2-PG) 2-phosphoglycerate; (PEP) phosphoenolpyruvate.

Cofactors: (ADP) adenosine diphosphate; (ATP), adenosine triphosphate; (NAD) nicotinamide adenine dinucleotide; (NADH) reduced nicotinamide adenine dinucleotide; (NADP) nicotinamide adenine dinucleotide phosphate; (NADPH) reduced nicotinamide adenine dinucleotide phosphate.

Enzymes are shown in boxes: (HK) hexokinase; (G6PD) glucose 6 phosphate dehydrogenase; (GPI) glucosephosphate isomerase; (PFK) phosphofructokinase; (TPI) triosephosphate isomerase; (G3PD) glyceraldehyde-3-phosphate dehydrogenase; (PGK) phosphoglycerate kinase; (DPGM) diphosphoglycerate mutase; (DPGP) diphosphoglycerate phosphatase; (PGM) phosphoglycerate mutase; (PK) pyruvate kinase; (LDH) lactate dehydrogenase. (From Glader B. [66]. Reproduced with permission.)

tripeptide that serves as an intracellular antioxidant, neutralizing peroxides that form during metabolism or are introduced directly from the extracellular environment. In contrast, G6PD-deficient RBCs have a limited capacity to regenerate GSH from oxidized glutathione, and in the absence of GSH, are vulnerable to oxidant injury (see Fig. 10.3). The effects of oxidants on RBCs are multifocal. Denatured globin precipitates, termed Heinz bodies, bind to the cell membrane, unfavourably altering its structure and function. Membrane lipid

peroxidation may contribute to altered function. The ultimate result of these insults is hemolysis.

The clinical heterogeneity of G6PD deficiency is due to the very large number of different mutations, usually single amino-acid substitutions, that lead to altered enzyme function [67] (see www .bioinf.org.uk/g6pd/). The normal or wild-type enzyme is referred to as G6PD B, and many variant G6PD enzymes have been identified and characterized on the basis of biochemical properties. The World Health Organization (WHO) has further classified these different G6PD variants on the magnitude of enzyme deficiency and also the severity of hemolysis (Table 10.3) [68, 69]. Class I variant patients have severe enzyme deficiency, associated with chronic hemolysis, but these individuals are very rare. Class II variant patients also have severe enzyme deficiency (<10% activity). A common class II variant G6PD^{Mediterranean}, (563 C>T) found in those whose origins are in the Mediterranean area, the Near East and South Asia. For class II variants, oxidant-hemolysis may be quite severe and the hemoglobin may fall to life-threatening levels. Moreover, severe hemolysis can occur in children with class II G6PD variants following exposure to fava (broad) beans. Class III variant people have moderate enzyme deficiency (10%–60% of normal) with intermittent hemolysis, usually associated with infection or drugs. A very common variant in this class is G6PD^{A-} (202 G>A/376A>G), found in 10%–15% of African Americans and with similar frequencies in western and central Africa. Hemolysis in children with class III variants usually is milder than class II and is self-limited.

In China, three major variants are recognized [70]. The most common is G6PD Canton (1376 G>T), which is usually reported to be a class II variant, although sometimes it is considered to be in class III. Another common variant is G6PD Kaiping (1388 G>A), which is usually classified as a class III variant although occasionally considered to be in class II. A third variant is G6PD Gaohe (95

Table 10.4 Drugs and chemicals associated with hemolysis in G6PD deficiency

Unsafe (class I, II, and III G6PD variants)	
Acetanilid	Thiazolesulfone
Diaminodiphenyl sulfone (dapsone)	Phenazopyridine (pyridium)
Furazolidone (furoxone)	Phenylhydrazine
Glibenclamide	Primaquine
Henna (lawsone)	Sulfacetamide
Isobutyl nitrate	Sulfanilamide
Methylene blue	Sulfapyridine
Nalidixic acid (neggram)	Thiazolesulfone
Naphthalene (mothballs)	Trinitrotoluene (TNT)
Niridazole (ambilhar)	Urate oxidase (rasburicase)
Nitrofurantoin (furadantin)	

A>G), which is usually considered to be a class II variant. These three variants account for over 70 percent of G6PD deficiency cases in China. The most common variant in Southeast Asia is G6PD Mahidol (487 G>A), a class III variant.

The recognition of G6PD deficiency in older children is suggested by the sudden onset of non-immune hemolytic anemia associated with infection, fava bean ingestion, or the exposure to certain drugs and chemicals (see Table 10.4). Cells that appear as if a "bite" had been taken from them (due to splenic removal of Heinz bodies) and "blister cells" with hemoglobin puddled to one side may be seen on the peripheral blood smear. Although screening tests are available, definitive diagnosis requires assay of RBC G6PD activity. The diagnosis occasionally may be complicated in the setting of a high reticulocyte count, as is observed following a hemolytic crisis, because the population of deficient cells has been eliminated or, in transfused patients, because of the presence of normal, enzyme-replete RBC. Repeating the enzyme assay after at least 3 months ensures that any transfused cells are gone and that the population of deficient cells has been regenerated so that a more accurate determination of the presence of G6PD deficiency can be made. In some cases, specific G6PD mutations can be identified by DNA analysis, but this is used rarely in routine diagnosis.

Hemolysis resulting from G6PD deficiency is well documented in the newborn period [71], and may occur in utero [72]. However, the major

Table 10.3 WHO classificaton of glucose-6-phosphate dehydrogenase variants

Variant type	Residual enzyme activity	Clinical findings
Class I	Severe deficiency <10% normal	Chronic hemolytic anemia
Class II	Severe deficiency <10% normal	Episodic moderate–severe hemolysis with oxidative triggers
Class III	Moderate deficiency 10%–60% normal	Episodic mild–moderate hemolysis with oxidative triggers
Class IV	Normal activity >60%	None

consequence of G6PD deficiency in the newborn period is not hemolysis, but rather it is hyperbilirubinemia. Neonates with the rare class I variants are at greatest risk of neonatal jaundice, but these cases are rare. Most encountered infants with hyperbilirubinemia due to G6PD deficiency have one of the more common variants and come from the Mediterranean region or Asia, and to a lesser extent those with the G6PD A- variant. The degree of jaundice is quite variable; and in severe cases, there is a risk of bilirubin-induced neurologic dysfunction and kernicterus with permanent neurologic damage if the patient is not treated aggressively [73]. In neonates with Class II or III G6PD-deficiency, jaundice is rarely present at birth with the peak of onset occurring 2 to 3 days after birth. Jaundice is more prominent than anemia, which is rarely severe. Monitoring of jaundice and serum bilirubin levels in infants known to be G6PD-deficient is critical. [72, 74–76]. Of interest, African American infants with G6PD A⁻ appear to be at lesser risk, although infants with the same G6PD variant in Africa have an increased incidence of neonatal hyperbilirubinemia [74, 77]. Moreover, in the latter group, untreated hyperbilirubinemia frequently leads to kernicterus with severe neurologic injury or death [77, 78]. Since black Africans and African Americans have the same G6PD A− genotypes, the adverse outcomes in Africa are thought to relate to local customs and differences in oxidant exposure [77, 78]. Herbs used in traditional Chinese medicine and clothing impregnated with naphthalene also are examples of covert oxidants to which susceptible infants may be exposed. Moreover, drugs (e.g., some sulfonamides), and fava-bean ingestion by mothers in late gestation have been implicated as the inciting stimulus in G6PD deficient newborns [79].

A study from Nigeria has reported a much poorer outcome for G6PD-deficient infants born at home, presumably a reflection of delayed identification and treatment of hyperbilirubinemia [77]. In the USA, there is concern that changes in healthcare delivery with early discharge of newborn infants may have similar consequences. In support of this is the report of four newborn infants with G6PD deficiency (three African American, one mixed Peruvian/Chinese) who developed kernicterus following early hospital discharge [80]. This report is disturbing because kernicterus in the USA has been rare in recent

years and the adverse outcomes in these four cases occurred despite adherence to the early neonatal discharge guidelines of the American Academy of Pediatrics and the American College of Obstetricians and Gynecologists. Furthermore, in data from the USA Kernicterus Registry for the period from 1992 to 2004, over 30% of neonates requiring re-admission for hyperbilirubinemia and kernicterus were ultimately diagnosed with G6PD deficiency [73].

These disturbing findings have led some to suggest that universal neonatal testing programs for G6PD deficiency should be implemented [81]. Neonatal screening for G6PD deficiency has been very effective in reducing the incidence of favism later in life in Sardinia [82], and in other regions where this potentially fatal complication is common [71]. Thus, routine testing for G6PD deficiency is performed in many neonates with hyperbilirubinemia and/or those with less dramatic bilirubin elevations who are of Mediterranean, Nigerian, or East Asian ancestry. The American Academy of Pediatrics clinical guideline on the management of neonatal hyperbilirubinemia recognizes G6PD deficiency as a major etiologic risk factor for the development of severe hyperbilirubinemia and bilirubin-induced brain damage [83]. However, newborn screening for G6PD deficiency is only recommended for jaundiced newborns receiving phototherapy, whose family history, ethnicity, or geographic origin suggest the possibility of G6PD deficiency or for infants whose response to phototherapy is poor. Currently, in the USA the only newborn screening programs for G6PD deficiency are in the District of Columbia and the Pennsylvania newborn screening programs [84]. However, with changing immigrant populations, severe variants of G6PD deficiency nowadays are often found in many cities in the USA [85]. The need for point-of-care tests to be used on-site has been emphasized by various groups (e.g., prior to administration of antimalarial drugs). Similarly, for neonates, G6PD deficiency needs to be identified before an infant is discharged from the hospital. Since the maximum bilirubin does not occur until after 3 days of life, point-of-care enzyme testing in potentially affected infants is being assessed as a means of risk reduction for neonatal kernicterus [86].

In some cases, the hyperbilirubinemia seen in G6PD-deficient infants reflects accelerated red-cell breakdown, but more commonly there is no obvious RBC destruction or oxidant exposure. It has been suggested that hyperbilirubinemia may have another etiology, possibly related to impaired liver clearance of bilirubin. In support of this hypothesis are the observations that production of carboxyhemoglobin, a marker of hemolysis or RBC breakdown, is the same in G6PD^{Mediterranean}-deficient neonates with and without hyperbilirubinemia [87]. It is now thought that the variable degree of hyperbilirubinemia in G6PD-deficient neonates reflects the presence or absence of the variant form of uridine-diphosphoglucoronylsyl transferase responsible for Gilbert's syndrome [67].

The major therapy for neonatal hyperbilirubinemia resulting from G6PD deficiency includes phototherapy or exchange transfusion to prevent kernicterus. RBC transfusion for symptomatic anemia, removal of potential oxidants contributing to hemolysis, and treatment of associated infections also needs to be addressed. In infants known to be G6PD-deficient, prevention of severe hyperbilirubinemia by administration of a single intramuscular dose of Sn-mesoporphyrin, an inhibitor of heme oxygenase, appears highly effective and safe, although this therapy has not been widely adopted [88].

Routine blood-bank screening likewise appears to be unwarranted, and G6PD deficiency is not considered a problem in transfusion medicine. Even in areas where G6PD deficiency is endemic, screening of blood donors is not required. Several years ago, a careful evaluation of the recipients of G6PD-deficient blood uncovered no deleterious consequences [89]. However, in premature infants, simple transfusions with G6PD-deficient red cells have been associated with hemolysis and severe hyperbilirubinemia requiring exchange transfusion [90]. Also, massive intravascular hemolysis has occurred in a South Asian neonate following an exchange transfusion with G6PD-deficient blood [91]. In view of these occurrences, it has been recommended that in areas where class II variants are common, donor blood should be screened for G6PD deficiency before transfusing premature infants or using the blood for a neonatal exchange transfusion. Currently, this recommendation is not standard blood-banking practice.

Pyruvate Kinase Deficiency

Pyruvate kinase deficiency (PKD) is an autosomal recessive disorder that occurs in all ethnic groups [64, 92]. Although it is the most common of the glycolytic pathway defects, it is rare in comparison to G6PD deficiency. Several hundreds of cases have been identified in Europe, Japan, and the USA [93]. The actual prevalence of PKD is somewhat in question with estimates ranging from 3 to 50 per million in the general white population [94–96]. Pyruvate kinase is one of the two key enzymatic steps that generate ATP in RBCs. Because nonerythroid tissues have alternative means of generating ATP, clinical abnormalities in pyruvate kinase deficiency are limited to RBCs.

The hemolytic anemia associated with PK deficiency is due to homozygous or compound heterozygous mutations in the PKLR gene located on chromosome 1 (1q21). More than 300 PKLR mutations have been identified [96, 97]. Reflecting this genetic diversity, the severity of hemolytic anemia in PKD varies considerably. Most PKD individuals are compound heterozygotes for two different PKLR mutations. A particularly high frequency exists among the Pennsylvanian Amish people, in whom the disorder can be traced to a single immigrant couple [98, 99].

Data from the PKD Natural History Study reveal that perinatal complications are common, occurring in 28% (65 of 233 births) and these include preterm birth, prenatal anemia requiring in utero RBC transfusions, intrauterine growth retardation, and even hydrops [93]. Approximately 90% of PKD patients (207 of 230 patients) have a history of neonatal hyperbilirubinemia which required phototherapy (93%) and/or exchange transfusion (46%). Jaundice tends to appear early (on the first day of life) and may require exchange transfusion. Beyond the neonatal period PKD is characterized by chronic hemolysis often requiring red blood cell transfusions. The severity of hemolysis and need for transfusion is minimized by splenectomy after 5 years of age.

The possibility of pyruvate kinase deficiency should be considered in any jaundiced newborn infant with nonimmune hemolysis in the absence of infections and without evidence of an RBC membrane defect or G6PD deficiency. RBC morphology in PKD is normal, although a few dense cells with irregular margins (echinocytes) occasionally are present. Assay of PK enzyme activity is the most useful and rapid way to make the diagnosis of PKD [100, 101]. Any case of PK deficiency detected by biochemical assay should be confirmed by molecular testing that is available in several referral labs. This is important because there is evolving evidence that the type of mutation relates to clinical prognosis [93].

Heterozygotes with one PKLR mutation have roughly half the normal amount of RBC PK enzyme activity, although sometimes it is hard to distinguish from patients with PKD. In all cases, however, PK heterozygotes are clinically and hematologically normal with no evidence of hemolysis.

Failure to demonstrate PK deficiency in the face of chronic hemolysis necessitates considering some of the other less common enzymopathies that occur in children (Table 10.5). Glucose phosphate isomerase (GPI) deficiency is the second most common glycolytic enzymopathy associated with hemolysis. The clinical manifestations of this disorder are identical to those of pyruvate kinase deficiency. The severity of hemolysis varies considerably. Anemia and hyperbilirubinemia complicate the postnatal

course in many patients [102, 103]. Hydrops fetalis with death in neonates has been reported [104–106].

Phosphoglycerate kinase (PGK) deficiency is unique amongst glycolytic enzymopathies in that it is X-linked and most severely PGK deficient individuals with hemolysis also have neurologic abnormalities (seizures, mental retardation, aphasia, movement disorders) [107, 108].

Triose phosphate isomerase (TPI) deficiency associated with hemolytic anemia has been reported in several children. A unique feature of this enzymopathy is an early onset of a severe neurologic disorder characterized by spasticity, motor retardation, and hypotonia. Most affected patients die before they are 5 years old [109–111].

Hexokinase deficiency is a rare cause of hemolysis that has been identified in over 20 individuals [112, 113]. Splenectomy ameliorates but does not cure the hemolytic process.

Pyrimidine 5′nucleotidase (P5′N) deficiency is another rare enzyme abnormality associated with hereditary hemolytic anemia [114, 115]. Several kindred representing a wide geographic distribution have been reported, with a predisposition for people of Mediterranean, Jewish, and African ancestry. In all families studied, the disorder follows an autosomal recessive pattern. P5′N catalyzes the degradation of pyrimidine nucleotides to inorganic

Table 10.5 RBC enzymopathies other than G6PD deficiency

Enzymopathy	Approximate fraction of enzymopathies	Mode of inheritance	Effects of enzymopathy
Hexokinase (HK)	<1%	AR	mild/severe CNSHA
Glucosephosphate Isomerase (GPI)	3%–5%	AR	mod/severe CNSHA; +/− neurologic deficits
Phosphofructokinase (PFK)	<1%	AR	mild CNSHA; +/−myopathy
Aldolase	<1%	AR	mild/mod CNSHA; +/− myopathy
Triosephosphate isomerase (TPI)	<1%	AR	mod/severe CNSHA; neurologic deficits,
Phosphoglycerate kinase (PGK)	<1%	X-linked	mild/severe CNSHA; +/− neurologic deficits; +/− myopathy
Pyruvate kinase (PK)	>90%	AR	mod/severe CNSHA
Pyrimidine 5′nucleotidase (P5′N)	2%–3%	AR	moderate CNSHA
Adenylate kinase (AK)	<1%	AR	CNSHA

phosphate and the corresponding pyrimidine nucleoside [116, 117]. The most reasonable explanation for hemolysis in P5′N deficiency is that retained aggregates of ribosomes produce direct membrane injury, akin to that observed with Heinz bodies. There is mild to moderate anemia, reticulocytosis, and hyperbilirubinemia. RBC morphology is unique in that marked basophilic stippling is present. Basophilic stippling of RBCs is the morphologic equivalent of partially degraded ribosomes. Diagnosis requires a specific spectrophotometric enzyme assay.

Hemolysis Due to Hemoglobin Abnormalities

General Considerations

The earliest embryonic hemoglobins are composed of zeta globin chains (forerunners of alpha globin chains) and epsilon chains (forerunners of gamma globin and beta globin chains) (Fig. 10.4). The transition from zeta to alpha globin chains is complete by the end of the first trimester. Epsilon chains disappear more slowly and are replaced first by gamma globin and later by beta globin. Hemoglobin F (α2,γ2) is the hemoglobin found in fetuses after the first trimester, while Hb A (α2, β2) is the major hemoglobin in children and adults. At the time of birth, 60%–90% of hemoglobin found in normal term infants is Hb F. After birth, γ-globin synthesis declines as β-globin production increases, and by six months of age Hb F is approximately 5%. Only trace amounts of Hb A_2 (α2,δ2) and gamma globin chain tetramers (γ4) are present in cord blood. With postnatal maturation, hemoglobin A_2 increases gradually to the adult level of 2%–3.5%, while Hb Barts quickly disappears. In contrast to the major globin changes during development, heme is unchanged in structure in embryonic, fetal, and postnatal haemoglobins.

Hemolysis occurs with hereditary abnormalities due to decreased production of normal hemoglobins (thalassemia syndromes) or the production of qualitatively abnormal hemoglobins (sickle cell disorders, unstable hemoglobins). Those due to α-globin abnormalities are manifested at birth. In contrast, those due to β-globin abnormalities may not be apparent until four to six months of age when the switch from Hb F to Hb A synthesis reveals the defect. In contrast, rare gamma globin mutations are evident in fetal and neonatal life but

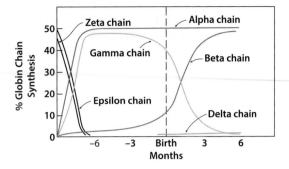

Hemoglobin	Birth	1 year ⟶ adult
F ($\alpha_2 \gamma_2$)	60–90%	<1%
A ($\alpha_2 \beta_2$)	15–40%	96–98%
A_2 ($\alpha_2 \delta_2$)	1%	2–3%

Fig. 10.4 Summary of fetal and infant hemoglobin synthesis. (Reproduced with permission from Benz E, Berliner N, Schiffman F. *Anemia: Pathophysiology, Diagnosis and Management* (Cambridge, UK: Cambridge University Press, 2018), fig. 5.1.)

disappear by three months of age when γ-globin synthesis is replaced by β-globin synthesis.

Thalassemia Syndromes

Thalassemia syndromes are characterized by diminished or absent production of normal α-globin polypeptides (α-thalassemia) or β-globin chains (β-thalassemia) [118]. Decreased globin synthesis causes a microcytic anemia, the severity of which depends upon the remaining number of functional α or β globin genes. However, since non-thalassemic globin chains are produced at a normal rate, the resulting imbalance of globin chain production also contributes to the pathophysiology. For example, in α-thalassemia, diminished synthesis of α-globin chains, leads to a relative excess of γ or β chains. In the fetus, excess gamma chains form tetramers (γ4), also known as Hb Barts, while beyond the neonatal period, the excess beta chains form tetramers (β4), also known as Hb H. The opposite is true of β-thalassemia in which α-globin chains accumulate, causing RBC membrane damage and hemolysis.

Alpha Thalassemia

Alpha thalassemia is of particular importance to neonatologists because its clinical manifestations are present in utero and at birth. These disorders

169

occur worldwide, with an increased frequency in Africa, the Mediterranean, and throughout Southeast Asia, where the more severe forms of α-thalassemia are found. The genes directing α-globin synthesis (α2 and α1) are duplicated on the short arm of chromosome 16. Thus, with two genes per chromosome there are four genes, (α2α1/α2α1) that control normal alpha globin production. However, the α2 locus produces 2–3 times more globin than α1 does. Most α-thalassemia syndromes are due to deletions of alpha globin genes, although nondeletion α-thalassemia also occurs. Moreover, because non-deletion mutations involve α2, these thalassemia disorders are more severe [119–121]. Since the non-thalassemia globin chains are produced at a normal rate, gamma globin tetramers (γ4 or Hb Barts) and beta globin tetramers (β4 or Hb H) appear in substantial quantity as the number of functional alpha globin genes decreases. In families with α-thalassemia, an infant can inherit one, two, three, or four alpha thalassemia gene deletions, giving rise to the following four clinical alpha thalassemia syndromes: silent carrier state, α-thalassemia trait, hemoglobin H disease, or homozygous α-thalassemia (Table 10.6).

The silent carrier state occurs in individuals lacking one functional alpha globin gene (−α/αα). In these cases, there are no clinical or haematological manifestations. At birth, the one distinguishing feature is a slightly increased concentration of Hb Barts (1%–3%) compared with that seen in normal neonates (less than 1%). Beyond the newborn period, there is no anemia or microcytosis, and the percentages of both Hb F and Hb A$_2$ are normal.

Alpha thalassemia trait is due to a deficiency of two α-globin genes. Deletion of two α-globin genes, in *cis* or *trans*, is associated with mild microcytic anemia, without hemolysis or reticulocytosis. Even neonates are microcytic (i.e., MCV less than 100 fl). The cord blood of infants with α-thalassemia trait usually contains 3%–10% Hb Barts. There are no significant clinical abnormalities associated with α-thalassemia trait, and beyond the newborn period this mild microcytic anemia can be mistaken for iron deficiency. In toddlers, the presumptive diagnosis of alpha thalassemia trait is made after iron deficiency, beta thalassemia trait, and hemoglobin E disorders have been ruled out. Definitive diagnosis is established by testing for the common α-globin gene mutations and/or α-globin gene sequencing. Of interest, alpha globin gene deletions occurring in Southeast Asians with α-thalassemia trait are in *cis*, or located on the same chromosome (−−/αα), whereas people of African descent with α-thalassemia trait have their gene deletions in *trans*, on different chromosomes (−α/−α). Consequently, the more serious alpha thalassemia disorders Hb H disease and homozygous α-thalassemia, (see below) almost exclusively are found in Southeast Asians and rarely in people of African ancestry.

Hemoglobin H (Hb H) disease occurs in individuals with one functional α-globin gene. In Southeast Asia, it has been estimated that 13,000–16,000 infants with Hb H are born annually, translating into nearly 700,000 affected individuals living with Hb H disease. This disorder occurs most commonly when there is a deletion of three genes (−−/−α), in which case

Table 10.6 Alpha thalassemia syndromes

Alpha thalassemia syndromes	Genotype	Clinical features
Normal	(αα/αα)	
Silent carrier	(−α/αα)	
Alpha thalassemia trait	(−−/αα) or (−α/−α)	Mild microcytic anemia
Hemoglobin H disease	(−−/−α)	Mild moderate hemolytic anemia
Homozygous alpha thalassemia	(−−/−−)	Severe anemia hydrops fetalis
Hemoglobin Constant Spring (Hb CS) syndromes		
Heterozygous Hb CS	(α^{CS}α/αα)	Similar to alpha thalassemia trait
Hb H disease with Hb CS	(α^{CS}α/−−)	Similar to Hb H disease
Homozygous Hb CS	(α^{CS}α/α^{CS}α)	Similar to Hb H disease

one parent usually has alpha thalassemia trait ($--/\alpha\alpha$) while the other parent is a silent carrier for alpha thalassemia ($\alpha\alpha/\alpha-$). Also, individuals who inherit the alpha thalassemia trait genotype on one chromosome and have a Hb Constant Spring gene on the other chromosome ($--/\alpha^{CS}\alpha$) also have hemoglobin H disease (see below). During the newborn period, Hb H disease is characterized by marked hypochromia, microcytosis, and increased concentration of Hb Barts (20%–30%). Beyond infancy, the imbalance in globin chain synthesis is associated with β-globin excess and the presence of Hb H. The latter appears as a rapidly migrating hemoglobin (5%–40% total Hb) on electrophoresis on cellulose acetate at alkaline pH or by other hemoglobin testing (HPLC, capillary electrophoresis). When erythrocytes from a patient with an intact spleen are incubated with the dye brilliant cresyl blue, small inclusions of precipitated Hb H are seen.

Infants with Hb H disease usually have minimal or no anemia; and beyond the newborn period there typically is a mild hemolytic anemia. Clinical features may include fatigue, and splenomegaly. Occasionally there are episodes of accelerated hemolysis in association with infections or exposure to oxidant agents. Parents of infants who have hemoglobin H disease should be instructed to avoid oxidant agents that can cause hemolysis (the same list that is given to patients with G6PD deficiency (see Table 10.4).

Homozygous alpha thalassemia (hydrops fetalis) is due to deletion of all four alpha globin structural genes ($--/--$). Family studies of children with homozygous alpha thalassemia reveal that both parents have alpha thalassemia trait ($--/\alpha\alpha$). The absence of functioning alpha globin genes is incompatible with extrauterine life. In those infants who are born, the anemia is severe (Hb 3–10 g/dl) and erythroblastosis is present [122]. The hemoglobins present in cord blood are tetramers of non-alpha globin chains, with approximately 70%–80% Hb Barts and smaller amounts of Hb H and Hb Portland ($\xi_2\gamma_2$). The reason some fetuses survive in utero may be due to persistent function of the embryonic Hb Portland which has normal oxygen affinity. In contrast, Hb Barts has an extremely high oxygen affinity that impairs oxygen delivery, thereby contributing to the pathophysiology of this disorder.

Physical findings in affected infants include marked pallor, edema, hepatosplenomegaly, and a variety of other congenital abnormalities [123]. Most fetuses with homozygous alpha thalassemia who are not aborted are usually stillborn, although some have been born alive, resuscitated, and placed on chronic RBC transfusion programs [124–126]. The natural history of the Hb Barts hydrops fetalis syndrome has been described in 65 infants in Thailand: 25% died in utero, 18% died during delivery, and 54% died within one hour of delivery [127]. Abnormalities noted at autopsy included gross enlargement of the placenta, heart, liver, spleen, and adrenal glands. Moreover, there was significant retardation of brain growth, and many were less than 60% of the expected weight for the gestational age. Also of interest was the observation that some infants had relatively few abnormalities at autopsy.

In addition to the fetal problems there also are significant maternal complications. The vast majority of mothers carrying fetuses with homozygous alpha thalassemia develop toxemia of pregnancy [128]; the reason for this is unknown. Also, vaginal delivery is complicated by the retention of large bulky placentas, and occasionally there is postpartum hemorrhage [128, 129]. It has been estimated that in the absence of obstetrical care, up to 50% of mothers carrying hydropic fetuses suffer lethal complications.

For all of the above reasons, it is important to identify those families at risk for bearing children with homozygous alpha thalassemia. Specifically, if one partner in a relationship is noted to have alpha thalassemia trait (microcytosis not related to iron deficiency, beta thalassemia trait, or Hb E), it then is important to assess the other partner [130]. Moreover, if alpha thalassemia trait is first noted in a child, then it is important to study both parents, since families may anticipate having more children [131]. Genetic counselling for these high-risk families should include a discussion of the risks to the fetus as well as to the mother. In families at risk who are already pregnant when first seen, prenatal diagnosis is available [132, 133]. Chorionic villus sampling (at 8–12 weeks) and amniocentesis (at 16–18 weeks) can provide fetal cells for DNA analysis [122, 132]. This approach also has been used to detect hemoglobin H disease during pregnancy [134]. More recently non-invasive prenatal testing

(NIPT) of chromosomal disorders has been accomplished by assessing cell free fetal DNA found in maternal plasma after 10 weeks' gestation. This has been very useful for detecting aneuploidies such as trisomy 21 [135]. However, the effectiveness of NIPT in monogenic autosomal recessive conditions is more challenging since 50% of the fetal DNA is the same as that inherited by the mother. NIPT for α- and β- thalassemia is now being validated [136, 140]. Ultrasound screening of at-risk pregnancies for fetal anemia, increased cardiothoracic ratio and placental thickness can detect affected pregnancies with a high sensitivity.

As noted previously, while most fetuses with homozygous alpha thalassemia are aborted or stillborn, some have been born alive, resuscitated, and placed on chronic RBC transfusion programs [124–126]. In other cases chronic intrauterine transfusions have been given followed by a bone marrow transplant after birth [141–144]. Also, treatment of homozygous alpha thalassemia by means of in utero hematopoietic stem-cell transplantation is currently being evaluated [145]. The rationale for this in utero therapy is to introduce donor cells into a naive host prior to immune maturation, thereby inducing donor-specific tolerance. This approach would have the advantage of not requiring the use myeloablative conditioning regimens with cytotoxic agents.

Hemoglobin Constant Spring (Hb CS) is due to a nondeletion mutation that alters the normal translation codon for terminating α-globin chain synthesis, thereby leading to the production of an elongated alpha globin variant (α^{CS} globin). This structural abnormality is associated with an α-thalassemia phenotype because the output of α^{CS} globin is less than 1% of normal; and the CS allele is found only on α2 while the α1 allele is normal ($\alpha^{CS}\alpha$) [146]. There are several different phenotypes associated with Hb CS [147]. Heterozygous Hb CS ($\alpha^{CS}\alpha/\alpha\alpha$) can appear like α-thalassemia silent carrier state or α-thalassemia trait, with minimal hematologic findings except for a small amount of Hb CS (1%–2%), detected by hemoglobin electrophoresis or HPLC. The simultaneous inheritance of an α^{CS} allele and alpha thalassemia trait ($\alpha^{CS}\alpha/--$) results in a phenotype that is similar to that seen in Hb H disease, characterized by a hemolytic anemia with 10%–15% Hb H and 2%–3% Hb CS. It is estimated that this variant of

Hb H disease in Southeast Asians may be as common as that due to deletion of three alpha globin gene. Individuals homozygous for Hb CS (α^{CS} α/ α^{CS} α) have a clinical syndrome more like that seen with Hb H disease. There is splenomegaly and a mild hemolytic anemia, RBCs are normocytic (not microcytic), and there is marked basophilic stippling. Moreover, beyond infancy, there is an accumulation of Hb Barts instead of Hb H. Homozygous Hb CS can cause severe fetal anemia and hydrops [148]. For unknown reasons the anemia improves after birth, somehow related to hemoglobin switching.

Beta Thalassemia

Like α-thalassemia, β-thalassemia is found in regions of the world where malaria was formerly endemic: Southeast Asia, India, Africa, and the Mediterranean basin [118]. The β-thalassemias are a consequence of mutations that impair normal beta globin chain production. There are two β globin genes, one located on each chromosome 11.

Heterozygous β-thalassemia (β-thalassemia trait) is due to inheritance of one beta thalassemia gene, resulting in a lifelong mild hypochromic microcytic anemia (Hb 8–11 g/dl) appearing at 3–6 months of age. The clinically important disorders seen in this population include homozygous β-thalassemia and Hb E/beta thalassemia.

Homozygous β-thalassemia is due to the inheritance of two β-thalassemia genes, leading to a marked reduction or absence of β-globin chain production. Although deletion of the beta globin locus is an occasional cause of β-thalassemia, most cases are due to point mutations that affect transcription, mRNA processing, or translation [149, 150]. There are two general types of homozygous beta thalassemia, β^0 and β^+. In β^0-thalassemia, no beta globin is produced by the thalassemia locus, whereas in β^+-thalassemia, there is reduced but measurable output of beta globin. The severity of homozygous β-thalassemia (or β-thalassemia major) is greatest when two β^0-thalassemia genes are inherited and is usually much milder when two β^+-thalassemia genes are inherited. Severe beta thalassemia is associated with lifelong hemolytic anemia, dependence on regular RBC transfusions for survival, and the gradual development of transfusion-associated hemosiderosis [118]. The clinical abnormalities of β-thalassemia are not evident at birth but first present after 3 to 6 months of age. Affected newborns have Hb F but little or no Hb A. The diagnosis of β^0 thalassemia can be made at birth when HPLC or other analyses fail to detect any Hb A. However, diagnosis of β^+-thalassemia by these techniques in neonates is more difficult because the reduced amount of Hb A produced overlaps the range for normal babies. Direct identification of beta thalassemia mutations by DNA diagnostic techniques is available and does allow the identification at newborn all infants with β-thalassemia major. Today, these techniques are particularly useful for prenatal diagnosis of beta thalassemia syndromes. Fetal DNA can be obtained during the first trimester from chorionic villi (at 9–11 weeks) or during mid trimester from fetal amniocytes (at 15–17 weeks); and the assay can be completed within a few days, allowing families to make informed decisions regarding the pregnancy [151]. Just as for α-thalassemia disorders, non-invasive prenatal testing of fetal DNA in maternal blood is under investigation.

The implementation of a strategy of carrier detection, genetic counseling, and prenatal diagnosis in countries where beta thalassemia is common has led to a striking reduction in the number of births of infants with beta thalassemia major [151].

Hemoglobin E/Beta Thalassemia

Hemoglobin E is the second most common hemoglobin variant in the world (Hb S being the most common) and occurs predominantly in people from Southeast Asia. At the border of Thailand, Laos, and Cambodia, there is a 20%–40% prevalence of Hb E. The structure of Hb E differs from Hb A by the replacement of lysine for glutamic acid at position 26 of the normal β-globin due to a DNA substitution of adenine for guanine at codon 26 of the β-globin gene. This mutation also alters RNA processing, thus resulting in decreased production of functional beta globin mRNA, reduced beta globin chains, and a mild thalassemia phenotype. Hemoglobin E carriers (Hb AE) are microcytic but do not have anemia. Even those who are homozygous for Hb E (Hb EE) have little or no anemia. However, coinheritance of hemoglobin E trait and β^0 thalassemia trait can give rise to a transfusion-dependent form of beta thalassemia major [152]. As with other types of β-thalassemia major, clinical abnormalities appear after 3 to 6 months of age.

However, the presence of hemoglobin E is readily detected at birth by hemoglobin electrophoresis or related techniques. Infants found to have an FE hemoglobin screening pattern need careful follow up to exclude the possibility of hemoglobin Eβ-thalassemia. Both hemoglobin electrophoresis and DNA analysis are used to confirm the diagnosis [153].

In Southeast Asia, Hb Eβ-thalassemia is much more common than homozygous beta thalassemia, and the same is true for refugees to the USA. During 2001–2004, of patients evaluated at the five largest thalassemia treatment centers in North America, Southeast Asians represented only 3% of patients with thalassemia major, while the same ethnic group represented 65% of those diagnosed with hemoglobin Eβ-thalassemia [154]. However, there also has been a marked decrease in the incidence of β-thalassemia major in other ethnic groups (e.g., Italians, Greeks) at high risk for having children with beta thalassemia major. The clinical course of Hb Eβ-thalassemia is quite variable. In some cases, the clinical features are identical to those seen in homozygous beta thalassemia and the anemia is sufficiently severe to require regular RBC transfusions, iron chelation therapy and, in some patients, stem-cell transplantation. In other cases, the anemia is milder, with Hb levels of 7–8 g/dl and no need for RBC transfusion therapy. One explanation for this difference, just as in the case for homozygous beta thalassemia, is the concomitant inheritance of α-thalassemia genes, which lessens the globin chain imbalance and, hence, the degree of RBC membrane damage and magnitude of hemolysis.

Gamma Thalassemia

Large deletions within the beta globin gene cluster may remove both gamma globin genes ($^A\gamma$ and $^G\gamma$) as well as the delta and beta globin genes. The resulting γδβ-thalassemia is lethal in the homozygous state, but in heterozygotes it produces a transient but moderately severe microcytic anemia in the newborn. Over the first few months of life, anemia improves without specific therapy and eventually the hematologic picture is that of beta thalassemia trait. At least eight different gamma delta beta deletions have been reported, all but one in families of European origin [150].

Sickle Cell Disease

The sickle hemoglobinopathies are beta globin mutations that, like beta thalassemia, do not become clinically evident until the infant is several months of age. Sickle hemoglobin (Hb S) is found throughout the world, with an increased incidence in central Africa, the Near East, the Mediterranean, and parts of India. From a practical perspective, four distinct sickle syndromes are recognized: sickle cell trait (Hb AS), homozygous sickle cell disease (Hb SS), hemoglobin SC disease, and hemoglobin Sβ-thalassemia. Beyond the neonatal period, hemoglobin electrophoresis on cellulose acetate at pH 8.6 has been the most practical test to differentiate the various sickling disorders. Under these conditions, hemoglobin S has a very distinct mobility, which distinguishes it clearly from Hb A, F, and C. At birth, as part of newborn screening programs, acid citrate agar electrophoresis allows for a better separation of Hbs A and F and, thus, a clearer definition of sickle trait versus sickle cell anemia. In recent years, high-performance liquid chromatography (HPLC) and isoelectric focusing have been used extensively and have been adopted by many states as the newborn screening test of choice [155]. Results of such screens are expressed as a pattern describing the hemoglobins present in order of descending concentration (Table 10.7). Newborn screening for hemoglobinopathies is further discussed in Chapter 6.

Sickle cell disease, the most severe of the disorders, is the result of inheritance of two β^S mutations

Table 10.7 Hemoglobin patterns observed in newborn screening

Hemoglobin screening pattern	Diagnosis
FA	Normal
FAS	Sickle trait
FS	Sickle cell anemia
FSA	Sickle beta thalassemia
FSC	Hb SC disease
F	Homozygous beta thalassemia
FAE	Hb E trait
FE	Hb EE
FEA	Hb E/β-thalassemia

Note: Patterns are reported by the hemoglobins that are present in order of decreasing concentration.

(substitution of valine for glutamic acid at the sixth amino acid on the beta globin chain), one from each parent. Sickle β^0-thalassemia, phenotypically similar to sickle cell anemia, is caused by inheritance of one β^S- and one β-thalassemia mutation. The third common form of sickle cell disease, hemoglobin SC disease, is somewhat milder than sickle cell anemia or sickle β^0-thalassemia. It is the consequence of inheritance of one β^S mutation and one β^c mutation (the substitution of lysine for glutamic acid at the sixth amino acid on the beta globin chain). Although no clinical abnormalities associated with sickle cell disease are present at birth, early diagnosis is important because two potentially fatal but largely preventable complications may occur during the first year of life [156]. The first is the splenic sequestration crisis, an unpredictable pooling of large numbers of RBCs in the spleen, which leads to a rapid decrease in hematocrit and, in the most severe cases, cardiovascular collapse and death. The second is overwhelming septicemia, usually caused by S. pneumoniae or H. influenzae. The unusually high susceptibility to infection with encapsulated organisms such as S. pneumoniae is the consequence of functional asplenia, which commonly appears by one year of age in sickle cell anemia or sickle β^0-thalassemia infants (but not until later in hemoglobin SC disease). Prompt treatment of splenic sequestration with RBC transfusions is lifesaving. As part of our practice parents are taught to recognize early manifestations such as splenic enlargement, lethargy, and pallor. Overwhelming sepsis can be prevented in most instances by early immunization with H. influenzae and conjugated pneumococcal vaccines, beginning at 2 months of age, and by institution of prophylactic penicillin at a dose of 125 mg twice daily [157]. It is the need to institute these prophylactic measures within the first 1–2 months of life that provided the compelling rationale for the development of newborn screening programs for sickle cell disease. Infant screening for sickle cell disease is mandatory in all 50 states and extensive experience and screening for infants has been accumulated in New York, Illinois, California [158], and elsewhere [159].

Infants born to mothers with sickle cell disease are more of a clinical problem than neonates who actually have sickle cell disease. Spontaneous abortion, intrauterine growth retardation, stillbirth, preterm labor and delivery, and perinatal mortality are all more frequent in infants of mothers with sickle cell anemia [160, 161]. These problems are due to abnormalities of the placenta, such as small size, infarction, and an increased incidence of placenta previa and abruptio placentae. These alterations appear to be the consequence of sickle vaso-occlusive events within the maternal side of the placental circulation.

Unstable Hemoglobinopathies

These disorders are due to amino-acid substitutions that decrease heme binding to globin and/or alter the normal tertiary structure of hemoglobin. As a consequence of these changes, hemoglobin is unstable as manifested by intracellular denaturation and Heinz body formation. Several unstable hemoglobins have been described, and generally, they are associated with mild to moderate hemolysis [162]. The overall clinical course may mimic G6PD deficiency. Specific diagnosis of unstable hemoglobinopathies is made by detecting hemoglobin instability at 50 °C or in the presence of isopropanol [163]. Neonatal problems due to unstable hemoglobins are unusual, since most described variants are due to beta globin chain abnormalities. Two unique hemoglobinopathies have been described in association with neonatal hemolysis: hemoglobin F-Poole and hemoglobin Hasharon. In all likelihood, however, some of the presently undiagnosed transient hemolytic anemias of infancy probably are due to unstable fetal hemoglobin variants.

Hemoglobin F-Poole [164], is a mutant fetal hemoglobin in which the 130th residue of the gamma globin chain contains glycine instead of tryptophane. As a consequence of this mutation, Hb F-Poole is unstable (heat and isopropanol instability) and associated with Heinz body hemolytic anemia during the first weeks of life. In the one reported case of this disorder, all signs of hemoglobin instability and hemolysis disappeared after 6 weeks of age.

Hemoglobin Hasharon differs from hemoglobin A by an amino-acid substitution at the 47th residue of the alpha globin chain (aspartic acid is replaced by histidine). Adults heterozygous for Hb Hasharon generally are asymptomatic although rarely there may be evidence of mild hemolysis [165]. A premature infant with this alpha chain mutation was reported to have moderate but persistent hemolytic disease throughout the first weeks of life [166]. Since hemolysis disappeared at the time beta globin synthesis became maximal, it was suggested that hemolysis may have been due to instability of the fetal form of this abnormal hemoglobin [167].

Methemoglobinemia

Although methemoglobinemia is not a hemolytic disorder, we have included a brief discussion of this problem here because maintaining low levels of methemoglobin is dependent on glycolysis for reduced nicotinamide adenine dinucleotide (NADH) production, and some of the congenital causes of this disorder are related closely to defects described elsewhere in this chapter. Methemoglobin is an oxidized derivative of hemoglobin in which heme iron is in the ferric (Fe^{3+}) or oxidized state rather than the ferrous (Fe^{2+}) or reduced state. Because methemoglobin is unable to bind oxygen, the presence of significant amounts of this respiratory pigment affects blood oxygen transport adversely. Normally, small amounts of methemoglobin are formed daily in vivo by the action of endogenous agents, which may include oxygen itself (auto-oxidation). However, as methemoglobin forms, it is reduced rapidly through the action of red-cell NADH and cytochrome b_5 reductase (also known as NADH-methemoglobin reductase), so that in normal individuals, levels of methemoglobin seldom exceed 1%. A second reduced nicotinamide adenine dinucleotide phosphate (NADPH)-methemoglobin reductase also is present in red cells but is not functional under normal physiologic conditions. The latter enzyme is activated only by certain redox compounds, and this is the basis for treatment of methemoglobinemia with methylene blue. Methemoglobinemia usually is a combined result of acquired environmental abnormalities, deficiency of cytochrome-b_5 reductase, and/or the presence of one of the M hemoglobins.

Acquired methemoglobinemia can occur in normal individuals following exposure to chemicals, such as aniline dyes, that readily oxidize hemoglobin iron. Newborns are particularly susceptible, because fetal hemoglobin is oxidized more readily to the ferric state than is hemoglobin A [168], and also because RBC cytochrome-b_5 reductase activity is low during the first few months of life [169]. Merely marking the diapers of newborns with aniline dyes has caused clinically significant methemoglobinemia.

The best known of the chemicals that cause methemoglobinemia are nitrites, either contained within ingested material or converted from nitrates by the action of intestinal bacteria. Fertilizers are rich in nitrites and the washout can contaminate well water and cause methemoglobinemia in infants [170, 171]. Also, foods with a high nitrate content (e.g., cabbage, spinach, beets, carrots) can produce methemoglobinemia in infants [172]. Diarrheal disorders during infancy have been associated with transient methemoglobinemia, possibly related to production of nitrites in the bowel [173–177]. Another nitrate association is the observation of methemoglobinemia following the administration of nitrous oxide to babies for treatment of persistent pulmonary hypertension [178].

Prilocaine administered before birth to provide local anesthesia can produce methemoglobinemia in both the mother and the infant [179]. Moreover, other local analgesics, including eutectic mixture of lidocaine and prilocaine (EMLA), can cause slight methemoglobinemia in the newborn, but usually this is not clinically significant and should not proscribe its use [180–183]. Other drugs, including over-the-counter medications and the dye henna also can cause methemoglobinemia [174, 181, 184]. During an 8-month period, Hjelt and coworkers studied 415 neonates in the neonatal intensive care unit (NICU) and 8% had methemoglobinemia. Prematurity, length of hospitalization, diarrheal illness, parenteral nutrition, and the use of antibiotics were associated strongly with the presence of methemoglobin [185].

Congenital methemoglobinemia is due to inherited disorders of hemoglobin structure or to a severe deficiency of cytochrome b_5 reductase (formerly called NADH methemoglobin reductase) activity [186–188]. The inherited abnormalities of hemoglobin structure that give rise to methemoglobinemia, known collectively as the hemoglobin M disorders, are rare autosomal dominant defects caused by point mutations that alter a single amino acid in the structure of normal globin. The altered conformation that ensues favors the persistence of the ferric rather than the ferrous form of heme iron. The normal methemoglobin reductive capacity of the RBC cannot compensate for such instability of ferrous heme. Of the 10 known hemoglobin M mutations, 3 affect the alpha globin chain, 5 alter the beta globin chain, and 2 involve the gamma chain. Most of these mutations are histidine-to-tyrosine mutations in the critical contact points of the heme moiety and the globin molecule. Only alpha and gamma globin chain mutations are associated with neonatal methemoglobinemia.s. Neonatal methemoglobinemia is transient when produced by one of the two gamma chain mutations, hemoglobin FM-Osaka [189, 190], or hemoglobin FM-Fort Ripley [191], because the normal developmental switch from fetal to adult hemoglobin eliminates all but a trace of the mutant hemoglobin. Hemoglobin M heterozygotes inheriting alpha or beta globin mutations appear cyanotic their entire life because of the increased methemoglobin levels present in their RBCs, but they are otherwise asymptomatic. No therapy is needed (and none is possible). The homozygous state is incompatible with life. Diagnosis of hemoglobin M disorders is made by hemoglobin spectroscopy.

NADH-methemoglobin reductase (cytochrome-b_5 reductase) deficiency is an uncommon autosomal recessive disorder. Heterozygotes are asymptomatic and do not have methemoglobinemia under normal circumstances. If challenged by drugs or chemicals that cause methemoglobinemia, however, patients become cyanotic and symptomatic at doses that have no effect in normal individuals. Homozygotes have lifelong methemoglobinemia at a level of 15%–40% and are cyanotic but otherwise asymptomatic, unless exposed to toxic agents. Two different types of hereditary NADH-cytochrome b_5 reductase deficiency are recognized. Type I deficiency is limited to RBCs and is manifested by methemoglobinemia only. Type II deficiency is due to a widespread enzyme deficiency and is characterized by mental retardation in addition to methemoglobinemia. The genefor NADH-cytochrome b_5 reductase is located on chromosome 22. Many different NADH-cytochrome b_5 reductase mutations, mostly missense, have been described in the two recognized types of enzyme deficiency [187]. Diagnosis of cytochrome b_5 reductase deficiency is by assay of the RBC enzyme activity, a procedure available only in specialized hematology laboratories. Confirmation of diagnosis is made by molecular diagnostic testing for CYB5 R mutations.

The main clinical manifestation of methemoglobinemia is cyanosis not resulting from cardiac or respiratory disease. Cyanosis present at birth suggests hereditary methemoglobinemia, whereas that appearing suddenly in an otherwise asymptomatic infant is more consistent with acquired methemoglobinemia. The blood is dark and, unlike deoxygenated venous blood, does not turn red when exposed to air. Rapid screening for methemoglobinemia is done by placing a drop of blood on filter paper and then waving the filter paper in the air to allow the blood to dry. Deoxygenated normal hemoglobin turns red, whereas methemoglobin remains brown. Using this technique, methemoglobin levels of 10% or more can be detected [192]. More accurate determination of methemoglobin levels are accomplished in the blood-gas laboratory by co-oximetry or in the clinical laboratory using a spectrophotometer. Cyanosis is first clinically evident when methemoglobin levels reach approximately 10% (1.5 g/dl), but symptoms attributable to hypoxemia and diminished oxygen transport do not appear until levels increase to 30%–40% of total hemoglobin. Death occurs at levels of 70% or greater. Methemoglobinemia is not associated with anemia, hemolysis, or other hematologic abnormalities.

In newborns, treatment with intravenous methylene blue (1 mg/kg as a 1% solution in normal saline) is indicated when methemoglobin levels are greater than 15%–20%. The response to methylene blue is both therapeutic and diagnostic. Methemoglobin levels decrease rapidly, within one to two hours, if methemoglobinemia is caused by a toxic agent or by a deficiency of cytochrome b5 reductase. In contrast, the hemoglobin M disorders do not respond to methylene blue. Reappearance of methemoglobinemia after an initial response to methylene blue suggests a deficiency of cytochrome b5 reductase or the persistence of an occult oxidant. A poor response to methylene blue also is seen in G6PD-deficient individuals; this occurs because G6PD is responsible for generation of NADPH, the required cofactor for the reduction of methemoglobin by methylene blue. In general, most infants with hereditary methemoglobinemia are asymptomatic and require no therapy. Older children are sometimes given daily administration of oral ascorbic acid or methylene blue to decrease cyanosis for cosmetic reasons. Methylene blue produces blue urine, but this is harmless.

References

1. Pearson HA. Life-span of the fetal red blood cell. *J Pediatr* 1967;**70**(2):166–71.

2. Oski FA, Naiman JL. *Hematologic Problems in the Newborn*, 3rd ed. (Philadelphia, PA: W. B. Saunders, 1982), pp. 1–360.

3. Matovcik LM, Mentzer WC. The membrane of the human neonatal red cell. *Clin Haematol* 1985;**14**(1):203–21.

4. Matovcik LM, Chiu D, LubinB, et al. The aging process of human neonatal erythrocytes. *Pediatr Res* 1986;**20**(11):1091–6.

5. Advani R, Mentzer W, Andrews D, Schrier S. Oxidation of hemoglobin F is associated with the aging process of neonatal red blood cells. *Pediatr Res* 1992;**32**(2):165–8.

6. Widness JA, Kuruvilla DJ, Mock DM, et al. autologous infant and allogeneic adult red cells demonstrate similar concurrent post-transfusion survival in very low birth weight neonates. *J Pediatr* 2015;**167**(5):1001–6.

7. Kuruvilla DJ, Widness JA, Nalbant D, et al. Estimation of adult and neonatal RBC lifespans in anemic neonates using RBCs labeled at several discrete biotin densities. *Pediatr Res* 2017;**81**(6):905–10.

8. Geaghan SM. Hematologic values and appearances in the healthy fetus, neonate, and child. *Clin Lab Med* 1999;**19**(1):1–37, v.

9. Holroyde CP, Oski FA, Gardner FH. The pocked erythrocyte red-cell surface alterations in reticuloendothelial immaturity of the neonate. *N Engl J Med* 1969;**281**(10):516–20.

10. Padmanabhan J, Risemberg HM, Rowe RD Howell-Jolly bodies in the peripheral blood of full-term and premature neonates. *Johns Hopkins Med J* 1973;**132**(3):146–50.

11. Maisels MJ, Pathak ANelson NM, Nathan DG, Smith CA. Endogenous production of carbon monoxide in normal and erythroblastotic newborn infants. *J Clin Invest* 1971;**50**(1):1–8.

12. Arias IM. The pathogenesis of physiologic jaundice of the newborn: A reevaluation. *Birth Defects Orig Artic Ser* 1970;**6**(2):55–9.

13. Bhutani VK, Johnson L, Sivieri EM. Predictive ability of a predischarge hour-specific serum bilirubin for subsequent significant hyperbilirubinemia in healthy term and near-term newborns. *Pediatrics* 1999;**103**(1):6–14.

14. Necheles TF, Rai US, Valaes T. The role of haemolysis in neonatal hyperbilirubinaemia as reflected in carboxyhaemoglobin levels. *Acta Paediatr Scand* 1976;**65**(3):361–7.

15. Coburn RF, Williams WJ, Kahn SB. Endogenous carbon monoxide production in patients with hemolytic anemia. *J Clin Invest* 1966;**45**(4):460–8.

16. Coburn RF. Endogenous carbon monoxide production. *N Engl J Med* 1970;**282**(4):207–9.

17. Smith DW, Inguillo D, Martin D, et al. Use of noninvasive tests to predict significant jaundice in full-term infants: Preliminary studies. *Pediatrics* 1985;**75**(2):278–80.

18. Stevenson DK, Vreman HJ. Carbon monoxide and bilirubin production in neonates. *Pediatrics* 1997;**100**(2 Pt 1):252–4.

19. Salmi TT Haptoglobin levels in the plasma of newborn infants with special reference to infections. *Acta Paediatr Scand Suppl* 1973;**241**:1–55.

20. Freda VJ, Gorman JG, Pollack W, Bowe E. Prevention of Rh hemolytic disease–ten years' clinical experience with Rh immune globulin. *N Engl J Med* 1975;**292**(19):1014–16.

21. Baumann R, Rubin H. Autoimmune hemolytic anemia during pregnancy with hemolytic disease in the newborn. *Blood* 1973;**41**(2):293–7.

22. Hocking DR. Neonatal haemolytic disease due to dapsone. *Med J Aust* 1968;**1**(26):1130–1.

23. Durocher JR, Payne RC, Conrad ME. Role of sialic acid in erythrocyte survival. *Blood* 1975;**45**(1):11–20.

24. Batton, DG, Amanullah A, Comstock C. Fetal schistocytic hemolytic anemia and umbilical vein varix. *J Pediatr Hematol Oncol* 2000;**22**(3):259–61.

25. Oski FA, Barness LA. Vitamin E deficiency:a previously unrecognized cause of hemolytic anemia in the premature infant. *J Pediatr* 1967;**70**(2):211–20.

26. Ritchie JH, Fish MB, McMasters V, Grossman M. Edema and hemolytic anemia in premature infants A vitamin E deficiency syndrome. *N Engl J Med* 1968;**279**(22):1185–90.

27. Gomez-Pomar E, Hatfield E, Garlitz K, Westgate PM, Bada HS. Vitamin E in the preterm infant: A forgotten cause of hemolytic anemia. *Am J Perinatol* 2018;**35**(3):305–10.

28. Smith H. *Normal Values and Appearances: Diagnosis in Paediatric Haematology* (New York: Churchill Livingstone, 1996) p. 338.

29. Tuffy P, Brown AK, Zuelzer WW. Infantile pyknocytosis: A common erythrocyte abnormality of the first trimester. *AMA J Dis Child* 1959;**98**(2):227–41.

30. Zannos-Mariolea L, Kattamis C, Paidoucis M. Infantile pyknocytosis and glucose-6-phosphate dehydrogenase deficiency. *Br J Haematol* 1962;**8**:258–65.

31. Keimowitz R, Desforges JF. Infantile pyknocytosis. *N Engl J Med* 1965;**273**(21):1152–4.

32. Ackerman BD. Infantile pyknocytosis in Mexican-American infants. *Am J Dis Child* 1969;**117**(4):417–23.

33. Dabbous, IA, El Bahlawan L. Infantile pyknocytosis: A forgotten or a dead diagnosis? *J Pediatr Hematol Oncol* 2002;**24**(6):507.

34. Eyssette-Guerreau S, Bader-Meunier B, Garcon L, Guitton C, Cynober T. Infantile pyknocytosis: A cause of haemolytic anaemia of the newborn. *Br J Haematol* 200;6**133**(4):439–2.

35. Dahoui HA, Abboud MR, Saab R, et al. Familial infantile pyknocytosis in association with pulmonary hypertension. *Pediatr Blood Cancer* 2008;**51**(2):290–2.

36. Kraus D, Yacobovich J, Hoffer V, et al. Infantile pyknocytosis: A rare form of neonatal anemia. *Isr Med Assoc J* 2010;**12**(3):188–9.

37. Vos MJ, Martens D, van de Leur SJ, van Wijk R. Neonatal hemolytic anemia due to pyknocytosis. *Eur J Pediatr* 2014;**173**(12):1711–14.

38. Rees C, Lund K, Bain BJ. Infantile pyknocytosis. *Am J Hematol* 2019;**94**(4):489–90.

39. Gallagher PG. Abnormalities of the erythrocyte membrane. *Pediatr Clin North Am* 2013;**60**(6):1349–62.

40. Gallagher PG, Glader B. Hereditary spherocytosis, hereditary elliptocytosis, and other disorders associated with abnormalities of the erythrocyte membrane. In Greer JP, Rodgers GM, Glader B, et al., eds. *Wintrobe's Clinical Hematology* (Philadelphia PA: Wolters Kluwer/Lippincott Williams & Wilkins, 2019), pp. 720–41.

41. Morton NE, Mackinney AA, Kosower N, Schilling RF, GrayMP. Genetics of spherocytosis. *Am J Hum Genet* 1962;**14**:170–84.

42. Perrotta S, Gallagher PG, Mohandas N . Hereditary spherocytosis. *Lancet* 2008;**372**(9647):1411–26.

43. Agre P, Asimos A, Casella JF McMillan C. Inheritance pattern and clinical response to splenectomy as a reflection of erythrocyte spectrin deficiency in hereditary spherocytosis. *N Engl J Med* 1986;**315**(25):1579–83.

44. Eber SW, Pekrun A, Neufeldt A, Schroter W. Prevalence of increased osmotic fragility of erythrocytes in German blood donors: Screening using a modified glycerol lysis test. *Ann Hematol* 1992;**64**(2):88–92.

45. Palek J, Jarolim P. Clinical expression and laboratory detection of red blood cell membrane protein mutations. *Semin Hematol* 1993;**30**(4):249–83.

46. Stamey CC, Diamond LK. Congenital hemolytic anemia in the newborn: Relationship to kernicterus. *AMA J Dis Child* 1957;**94**(6):616–22.

47. Trucco JI, Brown AK. Neonatal manifestations of hereditary spherocytosis. *Am J Dis Child* 1967;**113**(2):263–70.

48. Rubins J, Young LE. Hereditary spherocytosis and glucose-6-phosphate dehydrogenase deficiency. *JAMA* 1977;**237**(8):797–8.

49. Christensen RD, Yaish HM, Gallagher PG. A pediatrician's practical guide to diagnosing and treating hereditary spherocytosis in neonates. *Pediatrics* 2015;**135**(6):1107–14.

50. King MJ, Behrens J, Rogers C, et al. Rapid flow cytometric test for the diagnosis of membrane cytoskeleton-associated haemolytic anaemia. *Br J Haematol* 2000;**111**(3):924–33.

51. Christensen RD, Agarwal AM, Nussenzveig RH, et al. Evaluating eosin-5-maleimide binding as a diagnostic test for hereditary spherocytosis in newborn infants. *J Perinatol* 2015;**35**(5):357–61.

52. Agarwal AM, Nussenzveig RH, Reading NS, et al. Clinical utility of next-generation sequencing in the diagnosis of hereditary haemolytic anaemias. *Br J Haematol* 2016;**174**(5):806–14.

53. Andolfo I, Russo R, Gambale A, Iolascon A. New insights on hereditary erythrocyte membrane defects. *Haematologica* 2016;**101**(11):1284–94.

54. Iolascon A, Faienza MF, Moretti A, Perrotta S, Miraglia del Giudice E. UGT1 promoter polymorphism accounts for increased neonatal appearance of hereditary spherocytosis. *Blood* 1998;**91**(3):1093.

55. Gallagher PG, Petruzzi MJ, Weed SA, et al. Mutation of a highly conserved residue of betaI spectrin associated with fatal and near-fatal neonatal hemolytic anemia. *J Clin Invest* 1997;**99**(2):267–277.

56. Delhommeau F, Cynober T, Schischmanoff PO, et al. Natural history of hereditary spherocytosis during the first year of life. *Blood* 2000;**95**(2):393–7.

57. Diamond LK. Splenectomy in childhood and the hazard of overwhelming infection. *Pediatrics* 1969;**43**(5):886–9.

58. Tracy ET, Rice HE. Partial splenectomy for hereditary spherocytosis. *Pediatr Clin North Am* 2008;**55**(2):503–19, x.

59. Niss O, Chonat S, Dagaonkar N, et al. Genotype-phenotype correlations in hereditary elliptocytosis and hereditary pyropoikilocytosis. *Blood Cells Mol Dis* 2016;**61**:4–9.

60. Austin RF, Desforges JF. Hereditary elliptocytosis: An unusual presentation of hemolysis in the newborn associated with transient morphologic abnormalities. *Pediatrics* 1969;**44**(2):196–200.

61. MacDougall LG, Moodley G, Quirk M. The pyropoikilocytosis-elliptocytosis syndrome in a black South African infant: Clinical and hematological features. *Am J Pediatr Hematol Oncol* 1982;**4**(3):344–9.

62. Mentzer WC, Jr, Iarocci TA, Mohandas N, et al. Modulation of erythrocyte membrane mechanical stability by 2,3-diphosphoglycerate in the neonatal poikilocytosis/elliptocytosis syndrome. *J Clin Invest* 1987;**79**(3):943–9.

63. Luzzatto L, Nannelli C, Notaro R. Glucose-6-phosphate dehydrogenase deficiency. *Hematol Oncol Clin North Am* 2016;**30**(2):373–93.

64. Grace RF, Glader B. Red blood cell enzyme disorders. *Pediatr Clin North Am* 2018;**65**(3):579–95.

65. Glader B, Grace RF. Hereditary hemolytic anemias due to red blood cell enzyme disorders. In Greer JP, Rodgers GM, Glader B, et al., eds. *Wintrobe's Clinical Hematology* (Philadelphia PA: Wolters Kluwer/Lippincott Williams & Wilkins, 2019), pp. 742–61.

66. Glader B. Hereditary hemolytic anemias due to red blood cell enzyme disorders. In Greer JP, FoersterJ, Lukens JN, et al., eds. *Wintrobe's Clinical Hematology* (Philadelphia PA: Wolters Kluwer/Lippincott Williams & Wilkins Health, 2003).

67. Cappellini, MD, Fiorelli G Glucose-6-phosphate dehydrogenase deficiency. *Lancet* 2008;**371**(9606):64–74.

68. WHO Working Group. Glucose-6-phosphate dehydrogenase deficiency. *Bull World Health Organ* 1989;**67**:601–11.

69. Beutler E. The molecular biology of enzymes of erythrocyte metabolism. In Stamatoyannopoulos G, ed. *The Molecular Basis of Blood Diseases* (Philadelphia PA: W.B. Saunders, 2001).

70. Jiang W, Yu G, Liu P, et al. Structure and function of glucose-6-phosphate dehydrogenase-deficient variants in Chinese population. *Hum Genet* 2006;**119**(5):463–78.

71. Valaes T. Severe neonatal jaundice associated with glucose-6-phosphate dehydrogenase deficiency: Pathogenesis and global epidemiology. *Acta Paediatr Suppl* 1994;**394**:58–76.

72. Kaplan M, Algur N, Hammerman C. Onset of jaundice in glucose-6-phosphate dehydrogenase-deficient neonates. *Pediatrics* 2001;**108**(4):956–9.

73. Johnson L, Bhutani VK, Karp K, Sivieri EM, Shapiro SM. Clinical report from the pilot USA Kernicterus Registry (1992 to 2004). *J Perinatol* 2009;**29**(Suppl 1):S25–45.

74. Bienzle U, Effiong C, Luzzatto L. Erythrocyte glucose 6-phosphate dehydrogenase deficiency (G6PD type A–) and neonatal jaundice. *Acta Paediatr Scand* 1976;**65**(6):701–3.

75. Kaplan M, Hammerman C, Feldman R, Brisk R. Predischarge bilirubin screening in

glucose-6-phosphate dehydrogenase-deficient neonates. *Pediatrics* 2000;**105**(3 Pt 1):533–7.

76. Kaplan M, Hammerman C, Beutler E. Hyperbilirubinaemia, glucose-6-phosphate dehydrogenase deficiency and Gilbert syndrome. *Eur J Pediatr* 2001;**160**(3):195.

77. Slusher TM, Vreman HJ, McLaren DW, et al. Glucose-6-phosphate dehydrogenase deficiency and carboxyhemoglobin concentrations associated with bilirubin-related morbidity and death in Nigerian infants. *J Pediatr* 1995;**126**(1):102–8.

78. Oyebola DD. Care of the neonate and management of neonatal jaundice as practised by Yoruba traditional healers of Nigeria. *J Trop Pediatr* 1983;**29**(1):18–22.

79. Mentzer WC, Collier E. Hydrops fetalis associated with erythrocyte G-6-PD deficiency and maternal ingestion of fava beans and ascorbic acid. *J Pediatr* 1975;**86**(4):565–7.

80. MacDonald MG. Hidden risks: Early discharge and bilirubin toxicity due to glucose 6-phosphate dehydrogenase deficiency. *Pediatrics* 1995;**96**(4 Pt 1):734–8.

81. Kaplan M, Hammerman C. The need for neonatal glucose-6-phosphate dehydrogenase screening: A global perspective. *J Perinatol* 2009;**29**(Suppl1):S46–52.

82. Meloni T, Forteleoni G, Meloni GF. Marked decline of favism after neonatal glucose-6-phosphate dehydrogenase screening and health education: The northern Sardinian experience. *Acta Haematol* 1992;**87**(1–2):29–31.

83. American Academy of Pediatrics Subcommittee on Hyperbilirubinemia Management of hyperbilirubinemia in the newborn infant 35 or more weeks of gestation. *Pediatrics* 2004;**114**(1):297–316.

84. Lin Z, Fontaine JM, Freer DE, Naylor EW. Alternative DNA-based newborn screening for glucose-6-phosphate dehydrogenase deficiency. *Mol Genet Metab* 2005;**86**(1–2):212–19.

85. Watchko JF, Kaplan M, Stark AR, Stevenson DK, Bhutani VK. Should we screen newborns for glucose-6-phosphate dehydrogenase deficiency in the United States? *J Perinatol* 2013;**33**:499.

86. Bhutani VK, Kaplan M, Glader B, et al. Point-of-care quantitative measure of glucose-6-phosphate dehydrogenase enzyme deficiency. *Pediatrics* 2015;**136**(5):e1268–75.

87. Kaplan M, Vreman HJ, Hammerman C, et al. Contribution of haemolysis to jaundice in Sephardic Jewish glucose-6-phosphate dehydrogenase deficient neonates. *Br J Haematol* 1996;**93**(4):822–7.

88. Kappas A, Drummond GS, Valaes T. A single dose of Sn-mesoporphyrin prevents development of severe hyperbilirubinemia in glucose-6-phosphate dehydrogenase-deficient newborns. *Pediatrics* 2001;**108**(1):25–30.

89. McCurdy PR, Morse EE. Glucose-6-phosphate dehydrogenase deficiency and blood transfusion. *Vox Sang* 1975;**28**(3):230–7.

90. Mimouni F, Shohat S, Reisner SH. G6PD-deficient donor blood as a cause of hemolysis in two preterm infants. *Isr J Med Sci* 1986;**22**(2):120–2.

91. Kumar P, Sarkar S, Narang A. Acute intravascular haemolysis following exchange transfusion with G-6-PD deficient blood. *Eur J Pediatr* 1994;**153**(2):98–9.

92. Grace RF, Zanella A, Neufeld EJ, et al. Erythrocyte pyruvate kinase deficiency: 2015 status report. *Am J Hematol* 2015;**90**(9):825–30.

93. Grace RF, Bianchi P, van Beers EJ, et al. Clinical spectrum of pyruvate kinase deficiency: Data from the Pyruvate Kinase Deficiency Natural History Study. *Blood* 2018;**131**(20):2183–92.

94. Beutler E, Gelbart T. Estimating the prevalence of pyruvate kinase deficiency from the gene frequency in the general white population. *Blood* 2000;**95**(11):3585–8.

95. Carey PJ, Chandler J, Hendrick A, et al. Prevalence of pyruvate kinase deficiency in northern European population in the north of England Northern Region Haematologists Group. *Blood* 2000;**96**(12):4005–6.

96. Zanella A, Fermo E, Bianchi P, Chiarelli LR, Valentini G. Pyruvate kinase deficiency: The genotype-phenotype association. *Blood Rev* 2007;**21**(4):217–31.

97. Grace RF, Layton DM, Barcellini W. How we manage patients with pyruvate kinase deficiency. *Br J Haematol* 2019;**189**:721–34.

98. Bowman HS, McKusick VA, Dronamraju KR. Pyruvate kinase deficient hemolytic anemia in an Amish isolate. *Am J Hum Genet* 1965;**17**:1–8.

99. Rider NL, Strauss, KA Brown K, et al. Erythrocyte pyruvate kinase deficiency in an old-order Amish cohort: Longitudinal risk and disease management. *Am J Hematol* 2011;**86**(10):827–34.

100. Gallagher PG, Glader B. Diagnosis of pyruvate kinase deficiency. *Pediatr Blood Cancer* 2016;**63**(5):771–2.

101. Bianchi P, Fermo E, Glader B, et al. Addressing the diagnostic gaps in pyruvate kinase deficiency: Consensus recommendations on the diagnosis of pyruvate kinase deficiency. *Am J Hematol* 2019;**94**(1):149–61.

102. Hutton JJ, Chilcote RR, Glucose phosphate isomerase deficiency with hereditary nonspherocytic hemolytic anemia. *J Pediatr* 1974;**85**(4):494–7.

103. Schroter W, Koch HH, Wonneberger B, et al. Glucose phosphate isomerase deficiency with congenital nonspherocytic hemolytic anemia: A new variant (type Nordhorn;IClinical and genetic studies. *Pediatr Res* 1974;**8**(1):18–25.

104. Van Biervliet JP, Van Milligen-Boersma L, Staal GE. A new variant of glucosephosphate isomerase deficiency (GPI-Utrecht). *Clin Chim Acta* 1975;**65**(2):157–65.

105. Ravindranath Y, Paglia DE, WarrierI, et al. Glucose phosphate isomerase deficiency as a cause of hydrops fetalis. *N Engl J Med* 1987;**316** (5):258–61.

106. Xu W, Beutler E. The characterization of gene mutations for human glucose phosphate isomerase deficiency associated with chronic hemolytic anemia. *J Clin Invest* 1994;**94** (6):2326–9.

107. Vora S. Isozymes of phosphofructokinase. *Isozymes Curr Top Biol Med Res* 1982;**6**:119–67.

108. Vora S, DiMauro S, Spear D, Harker D, Danon MJ. Characterization of the enzymatic defect in late-onset muscle phosphofructokinase deficiency: New subtype of glycogen storage disease type VII. *J Clin Invest* 1987;**80**(5):1479–85.

109. Schneider AS, Valentine WN, Hattori M, HeinsHL Jr. Hereditary hemolytic anemia with triosephosphate isomerase deficiency. *N Engl J Med* 1965;**272**:229–35.

110. Valentine WN, Hsieh HS, Paglia DE, et al. Hereditary hemolytic anemia: Association with phosphoglycerate kinase deficiency in erythrocytes and leukocytes. *Trans Assoc Am Physicians* 1968;**81**:49–65.

111. Schneider A, Westwood B, Yim C, et al. Triosephosphate isomerase deficiency: Repetitive occurrence of point mutation in amino acid 104 in multiple apparently unrelated families. *Am J Hematol* 1995;**50**(4):263–8.

112. Valentine WN, Oski FA, Paglia DE, et al. Hereditary hemolytic anemia with hexokinase deficiency: Role of hexokinase in erythrocyte aging. *N Engl J Med* 1967;**276**(1):1–11.

113. Kanno H. Hexokinase: Gene structure and mutations. *Baillieres Best Pract Res Clin Haematol* 2000;**13**(1):83–8.

114. Beutler E. Red cell enzyme defects as nondiseases and as diseases. *Blood* 1979;**54**(1):1–7.

115. Beutler E, Baranko PV, Feagler J, et al. Hemolytic anemia due to pyrimidine-5'-nucleotidase deficiency: Report of eight cases in six families. *Blood* 1980;**56**(2):251–5.

116. Paglia DE, Valentine WN. Hereditary and acquired defects in the pyrimidine nucleotidase of human erythrocytes. *Curr Top Hematol* 1980;**3**:75–109.

117. Paglia DE, Valentine WN, Keitt AS, Brockway RA, Nakatani M. Pyrimidine nucleotidase deficiency with active dephosphorylation of dTMP: Evidence for existence of thymidine nucleotidase in human erythrocytes. *Blood* 1983;**62**(5):1147–9.

118. Taher AT, Weatherall DJ, Cappellini MD. Thalassaemia. *Lancet* 2018;**391**(10116):155–67.

119. Vichinsky E. Advances in the treatment of alpha-thalassemia. *Blood Rev* 2012;**26** Suppl 1: S31–34.

120. Piel FB, Weatherall DJ. The alpha-thalassemias. *N Engl J Med* 2014;**371**(20):1908–16.

121. Singh SA, SarangiS, Appiah-Kubi A, et al. Hb Adana (HBA2 or HBA1:c.179 G > A) and alpha thalassemia: Genotype-phenotype correlation. *Pediatr Blood Cancer* 2018;**65**(9):e27220.

122. Chui DH, Waye JS. Hydrops fetalis caused by alpha-thalassemia: An emerging health care problem. *Blood* 1998;**91**(7):2213–22.

123. Liang ST, Wong VC, So WW, et al. Homozygous alpha-thalassaemia: Clinical presentation, diagnosis and management: A review of 46 cases. *Br J Obstet Gynaecol* 1985;**92**(7):680–4.

124. Beaudry MA, Ferguson DJ, Pearse K, et al. Survival of a hydropic infant with homozygous alpha-thalassemia-1. *J Pediatr* 1986;**108**(5 Pt 1):713–16.

125. Bianchi DW, Beyer EC, StarkAR, et al. Normal long-term survival with alpha-thalassemia. *J Pediatr* 1986;**108** (5 Pt 1):716–18.

126. Singer ST, Styles L, Bojanowski J, et al. Changing outcome of homozygous alpha-thalassemia: cautious optimism. *J Pediatr Hematol Oncol* 2000;**22**(6):539–42.

127. Chui DH. Alpha-thalassemia: Hb H disease and Hb Barts hydrops fetalis. *Ann N Y Acad Sci* 2005;**1054**:25–32.

128. Hsieh FJ, Ko TM, Chen HY. Hydrops fetalis caused by severe alpha-thalassemia. *Early Hum Dev* 1992;**29**(1–3):233–6.

129. Guy G, Coady DJ, Jansen V, Snyder J, Zinberg S. Alpha-thalassemia hydrops fetalis: Clinical and ultrasonographic considerations. *Am J Obstet Gynecol* 1985;**153**(5):500–4.

130. Stein J, Berg C, Jones JA, Detter JC. A screening protocol for a prenatal population at risk for

inherited hemoglobin disorders: Results of its application to a group of Southeast Asians and blacks. *Am J Obstet Gynecol* 1984;**150**(4):333–41.

131. Glader BE. Screening for anemia and erythrocyte disorders in children. *Pediatrics* 1986;**78** (2):368–9.

132. Chan V, Ghosh A, Chan TK, Wong V, Todd D. Prenatal diagnosis of homozygous alpha thalassaemia by direct DNA analysis of uncultured amniotic fluid cells. *Br Med J (Clin Res Ed)* 1984;**288**(6427):1327–9.

133. Fucharoen S, Winichagoon P, Thonglairoam V, et al. Prenatal diagnosis of thalassemia and hemoglobinopathies in Thailand: Experience from 100 pregnancies. *Southeast Asian J Trop Med Public Health* 1991;**22**(1):16–29.

134. Hsieh FJ, Chang FM, Ko TM, Chen HY Percutaneous ultrasound-guided fetal blood sampling in the management of nonimmune hydrops fetalis. *Am J Obstet Gynecol* 1987;**157** (1):44–9.

135. Jelin AC, Sagaser KG, Wilkins-Haug L. Prenatal genetic testing options. *Pediatr Clin North Am* 2019;**66**(2):281–93.

136. Winichagoon P, Sithongdee S, Kanokpongsakdi S, et al. Noninvasive prenatal diagnosis for hemoglobin Bart's hydrops fetalis. *Int J Hematol* 2005;**81**(5):396–9.

137. Tungwiwat W, Fucharoen S, Fucharoen G, Ratanasiri T, Sanchaisuriya K. Development and application of a real-time quantitative PCR for prenatal detection of fetal alpha(0)-thalassemia from maternal plasma. *Ann N Y Acad Sci* 2006;**1075**:103–7.

138. Ho SS, Chong SS, Koay ES, et al. Noninvasive prenatal exclusion of haemoglobin Bart's using foetal DNA from maternal plasma. *Prenat Diagn* 2009;**30**(1):65–73.

139. Hudecova I, Chiu RW. Non-invasive prenatal diagnosis of thalassemias using maternal plasma cell free DNA. *Best Pract Res Clin Obstet Gynaecol* 2017;**39**:63–73.

140. Yates A. *Prenatal Screening and Testing for Hemoglobinopathy* (Philadelphia PA: Wolters Kluwer, 2019).

141. Chik KW, Shing MM, Li CK, et al. Treatment of hemoglobin Bart's hydrops with bone marrow transplantation. *J Pediatr* 1998;**132** (6):1039–42.

142. Thornley I, Lehmann L, Ferguson WS, et al. Homozygous alpha-thalassemia treated with intrauterine transfusions and postnatal hematopoietic stem cell transplantation. *Bone Marrow Transplant* 2003;**32**(3):341–2.

143. Lucke T, Pfister S Durken M. Neurodevelopmental outcome and haematological course of a long-time survivor with homozygous alpha-thalassaemia: Case report and review of the literature. *Acta Paediatr* 2005;**94**(9):1330–3.

144. Yi JS, Moertel CL, Baker KS. Homozygous alpha-thalassemia treated with intrauterine transfusions and unrelated donor hematopoietic cell transplantation. *J Pediatr* 2009;**154**(5):766–8.

145. Derderian SC, Jeanty C, Walters MC, Vichinsky E, MacKenzie TC. In utero hematopoietic cell transplantation for hemoglobinopathies. *Front Pharmacol* 2014;**5**:278.

146. Higgs DR, Weatherall DJ. The alpha thalassaemias. *Cell Mol Life Sci* 2009;**66** (7):1154–62.

147. Jomoui W, Fucharoen G, Sanchaisuriya K, Nguyen VH, Fucharoen S. Hemoglobin Constant Spring among Southeast Asian populations: Haplotypic heterogeneities and phylogenetic analysis. *PLoS One* 2015;**10**(12):e0145230.

148. Sirilert S, Charoenkwan P, Sirichotiyakul S, et al. Prenatal diagnosis and management of homozygous hemoglobin Constant Spring disease. *J Perinatol* 2019;**39**(7):927–33.

149. Olivieri NF. The beta-thalassemias. *N Engl J Med* 1999;**341**(2):99–109.

150. Cunningham MJ, Sankaran VG, Nathan DG Orkin SH. The thalassemias. In Orkin SH, Nathan DG, Ginsburg D, et al., eds. *Nathan and Oski's Hematology of Infancy and Childhood* (Philadelphia PA: Saunders/ Elsevier,2009).

151. Cao A, Rosatelli MC, Monni G, Galanello R. Screening for thalassemia: A model of success. *Obstet Gynecol Clin North Am* 2002;**29** (2):305–28, vi–vii.

152. Olivieri NF, Muraca GM, O'Donnell A, et al. Studies in haemoglobin E beta-thalassaemia. *Br J Haematol* 2008;**141**(3):388–97.

153. Sirichotiyakul S, Saetung R, Sanguansermsri T. Prenatal diagnosis of beta-thalassemia/Hb E by hemoglobin typing compared to DNA analysis. *Hemoglobin* 2009;**33**(1):17–23.

154. Vichinsky EP, MacKlin EA, WayeJ S, Lorey F, Olivieri NF. Changes in the epidemiology of thalassemia in North America: A new minority disease. *Pediatrics* 2005;**116**(6):e818–825.

155. Lorey F, Cunningham G, Shafer F, Lubin B, Vichinsky E. Universal screening for hemoglobinopathies using high-performance liquid chromatography: Clinical results of

2.2 million screens. *Eur J Hum Genet* 1994;**2** (4):262–71.

156. Lenfant C. *The Management of Sickle Cell Disease* (Bethesda MD: National Insitutes of Health, 2002).

157. Gaston MH, VerterJ I, Woods G, et al. Prophylaxis with oral penicillin in children with sickle cell anemia. A randomized trial. *N Engl J Med* 1986;**314**(25):1593–99.

158. Michlitsch J, Azimi M, Hoppe C, et al. Newborn screening for hemoglobinopathies in California. *Pediatr Blood Cancer* 2009;**52**(4):486–90.

159. Wethers D, Pearson HA, Gaston M. Newborn screening for sickle cell disease and other hemoglobinopathies. *Pediatrics* 1989;**89** (5):813–14.

160. Koshy M, Burd L. Obstetric and gynecologic issues. In Embury S, Hebbel RP eds. *Sickle Cell Disease: Basic Principles and Clinical Practice* (New York: Raven Press, 1995), p. 689.

161. Villers MS, Jamison MG, De Castro LM, James AH. Morbidity associated with sickle cell disease in pregnancy. *Am J Obstet Gynecol* 2008;**199**(2):125,e121–5.

162. Williamson D. The unstable haemoglobins. *Blood Rev* 1993;**7**(3):146–63.

163. Carrell RW, Kay R. A simple method for the detection of unstable haemoglobins. *Br J Haematol* 1972;**23**(5):615–19.

164. Lee-Potter JP, Deacon-Smith RA, Simpkiss MJ, Kamuzora H, Lehmann H. A new cause of haemolytic anaemia in the newborn. A description of an unstable fetal haemoglobin: F Poole, alpha2-G-gamma2 130 tryptophan yields glycine. *J Clin Pathol* 1975;**28**(4):317–20.

165. Charache S, Mondzac AM, Gessner U. Hemoglobin Hasharon (alpha-2–47 his(CD5; beta-2): A hemoglobin found in low concentration. *J Clin Invest* 1969;**48**(5):834–47.

166. Levine RL, Lincoln DR, Buchholz WM, Gribble TJ Schwartz HC. Hemoglobin Hasharon in a premature infant with hemolytic anemia. *Pediatric Research* 1975;**9**(1):7–11.

167. Bender, JW, Reilly MP Asakura T. Molecular stability and function of hemoglobins Hasharon (alpha(2)47 (CD5)Asp–His beta 2) and Hasharon (alpha(2)47 (CD5)Asp–His delta 2). *Hemoglobin* 1984;**8**(1):61–73.

168. Martin H, Huisman TH. Formation of ferrihaemoglobin of isolated human haemoglobin types by sodium nitrite. *Nature* 1963;**200**:898–9.

169. Bartos HR, Desforges JF. Erythrocyte DPNH dependent diaphorase levels in infants. *Pediatrics* 1966;**37**(6):991–3.

170. Comly HH. Cyanosis in infants caused by nitrates in well water. *J Am Med Assoc* 1945;**129** (2):112–16.

171. Gelperin A, Jacobs EE, Kletke LS. The development of methemoglobin in mothers and newborn infants from nitrate in water supplies. *IMJ Ill Med J* 1971;**140**(1):42–4 passim.

172. Keating JP, Lell ME, Strauss AW, Zarkowsky H, Smith GE. Infantile methemoglobinemia caused by carrot juice. *N Engl J Med* 1973;**288**(16):824–6.

173. Yano SS, Danish EH, Hsia YE. Transient methemoglobinemia with acidosis in infants. *J Pediatr* 1982;**100**(3):415–18.

174. Avner JR, Henretig FM, McAneney CM. Acquired methemoglobinemia: The relationship of cause to course of illness. *Am J Dis Child* 1990;**144**(11):1229–30.

175. Kay MA, O'Brien W, Kessler B, et al. Transient organic aciduria and methemoglobinemia with acute gastroenteritis. *Pediatrics* 1990;**85** (4):589–92.

176. Pollack ES, Pollack CV, Jr. Incidence of subclinical methemoglobinemia in infants with diarrhea. *Ann Emerg Med* 1994;**24**(4):652–6.

177. Hanukoglu A, Danon PN. Endogenous methemoglobinemia associated with diarrheal disease in infancy. *J Pediatr Gastroenterol Nutr* 1996;**23**(1):1–7.

178. Wessel DL, Adatia I, Van MarterLJ, et al. Improved oxygenation in a randomized trial of inhaled nitric oxide for persistent pulmonary hypertension of the newborn. *Pediatrics* 1997;**100** (5):E7.

179. Climie CR, McLean S, Starmer GA, Thomas J. Methaemoglobinaemia in mother and foetus following continuous epidural analgesia with prilocaine: Clinical and experimental data. *Br J Anaesth* 1967;**39**(2):155–160.

180. Law RM, Halpern S, MartinsRF, et al. Measurement of methemoglobin after EMLA analgesia for newborn circumcision. *Biol Neonate* 1996;**70**(4):213–17.

181. Tush GM, Kuhn RJ. Methemoglobinemia induced by an over-the-counter medication. *Ann Pharmacother* 1996;**30**(11):1251–4.

182. Brisman M, Ljung BM, Otterbom I, Larsson LE, Andreasson SE. Methaemoglobin formation after the use of EMLA cream in term neonates. *Acta Paediatr* 1998;**87**(11):1191–4.

183. Essink-Tebbes CM, WuisEW, Liem KD, van Dongen RT, Hekster YA. Safety of lidocaine-prilocaine cream application four times a day in premature neonates:a pilot study. *Eur J Pediatr* 1999;**158**(5):421–3.

184. Kearns GL, Fiser DH. Metoclopramide-induced methemoglobinemia. *Pediatrics* 1988;**82**(3):364–6.

185. Hjelt K, Lund JT, Scherling B, et al. Methaemoglobinaemia among neonates in a neonatal intensive care unit. *Acta Paediatr* 1995;**84**(4):365–70.

186. Percy MJ, McFerran NV, Lappin TR. Disorders of oxidised haemoglobin. *Blood Rev* 2005;**19**(2):61–8.

187. Percy MJ, Lappin TR. Recessive congenital methaemoglobinaemia: Cytochrome b(5; reductase deficiency. *Br J Haematol* 2008;**141**(3):298–308.

188. Kutlar F, Hilliard LM, Zhuang L, et al. Hb M Dothan [beta 25/26 (B7/B8)/(GGT/GAG->GAG//Gly/Glu->Glu]; a new mechanism of unstable methemoglobin variant and molecular characteristics. *Blood Cells Mol Dis* 2009;**43**(3):235–8.

189. Hayashi A, Fujita T, Fujimura M, Titani K. A new abnormal fetal hemoglobin, Hb FM-Osaka (alpha 2 gamma 2 63His replaced by Tyr). *Hemoglobin* 1980;**4**(3–4):447–8.

190. Glader BE, Zwerdling D, Kutlar F, et al. Hb F-M-Osaka or alpha 2 G gamma 2 (63)(E7)His -- Tyr in a Caucasian male infant. *Hemoglobin* 1989;**13**(7–8):769–73.

191. Priest JR, Watterson J, Jones RT, Faassen AE, Hedlund, BE. Mutant fetal hemoglobin causing cyanosis in a newborn. *Pediatrics* 1989;**83**(5):734–6.

192. Harley JD, Celermajer JM. Neonatal methaemoglobinaemia and the red-brown screening-test. *Lancet* 1970;**2**(7685):1223–5.

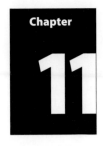

Polycythemia and Hyperviscosity in the Newborn

Chapter 11

Ted S. Rosenkrantz and William Oh

Introduction

Polycythemia of the newborn is first mentioned in the Bible as Esau and Jacob are described at the time of their birth. Esau appears to be the recipient of a twin-to-twin transfusion (Genesis 25:25: "The first one emerged red ..."). There is little in the modern medical literature concerning polycythemia in the newborn until the early 1970s [1–5]. During this time, there were a number of case reports and small series of infants with various symptoms that were thought to be secondary to an elevated hematocrit and blood viscosity. It was not until the 1980s that several investigators systematically examined the association between polycythemia, hyperviscosity of the blood, and organ-system dysfunction. These studies have done much to enlighten our understanding of the relationships between abnormalities of the hematocrit, blood viscosity, organ blood flow, and organ function. The dissemination of this knowledge has provided a clinical approach that is based on well-defined data and has clarified the role of polycythemia as an etiologic factor for organ dysfunction in the neonate.

Definitions

Definitions of polycythemia and hyperviscosity have varied by study and methodology. Common variables have been the source of the blood sample and the age of the infant at the time of measurement [6–11]. In many studies, a hematocrit value of 65% or above has been diagnostic for polycythemia. Using cord blood from appropriate-for-gestational-age (AGA) infants, Gross and colleagues defined hyperviscosity as a value that was two standard deviations greater than the mean (Fig. 11.1) [5]. Using blood samples from three different sites (peripheral vein, umbilical vein, and capillary), Ramamurthy and Brans defined hyperviscosity as a value that was three standard deviations from the mean [6]. This coincided with an umbilical venous hematocrit value of 63% or above. This study also found that

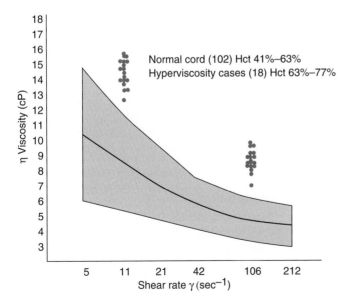

Fig. 11.1 The shaded area represents the viscosity of cord blood at shear rates from 2 to 212/s for 102 healthy full-term appropriate-for-gestational-age infants (mean ± 2 SD). Viscosity for 18 "symptomatic" infants is plotted at shear rates of 11/s and 106/s. Hematocrit (Hct) values for each group are indicated. (From Gross et al. [5] with permission.)

Normal cord (102) Hct 41%–63%
Hyperviscosity cases (18) Hct 63%–77%

Table 11.1 Factors that influence hematocrit in the perinatal period

Timing of cord clamping

Relative height of infant to placenta before cord clamping

Altitude

Sampling site

Postnatal age

Intrauterine growth

Fetal hypoxia

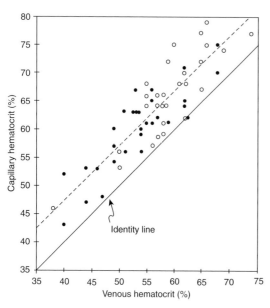

Fig. 11.2 Correlation between capillary and venous blood hematocrit in newborn infants. (○) 1–6 h; (●) 12–24 h. (From Rosenkrantz and Oh [68] with permission.)

capillary samples were higher than those from the peripheral vein, which in turn were greater than those from the umbilical vein. This is consistent with findings published previously by Oh and Lind [7]. In their study, the capillary hematocrit was consistently 10% higher than simultaneously obtained peripheral venous samples. Data from this study have been replotted and shown in Fig. 11.2. Based on population data from many sources, it is now accepted that polycythemia should be defined as a hematocrit value of 65% or above from a large, freely flowing peripheral vein. In a parallel manner, hyperviscosity should be defined as a value of more than two standard deviations from the mean.

Incidence

The incidence of polycythemia is 2%–5% of all infants born at term [6, 8–11]. Factors known to influence the hematocrit at birth are listed in Table 11.1. Delay in clamping of the umbilical cord will result in a significant increase in hematocrit and blood volume [12–15]. A recent Cochrane Review that included 12 trials and 3,139 infants show an increase of 0.49 mg/dL associated with delayed cord clamping and no infants with polycythemia [16]. From birth to 6–12 hours of age, the hematocrit will increase due to shifts in body water [11, 17]. By 24 hours of age, the hematocrit will become similar to the value at birth and will remain relatively stable. Infants who experience fetal distress, with abnormalities in fetal growth, with genetic abnormalities and of mothers with poorly controlled diabetes have an increased incidence of polycythemia. Acute fetal distress results in a shift of blood volume from the placenta to the fetus, leading to an increased blood volume and red-cell mass. Those infants who experience intrauterine growth retardation or fetal hyperglycemia exist in a relatively hypoxic intrauterine environment. This results in increased erythropoietin production, increased red-cell mass, and a greater likelihood of polycythemia. Birth at centers located at higher elevations also is associated with a greater incidence of polycythemia. This was documented in two studies by Wirth and colleagues [8, 9], who noted that the incidence of polycythemia in Denver, Colorado (1,610 m above sea level), was twice that in Norfolk, Virginia (sea level).

Viscosity

It is important to have an understanding of the physics of the flow of fluids to understand how blood viscosity affects blood flow in the newborn infant. It will also allow for the understanding of the clinical symptoms observed in infants with an elevated hematocrit.

Definition

Viscosity, as defined by Poiseuille, is the ratio of shear stress to shear rate, as demonstrated in the formula below [18]:

$$\eta = \frac{(p - p')r^4\pi}{8LQ} = \frac{\text{shear stress}}{\text{shear rate}},$$

in which η is blood viscosity (dyn·s/cm^2, or poise), $p - p'$ is the pressure gradient along the blood vessel, r is the radius, L is the length of the blood vessel, and Q is blood flow. The shear stress that represents the pressure gradient along the blood vessel is expressed in dyne [19]. The shear rate, which represents the velocity between two fluid planes, divided by the distance between them, is expressed as reciprocal seconds, s^{-1}.

As demonstrated in Poiseuille's original work, the ratio of shear stress to shear rate, or viscosity, of a fluid is constant. However, this is true only for homogeneous or Newtonian fluids. Blood is a suspension of particles in a solution and does not behave as a Newtonian fluid. The viscosity of blood does not remain constant with variations in shear stress and shear rate. This can be demonstrated in vitro using a cone/plate viscometer, such as that described by Wells and colleagues [20]. In this device, shear rate can be varied and the resultant shear stress measured.

Shear rates in large vessels such as the aorta are greater (100–300/s) than those observed in small vessels such as arterioles (11–25/s) [19]. Using the above formula, one would then predict that the viscosity of the blood would be lower in large vessels and higher in small blood vessels (see later in this chapter for exceptions to this rule). While knowing the shear rate in a particular vessel will allow an estimate of the blood viscosity and a microviscometer will allow in vitro measurement of blood viscosity, there are multiple factors that can vary the in vivo viscosity of the blood. These other factors are reviewed below.

Factors That Affect Blood Viscosity

It is pertinent to understand all of the factors that contribute to whole-blood viscosity, although the primary determinant of blood viscosity in the newborn is the red blood cell (RBC) concentration.

Hematocrit

The hematocrit, a reflection of the RBC concentration, has a logarithmic relationship with blood viscosity at shear rates (Fig. 11.3). The greatest changes occur at the lowest shear rates and at hematocrits that exceed 65% [17, 21].

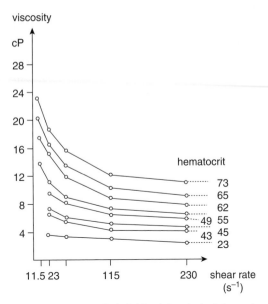

Fig. 11.3 Variation of whole-blood viscosity in eight newborn infants at different hematocrit values and shear rates. From Bergqvist [25] with permission.

Plasma Proteins

The plasma has a viscosity of 1.0–1.5 centipoise (cP), similar to the viscosity of water [22–24]. Water, with a viscosity of 1 cP, behaves as a Newtonian fluid, as the viscosity is constant at all shear rates. As such, the plasma protein contributes little to blood viscosity under normal conditions. Adult syndromes of hyperviscosity can be attributed to hyperproteinemia in conditions such as diabetes and Waldenstrom's macroglobulinemia. These are not conditions observed in the newborn [25–27].

Red Blood Cell Deformity

The RBC is the major contributor to whole-blood viscosity, because it is the most prominent particle suspended in the blood and because of its intrinsic properties. The RBC consists of a membrane that moves around a body of internal fluid, making it a dynamic particle [24, 28]. The surrounding membrane is quite deformable, with the RBC of the newborn having a greater degree of deformability than that of the adult [27, 29]. The viscosity of the internal fluid of the RBC will increase with cell age [30]. The internal viscosity also appears to increase with decreasing blood flow and external shear rate.

White Blood Cells

The white blood cell of the newborn is larger and less deformable than the RBC. It has been shown that extremely high concentrations of white blood cells, as observed in congenital leukemia, can increase the whole-blood viscosity [31–33].

Fibrinogen

Due to its low concentration in the blood of the newborn, fibrinogen contributes little to whole-blood viscosity [23].

Platelets

Although they are relatively inflexible particles, platelets do not appear to affect blood viscosity in the normal state. In adults with vaso-occlusive disease, platelet aggregates may affect the viscosity of the blood in narrowed vascular areas [22]. Platelet aggregates do not appear to be a factor in the blood viscosity of newborn infants with normal hematocrits or polycythemia.

Blood pH

Whole-blood viscosity increases with pH below 7.00 [22, 34]. This is due to a shift of the fluid into the RBCs with acidosis. This may be one of the factors responsible for an increase in blood viscosity in asphyxia, along with the associated placental transfusion that also increases the blood volume of the infant.

Vessel Size

In large blood vessels, such as the aorta, blood flow and shear rate (100–300/s) are high. Therefore, the apparent viscosity of the blood is low. The opposite is true in small blood vessels. Blood flow and shear rate are low (11–25/s) and viscosity is high. As shown in Fig. 11.3, changes in hematocrit cause the greatest changes in viscosity in the small blood vessels.

While blood behaves as a non-Newtonian fluid in large and small blood vessels, the opposite is true in the capillaries of most organs. The diameter of capillaries is in the range of 3–5 μm while the RBC has a diameter of 8.5 μm. As shown by Fahraeus and Lindqvist, viscosity actually decreases with diminishing size of the capillary (see Fig. 11.4) [35]. This phenomenon has been confirmed in vivo in capillaries as narrow as 3 μm [24]. The term "bolus flow" has been given to this phenomenon. It reflects high hemodynamic efficiency. Measurements of the viscosity in the

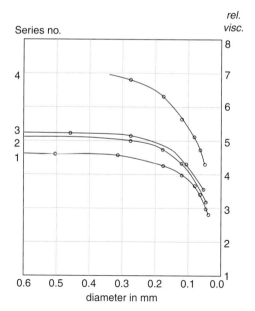

Fig. 11.4 Blood viscosity in small capillaries. (From Fahraeus and Lindqvist [35] with permission.)

capillary are in the range of 1.3 cP, similar to those of plasma and water. As observed in Fig. 11.4, the hematocrit of the blood does not affect the viscosity in the capillary. Thus, it is important to keep in mind that in vitro measurements of blood viscosity may not reflect the in vivo viscosity of the blood in the capillary. Dintenfass has suggested that viscosity may increase again as the capillary size decreases below 4 μm [22]. The variation in capillary size in different organs may therefore explain why changes in hematocrit and viscosity seem to have an effect on flow in some organs but no effect in others.

Hemodynamics

Many of the clinical problems observed in infants with polycythemia and hyperviscosity have been ascribed to disturbances in organ blood flow. Therefore, it is essential to understand how changes in hematocrit and blood viscosity affect the blood flow of the different organs of the newborn infant.

Cardiopulmonary Blood Flow and Function

The primary change in cardiac function is decreased output, which is associated with an increase in arterial oxygen content, no change in oxygen transport/delivery or consumption in the myocardium or whole body, and increased pulmonary and, to a lesser extent, systemic resistance [36–44]. These findings have been observed in both appropriate animal models and human newborn infants.

The decrease in cardiac output appears to be the result of a reduction in stroke volume and heart rate, or both [44]. In our own studies of polycythemic infants, we found that heart rate increased following a partial exchange transfusion (PET) with Plasmanate® to decrease the hematocrit and maintain blood volume [40]. Swetnam and colleagues found that following PET, there was an increase in heart rate, stroke volume, and cardiac output as well as systemic oxygen transport [44]. Studies of myocardial oxygenation have shown that polycythemia and changes in blood viscosity do affect blood flow but do not adversely affect oxygen transport and consumption [38].

The changes in systemic and pulmonary circulation with changes in hematocrit have been demonstrated in both newborn animal and human studies [39, 41]. Fouron and Hebert have shown in the newborn lamb model that pulmonary resistance increases to a greater extent than systemic resistance with increases in hematocrit [41]. At hematocrit values of 70%, pulmonary vascular resistance was equal to systemic resistance. The change in pulmonary resistance will also change the direction in blood flow through the ductus arteriosus if it is still patent. These findings are similar to those found in a study of human infants [45]. The change in pulmonary resistance with elevation of the hematocrit is thought to explain, in part, the cardiopulmonary symptoms that have been reported by Gatti and colleagues as well as the plethoric or cyanotic appearance observed by many clinicians [42].

Gastrointestinal Blood Flow and Oxygenation

Gastrointestinal blood flow has been studied in animal models [36, 43]. In the newborn piglet, polycythemia is associated with a decrease in blood flow but normal oxygen transport. However, oxygen extraction and uptake are reduced, suggesting abnormalities in local regulation of oxygen uptake that are not related to oxygen availability. The underlying etiology is unclear.

Liver and pancreatic function have been reported in the term newborn with polycythemia [46]. Compared with infants with normal hematocrit, the study found an elevated bile concentration in the serum and a low lipase and trypsin activity in duodenal juice on the first day of life. PET tended to normalize the bile acid and lipase concentrations. These findings suggest that polycythemia affects the enterohepatic circulation of bile acids and the exocrine pancreatic function during the first days of life. However, it should be noted that there were no clinical symptoms associated with these findings. Therefore, the implications for short- and long-term management as well as nutritional consequences are not clear.

Renal Blood Flow and Function

Kotagal and Kleinman studied renal function in a puppy model of normovolemic polycythemia [47]. Renal blood flow was unaffected by the elevation in hematocrit. However, the decrease in plasma volume resulted in a lower plasma flow and glomerular filtration rate (GFR). The urine output was also lower, as was the Na^+ and K^+ excretion. There was no change in systemic blood pressure or renal blood flow. Therefore, the calculated renal vascular resistance was not increased by the change in hematocrit. This suggests that the Fahraeus–Lindqvist effect (decreased viscosity as vessel size decreases) is present in the kidney.

In a study of renal function in normovolemic and hypervolemic newborn infants, Oh and colleagues found that renal function was affected by blood volume [12]. One group of infants had late cord clamping and a mean hematocrit of 62%, while those with immediate cord clamping had hematocrit of 50%. The group with late cord clamping had higher blood and RBC volume, mean arterial blood pressure, and renal blood flow as well as a greater GFR and urine output compared with the group with immediate cord clamping and normal blood volumes.

The apparent discrepancy between these two studies can be explained by the methodology. In the puppy model, blood volume was held constant so that plasma volume and flow were reduced in subjects with polycythemia. In the human study, the expanded blood volume was accompanied by a normal plasma volume and flow. Therefore, renal function in infants is a function of not only hematocrit but also blood volume. Infants with normovolemic polycythemia would be expected to have a reduction in renal function, while those with an increased blood volume should have normal renal function.

Carcass Blood Flow

Studies of isolated muscle in calf and dog models have shown that despite changes in blood flow associated with polycythemia, oxygen transport, and uptake are normal in resting and working muscle [48–51]. Studies of peripheral blood flow in newborn infants show an increase in blood flow following PET [44]. Transcutaneous oxygen measurements are normal in polycythemia [51]. These studies suggest that polycythemia and hyperviscosity do not adversely affect oxygenation of the carcass.

Brain Blood Flow and Oxygenation

In 1982, we published the first study to document changes in the cerebral circulation of polycythemic newborn infants using Doppler techniques [40]. Polycythemic infants were found to have a significant reduction in cerebral blood flow (CBF) velocity compared with similar term infants with normal hematocrit and blood viscosity values. Following PET to lower the hematocrit and blood viscosity, the CBF velocity measurements increased and were similar to those of the control infants.

Jones and colleagues demonstrated in newborn lambs that CBF was correlated inversely with the arterial oxygen content of the blood in studies in which hematocrit and oxygen levels were varied independently [52]. Viscosity, which was not measured, presumably varied with the changes in hematocrit. Since the blood viscosity was not measured, Jones and colleagues could not state conclusively that it played a role in the observed changes in blood flow. However, the study concluded that arterial oxygen content was the primary determinate of CBF when other variables, such as cerebral metabolic rate, are constant.

To answer the question about the role that blood viscosity might play in the cerebral circulation, we designed a study in newborn lambs in which arterial oxygen content and blood viscosity were varied independently [53]. Using isovolemic exchange transfusion of newborn lamb RBCs, we increased the hematocrit, arterial oxygen content, and blood viscosity. This was associated with a decrease in the CBF. Sodium nitrite was then infused to cause methemoglobin formation and to decrease the arterial oxygen content while maintaining the increased blood viscosity. The CBF values increased to control levels. Cerebral oxygen delivery was constant throughout the study. From this, we concluded that the decreased CBF observed with polycythemia and hyperviscosity is due to the associated increase in arterial oxygen content.

Following these studies, Goldstein and colleagues varied blood viscosity by increasing the concentration of fibrinogen in the blood to see whether this would affect CBF in a newborn-lamb model [54]. Again, it was found that CBF varied with the arterial oxygen content, and not with the blood viscosity. Lastly, we found in a study of newborn lambs that polycythemia does not affect the uptake of oxygen or the metabolic rate of the brain, as long as usual brain substrates are available [55].

In conclusion, brain blood flow is decreased in infants with polycythemia. Blood viscosity is not responsible for this reduction in blood flow. Therefore, it would appear that the Fahraeus–Lindqvist effect is functional in the vasculature of the brain. That is, classic cerebral autoregulation is intact in infants with polycythemia and who have not suffered from some type of brain injury such as brain hypoxia or trauma.

Fetal Blood Flow and Oxygenation

There is little information on the in utero effects of polycythemia and hyperviscosity on the fetus. Tenenbaum and colleagues performed isovolemic packed red cell transfusion on fetal lambs using adult sheep RBCs [56]. This resulted in an increase in hematocrit and viscosity, no change in venous oxygen content, and a decrease in umbilical blood flow and oxygen delivery. However, there was an increase in oxygen extraction, so that fetal oxygen uptake was not affected by the polycythemia. It should be noted that it is not clear what the effects of hypervolemic polycythemia might have on the fetus. This is an important point, as shifts in placental–fetal blood volume distribution are not uncommon (e.g., fetal hypoxia). In addition, there are no data on polycythemia and hyperviscosity and regional blood flow and oxygenation in the fetus.

Etiologies

There are three major categories of etiologies or clinical scenarios in which polycythemia and hyperviscosity may be observed. As outlined in Table 11.2, these include chronic fetal hypoxia, acute fetal hypoxia/asphyxia, and delayed clamping of the umbilical cord at delivery. Other less common causes and associations include maternal–fetal hemorrhage, fetofetal transfusion, and chromosomal abnormalities, including trisomy 21 and Beckwith–Wiedemann syndrome [2, 9, 13–15, 57–59].

In the past, the most common cause of polycythemia was placental–fetal transfusion via delayed clamping of the umbilical cord. To avoid this problem, the cord should be clamped within 60 seconds of delivery of the body [15].

As discussed earlier in this chapter, altitude of the external maternal environment and intrinsic oxygen concentration are important but uncontrollable causes of polycythemia [8, 9].

Perinatal asphyxia and fetal hypoxia remain significant causes of polycythemia. Philip and colleagues examined placental residual volumes and neonatal outcomes [60]. Small placental residual blood volume was associated with fetal distress and low Apgar scores. Similar observations were made by Flod and Ackerman and Yao and

Lind [61, 62]. Oh and colleagues demonstrated that intrauterine hypoxia resulted in a shift of blood from the placental compartment to the fetus [63]. There was a correlation between the length of the hypoxic event and the shift in blood volume. The data suggested that fetal vasodilatation associated with fetal hypoxia was part of the mechanism.

Fetuses with abnormal growth (small (SGA) or large (LGA) for gestational age) are at high risk for polycythemia [64]. This would appear to be secondary to chronic fetal hypoxia, which leads to increased erythropoietin levels, which in turn cause an increase in RBC production [65]. Over time, the red cell mass increases to increase the oxygen-carrying capacity and maintain a normal oxygen content in the face of a low PaO_2. Clinical examples include pregnancies complicated by placental insufficiency and increased fetal metabolism. Placental insufficiency frequently exists in pregnancy-induced hypertension, HELLP (hemolysis, elevated liver enzymes, and low platelets) syndrome, post-term pregnancy, and maternal cigarette smoking. Poorly controlled diabetes during pregnancy is associated with an increased fetal metabolic rate, as is fetal hyperthyroidism [66]. Hod and colleagues have documented that fetal hypoxia and polycythemia can be prevented by good glycemic control in the pregnant woman [67].

Table 11.2 Etiologies and syndromes associated with polycythemia

Acute hypoxia
Chronic hypoxia
Infant of diabetic mother
IUGR, SGA
Pre-eclampsia
Placental insufficiency
Neonatal thyrotoxicosis
Maternal smoking
High altitude
Intrauterine transfusion
Fetofetal transfusion
Maternal–fetal transfusion
Genetic syndromes
Trisomy 21, 18, 13
Beckwith–Wiedemann syndrome

Notes: IUGR, intrauterine growth retardation; SGA, small for gestational age

Symptoms

This section will attempt to sort the clinical symptoms associated with polycythemia by organ system and to provide a physiologic explanation for the symptomatology. Table 11.3 lists symptoms that have been observed in populations of newborn infants with polycythemia and their frequency, as reported in several different series [68]. In addition, Gatti and colleagues reported prospectively on a population of 629 infants; 25 were polycythemic but none had any symptoms [42].

Investigators have noted an increased incidence of polycythemia in the SGA population of infants. While some have attributed observed abnormalities to polycythemia, Hakanson and Oh found the incidence of abnormalities in SGA infants with a normal hematocrit to be similar to that in those with polycythemia [69]. This observation serves as an important point. Many of the symptoms observed in infants with polycythemia are attributable to other perinatal problems associated with

Table 11.3 Frequency of clinical symptoms observed in association with polycythemia

Clinical symptoms	Gross et al. [5] (n = 18) (%)	Ramamurthy and Brans [6] (n = 54) (%)	Black et al. [100] (n = 111) (%)	Goldberg et al. [98] (n = 20) (%)
Cyanosis	89	17	7	nr
Plethora	83	63	nr	nr
Tremulous/jittery	67	13	nr	nr
Abnormal EEG	33	nr	nr	nr
Seizures	28	0	0	nr
Respiratory distress	44	4	10	15
Cardiomegaly	17	nr	nr	85
Lethargy/poor feeding	nr	50	+	55
Hyperbilirubinemia	50	6	nr	5
Abnormal blood smear	50	nr	nr	nr
Thrombocytopenia	39	nr	nr	25
Hypoglycemia	33	nr	27	40
Hypocalcemia	6	nr	nr	0

Notes: EEG, electroencephalogram; nr, not reported or examined; +, greater incidence compared with control group

polycythemia, such as asphyxia and chronic hypoxia, and are not related directly to the polycythemia and hyperviscosity.

Abnormalities of Blood Volume

When the population of all polycythemic infants is studied, blood volume is increased for body weight at all gestational ages [12, 70, 71]. However, there is a fair amount of variability from infant to infant due to the multiple etiologies for the polycythemia. Saigal and Usher showed a significant relationship between infants with increased blood volume and infants with cardiorespiratory problems [57]. Brans and colleagues and Thorton and colleagues demonstrated that polycythemic infants do not differ from infants with normal hematocrits when total body water, mean extracellular water, mean intracellular water, and mean interstitial water are compared [71, 72]. Plasma volumes also appear to be normal.

Cardiopulmonary Symptoms

Cyanosis, tachypnea, cardiomegaly, and "plethora" of the lung fields on X-ray film of the chest are frequent findings reported in infants with polycythemia [4, 5, 42, 57, 73]. Although the PaO$_2$ may be normal, many of these infants have a red–blue color. The respiratory distress may be due, in part, to an elevated pulmonary vascular resistance and increased intrapulmonary shunting secondary to the increase in blood viscosity. Most investigators have reported complete resolution of the respiratory symptoms with PET.

In 1995, Scott and Evans reported on a set of monochorionic twins in which the recipient twin developed ischemia and gangrene of a lower leg [74]. We have observed a similar situation in a set of preterm monoamniotic twins. The recipient had an elevated hematocrit. Within an hour of birth, there was decreased perfusion of one leg. The systemic blood pressure was normal to elevated and cardiac performance was poor. An ultrasound examination revealed a clot in the distal aorta that extended into the iliac artery. The clot, causing aortic obstruction and increased afterload, was thought to be responsible for normal to increased systemic blood pressure and poor cardiac function. Various thrombolytic agents were not helpful, and the infant was too small to introduce a catheter into the aorta for perfusion of local thrombolytic therapy. The clinical picture was consistent with prenatal development of the clot. Recent literature warns of the risk of intraventricular hemorrhage (IVH) in such preterm twins.

Gastrointestinal Symptoms

Multiple investigators have reported on infants with polycythemia and poor feeding or vomiting [65, 75, 76]. In addition some studies have suggested an association between polycythemia and the development of necrotizing enterocolitis (NEC) [77, 78]. Many of these infants have other risks for the development of NEC, including intrauterine growth retardation, asphyxia, or both. A study by Martinez-Tallo and colleagues found no association between polycythemia and NEC [79]. Thus, it is unclear whether polycythemia is responsible for the development of the NEC or the other associated perinatal complications.

LeBlanc and colleagues created a model of polycythemia in the newborn puppy [80]. The incidence of intestinal histology that was consistent with NEC was 58%. The intestinal blood flow and oxygen uptake data published by Nowicki and colleagues suggest that the bowel may experience some hypoxia in the unfed state [36].

In a randomized study of infants with polycythemia, Black and colleagues found that 6% of the observed or untreated infants had serious gastrointestinal symptoms whereas 51% who received a PET exhibited serious gastrointestinal symptoms [81]. One-third of the treated infants had radiographic evidence of pneumatosis intestinalis. This study suggests that the most important risk factor for the development of NEC is an exchange transfusion to reduce the hematocrit, and not polycythemia. Of interest is that an isovolemic exchange transfusion with packed RBCs was used to increase the hematocrit in the experiments of both LeBlanc and Nowicki.

Renal Symptoms

Acute renal failure has been reported in a term infant with polycythemia [82]. The mechanism for alterations in renal function has been clarified by the studies of Oh and colleagues and Kotagal and Kleinman [12, 47]. In infants with a normal blood volume, plasma volume is decreased, as is renal plasma flow and GFR. In infants who are hypervolemic, the plasma volume, renal plasma flow, and GFR will be normal. The cause of renal dysfunction in any particular infant may be complicated further by acute tubular necrosis (ATN)

secondary to perinatal asphyxia. Therefore, the abnormalities in renal function in any individual infant with polycythemia may be multifactorial.

Hypoglycemia

Hypoglycemia is frequently a problem in infants with polycythemia, even after correcting for factors such as intrauterine growth retardation. Leake and colleagues and Creswell and colleagues have examined this problem utilizing the newborn lamb [83, 84]. Both groups speculated about decreased glucose production and increased glucose uptake, but a definitive conclusion could not be derived from their work; thus, there was no final explanation. Data from our own experiments in polycythemic lambs who were made hypoglycemic support the hypothesis that the hypoglycemia is secondary to a reduced plasma volume [85]. Glucose exists almost exclusively in the plasma. Therefore, the glucose-carrying capacity is reduced. Combined with decreased blood flow in many organs, extraction of glucose must be increased to meet the metabolic requirements of the body. Therefore, the plasma glucose concentration, especially the venous concentration, will be lower than normal.

Hematologic Symptoms

Both thrombocytopenia and low antithrombin III (AT-III) levels have been reported in infants with polycythemia [86–95]. Disseminated intravascular coagulation (DIC) has been reported by one investigator but not confirmed by others. Explanations for the low platelet count include impaired production secondary to tissue hypoxia, predominance in the marrow of erythropoietic cells, slow spleen blood flow, and decreased plasma fraction with normal concentrations. The platelet count consistently returns to normal in all of these infants.

Low AT-III is observed in asphyxiated infants. Therefore, the low concentrations may be secondary to asphyxia, which is also responsible for polycythemia.

Other Endocrine Symptoms

After correcting for other factors, hypocalcemia appears to be more common in infants with polycythemia. The etiology is unclear although abnormalities in calcitonin gene-related peptide as well as low levels of 1,25-cholecalciferol and 24,25-cholecalciferol have been documented [96, 97].

Neurologic Symptoms

Newborn Period

Numerous papers dating back to the 1950s have reported neurologic abnormalities in newborn infants with polycythemia and hyperviscosity. Symptoms have included lethargy, irritability, tremulousness, and seizures. Several papers have also reported cerebral infarction.

In a controlled study, Goldberg and colleagues demonstrated abnormalities in the Prechtl and Brazelton examinations in infants with polycythemia [98]. All of these infants improved spontaneously over time. Those infants that had hemodilution with PET improved at the same rate as those who did not receive any therapy. Van der Elst and colleagues also performed Brazelton examinations in a group of infants with polycythemia and in a control group [75]. The polycythemic infants were randomized to be observed or to receive a PET. At 10 days of age, the two polycythemic groups had similar Brazelton examinations. The control group had significantly better examinations than either of the polycythemic groups.

It would appear that polycythemic infants are different in their state behavior and neurologic function during the first week of life. Normalization of hematocrit and blood viscosity does not seem to affect the short-term outcome.

Long Term

There have been six series of patients that have been followed long term (8 months to 6 years) in order to obtain an understanding of the role that polycythemia in the newborn period might play in the long-term neurologic development. The first of the studies was by van der Elst and colleagues, who followed the group of infants described above to 8 months of age [75]. Both polycythemic groups and the control group had normal neurologic examinations and developmental scores (modified Griffith developmental score).

Goldberg and colleagues also re-examined their subjects at 8 months of age [98]. The Bayley scales of infant development, Milani-Comparetti postural

reflex examination, medical history, and neurologic and physical examinations were completed on all three groups of infants. There were no differences in the Bayley scales among the three groups. Neurologic abnormalities were found in all three groups, polycythemic-treated (67%), polycythemic-observed (50%), and controls (17%). While no statistical differences were found, the two polycythemic groups appeared to be very similar to each other but had more problems when compared with the control group. There was a high incidence of spastic diplegia in the two polycythemic groups.

Black and colleagues followed two populations of infants with polycythemia [99]. In the initial study, there were 111 polycythemic infants and 110 control infants [99]. Forty-two of the polycythemic infants received a PET to lower their hematocrit after birth. The decision to lower the hematocrit was not done by randomization; rather, the physician in the nursery made the decision. Sicker infants tended to be those who received the partial exchange transfusion. Follow-up examinations were done at one and three years and included the Bayley scales, the Denver developmental screening test, physical and neurologic examinations, and a medical history. There were no differences in the two polycythemic groups or control groups in mental performance, but a significant number of the polycythemic infants, independent of therapy, had motor delay compared with the control group. Twenty-five percent of all polycythemic infants had neurologic abnormalities, especially spastic diplegia. Forty-three percent of the treated infants and 35% of the observed polycythemic group had some handicap compared with 11% of the control group ($P <0.005$).

In a second study of polycythemic infants by Black and colleagues, in which the efficacy of PET was studied, 93 infants were randomized to treatment or observation [100]. There was no differentiation between infants who had symptoms in the newborn period and those who were asymptomatic. Eighty percent of infants were examined at one and/or two years of age (59% at 1 year, 61% at 2 years). No differences were detected between the two groups at the one-year follow-up. At 2 years of age, the treated group had fewer neurologic abnormalities. Forty-nine of the original 93 infants were evaluated again at school age (7 years of age) [101]. There were no differences between the treated and nontreated polycythemic children.

Host and Ulrich reported on a group of polycythemic infants who were part of a community health study [76]. At 2.5 years of age, a Denver developmental screen and a health questionnaire were administered. A second questionnaire was administered at 6 years of age. Eighty percent of the infants with a venous hematocrit of 65% or above completed the study. All were normal, except for one child who had hypocalcemic seizures.

Bada and colleagues studied a population of polycythemic infants who were randomized to receive a PET or observation along with a control group [102]. Follow-up at 30 months of age revealed no differences in the three groups. A multivariant analysis of the various perinatal risk factors was performed. The analysis revealed that outcome was related highly to perinatal risk factors other than polycythemia.

There are several points that become clear from a review of the data. Polycythemia appears to be part of the fetal adaptive process for acute and chronic hypoxia. Hypoxia is known to cause irreversible brain injury. Exchange transfusion to lower the hematocrit in the newborn period does not change long-term neurologic function in this population, although polycythemia is a marker for an increased risk of long-term neurologic dysfunction. The demographic data of Black and Bada indicate that infants who are symptomatic in the newborn period and have late sequelae are the same infants who experienced an adverse intrauterine environment or perinatal hypoxia or asphyxia [100–102]. Therefore, it would appear that it is the hypoxic–ischemic events that trigger the adaptive fetal response that increases the hematocrit and is responsible for the cerebral dysfunction. This would be consistent with the observation that PET to reduce the hematocrit in the newborn does not prevent long-term neurologic dysfunction.

Asymptomatic Newborn Infants

Most studies suggest that infants with an elevated hematocrit but who are asymptomatic are at a minimal and nonquantifiable risk for adverse outcome. A recent meta-analysis by Dempsey and Barrington confirm this finding as well as the observation that PET does not change neurologic outcome [103]. In light of our current understanding of the pathophysiology of the etiology of the neurologic dysfunction in polycythemia, there does not appear to be sufficient evidence to recommend exchange transfusion in this population.

Management

Partial exchange transfusion to reduce the hematocrit should be reserved for newborns with symptoms that can be attributable directly to the elevation in hematocrit and in which there is evidence that the reduction of the hematocrit will correct the observed problems. Such clinical conditions include respiratory distress with cyanosis, renal failure, and hypoglycemia. Before the exchange transfusion is performed, other explanations for the observed symptoms should be explored. Once it is clear that polycythemia appears to be the etiologic explanation for the infant's problems, then a PET should be undertaken. Colloidal fluids and crystalline fluids appear to have equal efficacy in PET [104, 105]. To determine the volume of the exchange transfusion, the following formula may be used [106]:

$$\frac{[\text{hematocrit(observed)} - \text{hematocrit(desired)}] \times \text{blood volume}}{\text{hematocrit(observed)}}.$$

Summary

The incidence of neonatal polycythemia and hyperviscosity is between 1% and 5%, making it a common occurrence. However, it has become a less common problem in the practice of newborn medicine, as timely cord clamping is now standard obstetric practice and the American Academy of Pediatrics no longer recommends screening the hematocrit in otherwise normal infants [107]. PET should be employed to correct problems that are clearly attributable to polycythemia and hyperviscosity. It should be emphasized that there is no clear evidence that PET will affect the long-term developmental and neurologic outcome of infants born with polycythemia and hyperviscosity.

References

1. Wood JL. Plethora in the newborn infant associated with cyanosis and convulsions. *J Pediatr* 1952;**54**:143–51.

2. Michael AF, Mauer AM. Maternal-fetal transfusion as a cause of plethora in the neonatal period. *Pediatrics* 1961;**28**:458–61.

3. Minkowski A. Acute cardiac failure in connection with neonatal polycythemia (in monovular twins and single newborn infants). *Biol Neonate* 1962;**4**:61–74.

4. Danks DM, Stevens LH. Neonatal respiratory distress with a high hematocrit. *Lancet* 1964;**2**:499–500.

5. Gross GP, Hathaway WE, McGaughey HR. Hyperviscosity in the neonate. *J Pediatr* 1973;**82**:1004–12.

6. Ramamurthy RS, Brans YW. Neonatal polycythemia. I. Criteria for diagnosis and treatment. *Pediatrics* 1981;**68**:168–74.

7. Oh W, Lind J. Venous and capillary hematocrit in newborn infants and placental transfusion. *Acta Paediatr Scand* 1966;**55**:38–40.

8. Wirth FH, Goldberg KE, Lubchenco LO. Neonatal hyperviscosity. I. Incidence. *Pediatrics* 1979;**63**:833–6.

9. Stevens K, Wirth FH. Incidence of neonatal hyperviscosity at sea level. *J Pediatr* 1980;**97**:118–19.

10. Brooks GI, Backes CR. Hyperviscosity secondary to polycythemia in the appropriate for gestational age neonate. *J Am Obstet Assoc* 1981;**80**:415–18.

11. Reisner SH, Mor N, Levy Y, Merlob P. Incidence of neonatal polycythemia. *Isr J Med Sci* 1983;**19**:848–9.

12. Oh W, Oh MA, Lind J. Renal function and blood volume in newborn infants related to placental transfusion. *Acta Paediatr Scand* 1966;**56**:197–210.

13. Oh W, Blankenship W, Lind J. Further study of neonatal blood volume in relation to placental transfusion. *Ann Paediatr* 1996;**207**:147–59.

14. Yao AC, Moinian M, Lind J. Distribution of blood between infants and placenta after birth. *Lancet* 1969;**2**:871–3.

15. Linderkamp O. Placental transfusion: determinants and effects. *Clin Perinatol* 1982;**9**:559–92.

16. McDonald SJ, Midddleton P, Dowswell T, Morris PS. Cochrane in context: Effect of timing of umbilical cord clamping in term infants on maternal and neonatal outcomes. *Evidence-based child Health: A Cochrane Review Journal* 2014;**9**:198–400.

17. Shohat M, Teisner SH, Mimoini F, Merlob P. Neonatal polycythemia. II. Definition related to time of sampling. *Pediatrics* 1984;**73**:11–13.

18. Poiseuille JLM. Recherches experimentales sur le mouvement des liquides dans les tubes de tres petits diametres. *C R Acad Sci* 1840;**11**:961–1041.

19. Van der Elst CW, Malan AF, de V Heese H. Blood viscosity in modern medicine. *S Afr Med J* 1977;**52**:526–8.

20. Wells RE, Pento R, Merrill EW. Measurements of viscosity of biologic fluids by core plate viscometer. *J Lab Clin Med* 1961;**57**:646–56.

21. Wells RE, Merrill EW. Influence of flow properties of blood upon viscosity–hematocrit relationships. *J Clin Invest* 1961;**41**:1591–8.

22. Dintenfass L. Blood viscosity, internal fluidity of the red cell, dynamic coagulation and the critical capillary radius as factors in the physiology and pathology of circulation and microcirculation. *Med J Aust* 1968;**1**:688–96.

23. Linderkamp O, Versmold HT, Riegel KP, Betke K. Contributions of red cells and plasma to blood viscosity in preterm and full-term infants and adults. *Pediatrics* 1984;**74**:45–51.

24. Burton AC. Role of geometry, of size and shape, in the microcirculation. *Fed Proc* 1966;**25**:1753–60.

25. Bergqvist G. Viscosity of the blood in the newborn infants. *Acta Paediatr Scand* 1974;**63**:858–64.

26. Wells R. Syndromes of hyperviscosity. *N Engl J Med* 1970;**283**:183–6.

27. Somer T, Ditze J. Clinical and rheological studies in a patient with hyperviscosity syndrome due to Waldenstrom's macroglobulinemia. *Bibl Haematol* 1981;**47**:242–6.

28. Charm SE, Kurland GS. *Blood Flow and Microcirculation* (New York: John Wiley & Sons, 1974).

29. Smith CM, Prasler WJ, Tukey DP, et al. Fetal red cells are more deformable than adult red cells. *Blood* 1981;**58**:35a.

30. Linderkamp O, Wu PYK, Meiselman HJ. Deformability of density separated red blood cells in normal newborn infants and adults. *Pediatr Res* 1982;**16**:964–8.

31. Lichtman MA. Cellular deformability during maturation of the myeloblast. *N Engl J Med* 1970;**283**:943–8.

32. Lichtman MA. Rheology of leukocytes, leukocyte suspensions, and blood in leukemia. *J Clin Invest* 1973;**52**:350–8.

33. Miller ME. Developmental maturation of human neutrophil motility and its relationship to membrane deformability. In Bellanti, JA, Dayton, DH, eds. *The Phagocytic Cell in Host Resistance* (New York: Raven Press, 1975), p. 295.

34. Rand PW, Austin WH, Lacombe E, Barker N. pH and blood viscosity. *J Appl Physiol* 1968;**25**:550–9.

35. Fahraeus R, Lindqvist T. The viscosity of the blood in narrow capillary tubes. *Am J Physiol* 1931;**96**:562–8.

36. Nowicki P, Oh W, Yao A, Hansen NB, Stonestreet SS. Effect of polycythemia on gastrointestinal blood flow and oxygenation in piglets. *Am J Physiol* 1984;**247**:G220–G225.

37. LeBlanc MH, Kotagal VR, Kleinman LI. Physiological effects of hypervolemic polycythemia in newborn dogs. *J Appl Physiol* 1982;**53**:865–72.

38. Surjadhana A, Rouleau J, Boerboom L, Hoffman JIE. Myocardial blood flow and its distribution in anesthetized polycythemic dogs. *Circ Res* 1978;**43**:619–31.

39. Brashear RE. Effects of acute plasma for blood exchange in experimental polycythemia. *Respiration* 1980;**40**:297–306.

40. Rosenkrantz TS, Oh W. Cerebral blood flow velocity in infants with polycythemia and hyperviscosity: Effects of partial exchange transfusion with Plamanate. *J Pediatr* 1982;**101**:94–8.

41. Fouron JC, Hebert F. The circulatory effects of hematocrit variations in normovolemic newborn lambs. *J Pediatr* 1973;**82**:995–1003.

42. Gatti RA, Muister AJ, Cole RB, Paul MH. Neonatal polycythemia with transient cyanosis and cardiorespiratory abnormalities. *J Pediatr* 1966;**69**:1063–72.

43. Kotagal VR, Keenan WJ, Reuter JH, et al. Regional blood flow in polycythemia and hypervolemia. *Pediatr Res* 1977;**11**:394A.

44. Swetnam SM, Yabek SM, Alverson DC. Hemodynamic consequences of neonatal polycythemia. *J Pediatr* 1987;**110**:443–7.

45. Murphy DJ, Jr., Reller MD, Meyer RA, Kaplan S. Effects of neonatal polycythemia and partial exchange transfusion on cardiac function: An echocardiographic study. *Pediatrics* 1985;**76**:909–13.

46. Boehm G, Delitzsch AK, Senger H, et al. Postnatal development of liver and exocrine pancreas in polycythemic newborn infants. *J Pediatr Gastroenterol Nutr* 1992; **15**:310–14.

47. Kotagal VR, Kleinman LI. Effect of acute polycythemia on newborn renal hemodynamics and function. *Pediatr Res* 1982;**16**:14851.

48. Bergqvist G, Zetterman R. Blood viscosity and peripheral circulation in newborn infants. *Acta Paediatr Scand* 1974;**63**:865–8.

49. Linderkamp O, Strohhacker I, Versmold HT, et al. Peripheral circulation in the newborn: Interaction of peripheral blood flow, blood pressure, blood volume and blood viscosity. *Eur J Pediatr* 1978;**129**:73–81.

50. Gustafsson L, Applegren L, Myrvold HE. The effect of polycythemia on blood flow in working and non-working skeletal muscle. *Acta Physiol Scand* 1980;**109**:143–8.

51. Waffarn F, Cole CD, Huxtable RF. Effects of polycythemia and hyperviscosity on cutaneous blood flow and transcutaneous pO_2 and pCO_2 in neonate. *Pediatrics* 1984;**74**:389–94.

52. Jones MD, Traystman RJ, Simmons MA, Molteni RA. Effects of changes in arterial O_2 content on cerebral blood flow in the lamb. *Am J Physiol* 1981;**240**:H209–H215.

53. Rosenkrantz TS, Stonestreet BS, Hansen NB, et al. Cerebral blood flow in the newborn lamb with polycythemia and hyperviscosity. *J Pediatr* 1984;**104**:276–80.

54 Goldstein M, Stonestreet BS, Brann BS, 4th, Oh W. Cerebral cortical blood flow and oxygen metabolism in normocythemic hyperviscous newborn piglets. *Pediatr Res* 1988;**24**:486–9.

55. Rosenkrantz TS, Philipps AF, Skrzypczak PS, Raye JR. Cerebral metabolism in the newborn lamb with polythemia. *Pediatr Res* 1985;**23**:329–33.

56. Tenenbaum DG, Piasecki GJ, Oh W, Rosenkrantz TS, Jackson BT. Fetal polycythemia and hyperviscosity: effect in umbilical blood flow and fetal oxygen consumption. *Am J Obstet Gynecol* 1983;**147**:48–51.

57. Saigal S, Usher RH. Symptomatic neonatal plethora. *Biol Neonate* 1977;**32**:62–72.

58. Sacks MO. Occurrence of anemia and polycythemia in phenotypically dissimilar single ovum human twins. *Pediatrics* 1959;**24**:604–8.

59. Schwartz JL, Maniscalco WM, Lane AT, Currao WJ. Twin transfusion syndrome causing cutaneous erythropoiesis. *Pediatrics* 1984;**74**:527–9.

60. Philip AGS, Yee AB, Rosy M, et al. Placental transfusion as an intrauterine phenomenon in deliveries complicated by fetal distress. *Br Med J* 1969;**2**:11–13.

61 Flod NE, Ackerman BD. Perinatal asphyxia and residual placental blood volume. *Acta Paediatr Scand* 1971;**60**:433–6.

62. Yao AC, Lind J. Effect of gravity on placental transfusion. *Lancet* 1969;**2**:505–6.

63. Oh W, Omori K, Emmanouilides GC, Phelps DI. Placenta to lamb fetus transfusion in utero during acute hypoxia. *Am J Obstet Gynecol* 1975;**122**:316–21.

64. Humbert JR, Abelson H, Hathaway WE, Battaglia FC. Polycythemia in small for gestational age infants. *J Pediatr* 1969;**75**:812–19.

65. Widness JA, Garcia JA, Oh W, Schwartz R. Cord serum erythropoietin values and disappearance rates after birth in polycythemic newborns. *Pediatr Res* 1982;**16**:218A.

66. Philipps AF, Dubin, JW, Matty PJ, Raye JR. Arterial hypoxemia and hyperinsulinemia in the chronically hyperglycemic fetal lamb. *Pediatr Res* 1982;**16**:653–8.

67. Hod M, Merlob P, Friedman S. Prevalence of congenital anomalies and neonatal complications in the offspring of diabetic mothers in Israel. *Isr J Med Sci* 1991;**27**:498–502.

68. Rosenkrantz TS, Oh W. Neonatal polycythemia and hyperviscosity. In Milunsky A, Friedman EA, Gluck L, eds. *Advances in Perinatal Medicine*, vol. 5. (New York: Plenum Medical Book Co., 1986), pp. 93–123.

69. Hakanson DO, Oh W. Hyperviscosity in the small-for-gestational age infant. *Biol Neonate* 1980;**37**:109–12.

70. Rawlings JS, Pettet G, Wiswell TE, Clapper J. Estimated blood volumes in polycythemic neonates as a function of birth weight. *J Pediatr* 1982;**101**:594.

71. Brans YW, Shannon DL, Ramamurthy RS. Neonatal polycythemia. II. Plasma, blood and red cell volume estimates in relation to hematocrit levels and quality of intrauterine growth. *Pediatrics* 1981;**68**:175–82.

72. Thorton CJ, Shanno DL, Hunter MA, Ramamurthy RS, Brans YW. Body water estimates in neonatal polycythemia. *J Pediatr* 1983;**102**:113–17.

73. Oh W, Wallgren G, Hanson JS, Lind J. The effects of placental transfusion on respiratory mechanics of normal term newborn infants. *Pediatrics* 1967;**40**:6–12.

74. Scott F, Evans N. Distal gangrene in a polycythemic recipient fetus in twin-twin transfusion. *Obstet Gynecol* 1995;**86**:677–9.

75. Van der Elst CW, Moteno CD, Malan AF, de V Heese H. The management of polycythemia in the newborn infant. *Early Hum Dev* 1980;**4**:393–403.

76. Host A, Ulrich M. Late prognosis in untreated neonatal polycythemia with minor or no symptoms. *Acta Paediatr Scand* 1982;**71**:629–33.

77. Leake RD, Thanopoulos B, Nieberg R. Hyperviscosity syndrome associated with necrotizing enterocolitis. *Am J Dis Child* 1975;**129**:1192–4.

78. Hakanson DO, Oh W. Necrotizing enterocolitis and hyperviscosity in the newborn infant. *J Pediatr* 1977;**90**:458–61.

79. Martinez-Tallo E, Claure N, Bancalari E. Necrotizing enterocolitis in full term or near term infants: Risk factors. *Biol Neonate* 1997;**71**:292–8.

80. LeBlanc MH, D'Cruz C, Pate K. Necrotizing enterocolitis can be caused by polycythemic hyperviscosity in the newborn dog. *J Pediatr* 1984;**105**:804–9.

81. Black VD, Rumack CM, Lubchenco LO, Koops BL. Gastrointestinal injury in polycythemic term infants. *Pediatrics* 1985;**76**:225–31.

82. Herson VC, Raye JR, Rowe JC, Philipps AF. Acute renal failure associated with polycythemia in a neonate. *J Pediatr* 1982;**100**:137–9.

83. Leake RD, Chan GM, Zakauddin S, et al. Glucose perturbation in experimental hyperviscosity. *Pediatr Res* 1980;**14**:1320–3.

84. Creswell JS, Warburton D, Susa JB, et al. Hyperviscosity in the newborn lamb produces perturbation in glucose homeostasis. *Pediatrics* 1981;**15**:1348–50.

85. Rosenkrantz TS, Philipps AF, Knox I, et al. Regulation of cerebral glucose metabolism in normal and polycythemic newborns. *J Cereb Blood Flow Metab* 1992;**12**:856–65.

86. Rivers RPA. Coagulation changes associated with a high haematocrit in the newborn infant. *Acta Paediatr Scand* 1975;**64**:449–56.

87. Katz J, Rodriquez E, Mandini G, Branson HE. Normal coagulation findings, thrombocytopenia, and peripheral hemoconcentration in neonatal polycythemia. *J Pediatr* 1982;**101**:99–102.

88. Henriksson P. Hyperviscosity of the blood and haemostasis in the newborn infant. *Acta Paediatr Scand* 1979;**68**:701–4.

89. Shaikh BS, Erslev AJ. Thrombocytopenia in polycythemic mice. *J Lab Clin Med* 1978;**92**:765–71.

90. Jackson CW, Smith PJ, Edwards CC, Whidden MA. Relationship between packed cell volume, platelets and platelet survival in red blood cell-hypertransfused mice. *J Lab Clin Med* 1979;**94**:500–9.

91. Meberg A. Transitory thrombocytopenia in newborn mice after intrauterine hypoxia. *Pediatr Res* 1980;**14**:1071–3.

92. Voorhies TM, Lipper EG, Lee BCP, et al. Occlusive vascular disease in asphyxiated newborn infants. *J Pediatr* 1984;**105**:92.

93. Peters M, Ten Cate JW, Koo LH, Breederveld C. Persistent antithrombin III deficiency: Risk factor for thromboembolic complication in neonates small for gestational age. *J Pediatr* 1984;**105**:310–14.

94. Merchant RH, Agarwal MB, Joshi NC, Parekh SR. Neonatal polycythemia: A potentially serious disorder. *Indian J Pediatr* 1983;**50**:149–52.

95. Amit M, Camfield PR. Neonatal polycythemia causing multiple cerebral infarcts. *Arch Neurol* 1980;**37**:109–10.

96. Saggese G, Bertelloni S, Baroncelli GI, et al. Elevated calcitonin gene related peptide in polycythemic newborn infants. *Acta Pediatr* 1992;**81**:966–8.

97. Alkalay A, Pomerance JJ, Prause J, et al. Cholecalciferol metabolites in polycythemic newborns. *Isr J Med Sci* 1985;**21**:95–7.

98. Goldberg K, Wirth FH, Hathaway WE. Neonatal hyperviscosity. II. Effect of partial plasma exchange transfusion. *Pediatrics* 1982;**69**:419–25.

99. Black VD, Lubchenco LD, Luckey DW, et al. Developmental and neurologic sequelae of neonatal hyperviscosity syndrome. *Pediatrics* 1982;**69**:426–31.

100. Black VD, Lubchenco LO, Koops BL, Poland RL, Powell DP. Neonatal hyperviscosity: Randomized study of effect of partial plasma exchange on long-term outcome. *Pediatrics* 1985;**75**:1048–53.

101. Black VD, Camp BW, Lubchenco LO, et al. Neonatal hyperviscosity is associated with lower achievement and IQ scores at school age. *Pediatr Res* 1988;**23**:442A.

102. Bada HS, Korones SB, Pourcyrous M, et al. Asymptomatic syndrome of polycythemic hyperviscosity: Effect of partial plasma exchange transfusion. *J Pediatr* 1992;**120**:579–85.

103. Dempsey EM, Barrington K. Short and long term outcomes following partial exchange transfusion in the polycythemic newborn: A systematic review. *Arch Dis Child Fetal Neonatal Ed* 2006;**91**(1):F2–F6.

104. Supapannachart S, Siripoonya P, Boonwattanasoontorn W, Kanjanavanit S. Neonatal polycythemia: Effects of partial exchange transfusion using fresh frozen plasma, Haemaccel and normal saline. *Med Assoc Thai* 1999;**82**(Suppl1):S82–S86.

105. Wong W, Fok TF, Lee CH, et al. Randomised controlled trial: comparison of colloid or crystalloid for partial exchange transfusion for treatment of neonatal polycythaemia. *Arch Dis Child Fetal Neonatal Ed* 1997;**77**:F115–F118.

106. Glader B. Erythrocyte disorders in infancy. In Schaffer AJ, Avery ME, eds. *Diseases of the Newborn* (Philadelphia, PA: W. B. Saunders, 1977), p. 625.

107. American Academy of Pediatrics Committee on Fetus and Newborn. Routine evaluation of blood pressure, hematocrit, and glucose in newborns. *Pediatrics* 1993;**92**:474–6.

Chapter

12

Approach to the Thrombocytopenic Neonate

Emöke Deschmann and Martha C. Sola-Visner

Introduction

Over the last decades, as the survival of neonates admitted to the neonatal intensive care unit (NICU) improved, thrombocytopenia became an increasingly important problem in the care of sick term and particularly preterm neonates. In this population, the majority of thrombocytopenias are due to acquired processes, and most resolve with time and/or treatment of the underlying illness. Frequently, however, the etiology of the thrombocytopenia poses a diagnostic dilemma, and – if severe enough – may place the affected neonate at risk of bleeding.

In this chapter, we review the incidence of neonatal thrombocytopenia and propose a classification and diagnostic approach based on timing and clinical presentation, as well as on novel tests of platelet production. Next, we discuss the risks and benefits associated with platelet transfusions. Acquired, immune, and congenital varieties of neonatal thrombocytopenia are discussed in detail in Chapters 13, 14, and 15, respectively.

Definition and Incidence of Neonatal Thrombocytopenia

In general, at the time of birth, the platelet count in neonates is similar to that in older children and adults, ranging from 150 to 450×10^9/L [1–3]. Aballi and colleagues reported a mean platelet count in full-term newborns of 250×10^9/L, with a range from 117 to 450×10^9/L [1]. Ablin and colleagues [2] reported a mean platelet count of 190×10^9/L, with a range from 84 to 478×10^9/L. In that study, 4% of full-term babies had a platelet count below 150×10^9/L. Sell and Corrigan [3] reported a mean platelet count in full-term newborns of 325×10^9/L, with a standard error of $50 \times$ 10^9/L. Premature infants at birth, in general, also have mean platelet counts within the normal range of older children or adults, although platelet counts $<150 \times 10^9$/L are more frequent among preterm than among term infants. In the series by Aballi and colleagues, 14% of preterm infants had a platelet count below 150×10^9/L [1].

In a recent very large population study involving 47,291 neonates from a multi-hospital system, reference ranges for platelet counts at different gestational and post-conceptional ages were determined by excluding the top and lower 5th percentile of all platelet counts [4]. Using this approach, the lowest limit (5th percentile) of platelet counts for infants <32 weeks' gestation at birth was found to be 104×10^9/L, compared to 123×10^9/L for late preterm/term neonates (>32 weeks) (Fig. 12.1a). While this is the largest study of platelet counts in neonates published to date, it is important to keep in mind that ill neonates were not excluded from this study, so that these values should be regarded as epidemiological "reference ranges" for neonates admitted to the neonatal intensive care unit (NICU), rather than as "normal ranges" for this population.

An additional finding from this study was a strong correlation between the gestational age at birth and the time required postnatally before the platelet count began to increase and reached values similar to those of term infants. Specifically, the investigators noticed that the mean postnatal platelet counts of infants born at 29 to 34 weeks increased steadily over the first 2–4 weeks of life, and then stabilized at levels similar to those of term infants. In contrast, the postnatal platelet counts of infants born between 22 and 27 weeks did not begin to increase until they reached a post-conceptional age

Neonatal Hematology, Pathogenesis, Diagnosis, and Management of Hematologic Problems, 3rd edition, ed. Pedro A. de Alarcón, Eric J. Werner, Robert D. Christensen, and Martha C. Sola-Visner. Published by Cambridge University Press. © Cambridge University Press 2021.

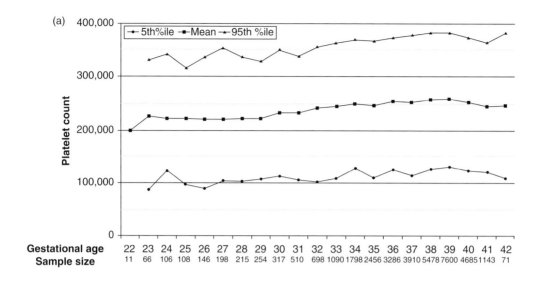

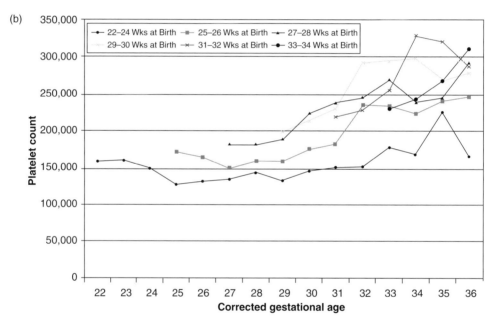

Fig. 12.1 (a) First recorded platelet counts obtained in the first 3 days after birth in neonates 22 to 42 weeks' gestation. The red line represents the mean values and the blue and green lines represent the 5th and 95th percentiles, respectively. (b) Effects of postnatal age on mean platelet counts of premature infants. The mean platelet counts were plotted according to gestational age at birth. Data were grouped according to weeks of gestation completed at birth as follows: 22 to 24 weeks, 25 to 26 weeks, 27 to 28 weeks, 31 to 32 weeks, and 33 to 34 weeks. (Reproduced from: Wiedmeier et al., *J Perinatol* 2009;29:130–6, with permission [4].) (See plate section for color version.)

of approximately 29 weeks. Furthermore, the platelet counts of the most immature infants (born at 22–25 weeks) always remained below the mean levels measured in near-term and term infants (Fig. 12.1b). Similar findings were reported by McPherson and Juul in a study following platelet counts in infants born between 24 and 40 weeks'

gestation over the first 4 weeks of life [5]. The mechanisms underlying these observations are unknown, but it is likely that developmental differences between fetal, neonatal, and adult megakaryocytopoiesis play a role (see Chapter 13 for details).

Thrombocytopenia in neonates has traditionally been defined as a platelet count $<150 \times 10^9$/L, and has been classified as mild (100–150 × 10⁹/L), moderate (50–99 × 10⁹/L), and severe (<50 × 10⁹/L). Applying those definitions, large studies in unselected populations established an overall incidence of neonatal thrombocytopenia of 0.7 to 0.9% [6, 7]. In contrast, investigators focusing on neonates admitted to the NICU found a much higher incidence of thrombocytopenia, ranging from 18 to 35% [8–10]. Consistent with the observations of lower mean platelet counts in the most preterm infants, the incidence of neonatal thrombocytopenia has also been shown to be inversely related to gestational age, so that the most immature neonates are the most frequently affected. Christensen et al. conducted a study limited to extremely low birth weight neonates (ELBW, <1,000 g), and found that 73% had at least one recorded platelet count <150 × 10⁹/L [11].

Classification and Evaluation of Neonatal Thrombocytopenia

The timing of presentation of the thrombocytopenia is a helpful factor when narrowing the differential

diagnosis, although there is significant overlap and several conditions can present with thrombocytopenia of early- or late-onset (i.e., sepsis or thromboses). Congenital and immune (allo- and auto-immune) thrombocytopenias usually present during the first 72 hours of life, and are reviewed in detail in Chapters 13, 14 and 15. Thrombocytopenias presenting after 72 hours (late onset) are most commonly acquired and not mediated by immune mechanisms – these will be reviewed in Chapter 13. Algorithms describing the diagnostic approach to thrombocytopenic neonates with early onset or late onset thrombocytopenia are presented in Figs. 12.2 and 12.3.

Early-Onset Thrombocytopenia

In neonates with early-onset thrombocytopenia (<72 hours of life), the initial evaluation is based on the severity of thrombocytopenia, the clinical presentation, and the maternal history (see diagnostic algorithm in Fig. 12.2). A documented maternal history of pregnancy-induced hypertension, chronic hypertension,

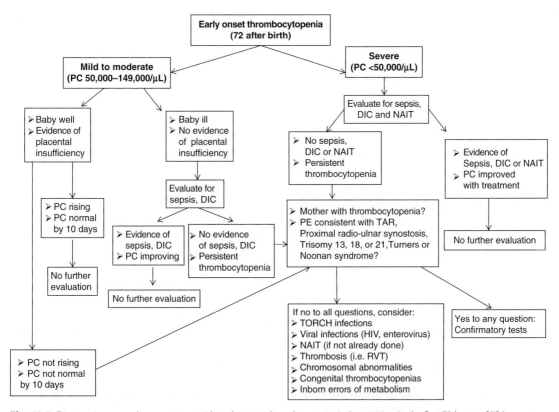

Fig. 12.2 Diagnostic approach to neonates with early-onset thrombocytopenia (presenting in the first 72 hours of life).

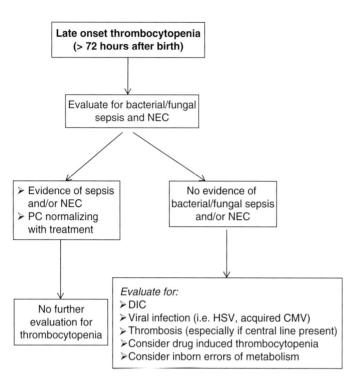

Fig. 12.3 Diagnostic approach to neonates with late-onset thrombocytopenia (presenting >72 hours after birth).

and/or intrauterine growth restriction (all of which are associated with placental insufficiency and chronic intrauterine hypoxia) is particularly helpful in narrowing the differential diagnosis. Placental insufficiency is the most common etiology of transient mild thrombocytopenia in non-septic appearing neonates (particularly those born preterm) and can be managed expectantly with close observation. However, either the development of severe thrombocytopenia or the lack of resolution within 10 days should prompt evaluation for other causes. Congenital viral or parasitic infections (i.e., CMV, or toxoplasma infections) and genetic disorders, in particular, can present with thrombocytopenia and intrauterine growth restriction as the most salient features in the neonatal period, and their diagnosis requires a high index of suspicion. Close monitoring of the clinical condition is also very important, since thrombocytopenia can be the first presenting sign of a serious condition (i.e., sepsis, hemophagocytic lymphohistiocytosis). For this reason, many clinicians choose to send blood cultures and closely monitor the clinical status of well-appearing neonates in whom the etiology of the thrombocytopenia is not yet clearly defined. *Severe* early-onset thrombocytopenia in an otherwise healthy or mildly symptomatic infant should trigger suspicion for immune-mediated thrombocytopenia, either autoimmune (i.e., the mother is also thrombocytopenic) or alloimmune (the mother has a normal platelet count). The evaluation and management of alloimmune thrombocytopenia is reviewed in detail in Chapter 14.

Early-onset thrombocytopenia (of any severity) in an ill-appearing term or preterm neonate or in a neonate with abnormal liver enzymes and/or coagulation tests should prompt evaluation for bacterial sepsis, viral or parasitic infections, or DIC (i.e., related to perinatal asphyxia). The physical exam is also extremely important in all patients with thrombocytopenia, since it can provide important clues to the diagnosis, such as subtle congenital anomalies in genetic disorders [12], hepatosplenomegaly in congenital viral infections [13] or in hemophagocytic lymphohistiocytosis (HLH), or a palpable abdominal mass in renal vein thrombosis (RVT) [14]. Appropriate tests should be sent, and treatment should be initiated based on index of suspicion. Many of these cases require hematology consultation for appropriate diagnosis and management, and presenting features and mechanisms are reviewed in Chapter 13 and 15.

Late-Onset Thrombocytopenia

Late-onset thrombocytopenia (≥72 hours after birth) should always prompt rapid evaluation and potential treatment for bacterial/fungal sepsis, necrotizing enterocolitis, or viral infections such as HSV, acquired CMV, or enteroviruses (Fig. 12.3). If these most common etiologies have been ruled out, other potential causes include inborn errors of metabolism, thromboses (i.e., catheter-associated thrombosis), or drug-induced thrombocytopenias (see Acquired Thrombocytopenias, Chapter 13).

Measurements of Neonatal Platelet Production

In cases where the etiology of the thrombocytopenia is unclear, assessing the platelet production can be very helpful to identify the mechanism of the thrombocytopenia (decreased platelet production vs. increased consumption vs. a combination of the two), narrow the differential diagnosis and predict the course of the thrombocytopenia. In adults, bone marrow biopsy is the gold standard test for the mechanistic evaluation of thrombocytopenia. In neonates, however, this procedure is technically difficult, and is frequently postponed until the infant is larger and/or out of the neonatal period. With the hope of overcoming this limitation, a number of potentially useful indirect measurements of platelet production were developed, including plasma or serum thrombopoietin (Tpo) concentrations, circulating megakaryocyte (MK) progenitors, and reticulated platelet percentages (RP%). The circulating Tpo concentrations reflect the balance between Tpo production and Tpo binding to available receptors [15]. Thus, elevated levels are seen in cases of up-regulated Tpo production, such as during infection, or in cases of bone marrow suppression and decreased megakaryocytes, such as in congenital amegakaryocytic thrombocytopenia or infiltrative bone marrow diseases [16]. Circulating MK progenitors have been used as a reflection of bone marrow MKs [17, 18], although no studies to date have directly correlated these measures in neonates. Reticulated platelets are platelets recently released from the bone marrow (<24 hours old), which can be identified by their high RNA content [19]. In a manner similar to reticulocytes in anemia, the reticulated platelet percentage is elevated in consumptive

thrombocytopenias, and is low in thrombocytopenias due to decreased platelet production [20]. Four studies evaluated the RP% in fetuses and neonates, with three of the four demonstrating similar to higher RP% in neonates compared to adults [21–24].

Until recently, all of these tests were only available in the research setting. However, a test similar to the RP% was recently developed for clinical use. This RP% equivalent, termed the immature platelet fraction (IPF) can be measured in Sysmex standard hematology analyzers (Sysmex, Kobe, Japan) as part of a routine complete blood count. Similarly to the RP%, the IPF% is elevated in thrombocytopenic conditions associated with increased platelet destruction (e.g., immune thrombocytopenic purpura, ITP), and decreased in thrombocytopenias due to decreased platelet production (e.g., aplastic anemia) [25]. Only a few studies so far have evaluated IPF values in neonates. Cremer and collaborators were the first to report the IPF in non-thrombocytopenic infants and in neonates with early-onset thrombocytopenia [26]. Based on their findings, these investigators suggested that the IPF could be used to predict recovery of the platelet count within the next 24 hours [26]. Ko and collaborators generated IPF reference ranges for full term neonates using cord blood samples and found that they were similar to adult reference ranges [27]. More recently, two groups examined the IPF in preterm neonates [28, 29]. In the largest IPF study published to date, MacQueen et al. examined 24,372 platelet counts and IPF percentages from 9,172 term and preterm neonates 0–90 days old [29]. Data from non-thrombocytopenic infants in this cohort were used to generate age-specific reference intervals for IPF% and immature platelet counts (IPC, calculated as IPF% × platelet count) (Fig. 12.4) [29]. As seen in the figure, the IPF at the time of birth was higher in preterm infants, and decreased trough gestation until 32 weeks, at which time the IPF stabilized at full-term values. Postnatally, the IPF increased progressively over the first 2 weeks of life and returned to baseline by 1 month in all gestational ages. Importantly, this study also assessed IPF percentages in neonates with thrombocytopenia, and found significantly higher values in neonates with consumptive etiologies compared to those with thrombocytopenia secondary to decreased production (Table 12.1). Thus, when available, the IPF can be a useful clinical tool in neonates, in whom it may help discern the underlying mechanisms of thrombocytopenia, narrow the differential diagnosis, and predict platelet recovery.

Platelet Transfusions in the NICU

Several surveys [30, 31] and observational studies over the last decade revealed a great deal of variability in platelet transfusion thresholds used by neonatologists worldwide [32–35]. While the causes for this diversity are multifactorial, the lack of solid evidence to guide neonatal platelet transfusion decisions has likely been a major contributing factor. Until recently, there had only been one prospective, randomized trial (published in 1993) comparing platelet transfusion thresholds in neonates [36]. This study, which enrolled 152 thrombocytopenic very low birth weight (VLBW) infants and followed them for the first week of life found no differences in the incidence

or severity of intraventricular hemorrhages (IVH) between infants randomized to receive platelet transfusions when the platelet count fell below 150×10^9/L (treated group) vs. when it fell below 50×10^9/L or there were clinical indications (control group) [36]. Thus, the authors concluded that the administration of platelet transfusions to VLBW infants with platelet counts greater than 50×10^9/L during the first week of life did not decrease the incidence or severity of intracranial hemorrhages.

The recently published PlaNeT-2 multicenter trial, the largest neonatal platelet transfusion trial to date, randomized 660 thrombocytopenic neonates with a median gestational age of 26.6 weeks and a median birth weight of 740 grams to receive platelet transfusions at a platelet count threshold of $<50 \times 10^9$/L (<50 group) or at $<25 \times 10^9$/L (<25 group) [37]. The primary outcome was a composite of death or new major bleeding within 28 days of randomization. Ninety percent of infants in the <50 group and 53% in the <25 group received at least one platelet transfusion, and infants in the <50 group had a significantly *higher* rate of mortality or major bleeding within 28 days of randomization compared to those in the <25 group (26% vs. 19%, respectively; odds ratio 1.57, 95%CI 1.06–2.32). In a subgroup analysis, findings were similar for neonates <28 weeks' gestation, the group at highest risk of bleeding and death [38]. Among secondary outcomes, infants in the liberal group (<50 group) also had a higher incidence of chronic lung disease. While these findings might have seemed surprising at first, they were in fact consistent with a growing body of literature describing

Table 12.1 Immature platelet fraction values in neonates with thrombocytopenia of different etiologies

Mechanism of thrombocytopenia	N	IPF%
Hypoproliferative*	92	10.4 ± 2.9
Consumptive**	98	20.9 ± 7.9
Both	76	17.9 ± 5.9
Indeterminate***	14	12.8 ± 8.1

Notes: *SGA, birth asphyxia or a syndrome associated with hypoproliferative thrombocytopenia;

**Immune-mediated, NEC, sepsis, or DIC;

***None of the above diagnoses.

(Adapted from: MacQueen et al., *J Perinatol* 37, 2017 [29].)

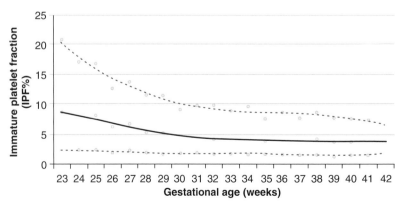

Fig. 12.4 Immature platelet fraction (IPF%) on the day of birth, according to gestational age. The lower and upper dashed lines represent the 5th and 95th percentile reference intervals, and the solid black line represents the median. Light circles are the actual medians for 5th, median and 95th percentile each day. The dashed and solid lines were generated by smoothing the values in the circles. (Reproduced from MacQueen et al., J Perinatol 2017;37: 834–8, with permission [29].)

a poor association between platelet counts and bleeding [38–40], a lack of effectiveness of platelet transfusions to prevent bleeding [39, 41, 42], and the potential of platelet transfusions to cause harm to neonates through various possible mechanisms [33, 34, 43–46].

The results of PlaNeT-2 provided high-level evidence in support of these concepts. However, concerns that the benefits of the lower transfusion threshold would be limited to clinically stable infants with a low risk of bleeding and/or death led to initial skepticism. This question was largely addressed in a follow-up study in which a multivariable logistic regression model was developed (incorporating factors known to influence neonatal bleeding risk and mortality, such as gestational age) and used to predict the baseline bleeding/mortality risk of neonates enrolled in PlaNeT-2 [47]. Based on their model-predicted baseline risk, 653 neonates in PlaNeT-2 were divided into four quartiles (very low, low, moderate, and high risk) and the absolute risk difference between the <50 group and the <25 group was assessed within each quartile. Interestingly, the lower transfusion threshold was associated with an absolute risk reduction in all four groups, varying from 4.9% in the lowest to 12.3% in the highest risk group. These results suggested that using a lower (<25 × 10⁹/L) prophylactic platelet transfusion threshold is beneficial even in high risk neonates.

While these studies provided strong support for the use of lower platelet transfusion thresholds in non-bleeding preterm infants, PlaNeT-2 had some weaknesses. First, 37% of infants in the study were randomized by day of life 5 and 59% by day 10, the highest risk period for bleeding [48]. While this might have simply reflected the time of onset of thrombocytopenia, 39% of infants received one or more platelet transfusions prior to randomization (for unknown reasons), raising the question of whether these transfusions were given during the high-risk period for IVH. Second, the study required obtaining a head ultrasound within 6 hours of randomization, and excluded infants with a significant IVH for 72 hours (after which they could be randomized). Thus, by design, PlaNeT-2 did not assess the effects of a restrictive vs. liberal platelet transfusion threshold on the potential extension of an existing IVH.

Conclusion

In conclusion, thrombocytopenia is a common problem in the NICU, particularly among premature infants. Most cases are mild to moderate, and do not warrant aggressive treatment. However, 5%–6% of all NICU admissions develop severe thrombocytopenia, defined as a platelet count <50 × 10⁹/L. A thorough and stepwise approach to the neonate with thrombocytopenia is essential to reach the correct diagnosis and provide appropriate treatment while minimizing complications. The results of PlaNeT-2 made it clear that platelet transfusions may have deleterious effects in neonates, which could be mediated by various potential mechanisms. Thus, neonatologists should develop guidelines based on this new evidence aimed at minimizing unnecessary and potentially harmful platelet transfusions to neonates.

References

1. Aballi AJ, Puapondh Y, Desposito F. Platelet counts in thriving premature infants. *Pediatrics* 1968;**42** (4):685–9.

2. Ablin AR, Kushner JH, Murphy A, Zippin C. Platelet enumeration in the neonatal period. *Pediatrics* 1961;**28**:822–4.

3. Sell EJ, Corrigan JJ, Jr. Platelet counts, fibrinogen concentrations, and factor V and factor VIII levels in healthy infants according to gestational age. *J Pediatr* 1973;**82**(6):1028–32.

4. Wiedmeier SE, Henry E, Sola-Visner MC, Christensen RD. Platelet reference ranges for neonates, defined using data from over 47,000 patients in a multihospital healthcare system. *J Perinatol* 2009;**29**(2):130–6.

5. McPherson RJ, Juul S. Patterns of thrombocytosis and thrombocytopenia in hospitalized neonates. *J Perinatol* 2005;**25**(3):166–72.

6. Dreyfus M, Kaplan C, Verdy E, et al. Frequency of immune thrombocytopenia in newborns: A prospective study. *Blood* 1997;**89**(12):4402–6.

7. Uhrynowska M, Maslanka K, Zupanska B. Neonatal thrombocytopenia: Incidence, serological and clinical observations. *Am J Perinatol* 1997;**14** (7):415–18.

8. Castle V, Andrew M, Kelton J, et al. Frequency and mechanism of neonatal thrombocytopenia. *J Pediatr* 1986;**108**(5 Pt 1):749–55.

9. Mehta P, Vasa R, Neumann L, Karpatkin M. Thrombocytopenia in the high-risk infant. *J Pediatr* 1980;**97**(5):791–4.

10. Oren H, Irken G, Oren B, Olgun N, Ozkan H. Assessment of clinical impact and predisposing factors for neonatal thrombocytopenia. *Indian J Pediatr* 1994;**61**(5):551–8.

11. Christensen RD, Henry E, Wiedmeier SE, et al. Thrombocytopenia among extremely low birth weight neonates: Data from a multihospital healthcare system *J Perinatol* 2006;**26**(6):348–53.

12. Sola MC, Slayton WB, Rimsza LM, et al. A neonate with severe thrombocytopenia and radio-ulnar synostosis. *J Perinatol* 2004;**24**(8):528–30.

13. Tighe P, Rimsza LM, Christensen RD, Lew J, Sola MC. Severe thrombocytopenia in a neonate with congenital HIV infection. *J Pediatr* 2005;**146**(3):408–13.

14. Saxonhouse MA, Manco-Johnson MJ. The evaluation and management of neonatal coagulation disorders. *Semin Perinatol* 2009;**33**(1):52–65.

15. Kaushansky K. Lineage-specific hematopoietic growth factors. *N Engl J Med* 2006;**354**(19):2034–45.

16. Dame C. Thrombopoietin in thrombocytopenias of childhood. *Semin Thromb Hemost* 2001;**27**(3):215–28.

17. Murray NA, Roberts IA. Circulating megakaryocytes and their progenitors (BFU-MK and CFU-MK) in term and pre-term neonates. *Br J Haematol* 1995;**89**(1):41–6.

18. Murray NA, Roberts IA. Circulating megakaryocytes and their progenitors in early thrombocytopenia in preterm neonates. *Pediatr Res* 1996;**40**(1):112–19.

19. Ault KA, Knowles C. In vivo biotinylation demonstrates that reticulated platelets are the youngest platelets in circulation. *Exp Hematol* 1995;**23**(9):996–1001.

20. Ault KA, Rinder HM, Mitchell J, et al. The significance of platelets with increased RNA content (reticulated platelets). A measure of the rate of thrombopoiesis. *Am J Clin Path* 1992;**98**(6):637–46.

21. Joseph MA, Adams D, Maragos J, Saving KL. Flow cytometry of neonatal platelet RNA. *J Pediatr Hematol Oncol* 1996;**18**(3):277–81.

22. Peterec SM, Brennan SA, Rinder HM, Wnek JL, Beardsley DS. Reticulated platelet values in normal and thrombocytopenic neonates. *J Pediatr* 1996;**129**(2):269–74.

23. Saxonhouse MA, Sola MC, Pastos KM, et al. Reticulated platelet percentages in term and preterm neonates. *J Pediatr Hematol Oncol* 2004;**26**(12):797–802.

24. Jilma-Stohlawetz P, Homoncik M, Jilma B, et al. High levels of reticulated platelets and thrombopoietin characterize fetal thrombopoiesis. *Br J Haematol* 2001;**112**(2):466–8.

25. Briggs C, Kunka S, Hart D, Oguni S, Machin SJ. Assessment of an immature platelet fraction (IPF) in peripheral thrombocytopenia. *Br J Haematol* 2004;**126**(1):93–9.

26. Cremer M, Paetzold J, Schmalisch G, et al. Immature platelet fraction as novel laboratory parameter predicting the course of neonatal thrombocytopenia. *Br J Haematol* 2009;**144**(4):619–21.

27. Ko YJ, Hur M, Kim H, et al. Reference interval for immature platelet fraction on Sysmex XN hematology analyzer: A comparison study with Sysmex XE-2100. *Clin Chem Lab Med* 2015;**53**(7):1091–7.

28. Cremer M, Weimann A, Szekessy D, et al. Low immature platelet fraction suggests decreased megakaryopoiesis in neonates with sepsis or necrotizing enterocolitis. *J Perinatol* 2013;**33**(8):622–6.

29. MacQueen BC, Christensen RD, Henry E, et al. The immature platelet fraction: Creating neonatal reference intervals and using these to categorize neonatal thrombocytopenias. *J Perinatol* 2017;**37**(7):834–8.

30. Josephson CD, Su LL, Christensen RD, et al. Platelet transfusion practices among neonatologists in the United States and Canada: Results of a survey. *Pediatrics* 2009;**123**(1):278–85.

31. Cremer M, Sola-Visner M, Roll S, et al. Platelet transfusions in neonates: Practices in the United States vary significantly from those in Austria, Germany, and Switzerland. *Transfusion* 2011;**51**(12):2634–41.

32. Kahn DJ, Richardson DK, Billett HH. Inter-NICU variation in rates and management of thrombocytopenia among very low birth-weight infants. *J Perinatol* 2003;**23**(4):312–16.

33. Del Vecchio A, Sola MC, Theriaque DW, et al. Platelet transfusions in the neonatal intensive care unit: Factors predicting which patients will require multiple transfusions. *Transfusion* 2001;**41**(6):803–8.

34. Garcia MG, Duenas E, Sola MC, et al. Epidemiologic and outcome studies of patients who received platelet transfusions in the neonatal intensive care unit. *J Perinatol* 2001;**21**(7):415–20.

35. Murray NA, Howarth LJ, McCloy MP, Letsky EA, Roberts IA. Platelet transfusion in the management of severe thrombocytopenia in neonatal intensive care unit patients. *Transfus Med* 2002;**12**(1):35–41.

36. Andrew M, Vegh P, Caco C, et al. A randomized, controlled trial of platelet transfusions in thrombocytopenic premature infants. *J Pediatr* 1993;**123**(2):285–91.

37. Curley A, Stanworth SJ, Willoughby K, et al. Randomized trial of platelet-transfusion thresholds in neonates. *N Engl J Med* 2019;**380** (3):242–51.

38. Stanworth SJ, Clarke P, Watts T, et al. Prospective, observational study of outcomes in neonates with severe thrombocytopenia. *Pediatrics* 2009;**124**(5): e826–34.

39. Sparger KA, Assmann SF, Granger S, et al. Platelet transfusion practices among very-low-birth-weight infants. *JAMA Pediatr* 2016;**170**(7):687–94.

40. von Lindern JS, van den Bruele T, Lopriore E, Walther FJ. Thrombocytopenia in neonates and the risk of intraventricular hemorrhage: A retrospective cohort study. *BMC Pediatr* 2011;**11**:16.

41. von Lindern JS, Hulzebos CV, Bos AF, et al. Thrombocytopaenia and intraventricular haemorrhage in very premature infants: A tale of two cities. *Arch Dis Child Fetal Neonatal Ed* 2012;**97**(5):F348–52.

42. Sparger K, Deschmann E, Sola-Visner M. Platelet transfusions in the neonatal intensive care unit. *Clin Perinatol* 2015;**42**(3):613–23.

43. Baer VL, Lambert DK, Henry E, et al. Do platelet transfusions in the NICU adversely affect survival? Analysis of 1600 thrombocytopenic neonates in a multihospital healthcare system. *J Perinatol* 2007;**27**(12):790–6.

44. Kenton AB, Hegemier S, Smith EO, et al. Platelet transfusions in infants with necrotizing enterocolitis do not lower mortality but may increase morbidity. *J Perinatol* 2005;**25** (3):173–7.

45. Patel RM, Josephson CD, Shenvi N, et al. Platelet transfusions and mortality in necrotizing enterocolitis. *Transfusion* 2018;**59**(3):981–8.

46. Ferrer-Marin F, Chavda C, Lampa M, et al. Effects of in vitro adult platelet transfusions on neonatal hemostasis. *Thromb Haemost* 2011;**9** (5):1020–8.

47. Fustolo-Gunnink SF, Fijnvandraat K, van Klaveren D, et al. Preterm neonates benefit from low prophylactic platelet transfusion threshold despite varying risk of bleeding or death. *Blood.* 2019;**134**(26):2354–60.

48. Muthukumar P, Venkatesh V, Curley A, et al. Severe thrombocytopenia and patterns of bleeding in neonates: Results from a prospective observational study and implications for use of platelet transfusions. *Transfus Med* 2012;**22** (5):338–43.

Chapter 13

Acquired Thrombocytopenias

Patricia E. Davenport and Martha C. Sola-Visner

Introduction

In this chapter, we will focus exclusively on acquired thrombocytopenias that present in the neonatal period. We will discuss the mechanisms underlying some of the most common varieties of neonatal thrombocytopenia, and how the biological differences between neonatal and adult megakaryocytes might contribute to the susceptibility of neonates to develop thrombocytopenia. We will then review the presentation, pathophysiology, and management of the most common etiologies of neonatal early- and late-onset thrombocytopenia, including autoimmune neonatal thrombocytopenia. Alloimmune and congenital causes of neonatal thrombocytopenia will be discussed in detail in Chapters 14 and 15, respectively.

Neonatal Platelet Production

In this section, we will review the most important differences between neonatal and adult platelet production (Table 13.1) and will discuss how these differences might predispose neonates to develop thrombocytopenia during illness. The

process of platelet production in neonates, as in adults, can be schematically represented as consisting of four main steps (Fig. 13.1):

1. The production of thrombopoietin (Tpo), the most potent stimulator of platelet production, in the liver.
2. The proliferation of megakaryocyte (MK) progenitors (the cells that multiply and give rise to MKs).
3. The maturation of MKs.
4. The release of new platelets by mature MKs.

While in essence these steps are the same at all developmental stages, there are substantial differences between neonatal and adult MK biology. Specifically, plasma Tpo concentrations are higher in healthy neonates than in healthy adults [1–3]. Neonatal MK progenitors have a higher proliferative potential than adult progenitors, and generate more MKs per colony [4, 5] and approximately 10 times more MKs per progenitor cell than adult progenitors in vitro [6, 7]. However, neonatal MKs are significantly smaller and of lower ploidy than adult MKs [8, 9], and

Table 13.1 Differences in megakaryopoiesis between neonates and adults

	Adults	Neonates
Tpo concentrations	Very high in hyporegenerative thrombocytopenia	Not as high in SGA neonates as in thrombocytopenic adults
Megakaryocyte progenitors	Sparse in the blood Give rise to small colonies Less sensitive to Tpo	Abundant in the blood Give rise to large colonies More sensitive to Tpo
Megakaryocytes (MKs)	Large High ploidy levels Make more platelets per MK	Small Low ploidy levels Make less platelets per MK
MK response to Tpo	Increased MK size/ploidy	No increase in MK size/ploidy

Neonatal Hematology, Pathogenesis, Diagnosis, and Management of Hematologic Problems, 3rd edition, ed. Pedro A. de Alarcón, Eric J. Werner, Robert D. Christensen, and Martha C. Sola-Visner. Published by Cambridge University Press.

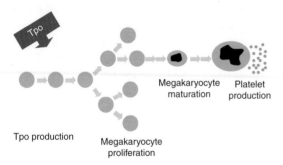

Tpo production

Megakaryocyte
proliferation

Megakaryocyte
maturation

Platelet
production

Fig.13.1 Schematic representation of the process of platelet production, as consisting of four steps: The production of Tpo, the proliferation of megakaryocyte progenitors, the maturation of megakaryocytes, and the release of new platelets into the circulation. (See plate section for color version.)

generate fewer platelets per cell [10]. Importantly, despite their small size and low ploidy, neonatal MKs have been shown to be cytoplasmically mature and contain all of the elements needed for platelet production [6].

Studies in thrombocytopenic adult patients and in animal models have shown that, under normal conditions, the adult bone marrow (BM) responds to increased platelet demand by first increasing the MK size and ploidy and then the MK number [11, 12]. These changes ultimately lead to a two- to eight-fold increase in MK mass. To determine whether thrombocytopenic neonates can mount a similar response when facing increased platelet consumption due to illness, our group evaluated the MK concentration and size in BM samples from thrombocytopenic and non-thrombocytopenic neonates and adults. In this study, thrombocytopenic neonates (unlike thrombocytopenic adults) did not increase the size of their MKs [13]. Similar results were obtained in a study using a murine model of fetal immune thrombocytopenia [14]. In this study, adult mice treated with an anti-platelet antibody (MWReg30) increased the number and size of their MKs as expected, while newborn mice exposed in utero to the same antibody did not increase their MK size. Consistent with these observations, a recent study showed significant differences in the response of newborn and adult mice to a single dose of the Tpo mimetic romiplostim [15]. While adult mice increased the number and size of MKs in the BM and spleen, newborn mice did not increase their MK size, which resulted in an attenuated platelet increment [15]. Taken together, these observations support the notion that MKs in neonates have a limited ability to increase their size

in response to increased platelet demand or to Tpo stimulation, which decreases their ability to upregulate platelet production and likely contributes to the predisposition of sick neonates to develop thrombocytopenia. Furthermore, the evidence suggests that platelet production in neonates is dependent on the proliferative potential of their MK progenitors, thus making them highly susceptible to factors that affect MK proliferation.

Neonatal Platelet Function

Multiple in-vitro studies evaluating platelet function in cord blood samples have shown that neonatal platelets are hyporesponsive to most platelet agonists, compared with platelets from adults [16, 17]. However, whole blood assays of hemostasis (such as the bleeding time, the Platelet Function Analyzer, PFA-100®, or the thromboelastogram) revealed that term neonates have normal to slightly *enhanced* hemostasis compared to adults [18, 19]. While the mechanisms underlying these apparently contradictory findings are not completely understood, it is currently accepted that the higher hematocrits, higher mean corpuscular volumes (MCVs), higher von Willebrand factor (vWF) levels, and presence of ultra large vWF polymers in neonates account for the apparent disparities between the results of platelet function assays and tests of primary hemostasis [20, 21]. Thus, it seems that the platelet hyporeactivity of full term infants should be viewed as part of a delicately balanced neonatal hemostatic system, rather than as a developmental deficiency.

Most of the studies mentioned above only included full term infants, and only a few evaluated preterm neonates at highest risk of bleeding. Bednarek et al. serially evaluated platelet function by flow cytometry in extremely low birth weight (ELBW) infants over the first 2 weeks of life [22]. These investigators showed that platelet responses to agonists and platelet pro-coagulant activity were significantly decreased in ELBW infants during the first days of life compared to adults, but improved significantly by day of life 10–14, to levels only slightly below those of adults [22]. Consistently, del Vecchio and collaborators found that bleeding times performed on day of life one were twice as high in infants born at 24–33 weeks' gestation compared to infants born at 38–41 weeks' gestation, but improved by day of life 10 [23]. These observations suggest that preterm neonates may have transient developmental deficiencies in primary hemostasis, but it remains unclear whether these contribute to the pathophysiology of intraventricular hemorrhages.

Specific Neonatal Diseases Causing Thrombocytopenia

Placental Insufficiency and Chronic Intrauterine Hypoxia

Chronic intrauterine hypoxia is the most frequent cause of early-onset thrombocytopenia (within the first 72 hours of life) in preterm neonates. Chronic intrauterine hypoxia is commonly seen in maternal conditions associated with placental insufficiency, such as pregnancy-induced hypertension and diabetes, and manifests in the fetus as intrauterine growth restriction resulting in small for gestational age (SGA) neonates and hematological abnormalities (i.e., thrombocytopenia, neutropenia, polycythemia). The thrombocytopenia associated with this condition is almost always mild to moderate, with platelet counts between 50 and 100×10^9/L. In a large study of SGA neonates with thrombocytopenia presumably due to placental insufficiency and chronic intrauterine hypoxia (i.e., without other identifiable cause), which the authors termed "thrombocytopenia of SGA," the mean nadir platelet count was 93×10^9/L [24]. In the same study, severely SGA neonates (birth weight <1st percentile for age) had lower platelet counts than less growth restricted infants (Fig. 13.2), and the nucleated red cell count at birth correlated with the severity of the thrombocytopenia. Severe thrombocytopenia

secondary to SGA is rare, however, and for that reason other causes of severe early onset thrombocytopenia (such as immune-mediated, infections, or genetic disorders) should be considered if the platelet count is $<50 \times 10^9$/L. The thrombocytopenia associated with chronic intrauterine hypoxia and intrauterine growth restriction also follows a well-characterized natural course, reaching its nadir by day of life 4, and typically resolving by days of life 10–14. Thus, persistence of the thrombocytopenia beyond this period should also trigger an evaluation for other causes.

The pathophysiology of thrombocytopenia in fetuses and neonates exposed to chronic intrauterine hypoxia is not completely understood, but studies have implicated decreased platelet production. Murray and Roberts observed that preterm neonates with early-onset thrombocytopenia had decreased concentrations of circulating MK progenitors compared to their non-thrombocytopenic counterparts [1, 25]. Similarly, Sola and collaborators reported decreased numbers of MKs in the BM of three thrombocytopenic preterm neonates born from pregnancies complicated by placental insufficiency [2]. Contrary to what would be expected, both groups of investigators reported that plasma Tpo concentrations in these neonates were normal to minimally elevated, suggesting that an inadequate up-regulation of Tpo production could contribute to the thrombocytopenia.

The effects of chronic hypoxia on thrombopoiesis in vivo have also been studied in animal models. These studies confirmed the association between chronic hypoxia and thrombocytopenia, and showed

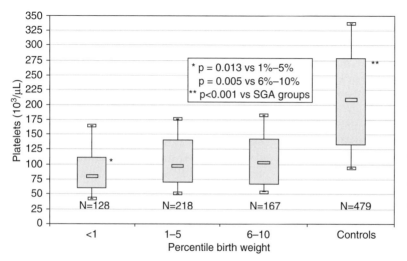

Fig. 13.2 Platelet counts measured on day of life 4 (the mean nadir of platelet count) in SGA neonates according to birth weight percentile. Counts are grouped as neonates <1st percentile, 1st to 5th percentile, 6th to 10th percentile, and 11th to 99th percentile for gestational age ("controls"). In each weight category, the median platelet count is shown, along with the first and third interquartile range (box), and the 10th percentile and 90th percentile values (whiskers). (Reproduced from Christensen et al., *Pediatrics* 2015;136:e361–e370, with permission [24].)

reduced MK differentiation of hematopoietic precursors resulting in decreased MK numbers in both adult and newborn animals exposed to hypoxia [26, 27]. Subsequent in vitro studies demonstrated that MK progenitors are not directly damaged by hypoxia, but rather the effects seem to be mediated by non-progenitor cells [28]. Consistently, hypoxia was shown to alter the effects of cytokines on MK progenitors without damaging the MK cells directly [29]. Taken together, these findings suggest that chronic intrauterine hypoxia alters the MK response to cytokines leading to decreased MK production, which improves once the infant is exposed to the normoxic extrauterine environment. This explains the spontaneous resolution of this thrombocytopenia starting on day of life 4–5. Typically, no intervention is needed for the thrombocytopenia in affected infants, but it is important to document the normalization of the platelet count to rule out other possible causes.

Autoimmune Neonatal Thrombocytopenia (Secondary to Maternal ITP)

Early onset thrombocytopenia can also be caused by the transplacental passage of anti-platelet antibodies from the mother to the fetus. Most commonly, these are alloantibodies that react against the fetal platelets, but not the maternal platelets, so that the mother is not thrombocytopenic herself (fetal/neonatal alloimmune thrombocytopenia). The pathophysiology, evaluation and management of this variety of thrombocytopenia are reviewed in detail in Chapter 14.

Other times the neonatal thrombocytopenia is secondary to the passage of antibodies from a mother with immune thrombocytopenic purpura (ITP), or other autoimmune condition associated with anti-platelet antibodies. Several large observational studies published in the 1990s concluded that infants born to mothers with ITP are at low risk of developing severe thrombocytopenia. In one of the earliest studies, Burrows and Kelton found a platelet count $<50 \times 10^9$/L in 10% of infants born to a mother with ITP, and a platelet count $<25 \times 10^9$/L in 4.2% [30]. In that study, encompassing 288 infants, no infant suffered an intracranial hemorrhage (ICH) [30]. Other studies reported similarly low incidences of severe thrombocytopenia (defined as a platelet count $<50 \times 10^9$/

L) in neonates born to mothers with ITP, ranging from 8.9% to 14.7%, with ICH occurring in 0% to 1.5% of thrombocytopenic infants [31–33]. In a recent national cohort study conducted in the UK including 107 pregnancies with ITP, no neonates required treatment for thrombocytopenia and there were no cases of neonatal intracranial bleeding. However, the mothers with ITP were at increased risk of severe post-partum hemorrhage compared to the general population [34].

Several studies have tried to identify antenatal predictors of severe thrombocytopenia in the offspring of mothers with ITP. Unfortunately, the fetal or neonatal platelet count cannot be reliably predicted by maternal platelet count, platelet antibody levels, or history of maternal splenectomy. Neonates born to a mother with history of delivering an infant with thrombocytopenia are usually as affected as the first. Attempts to measure the fetal platelet count prior to delivery carry risk and are not recommended. There is also no evidence that cesarean section is safer for the fetus than uncomplicated vaginal delivery (although forceps or vacuum assist deliveries should be avoided), and thus the current recommendation is to treat the maternal ITP appropriately, but to use only obstetrical indications for cesarean delivery. Interestingly, a recent study reported the use of a novel recombinant human thrombopoietin (rTPO) to manage ITP during pregnancy. In this study of 31 patients, 74% responded. Furthermore, rTPO was well tolerated and no problems were observed in the infants born to treated mothers [35]. This paved the way for the use of a new potential therapy to manage ITP during pregnancy.

While only a small percentage of neonates are born with severe thrombocytopenia in the setting of maternal ITP, mild to moderate thrombocytopenia is more common. Importantly, the platelet count typically decreases after birth, reaching a nadir between days 2 and 5 [36]. For that reason, the recommendation is to obtain a platelet count immediately after delivery (from the cord or the baby), and to follow platelet counts in all infants with mild or moderate thrombocytopenia. A head ultrasound should be obtained on all infants with a platelet count $<50 \times 10^9$/L at birth. Recommendations from the International Consensus Report on Management of ITP are to treat neonates with either clinical bleeding or a platelet count $<20 \times 10^9$/L with a single dose of intravenous immunoglobulin (IVIG, 1 g/kg), which can be repeated if necessary

[32]. Major bleeding should be treated with platelet transfusions in addition to IVIG. Severe thrombocytopenia and major hemorrhage secondary to maternal ITP are rare, so evaluation for alloimmune thrombocytopenia or other causes of thrombocytopenia should be considered in those cases [32].

Neonatal thrombocytopenia secondary to maternal ITP can last for months and requires long-term monitoring and occasionally a second dose of IVIG at 4–6 weeks after birth. Interestingly, a recent study suggested that antiplatelet antibodies from ITP mothers are transferred to the fetus by breastmilk, and are associated with neonatal thrombocytopenia persisting more than 4 months, which disappears following discontinuation of breastfeeding [37].

Asphyxia

Several studies have established an association between perinatal asphyxia and thrombocytopenia [38, 39]. The thrombocytopenia is typically self-limited and mild to moderate, with platelet counts between 50 and 100×10^9/L that improve spontaneously and normalize by days 19 to 21 [40]. In a cohort of 171 neonates with perinatal asphyxia, Boutaybi et al. found early-onset thrombocytopenia (within the first 48 hours of life) in 51% [41]. Multiple logistic regression analysis identified a significant independent association between early-onset thrombocytopenia and prolonged PT and higher lactate levels, suggesting a correlation between the severity of the asphyxia and the severity of thrombocytopenia.

The mechanisms responsible for the decreased platelet count are not entirely clear. In a significant number of infants, severe perinatal asphyxia is associated with disseminated intravascular coagulation (DIC), thus providing a reasonable explanation for the thrombocytopenia in these cases. However, some asphyxiated neonates develop thrombocytopenia in the absence of coagulopathy and the mechanisms underlying the thrombocytopenia in these cases are less clear. Findings in a rabbit model suggest that shortened platelet survival following exposure to transient hypoxia might lead to thrombocytopenia [42]. In contrast, a recent study by Christensen and colleagues described the thrombocytopenia of asphyxia as likely hyporegenerative and as a separate entity from, but also co-occurring with, disseminated intravascular coagulation (DIC) [40].

Recently, total body cooling became a widely accepted intervention aimed at improving the neurodevelopmental outcome of neonates with moderate to severe perinatal asphyxia [43]. Multiple studies have described changes in coagulation and platelet function induced by hypothermia. Specifically, in response to hypothermia, there is an inhibition of platelet activation, adhesion and aggregation as well as changes in the platelets' surface antigen composition that can lead to their rapid removal from the circulation [44–46]. Boutaybi and coworkers compared thrombocytopenia due to asphyxia alone versus asphyxia treated with total body cooling and found there to be a three-times higher incidence of thrombocytopenia in infants treated with hypothermia [41, 47]. Importantly, this increase was in infants with only mild to moderate thrombocytopenia [41, 47]. Characterization of the time course of thrombocytopenia between the two cohorts showed that patients with asphyxia treated with hypothermia reached their nadir platelet count later than those with thrombocytopenia of asphyxia alone (day 5 versus day 3) [41, 47]. Christensen et al. also showed a significant lengthening of bleeding times and closure times measured with the Platelet Function Analyzer 100® (both measures of platelet function and primary hemostasis) during hypothermia, followed by rapid normalization after rewarming. This study suggests that the platelet functional impairment in asphyxiated neonates undergoing therapeutic hypothermia is transient [48].

The dysregulation of coagulation, platelet function, and the development of thrombocytopenia induced by both asphyxia and therapeutic hypothermia manifests clinically with a higher incidence of bleeding and coagulopathy [49–51]. A few studies have aimed at determining the modifiable risk factors for bleeding during therapeutic hypothermia. One study using thromboelastography (TEG) as a comprehensive assessment of coagulation reported an increased risk of coagulopathy with hypothermia, which was associated with specific measures of TEG but not with platelet counts [52]. Two separate studies found that, while platelet counts below 130×10^9/L or below 100×10^9/L were associated with an increased risk of minor bleeding, coagulopathy and hypofibrinogenemia were associated with severe bleeding [49, 53]. Together, these studies suggest that thrombocytopenia in the setting of perinatal asphyxia and therapeutic hypothermia may put infants at increased risk of mild bleeding, but coagulopathy and hypofibrinogenemia may be more important in the development of severe hemorrhage.

Infections

The association of thrombocytopenia with neonatal bacterial sepsis has been described by several groups of investigators, although the reported incidence varies depending on the definition of thrombocytopenia. For example, Guida and collaborators defined thrombocytopenia as a platelet count $<100 \times 10^9/L$, and observed it in 54% of sepsis episodes [54], while Manzoni et al. defined thrombocytopenia as a platelet count $<80 \times 10^9/L$, and detected it in 17.2% of septic infants [55]. Whether infections with certain organisms are more likely to induce thrombocytopenia than infections with other types (i.e., Gram positive vs Gram negative organisms) is controversial [54, 55], but it appears that virtually any bacterial organism capable of causing sepsis in a neonate is also capable of inducing thrombocytopenia. In modern NICUs, late-onset sepsis is the most common clinical condition underlying severe thrombocytopenia in neonates [56]. If the infection is treated appropriately, the thrombocytopenia usually lasts an average of 6 days (range 1–10 days) [54, 57]. However, a number of neonates with sepsis develop severe thrombocytopenia that persists longer than 2 weeks [56], and sepsis accounts for approximately one-third of NICU patients who qualify as very-high platelet users (i.e., >20 transfusions) [58].

The etiology of thrombocytopenia in bacterial sepsis is an active area of research. Prior studies assessing platelet production in neonates with sepsis and/or NEC showed a modest (2–3 fold) elevation in Tpo levels, circulating MK progenitors and reticulated platelet percentages (a measure of newly released platelets) [59], suggesting primarily a platelet consumptive etiology rather than decreased production. Interestingly, however, neonates with Gram-negative sepsis had only modest increases in thrombopoiesis, despite having more severe thrombocytopenia and more severe illness. This suggested that the thrombopoietic response in neonates can be dampened during severe illness, reaching a state of "relative hypoproliferation," defined as a less than two-fold increase in platelet production in response to consumptive thrombocytopenia [59].

Traditionally, sepsis-induced platelet consumption has been attributed to DIC, increased platelet aggregation, and adherence to the damaged endothelium with subsequent removal by the reticulo-endothelial system, and/or immune mediated platelet destruction. With new research evidencing a central role of platelets in innate and adaptive immune responses, it is likely that the sepsis-induced consumption of platelets is more complex than previously thought. Platelets express and/or release multiple immune mediators, including cytokines, chemokines, and receptors known to be required for the initiation of the immune response to infection [60, 61]. Andonegui and colleagues demonstrated the expression of TLR-4 (the LPS receptor) on platelets and showed that, in response to LPS binding, platelets accumulate in the lungs where they bind to adherent neutrophils [62]. Clark and colleagues studied this further and described that, once LPS stimulated platelets adhere to neutrophils in the lungs, they induce robust neutrophil activation and the release of neutrophil extracellular traps (NETS) used to ensnare bacteria [63]. Furthermore, a recent study revealed that bacteria like *Escherichia coli* and *Staphylococcus aureus* are able to induce apoptosis in platelets by producing alpha-hemolysin or alpha-toxin, respectively, both enzymes that induce rapid degradation of platelet Bcl-xL, an anti-apoptotic protein essential for platelet survival [64]. This in turn results in a rapid drop in platelet count.

Viral and parasitic infections also can cause thrombocytopenia. The specific mechanisms of thrombocytopenia in these infections are unclear, but likely involve a mixture of platelet destruction and suppression of platelet production. Cytomegalovirus (CMV), the most common cause of congenital viral infection, affects megakaryopoiesis by directly infecting bone marrow stromal cells [65] and MKs [66]. In addition, CMV-infected infants frequently exhibit splenomegaly and require repeated transfusions due to platelet sequestration in the spleen. In regard to other viruses, herpes viruses can cause suppression of MK colony formation in vitro [67]. Parvovirus B19 usually causes severe anemia leading to hydrops fetalis, but it can also cause thrombocytopenia. In vitro, parvovirus B19 suppresses MK colony formation [68], and Forestier and coworkers found thrombocytopenia in 11 of 13 fetuses with parvovirus B19 infection [69]. Neonatal enterovirus infection can also cause thrombocytopenia, especially in the presence of hepatitis and DIC [70]. HIV has been recently recognized as a cause of thrombocytopenia in neonates. Like CMV and parvovirus, HIV can directly infect megakaryocytes and cause impaired platelet release, a phenomenon known as "ineffective platelet production" [71]. Adenovirus, Epstein–Barr virus, and dengue virus have also been reported to cause neonatal thrombocytopenia, although these are rather uncommon infections in the neonatal period.

Necrotizing Enterocolitis

Necrotizing enterocolitis (NEC) is frequently associated with thrombocytopenia. In an early study published in 1976 assessing hematological abnormalities in infants with NEC, as many as 90% of infants with NEC had platelet counts below 150×10^9/L, and 55% had platelet counts below 50×10^9/L [72]. Of the latter, 55% had bleeding complications, one-third of these serious enough to be considered contributory to the infant's death. Six of 14 infants studied had evidence of DIC and the mean duration of thrombocytopenia was 7 days (range 1–31 days). A more recent study found that neonates with NEC and thrombocytopenia (platelet count $<60 \times 10^9$/L) had two-times more bleeding events than neonates with similar degree of thrombocytopenia not related to NEC, but the bleeds were minor in severity [73]. In reviewing 58 cases of NEC treated in their institution, Ververidis and coworkers found that thrombocytopenia and/or a rapid fall in the platelet count was a poor prognostic factor, and that the degree of the thrombocytopenia correlated with the severity of the disease [74].

The etiology of thrombocytopenia in NEC is an area of active research. The shortened survival of platelet transfusions in these infants suggests a platelet-consumptive process. This was corroborated in studies of both murine models and human neonates with NEC/sepsis, which found markers of increased megakaryopoiesis in association with thrombocytopenia [59, 75]. However, a study by Cremer and coworkers found a reduced immature platelet fraction (IPF, a measure of platelet production; see Chapter 12) in *severely* thrombocytopenic neonates with NEC, suggesting decreased platelet production in these infants [76]. Interestingly, this subset of infants with NEC, severe thrombocytopenia, and low IPF had

the highest mortality, suggesting that decreased IPF in the setting of severe thrombocytopenia could be a marker of illness severity and poor prognosis in NEC.

Platelets may also play an active role in the pathogenesis of NEC. Many pro-inflammatory cytokines are elevated in NEC, particularly platelet-activating factor (PAF), interleukin 1 (IL-1), and tumor necrosis factor (TNF) [77]. PAF, in particular, has been strongly implicated in the pathogenesis of NEC, based on animal studies demonstrating that the inhibition of PAF attenuates or prevents the development of NEC [78]. Interestingly, the levels of several pro-inflammatory cytokines (IL-1, IL-6, IL-8, TNF-alpha) increase in the supernatant of platelet units during storage in the blood bank, prior to platelets being transfused [79–83]. While most of these pro-inflammatory factors are released from leukocytes present in the platelet suspension, and thus levels are markedly reduced when the products are leuko-reduced prior to storage, bioactive factors and cytokines are also released from platelet granules during storage, which could potentially contribute to the pathophysiology of NEC [84]. In that regard, at least two studies have suggested an association between higher number/volume of transfusions in patients with NEC and increased morbidity (short bowel syndrome and/or cholestasis) [85] or mortality (30.3 vs. 6.0 transfusions per 100 infant days in infants with NEC who died vs. survived in an unadjusted analysis) [84]. Although the difference in number of platelet transfusions between infants who died and those who survived was no longer significant in the latter study after adjusting for birth weight and severity of illness, the results strongly suggested the potential for such association. Thus, platelet transfusions should be administered judiciously to infants with NEC (See Chapter 12 for more discussion on platelet transfusions).

Thromboses

Neonatal thromboses can occur either spontaneously (such as renal vein thrombosis or sagittal sinus thrombosis), or in association with an indwelling central catheter [86]. Thrombocytopenia is not a mandatory component of the clinical presentation of neonatal thromboses, but the presence of persistent thrombocytopenia with no clear etiology should raise suspicion for the potential of thrombus formation, particularly if predisposing factors are present (including perinatal asphyxia, congenital heart disease, maternal diabetes mellitus, polycythemia, dehydration, twin pregnancy, or presence of an indwelling catheter). In recent reviews, thrombocytopenia/anemia or both were present in 51% of cases of renal vein thrombosis [87], but the classic triad of gross hematuria, palpable kidneys, and thrombocytopenia was found in only 13% [88]. Thus, a high index of suspicion is required to make an early diagnosis. While arterial thrombosis is less frequent than venous thrombosis in neonates [89, 90], a recent study in adults with consumptive platelet disorders, specifically heparin-induced thrombocytopenia and thrombotic thrombocytopenic purpura, found that platelet transfusion increased the risk for arterial thromboses [91]. While this study did not include neonates, the findings suggest that further study is warranted in this population. Further discussion of pathogenesis, presentation and treatment of neonatal thromboses can be found in Chapter 19.

Disseminated Intravascular Coagulation/ Malformations

Disseminated intravascular coagulation (DIC) is a thrombo-hemorrhagic disorder in which there is systemic activation of the coagulation system, simultaneously causing intravascular thrombi formation (compromising blood supply to organs) and depletion of platelets and coagulation factors, resulting in bleeding. DIC is not a primary pathological process, it is always secondary to an underlying disorder such as sepsis, trauma, vascular abnormalities, or hypoxic ischemic encephalopathy [92]. Laboratory parameters associated with DIC include thrombocytopenia as well as deficits in coagulation factors that prompt frequent transfusions of blood products. The thrombocytopenia in DIC is secondary to thrombin-induced platelet aggregation [93]. Neonates have an increased incidence of DIC compared to pediatric or adult patients [94–96] which has been attributed to their dynamically evolving hemostatic system after birth [97–99].

Thrombocytopenia is one of the features of the Kasabach–Merritt syndrome (KMS), also known as "hemangioma thrombocytopenia syndrome." It is now clear that the vascular tumors associated with the KMS are not true childhood hemangiomas, but rather hemangioendotheliomas [100]. Typically, the thrombocytopenia of KMS is preceded by enlargement and hardening of the vascular tumor. The primary mechanism is local consumption of platelets and clot formation, but platelets that have been damaged within the vascular abnormality are also removed in the spleen. KMS is refractory to transfused platelets and, if administered, they can result in painful tumor engorgement [101]. As a result, platelet transfusions are only indicated for active bleeding or immediately prior to surgery [102].

Drug-Induced Thrombocytopenia

A few drugs administered to pregnant women have been reported to cause thrombocytopenia in the mothers and their fetuses. However, only a small percentage of mothers who receive the particular drug have thrombocytopenia, thus making the firm establishment of this association difficult. Nevertheless, quinine, thiazide diuretics, hydralazine, and tolbutamide have been implicated as causes of fetal/neonatal thrombocytopenia when administered to pregnant women.

In addition, the development of moderate to severe late-onset thrombocytopenia in a well-appearing infant in whom infection, NEC, thromboses and DIC have been ruled out should trigger suspicion for drug-induced thrombocytopenia. The literature regarding drug-induced thrombocytopenia in neonates mostly consists of isolated case reports. However, there is a significant number of medications known to cause drug-induced thrombocytopenia that are also commonly used in neonates, including antibiotics (penicillins, linezolid, ciprofloxacin, cephalosporins, metronidazole, vancomycin, and rifampin), ibuprofen, acetaminophen, famotidine, cimetidine, hydrochlorotiazide, phenobarbital, and phenytoin [103]. If a neonate develops thrombocytopenia shortly after one of these medications has been started, and if other (more common) etiologies of thrombocytopenia have been ruled out, removal of the suspected medication should be considered.

One of the medications most frequently associated with thrombocytopenia among hospitalized patients is heparin, particularly unfractionated heparin. Heparin-induced thrombocytopenia (HIT) is an immune-mediated response to heparin administration. The incidence of HIT among neonates has been found to range from 0% to 1.5% [104, 105]. The incidence is slightly higher in pediatric ICU patients, particularly among those receiving therapeutic doses of unfractionated heparin for the treatment of thromboses or following cardiac surgery [106]. Unfractionated heparin in prophylactic doses [105] and low-molecular weight heparin are rare causes of HIT in pediatric patients [106].

HIT is a clinicopathological syndrome, which means that both clinical and laboratory characteristics have to be fulfilled in order to make the diagnosis. These include the presence of heparin, a fall in the platelet count by 50% or more, the correct time of onset (approximately 5–10 days after the initial exposure to heparin), and the presence of heparin dependent antibodies. There are two types of antibody assays used to diagnose HIT: antigen assays, which simply determine the presence of antibodies directed against the HIT-specific epitopes on platelet factor 4 (PF4), and functional assays, which determine the platelet-activating properties of the antibodies in a patient's serum. The latter represent the gold standard in HIT antibody testing, because they detect the clinically significant HIT antibodies. However, they are technically demanding and are only carried out by large laboratories. Furthermore, it is unclear whether these assays need to be modified for use in neonates.

If HIT is strongly suspected or confirmed, heparin therapy should be discontinued, and alternative anticoagulants such as lepirudin and argatroban should be considered to avoid the thrombotic manifestations of HIT. However, data regarding the use of these anticoagulants in the neonatal population is sparse [107], and therefore their potential benefits need to be carefully balanced against the potential risks. For more information on HIT in neonates and children, the reader is referred to the excellent review by Risch et al. [106].

Liver Failure

At least two studies of neonatal thrombocytopenia have linked liver failure with prolonged thrombocytopenia [108, 109], and it has been suggested that neonates with this presentation would be good candidates for therapy with thrombopoietic factors. The main mechanism responsible for this thrombocytopenia is likely decreased platelet production secondary to insufficient Tpo production in the liver (the main site of Tpo production). In

adults, this mechanism has been supported by the observation of increasing Tpo concentrations and reticulated platelet percentages following liver transplants [110, 111]. A second proposed mechanism involves the loss of liver cell function causing a reduction in the hepatic vascular bed and increasing the splanchnic inflow, ultimately resulting in elevated portal venous pressure, splenomegaly, and platelet sequestration in the spleen [112]. Adult studies have questioned the importance of this mechanism since interventions that reverse the portal hypertension do not reliably correct the thrombocytopenia. The mechanism of thrombocytopenia in neonatal liver failure has never been specifically studied.

Other Disorders

Other neonatal conditions in which thrombocytopenia occurs include polycythemia vera, extracorporeal membrane oxygenation, cyanotic congenital heart disease, metabolic disorders (organic acidemias), Down syndrome transient myeloproliferative disorder, congenital leukemia, osteopetrosis, and the histiocytoses, particularly hemophagocytic lymphohistiocytosis (HLH).

References

1. Murray NA, Watts TL, Roberts IA. Endogenous thrombopoietin levels and effect of recombinant human thrombopoietin on megakaryocyte precursors in term and preterm babies. *Pediatr Res* 1998;**43**(1):148–51.

2. Sola MC, Calhoun DA, Hutson AD, Christensen RD. Plasma thrombopoietin concentrations in thrombocytopenic and non-thrombocytopenic patients in a neonatal intensive care unit. *Br J Haematol* 1999;**104**(1):90–2.

3. Walka MM, Sonntag J, Dudenhausen JW, Obladen M. Thrombopoietin concentration in umbilical cord blood of healthy term newborns is higher than in adult controls. *Biol Neonate* 1999;**75** (1):54–8.

4. Nishihira H, Toyoda Y, Miyazaki H, et al., Growth of macroscopic human megakaryocyte colonies from cord blood in culture with recombinant human thrombopoietin (c-mpl ligand) and the effects of gestational age on frequency of colonies. *Br J Haematol* 1996;**92**(1):23–8.

5. Olson TA, Levine RF, Mazur EM, et al., Megakaryocytes and megakaryocyte progenitors in human cord blood. *Am J Pediatr Hematol Oncol* 1992;**14**(3):241–7.

6. Liu ZJ, Italiano J Jr., Ferrer-Marin F, et al., Developmental differences in megakaryocytopoiesis are associated with up-regulated TPO signaling through mTOR and elevated GATA-1 levels in neonatal megakaryocytes. *Blood* 2011;**117**(15):4106–17.

7. Liu ZJ, Sola-Visner M. Neonatal and adult megakaryopoiesis. *Curr Opin Hematol* 2011;**18** (5):330–7.

8. de Alarcón PA Graeve JL. Analysis of megakaryocyte ploidy in fetal bone marrow biopsies using a new adaptation of the feulgen technique to measure DNA content and estimate megakaryocyte ploidy from biopsy specimens. *Pediatr Res* 1996;**39**(1):166–70.

9. Hegyi E, Nakazawa M, Debili N, et al. Developmental changes in human megakaryocyte ploidy. *Exp Hematol* 1991;**19**(2):87–94.

10. Mattia G, Vulcano F, Milazzo L, et al. Different ploidy levels of megakaryocytes generated from peripheral or cord blood CD34+ cells are correlated with different levels of platelet release. *Blood* 2002;**99**(3):888–97.

11. Harker LA. Kinetics of thrombopoiesis. *J Clin Invest* 1968;**47**(3):458–65.

12. Harker LA, Finch CA. Thrombokinetics in man. *J Clin Invest* 1969;**48**(6):963–74.

13. Sola-Visner MC, Christensen RD, Hutson AD, et al. Megakaryocyte size and concentration in the bone marrow of thrombocytopenic and nonthrombocytopenic neonates. *Pediatr Res*, 2007;**61**(4):479–84.

14. Hu Z, Slayton WB, Rimsza LM, et al. Differences between newborn and adult mice in their response to immune thrombocytopenia. *Neonatology* 2010;**98**(1):100–8.

15. Sparger KA, Ramsey H, Lorenz V, et al. Developmental differences between newborn and adult mice in response to romiplostim. *Platelets* 2017:1–8.

16. Israels SJ, Odaibo FS, Robertson C, et al. Deficient thromboxane synthesis and response in platelets from premature infants. *Pediatr Res* 1997;**41** (2):218–23.

17. Rajasekhar D, Kestin AS, Bednarek FJ, et al. Neonatal platelets are less reactive than adult platelets to physiological agonists in whole blood. *Thromb Haemost* 1994;**72**(6):957–63.

18. Andrew M, Castle V, Mitchell L, et al. Modified bleeding time in the infant. *Am J Hematol* 1989;**30** (3):190–1.

19. Boudewijns M, Raes M, Peeters V, et al. Evaluation of platelet function on cord blood in 80 healthy term neonates using the Platelet Function Analyser (PFA-100); shorter in vitro bleeding times in neonates than adults. *Eur J Pediatr* 2003;**162**(3):212–13.

20. Israels SJ, Cheang T, McMillan-Ward EM, et al. Evaluation of primary hemostasis in neonates with a new in vitro platelet function analyzer. *J Pediatr* 2001;**138**(1):116–19.

21. Roschitz B, Sudi K, Kostenberger M, et al. Shorter PFA-100 closure times in neonates than in adults: role of red cells, white cells, platelets and von Willebrand factor. *Acta Paediatr* 2001;**90** (6):664–70.

22. Bednarek FJ, Bean S, Barnard MR, et al. The platelet hyporeactivity of extremely low birth weight neonates is age-dependent. *Thromb Res* 2009;**124**(1):42–5.

23. Del Vecchio A, Latini G, Henry E, et al. Template bleeding times of 240 neonates born at 24 to 41 weeks' gestation. *J Perinatol* 2008;**28**(6):427–31.

24. Christensen RD, Baer VL, Henry E, et al. Thrombocytopenia in small-for-gestational-age infants. *Pediatrics* 2015;**136**(2):e361–70.

25. Murray NA, Roberts IA. Circulating megakaryocytes and their progenitors in early thrombocytopenia in preterm neonates. *Pediatr Res* 1996;**40**(1):112–19.

26. McDonald TP, Cottrell MB, Steward SA, et al. Comparison of platelet production in two strains of mice with different modal megakaryocyte DNA ploidies after exposure to hypoxia. *Exp Hematol* 1992;**20**(1):51–6.

27. Meberg A. Transitory thrombocytopenia in newborn mice after intrauterine hypoxia. *Pediatr Res* 1980;**14**(9):1071–3.

28. Saxonhouse MA, Rimsza LM, Christensen RD, et al. Effects of anoxia on megakaryocyte progenitors derived from cord blood CD34pos cells. *Eur J Haematol* 2003;**71**(5):359–65.

29. LaIuppa JA, Papoutsakis ET, Miller WM. Oxygen tension alters the effects of cytokines on the megakaryocyte, erythrocyte, and granulocyte lineages. *Exp Hematol* 1998;**26**(9):835–43.

30. Burrows RF, Kelton JG. Pregnancy in patients with idiopathic thrombocytopenic purpura: assessing the risks for the infant at delivery. *Obstet Gynecol Surv* 1993;**48**(12):781–8.

31. Samuels P, Bussel JB, Braitman LE, et al. Estimation of the risk of thrombocytopenia in the offspring of pregnant women with presumed immune thrombocytopenic purpura. *N Engl J Med* 1990;**323**(4):229–35.

32. Provan D, Stasi R, Newland AC, et al. International consensus report on the investigation and management of primary

immune thrombocytopenia. *Blood* 2010;**115**(2):168–86.

33. Kaplan C, Daffos F, Forestier F, et al. Fetal platelet counts in thrombocytopenic pregnancy. *Lancet* 1990;**336**(8721):979–82.

34. Care A, Pavord S, Knight M, et al. Severe primary autoimmune thrombocytopenia in pregnancy: a national cohort study. *BJOG* 2018;**125**(5):604–12.

35. Kong Z, Qin P, Xiao S, et al. A novel recombinant human thrombopoietin therapy for the management of immune thrombocytopenia in pregnancy. *Blood* 2017;**130**(9):1097–103.

36. Burrows RF, Kelton JG. Low fetal risks in pregnancies associated with idiopathic thrombocytopenic purpura. *Am J Obstet Gynecol* 1990;**163**(4 Pt 1):1147–50.

37. Hauschner H, Rosenberg N, Seligsohn U, et al. Persistent neonatal thrombocytopenia can be caused by IgA antiplatelet antibodies in breast milk of immune thrombocytopenic mothers. *Blood* 2015;**126**(5):661–4.

38. Castle V, Andrew M, Kelton J, et al. Frequency and mechanism of neonatal thrombocytopenia. *J Pediatr* 1986;**108**(5 Pt 1):749–55.

39. Ropert JC, Dreyfus M, Dehan M, Tchernia G. Severe neonatal thrombopenia. Analysis of the etiologic data on 64 cases [in French]. *Arch Fr Pediatr* 1984;**41**(2):85–90.

40. Christensen RD, Baer VL, Yaish HM. Thrombocytopenia in late preterm and term neonates after perinatal asphyxia. *Transfusion* 2015;**55**(1):187–96.

41. Boutaybi N, Steggerda SJ, Smits-Wintjens VE, et al. Early-onset thrombocytopenia in near-term and term infants with perinatal asphyxia. *Vox Sang* 2014;**106**(4):361–7.

42. Castle V, Coates G, Mitchell LG, O'Brodovich H, Andrew M. The effect of hypoxia on platelet survival and site of sequestration in the newborn rabbit. *Thromb Haemost* 1988;**59**(1):45–8.

43. Shankaran S, Laptook AR, Ehrenkranz RA, et al. Whole-body hypothermia for neonates with hypoxic–ischemic encephalopathy. *N Engl J Med* 2005;**353**(15):1574–84.

44. Wolberg AS, Meng Z, Monroe D, Hoffman M. A systematic evaluation of the effect of temperature on coagulation enzyme activity and platelet function. *J Trauma* 2004;**56**(6):1221–8.

45. Michelson AD, Barnard M, Khuri S, et al. The effects of aspirin and hypothermia on platelet function in vivo. *Br J Haematol* 1999;**104**(1):64–8.

46. Valeri CR, Feingold H, Cassidy G, et al. Hypothermia-induced reversible platelet dysfunction. *Ann Surg* 1987;**205**(2):175–81.

47. Boutaybi N, Razenberg F, Smits-Wintjens VE, et al. Neonatal thrombocytopenia after perinatal asphyxia treated with hypothermia: a retrospective case control study. *Int J Pediatr* 2014;**2014**:760654.

48. Christensen RD, Sheffield M, Lambert D, Baer V. Effect of therapeutic hypothermia in neonates with hypoxic-ischemic encephalopathy on platelet function. *Neonatology* 2012;**101**(2):91–4.

49. Forman KR, Diab Y, Wong EC, et al. Coagulopathy in newborns with hypoxic ischemic encephalopathy (HIE) treated with therapeutic hypothermia: A retrospective case-control study. *BMC Pediatr* 2014;**14**:277.

50. Shankaran S, Pappas A, Laptook AR, et al. Outcomes of safety and effectiveness in a multicenter randomized, controlled trial of whole-body hypothermia for neonatal hypoxic-ischemic encephalopathy. *Pediatrics* 2008;**122**(4):e791–8.

51. Gluckman PD, Wyatt JS, Azzopardi D, et al. Selective head cooling with mild systemic hypothermia after neonatal encephalopathy: Multicentre randomised trial. *Lancet* 2005;**365**(9460):663–70.

52. Forman KR, Wong E, Gallagher M, et al. Effect of temperature on thromboelastography and implications for clinical use in newborns undergoing therapeutic hypothermia. *Pediatr Res* 2014;**75**(5):663–9.

53. Pakvasa MA, Winkler AM, Hamrick SE, Josephson CD, Patel RM. Observational study of haemostatic dysfunction and bleeding in neonates with hypoxic-ischaemic encephalopathy. *BMJ Open* 2017;**7**(2):e013787.

54. Guida JD, Kunig AM, Leef KH, McKenzie SE, Paul DA. Platelet count and sepsis in very low birth weight neonates: Is there an organism-specific response? *Pediatrics* 2003;**111**(6 Pt 1):1411–15.

55. Manzoni P, Mostert M, Galletto P, et al. Is thrombocytopenia suggestive of organism-specific response in neonatal sepsis? *Pediatr Int* 2009;**51**(2):206–10.

56. Murray NA, Howarth LJ, McCloy MP, Letsky EA, Roberts IAG. Platelet transfusion in the management of severe thrombocytopenia in neonatal intensive care unit patients. *Transfus Med* 2002;**12**(1):35–41.

57. Modanlou HD, Ortiz OB. Thrombocytopenia in neonatal infection. *Clin Pediatr (Phila)* 1981;**20**(6):402–7.

58. Dohner ML, Wiedmeier SE, Stoddard RA, et al. Very high users of platelet transfusions in the neonatal intensive care unit. *Transfusion* 2009;**49** (5):869–72.

59. Brown RE, Rimsza LM, Pastos K, et al. Effects of sepsis on neonatal thrombopoiesis. *Pediatr Res* 2008;**64**(4):399–404.

60. Haselmayer P, Grosse-Hovest L, von Landenberg P, Schild H, Radsak MP. TREM-1 ligand expression on platelets enhances neutrophil activation. *Blood* 2007;**110**(3):1029–35.

61. Semple JW, Italiano JE Jr., Freedman J. Platelets and the immune continuum. *Nat Rev Immunol* 2011;**11**(4):264–74.

62. Andonegui G, Kerfoot SM, McNagny K, et al. Platelets express functional Toll-like receptor-4. *Blood* 2005;**106**(7):2417–23.

63. Clark SR, Ma A, Tavener S, et al. Platelet TLR4 activates neutrophil extracellular traps to ensnare bacteria in septic blood. *Nat Med* 2007;**13**(4):463–9.

64. Kraemer BF, Campbell RA, Schwertz H, et al. Bacteria differentially induce degradation of Bcl-xL, a survival protein, by human platelets. *Blood* 2012;**120**(25):5014–20.

65. Steinberg HN, Anderson J Jr., Lim B, Chatis PA. Cytomegalovirus infection of the BS-1 human stroma cell line: effect on murine hemopoiesis. *Virology* 1993;**196**(2):427–32.

66. Crapnell K, Zanjani ED, Chaudhuri A, et al. In vitro infection of megakaryocytes and their precursors by human cytomegalovirus. *Blood* 2000;**95**(2):487–93.

67. Isomura H, Yoshida M, Namba H, Yamada M. Interaction of human herpesvirus 6 with human CD34 positive cells. *J Med Virol* 2003;**70**(3):444–50.

68. Srivastava A, Bruno E, Briddell R, et al. Parvovirus B19-induced perturbation of human megakaryocytopoiesis in vitro. *Blood* 1990;**76** (10):1997–2004.

69. Forestier F, Tissot JD, Vial Y, Daffos F, Hohlfeld P. Haematological parameters of parvovirus B19 infection in 13 fetuses with hydrops fetalis. *Br J Haematol* 1999;**104**(4):925–7.

70. Abzug MJ. Prognosis for neonates with enterovirus hepatitis and coagulopathy. *Pediatr Infect Dis J* 2001;**20**(8):758–63.

71. Tighe P, Rimsza LM, Christensen RD, Lew J, Sola MC. Severe thrombocytopenia in a neonate with congenital HIV infection. *J Pediatr* 2005;**146** (3):408–13.

72. Hutter JJ Jr., Hathaway WE, Wayne ER. Hematologic abnormalities in severe neonatal necrotizing enterocolitis. *J Pediatr* 1976;**88** (6):1026–31.

73. Muthukumar P, Venkatesh V, Curley A, et al. Severe thrombocytopenia and patterns of bleeding in neonates: Results from a prospective observational study and implications for use of platelet transfusions. *Transfus Med* 2012;**22** (5):338–43.

74. Ververidis M, Kiely EM, Spitz L, et al. The clinical significance of thrombocytopenia in neonates with necrotizing enterocolitis. *J Pediatr Surg* 2001;**36** (5):799–803.

75. Namachivayam K, MohanKumar K, Garg L, Torres BA, Maheshwari A. Neonatal mice with necrotizing enterocolitis-like injury develop thrombocytopenia despite increased megakaryopoiesis. *Pediatr Res* 2017;**81**(5):817–24.

76. Cremer M, Weimann A, Szekessy D, et al. Low immature platelet fraction suggests decreased megakaryopoiesis in neonates with sepsis or necrotizing enterocolitis. *J Perinatol* 2013;**33** (8):622–6.

77. Frost BL, Jilling T, Caplan MS. The importance of pro-inflammatory signaling in neonatal necrotizing enterocolitis. *Semin Perinatol* 2008;**32**(2):100–6.

78. Caplan MS, Hedlund E, Adler L, Lickerman M, Hsueh, W. The platelet-activating factor receptor antagonist WEB 2170 prevents neonatal necrotizing enterocolitis in rats. *J Pediatr Gastroenterol Nutr* 1997;**24** (3):296–301.

79. Markel TA, Crisostomo PR, Wairiuko GM, et al. Cytokines in necrotizing enterocolitis. *Shock* 2006;**25**(4):329–37.

80. Bubel S, Wilhelm D, Entelmann M, Kirchner H, Kluter H. Chemokines in stored platelet concentrates. *Transfusion* 1996;**36**(5):445–9.

81. Kluter H, Bubel S, Kirchner H, Wilhelm D. Febrile and allergic transfusion reactions after the transfusion of white cell-poor platelet preparations. *Transfusion* 1999;**39**(11–12):1179–84.

82. Fujihara M, Ikebuchi K, Wakamoto S, Sekiguchi S. Effects of filtration and gamma radiation on the accumulation of RANTES and transforming growth factor-beta1 in apheresis platelet concentrates during storage. *Transfusion* 1999;**39**(5):498–505.

83. Sellberg F, Berglund E, Ronaghi M, et al. Composition of growth factors and cytokines in lysates obtained from fresh versus stored pathogen-inactivated platelet units. *Transfus Apher Sci* 2016;**55**(3):333–7.

84. Patel RM, Josephson CD, Shenvi N, et al. Platelet transfusions and mortality in necrotizing enterocolitis. *Transfusion* 2019;**59**(3):981–8.

85. Kenton AB, Hegemier S, Smith EO, et al. Platelet transfusions in infants with necrotizing

enterocolitis do not lower mortality but may increase morbidity. *J Perinatol* 2005;**25**(3):173–7.

86. Saxonhouse MA, Manco-Johnson MJ. The evaluation and management of neonatal coagulation disorders. *Semin Perinatol* 2009;**33**(1):52–65.

87. Marks SD, Massicotte MP, Steeleet BT, et al. Neonatal renal venous thrombosis: Clinical outcomes and prevalence of prothrombotic disorders. *J Pediatr* 2005;**146**(6):811–16.

88. Zigman A, Yazbeck S, Emil S, Nguyen L. Renal vein thrombosis: A 10-year review. *J Pediatr Surg* 2000;**35**(11):1540–2.

89. Nowak-Gottl U, Kosch A, Schlegel N. Neonatal thromboembolism. *Semin Thromb Hemost* 2003; **29**(2):227–34.

90. Nowak-Gottl U, von Kries R, Gobel U. Neonatal symptomatic thromboembolism in Germany: Two-year survey. *Arch Dis Child Fetal Neonatal Ed* 1997;**76**(3):F163–7.

91. Goel R, Ness PM, Takemoto CM, et al. Platelet transfusions in platelet consumptive disorders are associated with arterial thrombosis and in-hospital mortality. *Blood* 2015;**125**(9):1470–6.

92. Levi M, de Jonge E, Meijers J. The diagnosis of disseminated intravascular coagulation. *Blood Rev* 2002;**16**(4):217–23.

93. Neame PB, Kelton JG, Walker IR, et al. Thrombocytopenia in septicemia: The role of disseminated intravascular coagulation. *Blood* 1980;**56**(1):88–92.

94. Dairaku M, Sueishi K, Tanaka K. Disseminated intravascular coagulation in newborn infants. Prevalence in autopsies and significance as a cause of death. *Pathol Res Pract* 1982;**174**(1–2):106–15.

95. Arkhangel'skii AV, Masliakova GN. Frequency and morphology of DIC-syndrome in children in early neonatal period [in Russian]. *Arkh Patol* 1996;**58**(5):61–3.

96. Schmidt B, Vegh P, Johnston M, Andrew M, Weitz J. Do coagulation screening tests detect increased generation of thrombin and plasmin in sick newborn infants? *Thromb Haemost* 1993;**69** (5):418–21.

97. Sola-Visner M, Bercovitz RS. Neonatal platelet transfusions and future areas of research. *Transfus Med Rev* 2016;**30**(4):183–8.

98. Veldman A, Fischer D, Nold M, Wong F. Disseminated intravascular coagulation in term and preterm neonates. *Semin Thromb Hemost* 2010;**36**(4):419–28.

99. El Beshlawy A, Alaraby I, Abou Hussein H, et al. Study of protein C protein S and antithrombin III in newborns with sepsis. *Pediatr Crit Care Med* 2010;**11**(1):52–9.

100. Enjolras O, Wassef M, Mazoyer E, et al. Infants with Kasabach–Merritt syndrome do not have "true" hemangiomas. *J Pediatr* 1997;**130** (4):631–40.

101. Phillips WG, Marsden JR. Kasabach–Merritt syndrome exacerbated by platelet transfusion. *J R Soc Med* 1993;**86**(4):231–2.

102. Drolet BA, Trenor CC 3rd, Brandão LR, et al. Consensus-derived practice standards plan for complicated Kaposiform hemangioendothelioma. *J Pediatr* 2013;**163** (1):285–91.

103. Aster RH, Bougie DW. Drug-induced immune thrombocytopenia. *N Engl J Med* 2007;**357** (6):580–7.

104. Spadone D, Clark F, James E, et al. Heparin-induced thrombocytopenia in the newborn. *J Vasc Surg* 1992;**15**(2):306–11; discussion 311–12.

105. Klenner AF, Fusch C, Rakow A, et al. Benefit and risk of heparin for maintaining peripheral venous catheters in neonates: A placebo-controlled trial. *J Pediatr* 2003;**143**(6):741–5.

106. Risch L, Huber AR, Schmugge M. Diagnosis and treatment of heparin-induced thrombocytopenia in neonates and children. *Thromb Res* 2006;**118** (1):123–35.

107. Nguyen TN, Gal P, Ransom JL, Carlos R. Lepirudin use in a neonate with heparin-induced thrombocytopenia. *Ann Pharmacother* 2003;**37** (2):229–33.

108. Del Vecchio A, Sola MC, Theriaque DW, et al. Platelet transfusions in the neonatal intensive care unit: Factorspredicting which patients will require multiple transfusions. *Transfusion* 2001;**41**(6):803–8.

109. Garcia MG, Duenas E, Sola MC, et al. Epidemiologic and outcome studies of patients who received platelet transfusions in the neonatal intensive care unit. *J Perinatol* 2001;**21** (7):415–20.

110. Peck-Radosavljevic M, Wichlas M, Zacherl J, et al. Thrombopoietin induces rapid resolution of thrombocytopenia after orthotopic liver transplantation through increased platelet production. *Blood* 2000;**95**(3):795–801.

111. Rios R, Sangro B, Herrero I, Quiroga J, Prieto J. The role of thrombopoietin in the thrombocytopenia of patients with liver cirrhosis. *Am J Gastroenterol* 2005;**100** (6):1311–16.

112. Aster RH. Pooling of platelets in the spleen: role in the pathogenesis of "hypersplenic" thrombocytopenia. *J Clin Invest* 1966;**45** (5):645–57.

Fetal and Neonatal Alloimmune Thrombocytopenias

W. Beau Mitchell and James B. Bussel

Fetal and neonatal alloimmune thrombocytopenia (AIT) is the most common cause of severe thrombocytopenia in fetuses and neonates [1]. Maternal IgG alloantibodies against paternally derived fetal platelet antigens cross the placenta early in pregnancy and commonly result in severe thrombocytopenia. While the reported incidence varies somewhat with the assigned threshold of thrombocytopenia (50, 100, or 150×10^9/L), in most unselected populations, AIT affects 1 in 1,000 live births. Table 14.1 displays the studies of AIT in unselected populations, systematically screened. In its severe form, AIT has the potential for significant morbidity (including intracranial hemorrhage in utero) and mortality. In milder forms, there are either antibodies with no thrombocytopenia, or mild to moderate thrombocytopenia, that are identified only by a complete blood count obtained for another indication or in a screening study. While there have been extensive efforts made in the diagnosis and characterization of the disease, strategies for early detection and intervention remain controversial.

Pathogenesis

There are three requisite components of the pathogenesis of AIT. First, there must be an incompatibility between maternal and fetal "platelet-specific" antigens, which are inherited from the father. The second requirement, alloimmunization, is a maternal humoral immune response specific to these "foreign" fetal platelet antigens. Finally, maternal antiplatelet IgG alloantibodies must cross the placenta, bind to fetal platelet antigens, and cause fetal platelet destruction with resultant thrombocytopenia. Recent work suggests that antibodies to fetal platelets may also

Table 14.1 Incidence of neonatal thrombocytopenia

Population and number screened	Incidence of AIT	Reference
Pregnant women		
24,417	1 in 1,285 pregnancies	[17]
100,448	1 in 1,182 pregnancies	[59]
Neonates		
15,932	1 in 5,000 newborns*	[1]
5,632	1 in 1,000 newborns	[45]
9,142	1 in 1,800 newborns**	[16]
8,388	1 in 1,700 newborns	[58]
4,489	1 in 1,200 newborns	[47]
24,101	1 in 2,400 newborns**	[19]
5,632	1 in 1,000 newborns	[31]

Notes: Unless otherwise specified, neonatal thrombocytopenia is defined as a cord blood platelet count less than 150×10^9/L

* Platelet count $<50 \times 10^9$/L

** Platelet count $<100 \times 10^9$/L

react with fetal megakaryocytes making an important contribution to fetal thrombocytopenia. The term alloimmunization, therefore, implies that there is a parental antigen incompatibility, and that maternal antibodies are produced and are specific to the paternally inherited (and foreign to the mother) fetal platelet antigen. The predictability of this process, and its ability to cause fetal or neonatal thrombocytopenia, is well characterized serologically but perplexing in a number of areas, and warrants careful discussion.

Human Platelet-Specific Antigens

Platelets share several antigen systems with other cell types, including the HLA class I antigens, and the

Neonatal Hematology, Pathogenesis, Diagnosis, and Management of Hematologic Problems, 3rd edition, ed. Pedro A. de Alarcón, Eric J. Werner, Robert D. Christensen, and Martha C. Sola-Visner. Published by Cambridge University Press.
© Cambridge University Press 2021.

ABO blood group antigens [2, 3]. However, these two antigen systems have never been unequivocally implicated in AIT. The existence of AIT secondary to an HLA antigen mismatch remains controversial, although there are anecdotal reports purporting to illustrate such cases. Rather, AIT is caused by antibodies to platelet-specific antigens, which represent epitopes of the platelet surface glycoproteins. Currently there are at least 33 human platelet-specific antigens listed by the Working Party on Platelet Serology of the International Society of Blood Transfusion (ISBT), each with a different serologic frequency and ethnic distribution [2, 4–6]. In 1990, the ISBT Working Party on Platelet Serology formulated nomenclature for the human platelet antigen system, as an attempt to standardize an otherwise confusing system of antigen names and descriptions. Platelet-specific antigens are designated HPA for human platelet antigen. They are numbered in the order of their original description, and the alleles labeled alphabetically in the order of their serologic frequency [2, 4, 7]. DNA sequencing has permitted the genotyping of the specific amino acid changes associated with each allele. This genotyping system provides an additional nomenclature for describing human platelet-specific antigens. Each HPA type is biallelic, and autosomal co-dominant, differing in only one amino acid. It is important to note that there is overlap of certain alleles, as discussed by Newman [8], and that the naming of a certain allele implies an understanding of the molecular identity of that glycoprotein although knowledge of the full sequence is typically lacking. Table 14.2 contains the HPA type, the glycoprotein on which it is located, the previous antigen designations, the associated amino acid changes for each allele, and the frequency of each antigen in selected populations. This information is maintained and updated in an internet database available online at www.ebi.ac.uk/ipd/hpa/table1.html [9,10].

As discussed above, AIT has been reported after alloimmunization to numerous human platelet antigens (see Tables 14.3 and 14.4). In almost all large series, HPA1a incompatibility is not only the most common incompatibility resulting in AIT [11–19], but also an incompatibility that results in the most severe fetal and neonatal thrombocytopenia. Other severe incompatibilities result from HPA 3a and b incompatibility as well as that of HPA-9b. Studies suggest that HPA-5b incompatibility may be nearly as common as HPA-1a incompatibility, but severe

thrombocytopenia after HPA-5b alloimmunization is rare [20–22]. HPA-4 incompatibility, as well as those of HPA-6b and HPA-21b, are more common in East and South Asian populations. Of note, the initial description of a new human platelet antigen is frequently prompted by a severely affected patient with significant morbidity. Therefore, most non-HPA-1a incompatibilities have severe index cases, but incidences appear to be very low. Despite numerous reports of new, and potentially severe or frequent incompatibilities, it is clear that HPA-1a incompatibility remains by far the most common cause of severe AIT in Caucasian populations. HPA-9b and HPA-3a and 3b are the next most common severe causes of neonatal alloimmune thrombocytopenia (NAIT).

Alloimmunization

Fetal platelet antigens may be expressed as early as 16 weeks' gestation [23], and alloantibody formation with fetal platelet destruction may occur as early as 16 to 20 weeks of gestation [24, 25]. Alloimmunization is reported in up to 50% of severely thrombocytopenic newborns. This may be due in part to beta 3 integrin (GPIIIa) expression on syncytiotrophoblasts, although this has not been confirmed [26]. Antibodies have not been detected in primiparous women prior to 17 weeks' gestation [17]. In 46 sensitized HPA-1a negative women, Williamson et.al. reported that alloantibodies were detected before the 20th week of gestation in 59%, between 21 and 34 weeks in 17%, between 33 weeks and term in 6.5%, and on postnatal testing only in 6.5% [17].

Van Loghem et al. initially reported that 97% of North American and European/white express HPA-1a [27]. The Hardy–Weinberg law predicts the allelic frequency to be 0.83 for HPA-1a and 0.17 for HPA-1b. Therefore, in populations of northern European descent, the genotypic distribution is calculated to be 68.9% homozygosity for HPA-1a, 2.9% homozygosity for HPA-1b, and 28.2% heterozygosity (HPA-1a/HPA-1b) [28, 29]. The frequency of the HPA-1b genotype has been confirmed in several large population studies [17, 18, 30, 31]. Both the predicted and actual frequency of mothers at risk for HPA-1a incompatibility, by virtue of being homozygous for HPA-1b, is 2%–3%. The HPA-1b homozygous mother will be susceptible to alloimmunization in all cases if her

Table 14.2 Human platelet antigen nomenclature and frequency

HPA name	Other names	Glycoprotein	DNA allele (amino acid change)	Gene frequency (Caucasian)	Serologic frequency	
					White	Japanese
HPA-1a	Zw^a, PL^{A}1	GPIIIa	Leu$_{33}$	0.85	97.90%	99.90%
HPA-1b	Zw^b, PL^{A}2	GPIIIa	Pro$_{33}$	0.15	26.50%	3.70%
HPA-2a	Ko^b	GPIb	Thr$_{145}$	0.93	99.30%	NT*
HPA-2b	Ko^a, Sib^a	GPIb	Met$_{145}$	0.07	14.60%	35.40%
HPA-3a	Bak^a, Luk^a	GPIIb	Ile$_{843}$	0.61	87.70%	78.90%
HPA-3b	Bak^b	GPIIb	Ser$_{843}$	0.39	64.10%	NT
HPA-4a	Pen^a, Yuk^b	GPIIIa	Arg$_{143}$	1.00	99.90%	99.90%
HPA-4b	Pen^b, Yuk^a	GPIIIa	Gln$_{143}$	<0.01	0.20%	1.70%
HPA-5a	Br^b, Zav^b	GPIa	Glu$_{505}$	0.89	99.20%	NT
HPA-5b	Br^a, Zav^a, Hc^a	GPIa	Lys$_{505}$	0.11	20.60%	NT
HPA-6bw**	Ca^a, Tu^a	GPIIIa	Arg489Gln	0.85		
HPA-7bw	Mo^a	GPIIIa	Pro407Ala	0.85	<1	
HPA-8bw	Sr^a	GPIIIa	Arg636Cys	0.85		
HPA-9bw	Max^a	GPIIb	Met$_{837}$Val			
HPA-10bw	La^a	GPIIIb	Gln$_{62}$Arg			
HPA-11bw	Gro^a	GPIIIa	His$_{633}$Arg			
HPA-12bw	Iy^a	GPIb	Glu$_{15}$Gly			
HPA-13bw	Sit^a	Gpla	Met$_{799}$Thr			
HPA14bw	Oe^a	GPIIIa	Lys611del			
HPA-15a	Gov^b	CD109	Ser682	0.5		
HPA-15b	Gov^a	CD109	Tyr682	0.5		
HPA-16bw	Duv^a	GPIIIa	ThrT140Ile			
HPA-17bw	Va^a	GPIIb/IIIa	Thr195Met			
HPA-18bw	Cab^a	GPIa	Gln716His			
HPA-19bw	Sta	GPIIIa	Lys137Gln			
HPA-20bw	Kno	GPIIb	Thr619Met			
HPA-21bw	Nos	GPIIIa	Glu628Lys			
HPA-22bw	Sey	GPIIb	Lys164Thr			
HPA-23bw	Hug	GPIIIa	Arg622Trp			
HPA-24bw	Cab2^{a+}	GPIIb	Ser472Asn			
HPA-25bw	Swi^a	GPIa	Thr1087Met			
HPA-26bw	Sec^a	GPIIIa	Lys580Asn			
HPA-27bw	Cab3^{a+}	GPIIb	Leu841Met			
HPA-28bw	War	GPIIb	Val740Leu			
HPA-29bw	Kha^b	GPIIIa	Thr7Met			

Notes: *NT = Not Tested

** "w" indicates antigens for which an alloantibody against only one allele is identified

Table 14.3 Clinically significant AIT

Number of patients	Entry criteria	Bleeding symptoms	Antigen incompatibility	Reference
88	Thrombocytopenic* infants with AIT	Petechiae (90%) Hematomas (66%) Melena (28%) Intracranial hemorrhage (14%) Hemoptysis (8%) Hematuria (7%) Retinal extravasations (7%) Hematemesis (2%) Death (1%)** Platelet count <30 × 10⁹/L (95%)	HPA-1a	[12]
24	Infants with AIT	Petechiae (58%) Intracranial hemorrhage (21%) 1 patient died as a result of an ICH Petechiae, purpura (83%)	HPA-1a	[15]
46	Thrombocytopenic infants with AIT	Visceral bleeding (15%) Intracranial Hemorrhage (11%) Platelet count <50 × 10⁹/L (87%)	HPA-1a, HPA-1b, and HPA-5b	[14]

Notes:
* Thrombocytopenia defined as a platelet count less than 100 x 10⁹/L
** Died at 6 months of age from complications of the ICH

Table 14.4 Less common antigen incompatibilities in AIT

HPA type	Reference	Patients reported	Platelet nadir (× 10⁹ cells/L)	Hemorrhagic sequelae	Maternal HLA type
HPA-1b	43, 146–150	6 total	10–13 duration up to 6 days	Petechiae (2 patients) Schizencephaly (1 patient) Prolonged thrombocytopenia (1 patient)	No consistent association
HPA-2b	47	3*	Mild	None	
HPA-3a	80, 151	1 14	13	Purpura, Death from ICH** ICH (2 patients)	None reported
HPA-3b	47	4*	Mild <20	None	
HPA-4b	77	2 (sibs)	6–12	Petechiae (2 patients) Ecchymoses (2 patients) Scalp Hematoma (1 patient) In utero ICH (2 patients)	No consistent association
HPA-5b	12, 13, 16, 20, 21, 45, 47, 58, 152	39 total	<10 (4 patients) 10–30 (13 patients) >30 (22 patients)	No symptoms (59%) Purpura or hematoma (18%) Visceral hemorrhage (15%) ICH (8%) Death due to ICH (1 patient)	Associated with HLA-DR6
HPA-6b	45, 47, 153, 154	4 total		Mild	Associated with maternal HLA DRB*1501 DQA1*0102 DQB1*0602

Notes: * AIT suspected due to antigen incompatibility and thrombocytopenia, but there was no antibody detected.
**ICH = intracranial hemorrhage

partner is homozygous for HPA-1a (68.9%), or in half the offspring of a heterozygous partner (14.1%). Based on these gene frequencies, alloimmune thrombocytopenia as a result of HPA-1a incompatibility may develop in 1 of 42 pregnancies[29]. The actual incidence, as stated above, is 1 in 1,000 to 1 in 2,000. In fact, several prospective studies have shown that only 4%–14% of mothers homozygous for HPA-1b will produce anti-HPA-1a antibodies [11, 17, 31, 32].

The discrepancy between the expected and actual incidence of AIT can be explained, at least in part, by the efficiency of antigen presentation by different MHC subtypes. In 1981, Reznikoff-Etievant et al. reported that the immune response to HPA-1a is associated with the maternal HLA type B8DR3 [33].[a] Subsequently, several authors confirmed a strong association between the production of anti-HPA-1a antibodies and the HLADR3 locus [32, 34–39]. de Waal et al. later linked it to the supertypic HLA DRB3*0101 allele [40].

The HLA DRB3*0101 protein has a binding affinity for a peptide containing the Leu33 substitution on the integrin β3 (HPA-1a), but not for the corresponding peptide containing Pro33 (HPA-1b), demonstrating the importance of recognition of fetal peptides expressed on the β3 integrin by the maternal class II MHC proteins for antigen presentation [41, 42]. This genetic maternal restriction on the immune response to foreign fetal antigens accounts, in large part, for the relatively low number of HPA-1a negative mothers who develop alloantibodies against their HPA-1a positive fetus. The other not-well- clarified factor is maternal exposure to fetal platelets.

Williamson et al. studied HPA type, antibody production, and maternal HLA type in more than 24,000 consecutive pregnancies in Cambridge and East Anglia, England [17]. Among the 2.5% of women homozygous for HPA-1b, anti-HPA-1a antibodies were detected in 12%. All but one of the antibody producers was HLA DRB3*0101 positive, while the overall frequency of the allele was 31.9%. The presence of the HLA DRB3*0101 phenotype did not predict alloimmunization (positive predictive value of 35%), but the absence of the HLA DRB3*0101 precluded alloimmunization with very few exceptions (negative predictive value 99.6%). Finally, only a minority of antibody-formers will have severely thrombocytopenic fetuses/newborns.

Although not as well studied, alloantibody formation in cases of HPA-5b incompatibility has been associated with maternal HLA DRw6 positivity [20, 21, 43]. Other HPA incompatibilities resulting in alloimmunization may have similar HLA associations [44], but the low incidence of AIT due to these antigens makes study difficult.

Alloantibody Mediated Thrombocytopenia

Maternal alloimmunization to fetal platelet antigens is most likely necessary and usually, but not always, sufficient to induce immune thrombocytopenia in the fetus or newborn. There are a number of reported cases of high titer maternal antiplatelet alloantibodies in infants with normal platelet counts [17, 21, 30, 31, 45]. Maternal alloimmunization without neonatal thrombocytopenia may be as high as 32% [45]. In addition to maternal HLA MHC class II modulation of alloimmunization, there appears to be another regulatory step in AIT. The process of antibody-mediated platelet destruction may be inhibited by unknown factors specific to certain maternal–fetal pairs. One possibility is a so-called "blocking" antibody that might be anti-HLA; this has not been confirmed. Such an antibody could be directed against FcγR and thus block platelet destruction.

Conversely, there are reports of maternal–fetal HPA incompatibility with neonatal thrombocytopenia (presumed AIT), with no detectable maternal alloantibody [12, 16, 19, 45–47]. Newer techniques of antibody measurement have substantially improved detection but not entirely resolved this issue[48].

Careful and extensive study of AIT is largely limited to anti-HPA-1a antibodies as discussed above. The role of alloantibodies to other fetal platelet antigens is less clear. There are reports of suspected AIT with anti-HLA antibodies [12, 49–51, 52–54], anti-blood group antibodies [12, 55, 56], and antiplatelet–glycoprotein-specific

---

[a] The original description was of increased incidence of HLA type B8 in women producing anti-HPA-1a antibody. HLA B8 is in linkage disequilibrium with HLA DR3 [29].

antibodies [47, 57]. Of these less common causes of AIT, anti-HLA antibodies are perhaps the most considered but the least certain. King et. al. found no significant relationship between the formation of anti-HLA antibodies and neonatal thrombocytopenia [51]. It is possible that the presence of anti-HLA antibodies in infants with thrombocytopenia is coincidental, as anti-HLA antibodies will be absorbed by HLA antigens in the placenta or on WBCs, thus minimizing their effect on fetal platelets. At best the role of anti-HLA alloantibodies is unclear but, when present, they appear to have little effect on neonatal platelet counts [50, 51]. It is, of course, impossible to exclude that they might have a thrombocytopenic effect in individual cases. Resolution could be achieved by collecting sufficient platelets from cord blood to identify specificity of the antibodies in the eluate, but this technically would require a tour de force.

Clearly, the details of the genetic and immunologic controls governing the process of alloimmunization and its outcome have yet to be completely described. Our ability to predict the occurrence of alloimmunization in cases of fetomaternal platelet antigen incompatibility is limited, as is our ability to predict the presence and severity of thrombocytopenia after alloimmunization occurs.

Clinical Presentation

For newborns with unsuspected AIT, evaluation will commonly be initiated by the pediatrician or neonatologist after perinatal identification of petechiae or purpura, or by the incidental finding of thrombocytopenia on a complete blood count obtained for a different indication, e.g., suspected infection. When defined as either a cord blood or neonatal platelet count of $<100-150 \times 10^9/L$, neonatal thrombocytopenia is reported in 0.5%–0.9% of newborns, with severe thrombocytopenia (platelet count less than $50 \times 10^9/L$) in 0.14%–0.24% [1, 19, 31, 45, 47, 58] (See Table 14.1). Immune-mediated thrombocytopenia may account for as much as 30% of neonatal thrombocytopenias, occurring in 0.3% of all newborns [45]. A small additional subset of asymptomatic patients will be identified because of a sibling with AIT.

The frequency of hemorrhagic symptoms in AIT is likely overestimated in clinical studies not based on population screening, considering that a substantial proportion of patients with AIT

identified by screening will not have severe thrombocytopenia and go undetected [17, 59]. For those patients with clinically significant disease, or with neonatal platelet counts less than $50 \times 10^9/L$, the incidence of minor hemorrhagic diatheses (petechiae, ecchymoses, or hematomas) is as high as 80% [12, 15, 19]. The most frequent bleeding symptoms for AIT with clinically significant disease are listed in Tables 14.3 and 14.4.

AIT identified through routine screening is more likely to follow a benign course. In two large maternal screening studies of AIT, 65% of infants with persistent in utero exposure to maternal anti-HPA-1a alloantibodies had mild or no thrombocytopenia [17, 59]. While petechiae and ecchymoses are important markers of clinically significant disease, they occur in a minority of screened patients with AIT. On the other hand, a family history of fetal and neonatal AIT (FNAIT) without perinatal hemorrhagic symptoms should not prevent the consideration of hemorrhagic AIT in subsequent pregnancies. Additionally, some thrombocytopenic infants with proven AIT will have other perinatal problems (e.g. infection, poor feeding, low birth weight, cardiac problems, or respiratory problems), which may confuse the etiology of the thrombocytopenia [16, 60].

Neonatal platelet counts can vary from normal to less than $10 \times 10^9/L$. When looking at all infants with AIT, as many as 35% may have platelet counts less than $50 \times 10^9/L$ [17]. However, in series of clinically affected AIT cases identified because of bleeding symptoms, 90% will have platelet counts $<50 \times 10^9/L$ and 50% with have counts $<20 \times 10^9/L$. While this represents a minority of all cases of AIT, when present and when identified clinically rather than by screening, thrombocytopenia in AIT is usually severe [12, 16, 17]. In fact, AIT is the most common cause of severe thrombocytopenia and intracranial hemorrhage in term newborns in all studies to date [1, 16, 19].

Intracranial Hemorrhage

The mortality rate with AIT has been reported as high as 15%, but may be less even in clinically recognized cases. Almost all deaths are associated with intracranial hemorrhage (ICH) [12, 30]. ICH occurs in 10%–20% of affected neonates [12, 30, 61]. In a series of almost 50,000 unselected term neonates, the incidence of ICH was 1 in 1,500 live births. Twenty-five percent occurred in infants with AIT, making it the most common cause of severe ICH in term newborns [62, 63]. Intraventricular hemorrhages are most common in neonates, especially premature ones, but unifocal, multifocal, and large parenchymal hemorrhages are more commonly reported in AIT [12, 64–67]. The vascular distribution of ICH in alloimmune thrombocytopenia may be expected from the fact that normal hemostasis is maintained, in part, through interaction between platelets and the vascular endothelium. It is possible that glycoprotein-bound antiplatelet antibodies interfere with the ability of platelets to support the vascular endothelium [68]. It is also possible that minimal trauma can lead to devastating vascular hemorrhage in the developing thrombocytopenic fetus or neonate. Platelets also support normal angiogenesis, and defective angiogenesis leading to intracranial hemorrhage has been demonstrated in an animal model of anti-HPA-1a antibodies in NAIT [69].

More than 50% of all reported intracranial hemorrhages in AIT will occur antenatally [12, 30, 70]. Severe thrombocytopenia (platelet count <20 × 10^9/L) was present at the time of initial fetal sampling by 24 weeks of gestation in 50% of affected fetuses; thrombocytopenia has been reported as early as 13 to 16 weeks' gestation [13, 24, 25, 71]. In utero hemorrhages may present at any point after 18 weeks of gestation or in the newborn period, presenting with fetal distress or demise [72, 73], fetal or neonatal hydrocephalus [12, 73, 74], encephalomalacia, intracranial cysts [64, 65, 75], an abnormal neurological exam, or poor feeding [15, 62, 70, 75, 76]. ICH has been reported in association with almost all antigen incompatibilities [77, 78], but it is most commonly associated with HPA-1a incompatibility [12, 15, 70].

In vitro binding of autoantibodies to GPIIb/IIIa may rarely result in an acquired disorder in platelet function [68]. In patients homozygous for HPA-1a, alloantibodies to HPA-1a will completely eliminate platelet aggregation to all platelet agonists except ristocetin, but the effect is much less in heterozygous HPA-1a expression (as in all fetuses with AIT). The pathophysiology mediating this effect is not entirely clear. Glycoprotein IIb/IIIa is the most abundant glycoprotein on the platelet surface, and it is the site of fibrinogen binding. However, antibodies to HPA-1a do not appear to bind near enough to the fibrinogen-binding site to cause a steric hindrance [79]. The vascular distribution of some in utero hemorrhages has led to additional speculation about the possible role of antibodies to endothelial GPIIIa in the pathogenesis of intracranial hemorrhages [69]. However, if there is a seemingly equivalent rate of ICH in HPA-3b (GPIIb) incompatibility, this suggests that this may not be a prominent factor since GPIIb is not expressed on endothelial cells [80]. In summary, platelet counts less than 20 × 10^9/L in AIT are permissive but not sufficient for ICH. Anti HPA-1a antibodies do not likely cause substantial platelet dysfunction in the HPA-1a heterozygous fetus. However, anti-HPA-1a antibodies may negatively affect angiogenesis and contribute to ICH.

Predictors of Disease

A goal of recent screening protocols has been to define prognostic factors that may identify those patients at risk for ICH [17, 18, 81, 82]. As discussed earlier, the presence of maternal alloantibody does not predict thrombocytopenia. However, studies have suggested that high (greater than 1:32) third trimester maternal antibody titers [17, 18], and high titers of the IgG3 subclass [82], may predict severe thrombocytopenia. For HPA-5b incompatibilities, neither antibody titer nor subclass appears to predict disease [22].

More than 80% of subsequent siblings of AIT patients will be affected. Mildly affected or undiagnosed first-born children may have severely affected siblings. Initial fetal platelet counts of less than 20 × 10^9/L are reported in 50% of siblings of affected children. Forty-five percent of second siblings may have platelet counts of less than 20 × 10^9/L by 24 weeks' gestation. However, the only significant predictor of severe disease in subsequent affected siblings is antenatal ICH in the previous sibling [63, 71]. Recent studies have focused on the predictive value of HLA, e.g., combinations of DRB30101 and specific DRB4 alleles, but this is still preliminary. Other approaches have been to study the association of anti-HPA-1a antibody effect on in vitro megakaryocytopoiesis and neonatal platelet counts, and the role of anti-HPA-1a antibody fucosylation in induction of ICH.

Diagnosis

The diagnosis of AIT in a thrombocytopenic infant or fetus requires several laboratory observations.

There must be HPA incompatibility between mother and child (usually defined via paternal typing). Although not always identifiable, even with the most sensitive techniques, a firm diagnosis of AIT requires the identification of maternal antiplatelet alloantibodies. These antibodies should bind to paternal, but not maternal platelets, and they should be specific to the antigen incompatibility in question, including specificity for the glycoprotein on which the incompatible epitope is located.

Antigen Testing

Few facilities can do both DNA-based and serologic testing for the complete range of the most frequently encountered HPA antigens. With the development of oligonucleotide probes and the refinement of PCR techniques, it is possible to obtain platelet antigen typing on amniocytes and fetal leukocytes [83–85]. Techniques are also now available for platelet antigen genotyping from dried blood spots on cards to aide in rapid perinatal diagnosis [86]. Currently, free fetal DNA in the maternal circulation can be identified and HPA-1a/b genotype determined from maternal blood alone.

Several ELISA-based [87, 88] and fluorescence-based [89] techniques have been developed for rapid antigen typing on large numbers of samples. ELISA-based kits are also available to screen for common HPA antigens, and to allow accurate testing of the common antigens at smaller centers [88].

Alloantibody Testing

Early antibody testing was performed with the platelet suspension immunofluorescent test (PSIFT). The PSIFT technique detects antiplatelet antibodies bound to the surface of platelets, but is not specific for anti-HPA alloantibodies [90, 91]. In 1987, Kiefel et al. reported accurate alloantibody detection with an enzyme immunoassay, the monoclonal antibody immobilization of platelet glycoprotein assay (MAIPA) [92]. This technique, and subsequent refinements, now allows for the identification and quantification of glycoprotein-specific alloantibodies [92–94]. MAIPA can be both utilized during pregnancy to monitor antibody levels, and possibly adapted for large scale screening programs [95]. The MACE is a similar technique. Other techniques using surface plasmon resonance and expressing specific antigens on fibroblasts show promise for large scale screening programs [5, 96, 97].

Genotyping

DNA-based typing is now widely used to perform antigen typing [98]. One method uses polymerase chain reaction (PCR) to amplify genomic DNA encoding specific antigens using allele-specific primers, followed by electrophoresis and band visualization. Another method relies on fluorescent, allele-specific DNA probes that are quenched in solution but become fluorescent when hybridized to DNA from patient samples.

Who to Test

When evaluating the thrombocytopenic newborn, it is important to carefully consider the diagnosis of AIT; if nothing else because of the high rate of ICH with which it is associated and the high recurrence rate. AIT is the most common diagnosis resulting in severe neonatal thrombocytopenia, is likely to result in more severe thrombocytopenia in the mother's next pregnancy, and can also affect her female siblings and cousins. We believe that all infants with platelet counts less than 50×10^9/L should be tested for AIT and managed accordingly. Even in patients with mild thrombocytopenia, it is important to identify those with AIT, because of the implication for subsequent offspring, who may be more severely affected [99]. In general, any thrombocytopenic infant, even with a platelet count greater than 50×10^9/L, without evidence of asphyxia or sepsis, is deserving of evaluation. A high index of suspicion must be maintained even in the setting of other medical problems, as up to 30%, infants with AIT will also have other medical problems that confuse the diagnosis of AIT. Therefore, the diagnosis of other newborn diseases, regardless of whether or not they are independent causes of thrombocytopenia, should not prevent an evaluation for AIT. This is especially true with severe thrombocytopenia or ICH, since both are strongly associated with AIT. In premature infants, where an ICH is likely due to an underdeveloped germinal matrix, AIT should be considered if the ICH is associated with thrombocytopenia, or if there is a parenchymal bleed. Finally, any familial or transient neonatal thrombocytopenia should also be evaluated [99, 100].

Screening Programs

There is no consensus on obtaining routine neonatal platelet counts, or whether to perform prenatal maternal platelet antigen typing. While numerous series have performed neonatal and maternal screening, only Norway currently routinely screens all pregnancies for AIT. Alloimmune thrombocytopenia is a significant cause of prenatal and perinatal morbidity and mortality, the pathogenesis is relatively well understood, and early intervention can prevent adverse outcomes. Unfortunately, we lack specific biological markers of severe disease to justify treating if no family history is available (previous affected fetus), either at all or more aggressively knowing that the fetus will be severely affected.

The financial and technical burden of screening all mothers for HPA-1a1b would be difficult to deal with unless prevention was possible. Testing would have to be based on the ethnic distribution of the most likely antigen incompatibility, and the severity of the associated thrombocytopenia. For European/white populations this would require testing for the HPA-1a antigen. Such a program would miss incompatibilities among the less common human platelet antigens, some of which can lead to severe disease, but would not likely miss many cases of neonatal thrombocytopenia.

If a screening program were to identify a woman with the HPA-1b antigen, what would be the next step to determine the need for treatment? Testing for both anti-HPA-1a antibody and HLA-typing for DRB*30101 has been suggested. High anti-HPA-1a antibody titers may predict significant thrombocytopenia and certain studies suggest that low level or absent antibody may be predictive of less severe thrombocytopenia. In most cases of AIT, alloimmunization is eventually detected but it may require multiple antibody assays throughout the pregnancy and postnatal period. Additionally, there are at least three reported cases (including those in unpublished communications) of alloimmunization to HPA-1a in mothers that do not have the HLA DRB*30101 subtype, although these are rare. A recent publication suggests that they may be more common than we thought, but that they are milder than those in HPA-1b1b mothers with the DRB3 haplotype.

Screening programs have the potential to prevent the devastating or fatal hemorrhagic complications of AIT. However, there is almost no circumstance in which fetal blood samplings would be justified from a screening program. If we assume that there is a human-platelet antigen incompatibility in 1 in 40 pregnancies, and that 2% of these will have detectable alloimmunization [17, 30–32], then 1 in 2,000 pregnancies will result in alloimmunization. Only 35% of infants exposed to antiplatelet alloantibodies will develop moderate to severe thrombocytopenia [17], and only 10%–20% of these neonates with suffer an intracranial haemorrhage [12, 15, 61].

Two large, multicentered studies completed in northern Europe have explored these issues [59, 101]. Both studies exclusively screened for anti-HPA-1a antibodies, and neither study used fetal blood sampling or antenatal treatment. In both studies the majority of maternal–fetal pairs with anti-HPA-1a antibodies did not result in AIT. The Norway study used preterm caesarian-section delivery to reduce the risk of ICH, while the United Kingdom study did not report any intervention. In the United Kingdom study it was estimated that the cost to diagnose one case of AIT would be US$ 99,000, while preventing one episode of ICH would cost US$ 1.9 million.

Management

The goal of diagnosing and treating AIT is to prevent ICH, either antenatal or perinatal, and prevent the severe morbidity or mortality associated with ICH in this period. For those patients diagnosed in the neonatal period, early diagnosis and intervention may prevent or at least stabilize ICH [70]. Some cases will be diagnosed antenatally due to diagnosis of AIT in a first degree relative, or due to an in-utero ICH diagnosed on screening ultrasound. Effective management of the affected fetus can dramatically reduce the risk of ICH in those with history of previously affected pregnancies. While the rate of ICH may be small, its consequences may be devastating and thus aggressive evaluation and treatment measures are warranted.

Antenatal Management

Several factors are important to consider when developing antenatal therapy plans for fetuses suspected of having AIT. The natural history of fetal NAIT must be considered, with the potential for severe thrombocytopenia, and the increasing risk of ICH with declining platelet counts. The efficacy, morbidity, and mortality associated with the available therapies and procedures must also be considered. First-born children are rarely diagnosed before birth, unless part of a maternal antigen typing program. Thus, the most experience (and data) on management of AIT is derived from treatment of siblings of previously affected fetuses.

Severity of Disease

There are no reliable predictors of severe fetal thrombocytopenia other than an antenatal ICH in an older sibling. However, subsequent affected infants are likely to have at least as severe thrombocytopenia as their older siblings. In one study, up to 40% of pre-treatment fetal platelet counts were lower than the nadir of the previously affected infant. When measured, fetal platelet counts were noted to decrease, sometimes rapidly, even if initially adequate. Conversely, there have been no reported cases of spontaneous fetal platelet count increases in AIT. If fetal thrombocytopenia in previous pregnancies was not severe, the outcome in subsequent pregnancies is impossible to predict.

ICH

Neonatal and fetal ICH is very rare at platelet counts greater than $20 \times 10^9/L$. However, the risk of ICH at a given platelet count after vaginal birth and after cesarean section has not been studied in randomized controlled trials in AIT. Several early reports of ICH in thrombocytopenic infants after vaginal delivery prompted authors to advocate for scheduled "elective" cesarean section in severely thrombocytopenic infants [102, 103]. However, it is not clear if vaginal delivery is an independent risk factor for ICH in thrombocytopenic neonates since most ICHs occur antepartum [104, 105]. The safety of cesarean section vs. vaginal delivery in AIT has also not been well studied. Although it may seem that cesarean section would be safer, antenatal therapy may increase the fetal platelet count to greater than $50 \times 10^9/L$, making vaginal birth an option.

Therapeutic Procedures

In the past, monitoring the efficacy of therapeutic interventions in fetuses with AIT required fetal blood sampling using cordocentesis. There is a reported fetal loss rate of 0.2% to 7.2%, depending on the technique (free-hand technique, fixed-needle technique, or combined technique), operator experience, and underlying fetal disease [82, 106–109]. In otherwise healthy but thrombocytopenic fetuses, the risk of fetal loss is approximately 1%–6%[110, 111]. The data is mixed on whether fetal loss is related to fetal platelet count, with some authors finding a correlation between low fetal platelet counts and fetal demise[111], and others not [82]; our data is in favor of a correlation. Therefore transfusion of maternal or other matched antigen negative platelets was the standard of care, to be given in conjunction with fetal blood sampling even prior to availability of the fetal platelet count. There is no longer an expectation that fetal sampling should be a routine part of care except possibly very late in pregnancy to decide when and how to deliver.

Efficacy of Selected Therapies

Intrauterine Platelet Transfusions

Shortly following the description of the cordocentesis procedure, Daffos et al. described the use of washed maternal platelets injected into the umbilical vein of an infant with AIT [112]. Subsequent publications reported the efficacy of prophylactic HPA-1a negative platelet transfusions in maintaining fetal platelet counts and avoiding hemorrhagic complications [25, 113–115]. Unfortunately, transfused platelets have a short half-life and repeat transfusions are required every 5 to 7 days to maintain an adequate platelet count ($>20 \times 10^9/\mu l$) in a fetus with severe AIT. Repeated weekly fetal blood samplings for the purpose of platelet transfusions carry a greatly increased risk of fetal loss or distress and therefore this approach has almost entirely been abandoned.

Intravenous Immunoglobulin and Corticosteroids

While corticosteroids have shown limited benefit as single agents in AIT [116], with some efficacy as primary treatment in mildly affected cases, they are used primarily as adjunctive treatment with intravenous immunoglobulin (IVIG). The use of maternally administered intravenous immunoglobulin has had the greatest impact on restoration of adequate fetal platelet counts and prevention of ICH [117–121]. The mechanism of effect of IVIG is unclear, although IVIG is thought to most likely work by reducing the level of maternal anti-HPA-1a antibodies and especially by competitively inhibiting the binding of alloantibodies to the F_cRn receptor [120, 122]. IVIG administered at sufficient doses will block F_cRn receptors in the placenta, preventing endocytotic uptake of alloantibodies [123]; whether IVIG also affects the fetal mononuclear-phagocytic system, preventing alloantibody-mediated platelet destruction, is unknown [120, 122]. However, the same mechanism in mothers may lower the anti-HPA-1a titer in the maternal circulation. The former mechanism is indirectly supported by the observation that the levels of IgG in the maternal circulation after infusion of 1 gm/kg of IVIG are in the range that was shown to competitively inhibit the transport of 90% of anti-D in a placental perfusion model [121, 123]. Direct infusion of IVIG into the fetal circulation [124, 125] and peritoneum [25] has been reported without great success. Given the efficiency of maternal IVIG transfer across the placenta, and the theoretical benefit of F_cRn receptor blockade in the placenta, it is most likely unnecessary to directly infuse IVIG into the fetus. However, data on this approach are limited. Recent data suggest that IVIG blockade of antibody transfer to the fetus may have its greatest impact in the protection of fetal megakaryocytes [126].

In 15 of the first 18 maternal–fetal pairs treated with maternally administered IVIG (1 gram/kg weekly), there was a substantial increase in fetal platelet counts. None of the fetuses or newborns suffered an ICH, even when an antenatal ICH was reported in an older sibling. Almost all of the infants had higher birth platelet counts than did their older siblings. However, in these first cases when IVIG was used in combination with 3 to 5 mg/kg per day of dexamethasone, 4 of 5 patients developed oligohydramnios [118, 120]. In 1992, Lynch et al. reported that the use of IVIG alone seemed inferior to that of IVIG and steroids [120]. Therefore, a treatment protocol with IVIG plus 1.5 mg/kg per day of dexamethasone was piloted. At this lower dose of dexamethasone, there was no reported oligohydramnios [100, 120]. However, a randomized trial failed to demonstrate benefit of combined IVIG and dexamethasone (1.5 mg/kg) over IVIG alone [100].

There are a number of reports of refractory fetal thrombocytopenia despite administration of maternal IVIG [25, 120, 127–129]. The addition of high dose prednisone (60 mg/day) to weekly IVIG tended to be effective in patients who do not respond to IVIG alone. This dose of prednisone in combination with IVIG did not cause oligohydramnios [100].

Weekly antenatal IVIG appears to be an effective therapy in preventing in utero and perinatal ICH. It is important that the intensity of therapy be matched to the perceived risk to the fetus so that there is no need to perform a fetal blood sampling since virtually all fetuses will be successfully treated. This means over-treating some fetuses to be sure to successfully treat almost all fetuses. Again, the risk of fetal blood sampling in potentially severe thrombocytopenia is too great to recommend its routine use.

Specific Management Strategies

For the purpose of defining the most safe and effective management strategies for fetuses with known AIT, it is helpful to consider the following: second affected fetuses from the same parents have comparable or more severe disease than their older sibling; thrombocytopenia worsens as the pregnancy progresses; fetal blood sampling is the only way to document a response to therapy; maintenance of a fetal platelet count above 20×10^9/L is likely necessary to reduce the risk of ICH; and maintenance of a platelet count above 50×10^9/L is likely necessary for a safe vaginal delivery. To translate these considerations into specific management strategies, our current protocol employs the following grading system: extremely high risk, very high risk, high risk, standard risk, and unknown risk (see Table 14.5). These are summarized in an algorithm [130].

Extremely High Risk

Patients are at extremely high risk for an adverse outcome if they are the antigen-positive sibling of a fetus who suffered an antenatal ICH before 28 weeks' gestation. For this group, 2 g/kg per week (in 2 doses) of maternal IVIG starting at 12 weeks' gestation may be more effective than 1 g/kg per week with prednisone empirically added at 20 weeks. Delivery could be chosen to be early at 32 weeks by cesarean section [102, 103].

Very High Risk

Fetuses are at very high risk for an adverse outcome if they are antigen positive and have a sibling who suffered an antenatal ICH between

Table 14.5 Risk stratification and initial therapy

Level of risk	Conditions	Initial treatment
Unknown risk	Antigen incompatibility, but other factors unknown	See text
Standard risk	Known AIT, platelet count >20 × 10^9, and no history of sibling* with ICH	IVIg 0.5 g to 1 g/kg per week
High risk	History of sibling with perinatal ICH	IVIg 1 g/kg per week, and consider prednisolone 1mg/kg per day
Very high risk	Sibling with ICH between 28 and 36 weeks' gestation	IVIg 2 g/kg per week, to start at 12 weeks' gestation
Extremely high risk	Sibling with ICH occurring before 28 weeks' gestation	IVIg 2 g/kg per week, to start at 12 weeks' gestation

*Note: * Refers to antigen positive sibling with suspected or confirmed AIT.*

28 and 36 weeks' gestation. IVIG at 2 g/kg per week starting at 12 weeks' gestation is often sufficient as initial treatment in preventing ICH in this group, but then adding 1 mg/kg per day prednisone starting at 24–28 weeks is mandatory. Delivery in this group could also be chosen to be early at 32 weeks by cesarean section.

High Risk

Fetuses with a sibling who suffered a perinatal ICH *or* fetuses with a platelet count less than 20 × 10^9/L are at high risk for an adverse outcome. Our study using initial fetal blood sampling, showed that 1 gm/kg per week IVIG and 0.5 mg/kg per day prednisone is more effective to increase the fetal platelet count than IVIG alone in fetuses with initial platelet counts < 10 × 10^9/L. This means that IVIG 1 g/kg per week alone is not sufficient for the fetuses that need treatment the most, i.e., whose counts are the lowest.

Standard Risk

Fetuses affected by AIT who have no history of a sibling ICH, *and* have a platelet count greater than 20 × 10^9/L, have a lesser risk of an adverse outcome. In the absence of fetal blood sampling, high risk and standard risk are collapsed into standard risk. Therefore, treatment of all mother–fetus pairs must be sufficient to successfully treat the fetuses (25% in our previous study) who had platelet counts ≤10 × 10^9/L. Therefore, in our current study, two treatment regimens were randomized: IVIG 1 g/kg twice a week compared to IVIG 1 g/kg once a week and prednisone 0.5 mg/kg per day. The two arms were comparable but both resulted in 20% of fetal platelet counts <50 × 10^9/L. Therefore, our current recommendation is to

start with either arm but then to empirically escalate treatment at 32 weeks so that all patients receive IVIG 1 gm/kg infusion twice a week and prednisone 0.5 mg/kg per day. Recent data suggest that approximately 1%–3% of neonates will have platelet counts <50 × 10^9/L and none will have grade 2 or higher ICH [131].

Unknown Risk

When there is maternal–fetal antigen incompatibility without alloantibody formation, there is an unknown but generally small risk of an adverse outcome. However, there are no absolute indications for antenatal intervention in patients referred with a history of a first or second degree relative with AIT, or in HPA-1a antigen negative primiparous women, even with an affected fetus, unless the fetal platelet count is known to be low. Given the low incidence of alloimmunization in HPA-1a negative mothers, the low incidence of severe thrombocytopenia after alloimmunization [17] and, consequently, the low incidence of ICH, management in the case where there is not a previous affected sibling is not well established. Paternal phenotype should be ascertained to determine the potential fetal genotype. If the father is heterozygous for the HPA-1a antigen, fetal genotype should be determined. This is typically done by amniocentesis. However, recent advances have been made in non-invasive fetal HPA-1a typing using highly sensitive techniques, such as coamplification at lower denaturation temperature PCR (COLD-PCR), to determine the fetal genotype analyzing cell-free DNA from HPA-1b1b pregnant women [132, 133]. If the following conditions are met (in the absence of a history of AIT in a first degree relative): (1) there is an HPA-1a antigen incompatibility between mother and fetus (by amniocentesis or non-invasive free fetal DNA testing, or if the mother is HPA-1b1b positive and the father is homozygous for HPA-1a), and (2) a maternal alloantibody is detected, then the safest course would be institution of antenatal treatment. A variation might be to consider the anti-HPA-1a titer higher than a certain cutoff (depending upon the laboratory). If there is no antibody detected, maternal alloantibody titers should be tested every 1–3 months until positive, or until 1–2 months postpartum. Alloimmunization may occur at delivery, in which case antibody titers will not rise until the postpartum period, which puts subsequent siblings at risk for thrombocytopenia.

Special Considerations

If there are parental antigen incompatibilities and a specific maternal antibody but not directed against HPA-1a, the appropriate management strategy is not clear. There is really no information regarding the antenatal management of antigens other than HPA-1a. Only for HPA-5b incompatibility is there sufficient clinical information to even suggest that there is lesser severity and therefore possibly less need for aggressive antenatal management. Fortunately, the reason for the lack of information is that the need for antenatal management of these other incompatibilities is vanishingly infrequent.

Treatment in the Newborn

Early attempts to treat AIT consisted primarily of (matched) maternal platelet transfusions [134]. Maternal platelet transfusion or transfusion of HPA-1a negative platelets were considered the treatment of choice in severe cases. In the early 1980s there were reports of the successful use of IVIG to treat immune thrombocytopenia in the newborn [135–137]. However, it was recognized that IVIG may require 24–72 hours to increase the platelet count, which would be too slow in the setting of either an ongoing ICH or the very high risk of one. Corticosteroids are a third option, but are most effective when used in combination with IVIG. Also, corticosteroids carry additional risk of infection in the neonate.

As a result, more emphasis was placed on matched platelets from unrelated donors, but the ability to have a very active donor pool such that there were always HPA-1b1b platelets available was beyond the possibilities of all but a very few centers.

In 2006, a non-randomized study of 42 neonates with HPA-1a incompatibility showed that three quarters of patients had platelet responses to incompatible platelets with or without concomitant IVIG [138]. This and another study provided evidence for the use of random donor platelets; both demonstrated that most patients could be satisfactorily managed without matched platelets [139]. Random donor platelets are effective despite alloimmune destruction. This may be because of the immaturity of the neonatal reticuloendothelial system allowing more prolonged survival of antibody-coated platelets.

For most infants with presumed AIT, IVIG (1 g/kg per dose) and random donor platelets, 10–20 ml/kg, will be sufficient to restore a normal platelet count; repeat treatment might be needed depending upon the platelet count. The addition of methylprednisolone (1 mg IV every 8 hours) to IVIG may be better than IVIG alone; we believe this dose is low enough to be relatively safe [12, 71, 140]. For visceral bleeding, including ICH, patients should also receive HPA-1a negative platelets (maternal or single donor), in combination with IVIG, methylprednisolone, and random platelets, unless the random platelets are so effective that additional platelets are not required.

Future Treatment Modalities

It is possible that future antenatal management will be aided by inhibition of F_cRn. This approach is in its infancy [141]. Another possibility for the future is the use of thrombopoietin (Tpo) agents. Both of the two licensed ones are expected to cross the placenta into the fetus and, in very high-risk cases, may be helpful in increasing the fetal platelet count.

An entirely different approach being pursued is that of prophylaxis. The goal would be to screen all pregnancies for HPA-1 typing and then administer prophylactic anti-HPA-1a in a manner analogous to the use of anti-D in rhesus negative pregnant women. This approach has not yet been used clinically [142–145].

Conclusions

Alloimmune thrombocytopenia is a disease of varied presentation and course that may have a devastating impact on severely affected infants and their families. Treatment of the first neonate described in a family unfortunately has limited impact, since ICH may have occurred before diagnosis. While early treatment and intervention may prevent many of the potential adverse sequelae in the next pregnancy, the prescribed therapy itself is not without risk. The capacity exists to effectively treat a great majority of affected fetuses, but we unfortunately lack non-invasive means to sensitively and reliably assess disease severity or response to therapy. Fetal blood sampling has too many risks to be acceptable in other than the most unusual cases.

As understanding of the pathogenesis of this disease broadens, more effective and specific intervention may become available. Future efforts in the study of AIT will focus on mechanisms of immune modulation in affected and unaffected mismatched maternal–fetal pairs; biologic markers that better define the disease and risk groups; and effective, non-toxic, risk-based therapeutic interventions.

References

1. Burrows RF, Kelton JG. Fetal thrombocytopenia and its relation to maternal thrombocytopenia. *N Engl J Med* 1993;**329**(20):1463–6.

2. von dem Borne AE, Decary F. Nomenclature of platelet-specific antigens. *Transfusion* 1990;**30** (5):477.

3. Kelton JG, Smith JW, Horsewood P, et al. ABH antigens on human platelets: Expression on the glycosyl phosphatidylinositol-anchored protein CD109. *J Lab Clin Med* 1998;**132**(2):142–8.

4. von dem Borne AE, Decary F. ICSH/ISBT Working Party on platelet serology: Nomenclature of platelet-specific antigens. *Vox Sang* 1990;**58**(2):176.

5. Kunicki TJ, Newman PJ. The molecular immunology of human platelet proteins. *Blood* 1992;**80**(6):1386–404.

6. Skupski DW, Bussel JB. Alloimmune thrombocytopenia. *Clin Obstet Gynecol* 1999;**42** (2):335–48.

7. Metcalfe P, Watkins NA, Ouwehand WH, et al. Nomenclature of human platelet antigens. *Vox Sang* 2003;**85**(3):240–5.

8. Newman PJ. Nomenclature of human platelet alloantigens: A problem with the HPA system? *Blood* 1994;**83**(6):1447–51.

9. Robinson J, Waller MJ, Stoehr P, Marsh SG. IPD: The Immuno Polymorphism Database. *Nucleic Acids Res* 2005;**33**(Database issue): D523–526.

10. Robinson J, Halliwell JA, McWilliam H, Lopez R, Marsh SG. IPD: The Immuno Polymorphism Database. *Nucleic Acids Res* 2013;**41**(Database issue): D1234–40.

11. Blanchette VS, Peters MA, Pegg-Feige K. Alloimmune thrombocytopenia: Review from a neonatal intensive care unit. *Curr Stud Hematol Blood Transfus* 1986(52):87–96.

12. Mueller-Eckhardt C, Kiefel V, Grubert A, et al. 348 cases of suspected neonatal alloimmune thrombocytopenia. *Lancet* 1989;**1**(8634):363–6.

13. Hohlfeld P, Forestier F, Kaplan C, Tissot JD, Daffos F. Fetal thrombocytopenia: A retrospective survey of 5,194 fetal blood samplings. *Blood* 1994;**84**(6):1851–6.

14. Taaning E, Petersen S, Reinholdt J, Bock J, Svejgaard A. Neonatal immune thrombocytopenia due to allo-or autoantibodies: Clinical and immunological analysis of 83 cases. *Platelets* 1994;**5**(1):53–8.

15. Bonacossa IA, Jocelyn LJ. Alloimmune thrombocytopenia of the newborn: Neurodevelopmental sequelae. *Am J Perinatol* 1996;**13**(4):211–15.

16. Uhrynowska M, Maslanka K, Zupanska B. Neonatal thrombocytopenia: Incidence, serological and clinical observations. *Am J Perinatol* 1997;**14**(7):415–18.

17. Williamson LM, Hackett G, Rennie J, et al. The natural history of fetomaternal alloimmunization to the platelet-specific antigen HPA-1a (PlA1, Zwa) as determined by antenatal screening. *Blood* 1998;**92**(7):2280–7.

18. Jaegtvik S, Husebekk A, Aune B, Oian P, Dahl LB, Skogen B. Neonatal alloimmune thrombocytopenia due to anti-HPA 1a antibodies; the level of maternal antibodies predicts the severity of thrombocytopenia in the newborn. *BJOG* 2000;**107**(5):691–4.

19. Uhrynowska M, Niznikowska-Marks M, Zupanska B. Neonatal and maternal thrombocytopenia: Incidence and immune background. *Eur J Haematol* 2000;**64**(1):42–6.

20. Kaplan C, Morel-Kopp MC, Kroll H, et al. HPA-5b (Br(a)) neonatal alloimmune thrombocytopenia: Clinical and immunological analysis of 39 cases. *Br J Haematol* 1991;**78**(3):425–9.

21. Panzer S, Auerbach L, Cechova E, et al. Maternal alloimmunization against fetal platelet antigens: A prospective study. *Br J Haematol*. 1995;**90** (3):655–60.

22. Kurz M, Stockelle E, Eichelberger B, Panzer S. IgG titer, subclass, and light-chain phenotype of pregnancy-induced HPA-5b antibodies that cause

or do not cause neonatal alloimmune thrombocytopenia. *Transfusion* 1999;**39**(4):379–82.

23. Gruel Y, Boizard B, Daffos F, Forestier F, Caen J, Wautier JL. Determination of platelet antigens and glycoproteins in the human fetus. *Blood* 1986;**68**(2):488–92.

24. Giovangrandi Y, Daffos F, Kaplan C, Forestier F, Mac Aleese J, Moirot M. Very early intracranial haemorrhage in alloimmune fetal thrombocytopenia. *Lancet* 1990;**336**(8710):310.

25. Murphy MF, Metcalfe P, Waters AH, Ord J, Hambley H, Nicolaides K. Antenatal management of severe feto-maternal alloimmune thrombocytopenia: HLA incompatibility may affect responses to fetal platelet transfusions. *Blood* 1993;**81**(8):2174–9.

26. Kumpel BM, Sibley K, Jackson DJ, White G, Soothill PW. Ultrastructural localization of glycoprotein IIIa (GPIIIa, beta 3 integrin) on placental syncytiotrophoblast microvilli: Implications for platelet alloimmunization during pregnancy. *Transfusion* 2008;**48**(10):2077–86.

27. van Loghem JJ, Dorfmeijer H, van der Hart M, Schreuder F. Serological and genetical studies on a platelet antigen (Zw). *Vox Sang* 1959;**4**(2):161–9.

28. Schulman NR, Marder VJ, Heller MC, Collier EM. Platelet and leukocyte isoantigens and their antibodies: Serologic, physiologic, and clinical studies. *Prog Hematol* 1964;**4**:222–304.

29. Flug F, Karpatkin M, Karpatkin S. Should all pregnant women be tested for their platelet PLA (Zw, HPA-1) phenotype? *Br J Haematol* 1994;**86**(1):1–5.

30. Blanchette VS, Chen L, de Friedberg ZS, et al. Alloimmunization to the PlA1 platelet antigen: Results of a prospective study. *Br J Haematol* 1990;**74**(2):209–15.

31. Durand-Zaleski I, Schlegel N, Blum-Boisgard C, et al. Screening primiparous women and newborns for fetal/neonatal alloimmune thrombocytopenia: A prospective comparison of effectiveness and costs. Immune Thrombocytopenia Working Group. *Am J Perinatol* 1996;**13**(7):423–31.

32. Mueller-Eckhardt C, Mueller-Eckhardt G, Willen-Ohff H, et al. Immunogenicity of and immune response to the human platelet antigen Zwa is strongly associated with HLA-B8 and DR3. *Tissue Antigens* 1985;**26**(1):71–6.

33. Reznikoff-Etievant MF, Dangu C, Lobet R. HLA-B8 antigens and anti-PLa1 allo-immunization. *Tissue Antigens* 1981;**18**(1):66–8.

34. Eckhardt CM. Letter to the editor. *Tissue Antigens* 1982;**19**(2):154–4.

35. Taaning E, Antonsen H, Petersen S, Svejgaard A, Thomsen M. HLA antigens and maternal antibodies in allo-immune neonatal thrombocytopenia. *Tissue Antigens* 1983;**21**(5):351–9.

36. Decary F. Is HLA-DR3 a risk factor in PLA1-negative pregnant women? *Curr Stud Hematol Blood Transfus* 1986(52):78–86.

37. Valentin N, Vergracht A, Bignon JD, et al. HLA-DRw52a is involved in alloimmunization against PL-A1 antigen. *Hum Immunol* 1990;**27**(2):73–9.

38. Decary F, L'Abbe D, Tremblay L, Chartrand P. The immune response to the HPA-1a antigen: Association with HLA-DRw52a. *Transfus Med* 1991;**1**(1):55–62.

39. L'Abbe D, Tremblay L, Filion M, et al. Alloimmunization to platelet antigen HPA-1a (PIA1) is strongly associated with both HLA-DRB3*0101 and HLA-DQB1*0201. *Hum Immunol* 1992;**34**(2):107–14.

40. de Waal LP, van Dalen CM, Engelfriet CP, von dem Borne AE. Alloimmunization against the platelet-specific Zwa antigen, resulting in neonatal alloimmune thrombocytopenia or posttransfusion purpura, is associated with the supertypic DRw52 antigen including DR3 and DRw6. *Hum Immunol* 1986;**17**(1):45–53.

41. Ahlen MT, Husebekk A, Killie MK, Skogen B, Stuge TB. T-cell responses associated with neonatal alloimmune thrombocytopenia: Isolation of HPA-1a–specific, HLA-DRB3*0101–restricted CD4+ T cells. *Blood* 2009;**113**(16):3838–44.

42. Wu S, Maslanka K, Gorski J. An integrin polymorphism that defines reactivity with alloantibodies generates an anchor for MHC class II peptide binding: A model for unidirectional alloimmune responses. *J Immunol* 1997;**158**(7):3221–6.

43. Mueller-Eckhardt C, Becker T, Weisheit M, Witz C, Santoso S. Neonatal alloimmune thrombocytopenia due to fetomaternal Zwb incompatibility. *Vox Sang* 1986;**50**(2):94–6.

44. Westman P, Hashemi-Tavoularis S, Blanchette V, et al. Maternal DRB1*1501, DQA1*0102, DQB1*0602 haplotype in fetomaternal alloimmunization against human platelet alloantigen HPA-6b (GPIIIa-Gln489). *Tissue Antigens* 1997;**50**(2):113–18.

45. Dreyfus M, Kaplan C, Verdy E, Schlegel N, Durand-Zaleski I, Tchernia G. Frequency of immune thrombocytopenia in newborns: A prospective study. Immune Thrombocytopenia Working Group. *Blood* 1997;**89**(12):4402–6.

46. Mueller-Eckhardt C, Marks HJ, Baur MP, Mueller-Eckhardt G. Immunogenetic studies of the platelet-specific antigen P1A1 (Zw(a)). *Immunobiology* 1982;**160**(5):375–81.

47. Sainio S, Jarvenpaa AL, Renlund M, et al. Thrombocytopenia in term infants: A population-based study. *Obstet Gynecol* 2000;**95**(3):441–6.

48. Ghevaert C, Rankin A, Huiskes E, et al. Alloantibodies against low-frequency human platelet antigens do not account for a significant proportion of cases of fetomaternal alloimmune thrombocytopenia: Evidence from 1054 cases. *Transfusion* 2009;**49**(10):2084–9.

49. Sharon R, Amar A. Maternal anit-HLA antibodies and neonatal thrombocytopenia. *Lancet* 1981;**1**(8233):1313.

50. Marshall LR, Brogden FE, Roper TS, Barr AL. Antenatal platelet antibody testing by flow cytometry: Results of a pilot study. *Transfusion.* 1994;**34**(11):961–5.

51. King KE, Kao KJ, Bray PF, et al. The role of HLA antibodies in neonatal thrombocytopenia: A prospective study. *Tissue Antigens* 1996;**47**(3):206–11.

52. Saito S, Ota M, Komatsu Y, et al. Serologic analysis of three cases of neonatal alloimmune thrombocytopenia associated with HLA antibodies. *Transfusion* 2003;**43**(7):908–17.

53. Moncharmont P, Dubois V, Obegi C, et al. HLA antibodies and neonatal alloimmune thrombocytopenia. *Acta Haematol* 2004;**111**(4):215–20.

54. Thude H, Schorner U, Helfricht C, et al. Neonatal alloimmune thrombocytopenia caused by human leucocyte antigen-B27 antibody. *Transfus Med* 2006;**16**(2):143–9.

55. Curtis BR, Edwards JT, Hessner MJ, Klein JP, Aster RH. Blood group A and B antigens are strongly expressed on platelets of some individuals. *Blood* 2000;**96**(4):1574–81.

56. Ogasawara K, Ueki J, Takenaka M, Furihata K. Study on the expression of ABH antigens on platelets. *Blood* 1993;**82**(3):993–9.

57. Curtis BR, Ali S, Glazier AM, et al. Isoimmunization against CD36 (glycoprotein IV): Description of four cases of neonatal isoimmune thrombocytopenia and brief review of the literature. *Transfusion* 2002;**42**(9):1173–9.

58. de Moerloose P, Boehlen F, Extermann P, Hohfeld P. Neonatal thrombocytopenia: Incidence and characterization of maternal antiplatelet antibodies by MAIPA assay. *Br J Haematol* 1998;**100**(4):735–40.

59. Kjeldsen-Kragh J, Killie MK, Tomter G, et al. A screening and intervention program aimed to reduce mortality and serious morbidity associated with severe neonatal alloimmune thrombocytopenia. *Blood* 2007;**110**(3):833–9.

60. Bussel JB, Zacharoulis S, Kramer K, et al. Clinical and diagnostic comparison of neonatal alloimmune thrombocytopenia to non-immune cases of thrombocytopenia. *Pediatr Blood Cancer* 2005;**45**(2):176–83.

61. Pearson HA, Shulman NR, Marder VJ, Cone TE, Jr. Isoimmune neonatal thrombocytopenic purpura: Clinical and therapeutic considerations. *Blood* 1964;**23**:154–77.

62. Chaoying M, Junwu G, Chituwo B. Intraventricular haemorrhage and its prognosis, prevention and treatment in term infants. *J Trop Pediatr* 1999;**45**(4):237–40.

63. Bussel J. Diagnosis and management of the fetus and neonate with alloimmune thrombocytopenia. *J Thromb Haemost* 2009;7 Suppl 1:253–7.

64. Naidu S, Messmore H, Caserta V, Fine M. CNs lesions in neonatal isoimmune thrombocytopenia. *Arch Neurol* 1983;**40**(9):552–4.

65. Dean LM, McLeary M, Taylor GA. Cerebral hemorrhage in alloimmune thrombocytopenia. *Pediatr Radiol* 1995;**25**(6):444–5.

66. Johnson J-AM, Ryan G, Al-Musa A, Farkas S, Blanchette VS. Prenatal diagnosis and management of neonatal alloimmune thrombocytopenia. *Semin Perinat* 1997;**21**(1):45–52.

67. Sherer DM, Anyaegbunam A, Onyeije C. Antepartum fetal intracranial hemorrhage, predisposing factors and prenatal sonography: A review. *Am J Perinatol* 1998;**15**(7):431–41.

68. Meyer M, Kirchmaier CM, Schirmer A, Spangenberg P, Strohl C, Breddin K. Acquired disorder of platelet function associated with autoantibodies against membrane glycoprotein IIb-IIIa complex–1. Glycoprotein analysis. *Thromb Haemost* 1991;**65**(5):491–6.

69. Yougbare I, Lang S, Yang H, et al. Maternal antiplatelet beta3 integrins impair angiogenesis and cause intracranial hemorrhage. *J Clin Invest* 2015;**125**(4):1545–56.

70. Bussel JB, Tanli S, Peterson HC. Favorable neurological outcome in 7 cases of perinatal intracranial hemorrhage due to immune thrombocytopenia. *Am J Pediatr Hematol Oncol* 1991;**13**(2):156–9.

71. Bussel JB, Zabusky MR, Berkowitz RL, McFarland JG. Fetal alloimmune

thrombocytopenia. *N Engl J Med* 1997;**337** (1):22–6.

72. Khouzami AN, Kickler TS, Callan NA, et al. Devastating sequelae of alloimmune thrombocytopenia: An entity that deserves more attention. *J Matern Fetal Med* 1996;**5**(3):137–41.

73. Murphy MF, Hambley H, Nicolaides K, Waters AH. Severe fetomaternal alloimmune thrombocytopenia presenting with fetal hydrocephalus. *Prenat Diagn* 1996;**16**(12):1152–5.

74. Zalneraitis EL, Young RS, Krishnamoorthy KS. Intracranial hemorrhage in utero as a complication of isoimmune thrombocytopenia. *J Pediatr* 1979;**95**(4):611–14.

75. Herman JH, Jumbelic MI, Ancona RJ, Kickler TS. In utero cerebral hemorrhage in alloimmune thrombocytopenia. *Am J Pediatr Hematol Oncol* 1986;**8**(4):312–17.

76. Morales WJ, Stroup M. Intracranial hemorrhage in utero due to isoimmune neonatal thrombocytopenia. *Obstet Gynecol* 1985;**65**(3 Suppl):20S–21S.

77. Friedman JM, Aster RH. Neonatal alloimmune thrombocytopenic purpura and congenital porencephaly in two siblings associated with a "new" maternal antiplatelet antibody. *Blood* 1985;**65**(6):1412–15.

78. Jesurun CA, Levin GS, Sullivan WR, Stevens D. Intracranial hemorrhage in utero re thrombocytopenia. *J Pediatr* 1980;**97**(4):695–6.

79. Beadling WV, Herman JH, Stuart MJ, Keashen-Schnell M, Miller JL. Fetal bleeding in neonatal alloimmune thrombocytopenia mediated by anti-PlAl is not associated with inhibition of fibrinogen binding to platelet GPIIb/IIIa. *Am J Clin Pathol* 1995;**103**(5):636–41.

80. Glade-Bender J, McFarland JG, Kaplan C, Porcelijn L, Bussel JB. Anti-HPA-3A induces severe neonatal alloimmune thrombocytopenia. *J Pediatr* 2001;**138**(6):862–7.

81. Proulx C, Filion M, Goldman M, et al. Analysis of immunoglobulin class, IgG subclass and titre of HPA-1a antibodies in alloimmunized mothers giving birth to babies with or without neonatal alloimmune thrombocytopenia. *Br J Haematol* 1994;**87**(4):813–17.

82. Mawas F, Wiener E, Williamson LM, Rodeck CH. Immunoglobulin G subclasses of anti-human platelet antigen 1a in maternal sera: Relation to the severity of neonatal alloimmune thrombocytopenia. *Eur J Haematol* 1997;**59** (5):287–92.

83. McFarland JG, Aster RH, Bussel JB, et al. Prenatal diagnosis of neonatal alloimmune

thrombocytopenia using allele-specific oligonucleotide probes. *Blood* 1991;**78**(9):2276–82.

84. Skogen B, Bellissimo DB, Hessner MJ, et al. Rapid determination of platelet alloantigen genotypes by polymerase chain reaction using allele-specific primers. *Transfusion* 1994;**34**(11):955–60.

85. Avent ND. Antenatal genotyping of the blood groups of the fetus. *Vox Sang* 1998;**74** Suppl 2:365–74.

86. Hughes D, Hurd C, Williamson LM. Genotyping for human platelet antigen-1 directly from dried blood spots on cards. *Blood* 1996;**88**(8):3242–3.

87. Bessos H, Mirza S, McGill A, et al. A whole blood assay for platelet HPA1 (PLA1) phenotyping applicable to large-scale screening. *Br J Haematol* 1996;**92**(1):221–5.

88. Bessos H, Hofner M, Salamat A, Wilson D, Urbaniak S, Turner ML. An international trial demonstrates suitability of a newly developed whole-blood ELISA kit for multicentre platelet HPA-1 phenotyping. *Vox Sang* 1999;**77**(2):103–6.

89. Quintanar A, Jallu V, Legros Y, Kaplan C. Human platelet antigen genotyping using a fluorescent SSCP technique with an automatic sequencer. *Br J Haematol* 1998;**103**(2):437–44.

90. von dem Borne AE, Verheugt FW, Oosterhof F, et al. A simple immunofluorescence test for the detection of platelet antibodies. *Br J Haematol* 1978;**39**(2):195–207.

91. von dem Borne AE, van Leeuwen EF, von Riesz LE, van Boxtel CJ, Engelfriet CP. Neonatal alloimmune thrombocytopenia: Detection and characterization of the responsible antibodies by the platelet immunofluorescence test. *Blood* 1981;**57**(4):649–56.

92. Kiefel V, Santoso S, Weisheit M, Mueller-Eckhardt C. Monoclonal antibody-specific immobilization of platelet antigens (MAIPA): A new tool for the identification of platelet-reactive antibodies. *Blood* 1987;**70** (6):1722–6.

93. Morel-Kopp MC, Kaplan C. Modification of the MAIPA technique to detect and identify antiplatelet glycoprotein auto-antibodies. *Platelets* 1994;**5**:285.

94. Joutsi L, Kekomaki R. Comparison of the direct platelet immunofluorescence test (direct PIFT) with a modified direct monoclonal antibody-specific immobilization of platelet antigens (direct MAIPA) in detection of platelet-associated IgG. *Br J Haematol* 1997;**96**(1):204–9.

95. Dawkins B. Monitoring anti-HPA-1a platelet antibody levels during pregnancy using the MAIPA test. *Vox Sang* 1995;**68**(1):27–34.

96. Metcalfe P, Doughty HA, Murphy MF, Waters AH. A simplified method for large-scale HPA-1a phenotyping for antenatal screening. *Transfus Med* 1994;**4**(1):21–4.

97. Curtis BR, McFarland JG. Detection and identification of platelet antibodies and antigens in the clinical laboratory. *Immunohematology* 2009;**25**(3):125–35.

98. Curtis BR. Genotyping for human platelet alloantigen polymorphisms: Applications in the diagnosis of alloimmune platelet disorders. *Semin Thromb Hemost* 2008;**34**(6):539–48.

99. Bussel JB, Sola-Visner M. Current approaches to the evaluation and management of the fetus and neonate with immune thrombocytopenia. *Semin Perinatol* 2009;**33**(1):35–42.

100. Bussel JB, Berkowitz RL, Lynch L, et al. Antenatal management of alloimmune thrombocytopenia with intravenous gamma-globulin: A randomized trial of the addition of low-dose steroid to intravenous gamma-globulin. *Am J Obstet Gynecol* 1996;**174**(5):1414–23.

101. Turner ML, Bessos H, Fagge T, et al. Prospective epidemiologic study of the outcome and cost-effectiveness of antenatal screening to detect neonatal alloimmune thrombocytopenia due to anti-HPA-1a. *Transfusion* 2005;**45**(12):1945–56.

102. Sitarz AL, Driscoll JM, Jr., Wolff JA. Management of isoimmune neonatal thrombocytopenia. *Am J Obstet Gynecol* 1976;**124**(1):39–42.

103. Murray JM, Harris RE. The management of the pregnant patient with idiopathic thrombocytopenic purpura. *Am J Obstet Gynecol* 1976;**126**(4):449–51.

104. Sia CG, Amigo NC, Harper RG, Farahani G, Kochen J. Failure of cesarean section to prevent intracranial hemorrhage in siblings with isoimmune neonatal thrombocytopenia. *Am J Obstet Gynecol* 1985;**153**(1):79–81.

105. Cook RL, Miller RC, Katz VL, Cefalo RC. Immune thrombocytopenic purpura in pregnancy: A reappraisal of management. *Obstet Gynecol* 1991;**78**(4):578–83.

106. Buscaglia M, Ghisoni L, Bellotti M, et al. Percutaneous umbilical blood sampling: Indication changes and procedure loss rate in a nine years' experience. *Fetal Diagn Ther* 1996;**11**(2):106–13.

107. Petrikovsky B, Schneider EP, Klein VR, Wyse LJ. Cordocentesis using the combined technique; needle guide-assisted and free-hand. *Fetal Diagn Ther* 1997;**12**(4):252–4.

108. Antsaklis A, Daskalakis G, Papantoniou N, Michalas S. Fetal blood sampling: Indication-related losses. *Prenat Diagn* 1998;**18**(9):934–40.

109. Tongsong T, Wanapirak C, Kunavikatikul C, et al. Cordocentesis at 16–24 weeks of gestation: Experience of 1,320 cases. *Prenat Diagn* 2000;**20**(3):224–8.

110. Pielet BW, Socol ML, MacGregor SN, Ney JA, Dooley SL. Cordocentesis: An appraisal of risks. *Am J Obstet Gyneco* 1988;**159**(6):1497–500.

111. Paidas MJ, Berkowitz RL, Lynch L, et al. Alloimmune thrombocytopenia: Fetal and neonatal losses related to cordocentesis. *Am J Obstet Gynecol* 1995;**172**(2 Pt 1):475–9.

112. Daffos F, Forestier F, Muller JY, et al. Prenatal treatment of alloimmune thrombocytopenia. *Lancet* 1984;**2**(8403):632.

113. Kaplan C, Daffos F, Forestier F, et al. Management of alloimmune thrombocytopenia: Antenatal diagnosis and in utero transfusion of maternal platelets. *Blood* 1988;**72**(1):340–3.

114. Nicolini U, Rodeck CH, Kochenour NK, et al. In-utero platelet transfusion for alloimmune thrombocytopenia. *Lancet* 1988;**2**(8609):506.

115. Murphy MF, Waters AH, Doughty HA, et al. Antenatal management of fetomaternal alloimmune thrombocytopenia–report of 15 affected pregnancies. *Transfus Med* 1994;**4**(4):281–92.

116. Daffos F, Forestier F, Kaplan C. Prenatal treatment of fetal alloimmune thrombocytopenia. *Lancet* 1988;**2**(8616):910.

117. Suarez CR, Anderson C. High-dose intravenous gammaglobulin (IVG) in neonatal immune thrombocytopenia. *Am J Hematol* 1987;**26**(3):247–53.

118. Bussel JB, Berkowitz RL, McFarland JG, Lynch L, Chitkara U. Antenatal treatment of neonatal alloimmune thrombocytopenia. *N Engl J Med* 1988;**319**(21):1374–8.

119. Wenstrom KD, Weiner CP, Williamson RA. Antenatal treatment of fetal alloimmune thrombocytopenia. *Obstet Gynecol* 1992;**80**(3 Pt 1):433–5.

120. Lynch L, Bussel JB, McFarland JG, Chitkara U, Berkowitz RL. Antenatal treatment of alloimmune thrombocytopenia. *Obstet Gynecol* 1992;**80**(1):67–71.

121. Bussel JB, Berkowitz RL, McFarland JG. Maternal IVIG in neonatal alloimmune thrombocytopenia. *Br J Haematol* 1997;**98**(2):493–4.

122. Debre M, Bonnet MC, Fridman WH, et al. Infusion of Fc gamma fragments for treatment of children with acute immune thrombocytopenic purpura. *Lancet* 1993;**342**(8877):945–9.

123. Urbaniak SJ, Duncan JI, Armstrong-Fisher SS, Abramovich DR, Page KR. Transfer of anti-D antibodies across the isolated perfused human placental lobule and inhibition by high-dose intravenous immunoglobulin: A possible mechanism of action. *Br J Haematol* 1997;**96**(1):186–93.

124. Bowman J, Harman C, Mentigolou S, Pollock J. Intravenous fetal transfusion of immunoglobulin for alloimmune thrombocytopenia. *Lancet* 1992;**340**(8826):1034–5.

125. Zimmermann R, Huch A. In-utero fetal therapy with immunoglobulin for alloimmune thrombocytopenia. *Lancet* 1992;**340**(8819):606.

126. Liu Z-J, Bussel JB, Lakkaraja M, et al. Suppression of in vitro megakaryopoiesis by maternal sera containing anti-HPA-1a antibodies. *Blood* 2015;**126**(10):1234–6.

127. Mir N, Samson D, House MJ, Kovar IZ. Failure of antenatal high-dose immunoglobulin to improve fetal platelet count in neonatal allo-immune thrombocytopenia. *Vox Sang* 1988;**55**(3):188–9.

128. Nicolini U, Tannirandorn Y, Gonzalez P, et al. Continuing controversy in alloimmune thrombocytopenia: Fetal hyperimmunoglobulinemia fails to prevent thrombocytopenia. *Am J Obstet Gynecol* 1990; **163**(4 Pt 1):1144–6.

129. Kroll H, Kiefel V, Giers G, et al. Maternal intravenous immunoglobulin treatment does not prevent intracranial haemorrhage in fetal alloimmune thrombocytopenia. *Transfus Med* 1994;**4**(4):293–6.

130. Bussel JB, Berkowitz RL, Hung C, et al. Intracranial hemorrhage in alloimmune thrombocytopenia: Stratified management to prevent recurrence in the subsequent affected fetus. *Am J Obstet Gynecol* 2010;**203**(2):135e131–114.

131. Lakkaraja M, Berkowitz RL, Vinograd CA, et al. Omission of fetal sampling in treatment of subsequent pregnancies in fetal-neonatal alloimmune thrombocytopenia. *Am J Obstet Gynecol* 2016;**215**(4):471.e1-9.

132. Ferro M, Macher HC, Fornés G, et al. Noninvasive prenatal diagnosis by cell-free DNA screening for fetomaternal HPA-1a platelet incompatibility. *Transfusion* 2018;**58**(10):2272–9.

133. Nogues N. Recent advances in non-invasive fetal HPA-1a typing. *Transfus Apher Sci* 2020;**59**(1):102708.

134. Adner MM, Fisch GR, Starobin SG, Aster RH. Use of "compatible" platelet transfusions in treatment of congenital isoimmune thrombocytopenic purpura. *N Engl J Med* 1969;**280**(5):244–7.

135. Sidiropoulos D, Straume B. The treatment of neonatal isoimmune thrombocytopenia with intravenous immunoglobin (IgG i.v.). *Blut* 1984;**48**(6):383–6.

136. Derycke M, Dreyfus M, Ropert JC, Tchernia G. Intravenous immunoglobulin for neonatal isoimmune thrombocytopenia. *Arch Dis Child* 1985;**60**(7):667–9.

137. Massey GV, McWilliams NB, Mueller DG, Napolitano A, Maurer HM. Intravenous immunoglobulin in treatment of neonatal isoimmune thrombocytopenia. *J Pediatr* 1987;**111**(1):133–5.

138. Kiefel V, Bassler D, Kroll H, et al. Antigen-positive platelet transfusion in neonatal alloimmune thrombocytopenia (NAIT). *Blood* 2006;**107**(9):3761–3.

139. Bakchoul T, Bassler D, Heckmann M, et al. Management of infants born with severe neonatal alloimmune thrombocytopenia: The role of platelet transfusions and intravenous immunoglobulin. *Transfusion* 2014;**54**(3):640–5.

140. Bussel J, Kaplan C, McFarland J. Recommendations for the evaluation and treatment of neonatal autoimmune and alloimmune thrombocytopenia. The Working Party on Neonatal Immune Thrombocytopenia of the Neonatal Hemostasis Subcommittee of the Scientific and Standardization Committee of the ISTH. *Thromb Haemost* 1991;**65**(5):631–4.

141. Mezo AR, McDonnell KA, Hehir CAT, et al. Reduction of IgG in nonhuman primates by a peptide antagonist of the neonatal Fc receptor FcRn. *Proc Natl Acad Sci USA* 2008;**105**(7):2337–42.

142. Tiller H, Killie MK, Chen P, et al. Toward a prophylaxis against fetal and neonatal alloimmune thrombocytopenia: Induction of antibody-mediated immune suppression and prevention of severe clinical complications in a murine model. *Transfusion* 2012;**52**(7):1446–57.

143. Stuge TB, Skogen B, Ahlen MT, et al. The cellular immunobiology associated with fetal and neonatal alloimmune thrombocytopenia. *Transfus Apher Sci* 2011;**45**(1):53–9.

144. Bakchoul T, Boylan B, Sachs UJ, et al. Blockade of maternal anti-HPA-1a-mediated platelet clearance by an HPA-1a epitope-specific F(ab') in an in vivo mouse model of alloimmune

thrombocytopenia. *Transfusion* 2009;**49** (2):265–70.

145. Bakchoul T, Greinacher A, Sachs UJ, et al. Inhibition of HPA-1a alloantibody-mediated platelet destruction by a deglycosylated anti-HPA-1a monoclonal antibody in mice: Toward targeted treatment of fetal-alloimmune thrombocytopenia. *Blood* 2013;**122**(3):321–7.

146. Maslanka K, Lucas GF, Gronkowska A, Davis JG, Zupanska B. A second case of neonatal alloimmune thrombocytopenia associated with anti-PlA2 (Zwb) antibodies. *Haematologia (Budap)* 1989;**22**(2):109–13.

147. Kuijpers RW, van den Anker JN, Baerts W, von dem Borne AE. A case of severe neonatal thrombocytopenia with schizencephaly associated with anti-HPA-1b and anti-HPA-2a. *Br J Haematol* 1994;**87**(3):576–9.

148. Mercier P, Chicheportiche C, Reviron D, et al. Neonatal thrombocytopenia in HLA-DR, -DQ, -DP-typed mother due to rare anti-HPA-1b (PLA2) (Zwb) fetomaternal immunization. *Vox Sang* 1994;**67**(1):46–51.

149. Van den Anker JN, Huiskes E, Porcelein L, von dem Borne AE. Anti-HPA-1b really causes neonatal thrombocytopenia. *Br J Haematol* 1995;**89**(2):428.

150. Winters JL, Jennings CD, Desai NS, Dickson LG, Ford RF. Neonatal alloimmune thrombocytopenia due to anti-HPA-1b (PLA2) (Zwb). A case report and review. *Vox Sang* 1998;**74**(4):256–9.

151. von dem Borne AE, von Riesz E, Verheugt FW, et al. Baka, a new platelet-specific antigen involved in neonatal allo-immune thrombocytopenia. *Vox Sang* 1980;**39**(2):113–20.

152. Kiefel V, Santoso S, Katzmann B, Mueller-Eckhardt C. A new platelet-specific alloantigen Bra. Report of 4 cases with neonatal alloimmune thrombocytopenia. *Vox Sang* 1988;**54**(2):101–6.

153. Kekomaki R, Jouhikainen T, Ollikainen J, Westman P, Laes M. A new platelet alloantigen, Tua, on glycoprotein IIIa associated with neonatal alloimmune thrombocytopenia in two families. *Br J Haematol* 1993;**83**(2):306–10.

154. McFarland JG, Blanchette V, Collins J, et al. Neonatal alloimmune thrombocytopenia due to a new platelet-specific alloantibody. *Blood* 1993;**81**(12):3318–23.

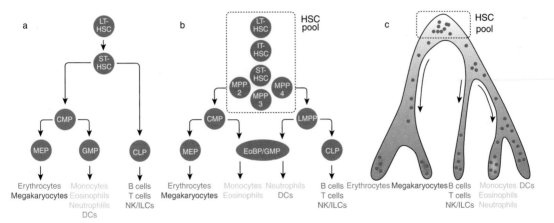

Fig. 2.2 Timeline of hierarchical models of hematopoiesis. (a) Visualization based on cutting-edge research around the year 2000: HSC are represented as a homogeneous population, downstream of which the first lineage bifurcation separates the myeloid and lymphoid branches via the common myeloid progenitor (CMP) and common lymphoid progenitor (CLP) populations. (b) During the years 2005–2015, this visualization incorporates new findings: The HSC pool is now accepted to be more heterogeneous both in terms of self-renewal (vertical axis) and differentiation properties (horizontal axis), the myeloid and lymphoid branches remain associated further down in the hierarchy via the lymphoid-primed multipotential progenitor (LMPP) population, the GMP compartment is shown to be fairly heterogeneous. (c) From 2016 onwards, single-cell transcriptomic snapshots indicate a continuum of differentiation. Each red dot represents a single cell and its localization along a differentiation trajectory. Abbreviations: DCs, dendritic cells; EoBP, eosinophil–basophil progenitor; GMP, granulocyte–monocyte progenitors; LT, long-term; ILCs, innate lymphoid cells; MEP, megakaryocyte–erythrocyte progenitors; NK, natural killer cells; ST, short-term. (From Laurenti E, Göttgens B. From haematopoietic stem cells to complex differentiation landscapes. *Nature* 2018; **553**(7689):418–26.)

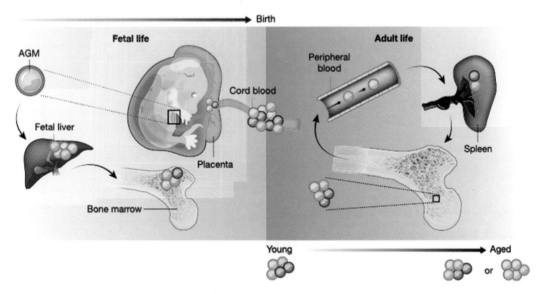

Fig. 2.3 The composition of the HSPC compartment changes in space and time. HSPCs are found in many organs in the body across a lifetime. Cells of different colors represent distinct HSPC subsets. It is unclear whether all HSPC subsets and differentiation trajectories are present in the same proportion in each of the organs. Current evidence suggests that age-related changes result from a combination of shifts in the composition of the HSPC pool, as well as phenotypic changes in particular cell types driven by intrinsic genetic or epigenetic changes and systemic alterations of the microenvironment. Abbreviation: AGM, aorta gonad mesonephros. (From Laurenti E, Göttgens B. From haematopoietic stem cells to complex differentiation landscapes. *Nature* 2018;**553** (7689):418–26.)

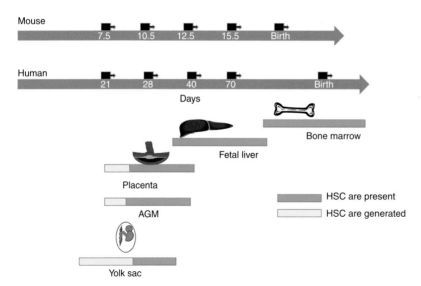

Fig. 3.1 Establishment of hematopoietic stem cells. Abbreviations: AGM, aorta gonad mesonephros, HSC, hematopoietic stem cells.

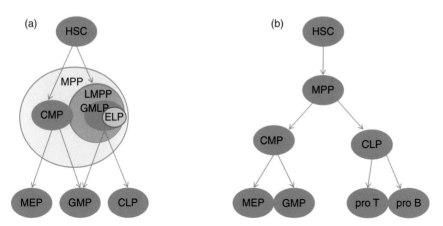

Fig. 3.2 Hematopoietic stem cell development. (a) Mouse hematopoietic hierarchy. (b) Human hematopoietic hierarchy. HSC, hematopoietic stem cell; MPP, multipotent progenitor; LMPP, lymphoid primed multipotent progenitor; CMP, common myeloid progenitor; GMLP, granulocyte monocyte lymphoid progenitor; GMP, granulocyte monocyte progenitor; CLP, common lymphoid progenitor; ELP, early lymphoid progenitor; MEP, megakaryocyte erythrocyte progenitor; pro T, pro T-cell; pro B, pro B-cell.

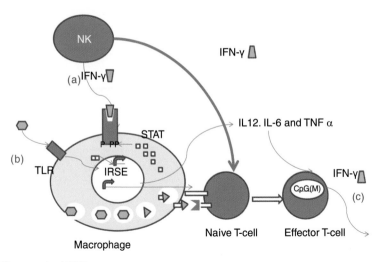

Fig. 3.3 Defects in neonatal innate immune signaling system. (a). Hypoactive response of nenonatal macrophages to activation by IFN-γ may be related to defective STAT posphorylation (b). Impaired response by neonatal monocytes to multiple TLR ligands (c). Diminished IFN-γ by neonatal lympocytes may be secondary to hypermethylationof IFN-γ promoter.

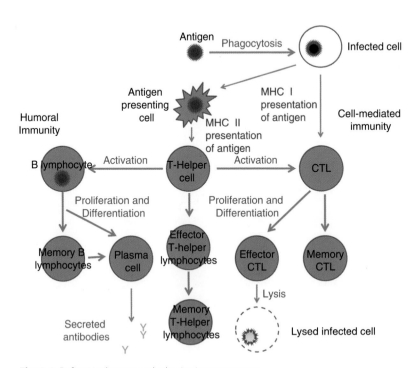

Fig. 3.4 Defects in the neonatal adaptive immune system.

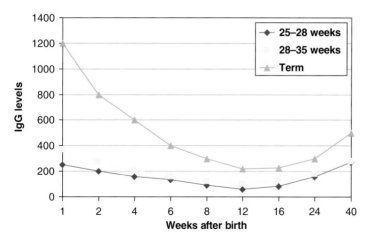

Fig. 5.1 Median IgG levels (*y*-axis) for term infants (triangle), preterm infants 28–35 weeks (square), and 25–28 weeks (diamond). Decay of maternal IgG over the first 40 weeks of life is shown on the *x*-axis. Modified from Ballow et al. [33].

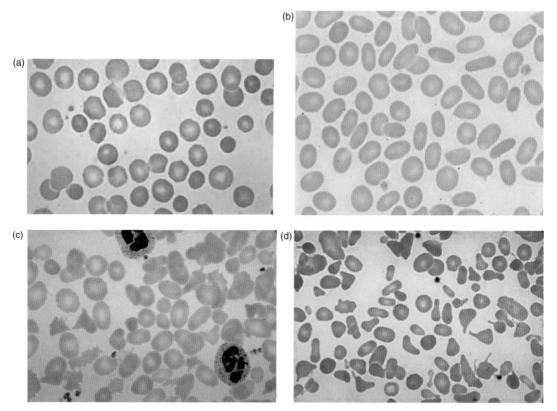

Fig. 10.1 Photomicrographs of blood smears from patients with different hereditary red blood cell (RBC) membrane disorders. (a) Hereditary spherocytosis; (b) mild, asymptomatic common hereditary elliptocytosis characterized by numerous elliptocytic cells; (c) hereditary elliptocytosis with chronic hemolysis with the presence of elliptocytes and rod-shaped cells and poikilocytes; (d) hereditary pyropoikilocytosis with a large number of microspherocytes and micropoikilocytes and relative paucity of elliptocytes.

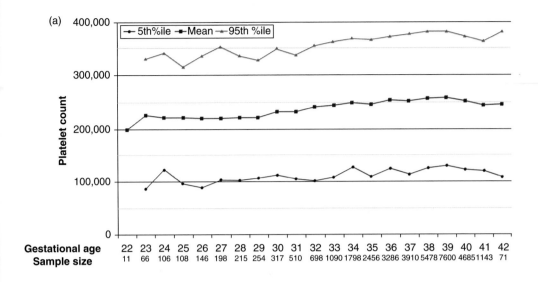

Gestational age   22 23 24 25 26 27 28 29 30 31 32 33 34 35 36 37 38 39 40 41 42
Sample size   11 66 106 108 146 198 215 254 317 510 698 1090 1798 2456 3286 3910 5478 7600 4685 1143 71

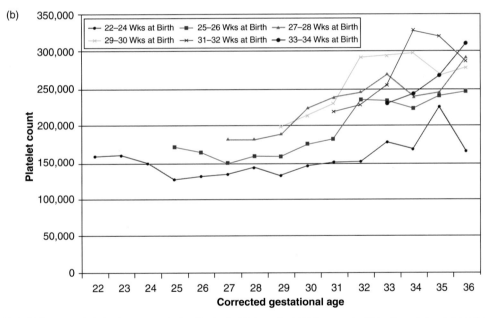

Fig. 12.1 (a) First recorded platelet counts obtained in the first 3 days after birth in neonates 22 to 42 weeks' gestation. The red line represents the mean values and the blue and green lines represent the 5th and 95th percentiles, respectively. (b) Effects of postnatal age on mean platelet counts of premature infants. The mean platelet counts were plotted according to gestational age at birth. Data were grouped according to weeks of gestation completed at birth as follows: 22 to 24 weeks, 25 to 26 weeks, 27 to 28 weeks, 31 to 32 weeks, and 33 to 34 weeks. (Reproduced from: Wiedmeier et al., *J Perinatol* 2009;29:130–6, with permission [4].)

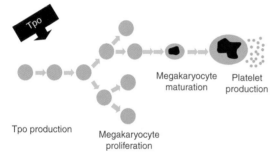

Tpo

Megakaryocyte
maturation

Platelet
production

Tpo production

Megakaryocyte
proliferation

Fig. 13.1 Schematic representation of the process of platelet production, as consisting of four steps: The production of Tpo, the proliferation of megakaryocyte progenitors, the maturation of megakaryocytes, and the release of new platelets into the circulation.

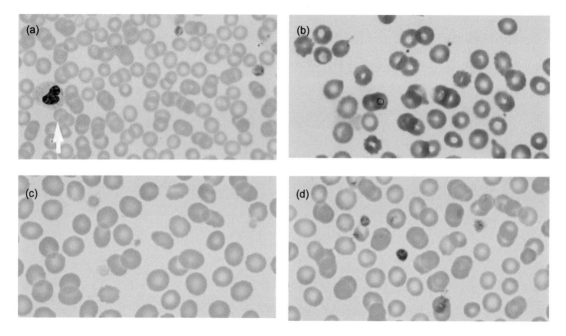

Fig. 15.1 Peripheral smear findings in representative inherited thrombocytopenia syndromes. (a) *MYH9*-related disorder. Arrow indicates neutrophil with a Dohle-like inclusion. (b) Small platelets in Wiskott–Aldrich syndrome. (c) Pale platelets in Gray platelet syndrome. (d) Large platelets in Bernard–Soulier syndrome. Magnification 100×. (Images courtesy of Alan Cantor.)

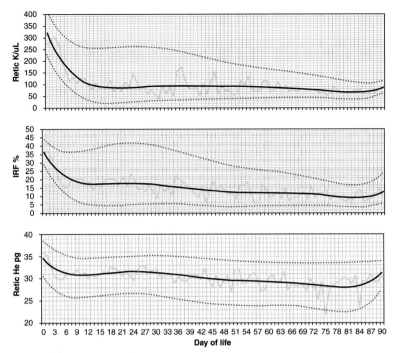

Fig. 24.10 Reference intervals for reticulocytes per microliter blood, immature reticulocyte fraction (IRF) (%), and RET-He (pg) over the first 90 days following birth. The lower line shows the 5th percentile values, the middle line shows the mean values and the upper line shows the 95th percentile values. (From [17], Christensen et al. Reference intervals for reticulocyte parameters of infants during their first 90 days after birth. *J Perinatol* 2016; **36**:61–66.)

(a)   Immature platelet fraction

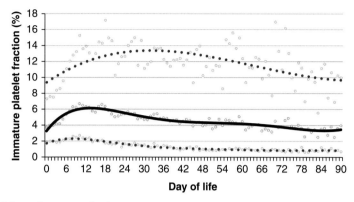

(b)   Immature platelet count

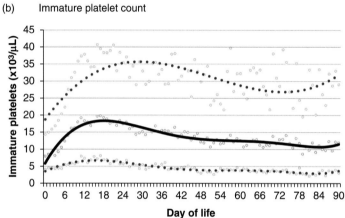

Fig. 24.28 Reference intervals of (a) immature platelet fraction (%) and (b) immature platelets/μL blood, over the first 90 days following birth. (From [65], MacQueen et al. The immature platelet fraction: creating neonatal reference intervals and using these to categorize neonatal thrombocytopenias. *J Perinatol* 2017;**37**:834–8.)

Chapter 15

Congenital Thrombocytopenias and Thrombocytopathies

Amy E. Geddis

Approach to Thrombocytopenia in the Newborn

Thrombocytopenia occurs in less than 1% of all newborns. However, thrombocytopenia is a common finding in the intensive-care nursery where it is present in 25%–35% of admitted infants [1, 2]. See Chapters 12 and 13 for a discussion of the approach to thrombocytopenia as well as acquired causes of thrombocytopenia in newborns. This chapter will focus primarily on the diagnosis and initial management of inherited thrombocytopenia disorders that present in infancy.

Acquired causes of thrombocytopenia are much more common than inherited ones at any age, and thus it can be challenging to recognize the rare situations when thrombocytopenia has a genetic basis. In general, an inherited condition can be suspected in newborns or infants if thrombocytopenia is persistent and unexplained, if there are characteristic findings on the peripheral blood smear, if there are associated congenital abnormalities, or if there is a family history suggestive of a thrombocytopenia syndrome. There are special challenges, however, in trying to identify inherited causes of thrombocytopenia in neonates. First, despite their individual rarity, there is a large number of genetic disorders associated with thrombocytopenia. Mutations in more than 30 different genes have been described in inherited thrombocytopenia syndromes [3]. Diagnosis can be challenging as the phenotype associated with a given mutant gene can vary from patient to patient, and in some disorders characteristic findings may not present until later in life. Laboratory studies can also be difficult to interpret in a young child. Although review of the peripheral blood smear is of key

importance in evaluating patients with thrombocytopenia, there are important caveats to consider when looking at a smear from a newborn. Acquired conditions that lead to increased platelet turnover can result in the finding of large platelets, and white cell inclusions may be seen in the setting of infection. Platelet clumping is a frequent artifact when blood is obtained from a heel stick. Normal ranges for measures such as the red blood cell MCV are higher in newborns than in older infants and adults, and von Willebrand antigen levels are increased due to the influence of maternal hormones. Time may be required to determine if specific findings are persistent. From a practical standpoint, it can be difficult to do an extensive workup on a small baby, due to either limitations in drawing blood or sedation risks, and in some cases it might be reasonable to either delay the evaluation or to try to establish the diagnosis from an affected parent. Finally, the use of genetic testing in young children is controversial: In general, if it will not affect clinical management of the child then one should consider delaying genetic testing until the child is old enough to understand its implications (A. Greinacher, personal communication). On the other hand, a timely genetic diagnosis may be important for counseling the parents about their risk of having another affected child; and may have implications for other family members. It is important that the family receive appropriate genetic counseling, particularly when considering diagnoses that include a risk for cancer. For these reasons and others, it may not be possible to establish a diagnosis of inherited thrombocytopenia in neonates. To allow a broader discussion, this chapter will consider thrombocytopenia in the newborn period and extending through infancy.

Neonatal Hematology, Pathogenesis, Diagnosis, and Management of Hematologic Problems, 3rd edition, ed. Pedro A. de Alarcón, Eric J. Werner, Robert D. Christensen, and Martha C. Sola-Visner. Published by Cambridge University Press.

With these caveats in mind, the approach to the diagnosis of inherited thrombocytopenia should begin with a review of the peripheral blood smear as well as a careful history and physical exam. These evaluations are readily available and can suggest the diagnosis and inform the subsequent workup.

Review of the Peripheral Smear

Review of the peripheral smear is an essential part of any thrombocytopenia evaluation, in particular noting platelet size and granularity, red cell morphology, and the presence or absence of white cell inclusions [4]. Inherited thrombocytopenia syndromes are classified by platelet size [5]. To gauge size on the peripheral smear, platelets can be compared to the diameter of a red blood cell. Platelets that are more than 50% of the diameter of a red cell are considered large, whereas platelets that are greater than the diameter of a red cell are referred to as giant. The mean platelet volume (MPV) reported on most automated cell analyzers is another readily available measure of platelet size, with the caveat that platelets that are very large or very small may be excluded from the analysis. If there are some large or giant platelets present on a background of small or normal sized platelets,

this suggests a state of increased platelet turnover such as is seen in immune thrombocytopenia, type 2B von Willebrand disease or thrombotic thrombocytopenic purpura. A pale or "gray" appearance to the platelets may indicate a deficiency in alpha granules. Platelet clumping may be an artifact, but it is also characteristic of von Willebrand disease type 2B. Red cell polychromasia suggests hemolysis. The presence of schistocytes suggests that hemolysis is due to a microangiopathic process such as thrombotic thrombocytopenic purpura, whereas stomatocytes should trigger consideration of sitosterolemia. Macrocytosis can be seen in the setting of underlying marrow failure syndromes such as Fanconi anemia, Diamond–Blackfan anemia or dyskeratosis congenita. Granulocytes should be carefully examined for the presence of Dohle-like inclusion bodies that are diagnostic of *MYH9*-related disorder. Representative peripheral smear findings are shown in Fig. 15.1.

Family History

A careful family history may establish the inheritance pattern as autosomal dominant, autosomal recessive, X-linked, or sporadic. If the parents are

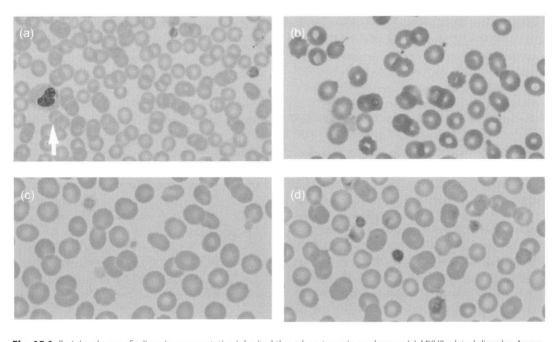

Fig. 15.1 Peripheral smear findings in representative inherited thrombocytopenia syndromes. (a) *MYH9*-related disorder. Arrow indicates neutrophil with a Dohle-like inclusion. (b) Small platelets in Wiskott–Aldrich syndrome. (c) Pale platelets in Gray platelet syndrome. (d) Large platelets in Bernard–Soulier syndrome. Magnification 100×. (Images courtesy of Alan Cantor.) (See plate section for color version.)

related or if they are from similar ethnic or religious backgrounds, the chances of an autosomal recessive condition are increased. Thrombocytopenia that is asymptomatic may be unrecognized, so it cannot always be assumed that a family member is unaffected if they have not been tested. In addition, some thrombocytopenia syndromes include a predisposition to complications that may not manifest until later in childhood or in adulthood, such as bone marrow failure, myelodysplasia or leukemia, renal failure, deafness, pulmonary or hepatic fibrosis, or other cancers. A detailed history that includes three generations may provide important clues to the diagnosis.

Exam Findings

While congenital abnormalities do not always accompany inherited thrombocytopenia syndromes, if present they may help to establish the diagnosis. It is important to examine the forearms carefully. Bilateral radial hypoplasia or aplasia is a feature of thrombocytopenia with absent radii. If thumbs are missing or otherwise abnormal, then Fanconi anemia should be considered. Radioulnar synostosis, which can be detected by the limitation of rotational movement of the forearm, has been associated with mutations in several genes, including *MECOM* and *HOXA11*. Plain X-rays of the forearms can be useful to detect subtle abnormalities. Additional anomalies, such as poor growth, renal or cardiac malformations, developmental delay, or hearing loss, may indicate the presence of a congenital syndrome associated with thrombocytopenia. Congenital abnormalities are frequent in inherited bone marrow failure syndromes such as Diamond–Blackfan anemia and Fanconi anemia. While Diamond–Blackfan anemia is classically thought to be a "pure red cell aplasia," thrombocytopenia or neutropenia may be present or even dominate the clinical picture, particularly in the newborn period [6]. Similarly, low platelets may be the first cytopenia to be recognized in children with Fanconi anemia. Thrombocytopenia is common in a range of other congenital disorders such as Paris-Trousseau syndrome, Noonan syndrome, del22q11.2 syndrome and trisomy 13, 18 or 21. In contrast, other inherited platelet disorders, such as congenital amegakaryocytic thrombocytopenia, are not associated with congenital abnormalities and may be initially difficult to differentiate from acquired causes of low platelets such as auto- or alloimmune thrombocytopenia.

Subsequent Evaluations and Supportive Care

Depending on the suspected diagnosis, additional evaluations may be appropriate (see Table 15.1).

Tools for the management of bleeding symptoms in children with inherited thrombocytopenia include platelet transfusions and antifibrinolytics. In infants, platelets are dosed at 10–15 milliliters per kilogram. Standard recommendations dictate that all blood products should be leukocyte reduced; leukocyte reduction minimizes the occurrence of febrile reactions, prevents transmission of CMV, and reduces alloimmunization. Irradiation of blood products should be performed if the donor is closely related, or if the recipient is suspected to have immunodeficiency. Irradiation of blood projects is also recommended for in utero transfusions and in patients who have received in utero transfusions (See Chapter 20 Transfusion Practices) [7]. Antifibrinolytics such as aminocaproic acid (Amicar) can be useful if bleeding involves a mucous membrane such as the nose or mouth; Amicar is contraindicated in the setting of urogenital tract bleeding. Specific diagnostic and management strategies will be discussed in the context of the individual diagnoses.

It is beyond the scope of this chapter to describe all of the genes now associated with inherited thrombocytopenia. The discussion that follows will focus on disorders that are likely to have implications for management in infancy, either for treatment of the child or counseling of the family. Disorders will be grouped as classical inherited thrombocytopenia syndromes, congenital syndromes with associated thrombocytopenia, and inherited disorders in which thrombocytopenia is related to abnormalities of vWF and increased platelet destruction. A comparison of diagnostic findings is summarized in Table 15.2.

Inherited Thrombocytopenia Syndromes

In these disorders, thrombocytopenia tends to be the presenting finding and mutations directly affect megakaryocyte or platelet production.

Wiskott–Aldrich Syndrome (MIM #301000)

Wiskott-Aldrich syndrome (WAS) is an X-linked disorder in which thrombocytopenia with small

Table 15.1 Common investigations used in the evaluation of inherited thrombocytopenia

Study	Useful to assess	Diagnostic implications
Complete blood count	Blood counts and parameters	All
Reticulocyte count	Red cell production	DBA, TTP
Immature platelet fraction	Platelet production	VWD2B, TTP
Peripheral smear	Morphology of blood cells	All
Bone marrow aspiration and biopsy	Marrow cellularity, megakaryocyte number, dysplasia, fibrosis, storage disorder	CAMT, RUSAT, FA and DC, GPS, RUNX1, ANKRD26, ETV6
Platelet aggregation	Platelet function	BSS, GT
Platelet electron microscopy	Platelet granules	GPS, PTS
Immunologic studies	Hypogammaglobulinemia, lymphopenia	WAS, DC, 22q11.2 deletion, RUSAT
Chromosomal breakage studies	DNA repair defect	FA
Cytogenetic studies	Numerical abnormalities, deletions or translocations of chromosomes	Trisomies, 22q11.2 deletion, PTS
von Willebrand assays	vWF activity, multimers	VWD2B, TTP
ADAMTS13 activity	Microangiopathic hemolytic anemia	TTP
Forearm xrays	Radial hypoplasia, radioulnar synostosis	TAR, RUSAT, FA
Echocardiogram	Congenital heart defects	FA, TAR, DBA, 22q11.2 del, PTS, NS
Abdominal US	Renal abnormalities	FA, DBA, TAR
Brain MRI	Cerebellar hypoplasia	DC/HHS
Genetic studies	Specific mutation analysis	All

Abbreviations: DBA (Diamond–Blackfan anemia), TTP (thrombotic thrombocytopenic purpura), vWD (von Willebrand disease), CAMT (congenital amegakaryocytic thrombocytopenia), RUSAT (radioulnar synostosis with amegakaryocytic thrombocytopenia), FA (Fanconi anemia), DC (dyskeratosis congenita), GPS (gray platelet syndrome), BSS (Bernard–Soulier syndrome), GT (Glanzmann thrombasthenia), PTS (Paris-Trousseau syndrome), WAS (Wiskott–Aldrich syndrome), NS (Noonan syndrome), HHS (Hoyeraal–Hreidarsson syndrome).

platelets is associated with eczema, immunodeficiency and a high risk of EBV-associated lymphoma [8–10]. Wiskott–Aldrich syndrome is rare, with an incidence of approximately one to four cases per 1,000,000 live male births, and an average age at diagnosis of 24 months in the absence of a known family history [11]. The disease is due to mutation in the *WAS* gene located on chromosome Xp11.23, encoding Wiskott–Aldrich associated protein (WASp), a protein that is important for actin polymerization and cytoskeletal rearrangement [12]. There is considerable variation in the clinical severity in patients with *WAS* mutations [13]. Thrombocytopenia may be mild or severe, with approximately half of affected boys having platelet counts <20,000/ul; bleeding symptoms generally correlate with the degree of thrombocytopenia and can include gastrointestinal and intracranial hemorrhage [11, 14]. Although eczema is considered part of the

classic presentation of WAS, it may not always be present or may develop later in childhood. In one series, fewer than 30% of patients had the complete triad of thrombocytopenia, eczema, and immunodeficiency, and 20% had thrombocytopenia alone [11]. *WAS* mutations that lead to isolated thrombocytopenia may be referred to as X-linked thrombocytopenia, although mutations in *GATA1* also cause thrombocytopenia with X-linked inheritance [15]. In addition to small platelets, laboratory findings that suggest WAS include reduced numbers of T-lymphocytes and abnormal immunoglobulins [16]. The diagnosis can be confirmed by flow cytometry showing reduced or absent expression of WASp in lymphocytes, or mutational analysis of the *WAS* gene [10]. Management of WAS must take into account not only the bleeding symptoms but also the significant risk for infection, autoimmune manifestations and EBV-associated lymphoma related to

Table 15.2 Comparison of findings in inherited thrombocytopenia syndromes

Diagnosis	Platelet size	Associated blood cell morphology	Inheritance	Associated Genes	Associated features in childhood
Wiskott–Aldrich Syndrome	Small		XLR	WASP	Immunodeficiency, eczema
Congenital amegakaryocytic thrombocytopenia	Normal		AR	c-MPL	Reduced or absent megakaryocytes
Thrombocytopenia with absent radii	Normal		Compound heterozygosity	RBM8A	Absent radii
Radioulnar synostosis with amegakaryocytic thrombocytopenia	Normal		AD	MECOM HOX11A	Radioulnar synostosis
Thrombocytopenia with predisposition to myeloid malignancy	Normal		AD	RUNX1 ANKRD26 ETV6	Family history of MDS or leukemia
Bernard–Soulier syndrome	Large		AR	GPIB, GP9	Platelet dysfunction
MYH9-related disease	Large	WBC inclusions	AD	MYH9	Family history of renal dysfunction, hearing loss, cataracts
Gray platelet syndrome	Large	Platelets with alpha granule deficiency	AR	NBEAL2	
GATA1 mutation	Large	Platelets with alpha granule deficiency	XLR	GATA1	Anemia
Sitosterolemia	Large	Red cell stomatocytes	AR	ABCG5, ABCG8	Hemolysis, high cholesterol
Fanconi anemia	Normal	Red cell macrocytosis	AR/XLR	Multiple	Congenital anomalies, abnormal chromosomal breakage
Dyskeratosis congenita	Normal	Red cell macrocytosis	AD/AR/XLR	Multiple	IUGR, cerebellar hypoplasia, immunodeficiency, lacrimal duct stenosis, nail dysplasia, shortened telomeres
Paris Trousseau syndrome	Normal	Platelets with fused alpha granules	Sporadic	Del11q23	Heart defects, developmental delay
Noonan syndrome	Normal		AD	PTPN11	Heart defects, lymphatic malformations
22q11.2 deletion syndrome	Large		Sporadic	Del 22q11.2	Heart defects, T-cell dysfunction
von Willebrand disease type 2B	Large	Platelet clumping	AD	VWF	von Willebrand factor deficiency
Platelet-type von Willebrand disease	Large	Platelet clumping	AD	GPIB	von Willebrand factor deficiency
Thrombotic thrombocytopenic purpura	Large	Schistocytes	AR	ADAMTS13	Hemolysis, renal insufficiency

the associated immunodeficiency [10, 11]. Patients should be referred for early consideration of hematopoietic stem cell transplant, which is the current standard for definitive therapy. Due to the associated immunodeficiency, transfused blood products including platelets should be irradiated to prevent transfusion-associated graft vs. host disease. Intravenous immunoglobulin therapy is unlikely to improve platelet counts [17], although it is important for prevention of infection and may improve symptoms related to autoimmunity. Splenectomy may improve platelet counts in patients with X-linked thrombocytopenia, although it has been associated with greater risk of bacteremia and death [11]; additionally splenectomy has been associated with an inferior outcome in patients who undergo hematopoietic stem cell transplant [18, 19]. The role of the newer thrombopoietin receptor agonists, such as Eltrombopag and Romiplostim, in patients with Wiskott–Aldrich syndrome remain unclear, though they may be a valuable adjunct as a bridge to transplant [20, 21].

Congenital Amegakaryocytic Thrombocytopenia (MIM #604498)

Congenital amegakaryocytic thrombocytopenia (CAMT) typically presents as thrombocytopenia in an otherwise well infant. CAMT is an autosomal recessive disease caused by mutations in the receptor for thrombopoietin, c-MPL. Thrombopoietin signaling is essential not only for megakaryocyte and platelet production but also for the maintenance of hematopoietic stem cells [22–24]. Fewer than 100 cases of CAMT have been reported in the literature, although more have certainly been diagnosed. At birth, most affected infants have isolated thrombocytopenia. Evaluation of the bone marrow shows a selective deficiency of megakaryocytes, although occasionally initial marrows may appear relatively normal [25]. Over time, most patients will progress to pancytopenia with trilineage marrow aplasia. An increased incidence of MDS and AML is also reported [26]. Genotype–phenotype correlation studies show that patients who have mutations resulting in absent expression of c-MPL (type I mutations) have persistent thrombocytopenia from birth and develop pancytopenia at a median age of 22 months. In comparison, patients whose mutations result in residual expression of c-MPL (type II mutations) may have transient improvement of their platelet counts after birth, followed by a recurrence of thrombocytopenia and a later onset of marrow failure at a median of 28 months [27]. While physical abnormalities have been described in patients with CAMT, there is no specific pattern associated with the diagnosis [27]. Neurologic abnormalities have been seen, including polymicrogyra, underdevelopment of the cerebellum and absence of the corpus callosum [27–29]; some findings might be attributable to

sequelae of intracranial hemorrhage [30]. Once suspected, the diagnosis of CAMT is confirmed by genetic testing. If clinically available, a serum thrombopoietin level can be helpful. In the setting of pathogenic c-MPL mutations, serum thrombopoietin levels are very high, often as much as tenfold above normal, due to absent thrombopoietin uptake and clearance from the circulation [31, 32]. If the clinical picture is consistent with CAMT but thrombopoietin levels are unexpectedly low, then mutations in the gene for thrombopoeitin itself can be investigated [33, 34]. Treatment of CAMT is initially supportive, but hematopoietic stem cell transplant is recommended once there is onset of trilineage marrow failure [27]. In the rare case that CAMT is due to a mutation in thrombopoietin, then treatment with recombinant thrombopoietin or a thrombopoietin receptor agonist may be effective [33].

Thrombocytopenia with Absent Radii (MIM #274000)

Thrombocytopenia with absent radii (TAR) is usually recognized at birth or even prenatally by the eponymous findings of thrombocytopenia and bilateral radial abnormalities [35–37]. The prevalence of TAR is estimated at 1:200,000–1:100,000. Radii may be hypoplastic or absent. Additional limb abnormalities may be seen, but importantly thumbs are present. Affected children may also have congenital heart or urogenital defects. Eosinophilia and cow's milk allergy are common, and exposure to cow's milk may exacerbate thrombocytopenia. Defects in platelet function may be present and lead to an increased severity of bleeding symptoms [38, 39]. Leukemoid reactions may occur, leading to concerns about malignant transformation. The differential diagnosis of thrombocytopenia in children with radial hypoplasia or aplasia includes Fanconi anemia. Thumbs are always present in TAR, whereas they may be absent or hypoplastic in Fanconi anemia. Radial aplasia has also been reported in the 22q11 deletion syndrome [40]. The genetic basis of TAR has only recently been elucidated [41, 42]. Affected patients have compound heterozygous mutations affecting the gene RBM8A, which encodes the exon-junction complex subunit member Y14 [43]. Typically, one mutation is a microdeletion on chromosome 1q21.1, encompassing the RBM8A gene, and the second mutation is a noncoding variant involving either the 5'UTR or first intron of the remaining *RBM8A* allele. Confirmation of the carrier status for the parents can be useful in counseling them regarding recurrence risks should they wish to have more children. Curiously, thrombocytopenia in patients with TAR but usually improves after the first year of life, so most patients can be managed with supportive care, including avoidance of cow's milk, until platelet counts improve. Data regarding long-term outcomes in patients with TAR are sparse but intermittent thrombocytopenia may recur. Leukemia, both lymphoid and myeloid, has been reported [44, 45].

Thrombocytopenia with Radioulnar Synostosis

Radioulnar synostosis with amegakaryocytic thrombocytopenia (RUSAT), has been attributed to mutations in *MECOM* (*RUSAT2*, MIM #616738) as well as *HOXA11* (*RUSAT1*, MIM #605432). *MECOM* encodes the zinc-finger transcription factor EVI1, which has an important role in hematopoietic stem cell renewal [46–48]. Heterozygous mutations in *MECOM* have been associated with a range of findings including thrombocytopenia, radioulnar synostosis, clinodactyly, cardiac or renal malformations, B-cell deficiency and hearing loss [49, 50]. Not all patients with *MECOM* mutations have radioulnar synostosis, and thus some authors suggest that the disease should be called *MECOM*-associated syndrome, to reflect the variety of clinical presentations [49]. Three patients from two families with thrombocytopenia and radioulnar synostosis were found to have heterozygous mutations in *HOXA11* [51]. Treatment of thrombocytopenia is generally supportive, however evolution to trilineage marrow failure or MDS is common [49, 51, 52], and thus identification of potential donors should occur early in the event that a hematopoietic stem cell transplant is needed.

Thrombocytopenia with Increased Risk of Leukemia

Autosomal dominant mutations in several genes are associated with thrombocytopenia with a markedly increased risk for development of myelodysplastic syndrome (MDS) or leukemia. Mutations in *RUNX1* (MIM #601399) were the first to be described as causing the syndrome of

Thrombocytopenia with Predisposition to Myeloid Malignancy [53], and subsequently mutations in *ANKRD26* (MIM #188000) and *ETV6* (MIM #616216) were also found to increase the risk for leukemia [54–56]. Thrombocytopenia can be mild and may not be recognized in the newborn period; the family history may lead to initial testing, or low platelets may be discovered incidentally. Patients with *RUNX1* mutations may have platelet dysfunction in addition to thrombocytopenia, which can exacerbate bleeding tendencies. The risk of developing MDS or acute myeloid leukemia (AML) may be as high as 50% in affected family members with *RUNX1* mutations, and although this most commonly occurs in adults it may occur at any age [53, 57]. Interesting, mutations in *RUNX1* are also associated with an increased risk for T-lymphoblastic lymphoma, and *ETV6* is associated with MDS, AML, and B-lymphoblastic leukemia [58–60]. Because acquired mutations in *RUNX1* and *ETV6* are common in MDS and leukemia, it is important to confirm the germline nature of mutations either by identification of the mutation in other family members or in DNA isolated from a non-hematologic tissue such as skin fibroblasts. Management of infants with *RUNX1*, *ANKRD26* or *ETV6* mutations includes supportive care for bleeding symptoms and genetic counseling. Older children and adults should have regular monitoring of blood counts and bone marrow studies to identify changes suggesting evolution towards malignancy which would be an indication for hematopoietic stem cell transplant [61]. Family members should receive genetic counseling and mutation testing should be considered regardless of their platelet counts; it is additionally important to clarify the mutational status of any family member being considered as a hematopoietic stem cell donor.

Bernard–Soulier Syndrome (MIM #231200)

Bernard–Soulier syndrome (BSS) is caused by mutations that affect the expression of the GPIB/IX/V complex on the platelet surface, which serves as the receptor for von Willebrand factor (vWF) [62, 63]. It is inherited as an autosomal recessive disorder, although rare cases of monozygous mutations have been described [64, 65]. The prevalence of BSS is estimated at 1:1,000,000. Patients with BSS have large platelets and bleeding symptoms that are out of proportion to the degree of thrombocytopenia, due to the impaired binding of platelets to vWF. It is important to recognize the platelet dysfunction in patients with BSS and not use the platelet count alone to make clinical decisions regarding hemostasis. Management is supportive; however, while platelet transfusions are effective, they should be reserved for clinically significant bleeding or major procedures due to the risk for alloimmunization, with development of anti-HLA or -GPIb/IX antibodies that might limit efficacy of future transfusions [66]. To minimize the risk for alloimmunization, transfused platelets should be leukocyte reduced and, if feasible, HLA matched. Antifibrinolytics can be particularly helpful as platelet-sparing agents in management of mucous membrane bleeding. Desmopressin or DDAVP, which may improve hemostasis in patients with patients with platelet function abnormalities, should not be used in infants due to the risk of hyponatremia. The role of rFVIIa is unclear, however there are reports supporting its efficacy in patients with BSS where platelets are not effective [67–69].

MYH9-Related Disease (MIM #155100)

Macrothrombocytopenia that is inherited in an autosomal dominant fashion is seen in MYH9-related disease [70]. The prevalence is unknown, though it is one of the more common causes of familial thrombocytopenia in the Italian registry [5]. The identification of mutations in MYH9, a non-muscle myosin heavy chain gene, allowed reclassification of several diseases, including May–Hegglin anomaly, Sebastian platelet syndrome, Fechtner syndrome, Epstein syndrome, and autosomal deafness *DFNA17*, as variants of a single disorder [71, 72]. In addition to large and frequently giant platelets, which may be larger than erythrocytes, careful evaluation of the peripheral smear may reveal Dohle-like white cell inclusions. Where available, detection of these inclusions is enhanced by the use of immunofluorescent staining techniques [4]. Genetic testing may not be necessary to make the diagnosis. Treatment of thrombocytopenia is supportive, however, the majority of the morbidity in *MYH9*-related disease comes not from bleeding symptoms but from the late onset of renal disease, sensorineural deafness, or cataracts. Renal

disease, characterized by progressive proteinuric nephropathy, develops in approximately 25% of patients and may progress to renal failure [73]. Although these complications are not anticipated during infancy, families should be educated about the importance of ongoing follow up. Parents should be referred for evaluation if they have not already been tested.

Gray Platelet Syndrome

Gray platelet syndrome can be suspected on the basis of laboratory findings, including thrombocytopenia with large platelets that are pale in appearance on a peripheral blood smear. The pale appearance of the platelets is due to lack of intracellular alpha granules, which contain a diverse array of compounds released on platelet activation such as vWF, thrombospondin, factor V, fibroblast growth factor and others [74]. The absence of platelet alpha granules can be confirmed by electron microscopy. Two different inheritance patterns have been associated with gray platelet syndrome. Mutations in *NBEAL2* (MIM #139090), encoding a protein important for intracellular vesicle trafficking, are inherited in an autosomal recessive fashion [75–77]. Mutations in the hematopoietic transcription factor *GATA1* (MIM #300367, #314050) are inherited as X-linked recessive traits [78]. *GATA1* regulates the expression of *NBEAL2* [79], thus explaining the overlapping phenotypes resulting from mutations in these different genes. As *GATA1* regulates genes critical for both megakaryopoiesis and erythropoiesis, it is not surprising that mutations in this transcription factor may also be associated with a variety of red cell abnormalities, including dyserythropoeisis, thalassemia, or even porphyria [15]. Because many of the components of the alpha granules have roles in hemostasis, platelet function in gray platelet syndrome is abnormal [80]. Bone marrow biopsy would not typically be pursued in the newborn period; however, marrows performed in older patients may show myelofibrosis and megakaryocyte emperipolesis [80, 81]. Management involves supportive care.

Congenital Syndromes with Associated Thrombocytopenia

In many of the inherited bone marrow failure syndromes, cytopenias are not typically present at birth but the diagnosis may be suspected on the basis of other congenital abnormalities or a family history [82]. Markers of stress erythropoiesis, such as elevated fetal hemoglobin or macrocytosis, which can be useful screening tools in older patients, are less helpful in newborns. In other congenital syndromes, not classified as marrow failure disorders, thrombocytopenia may be an associated finding.

Fanconi Anemia (MIM 607139)

Fanconi anemia is an inherited bone marrow failure syndrome caused by a defect in DNA repair (reviewed in [83]). In addition to cytopenias, patients with Fanconi anemia commonly have congenital abnormalities and are at a significantly increased risk for cancer. The prevalence of Fanconi anemia is estimated at 1–5 per million, and is more common in people of Ashekanzi Jewish descent, the Roma population of Spain and black South Africans due to the presence of founder mutations in those populations [84–86]. Bone marrow failure most commonly develops in the first decade of life, with a median age of 7 years, but occasionally may be seen in the newborn period. Thrombocytopenia may be the presenting hematologic abnormality [82]. More frequently, infants with Fanconi anemia are recognized on the basis of associated congenital anomalies such as poor growth, thumb or forearm abnormalities, café au lait spots, VACTERL syndrome (Vertebral defects, Anal atresia, Cardiac defects, Tracho-Esophageal fistula, Renal anomalies, and Limb abnormalities) and others. Fanconi anemia is diagnosed by demonstration of abnormal chromosomal breakage in the presence of clastogens such as diepoxybutane or mitomycin C. Mutations involving more than 18 genes have been identified [83], defining subypes of the disease. Eighty to 90% of cases are due to mutations in FANCA, FANCC, or FANCG. Inheritance is autosomal recessive, with the exception of FANCB which is inherited in an X-linked recessive pattern [87]. Although the diagnosis is made by demonstration of chromosomal fragility, confirmation of the subtype is important for counseling. Due to the increased risk for cancers, including hematologic and non-hematologic malignancies, patients with Fanconi anemia require ongoing follow up and screening to maximize opportunities for early detection when outcomes are best [83, 88].

Dyskeratosis Congenita

Dyskeratosis congenita is an inherited marrow failure syndrome caused by defects in telomere maintenance. The classic clinical triad consists of skin and nail abnormalities, oral leukoplakia and bone marrow failure, but in fact this triad is present in only a minority of patients; other symptoms such as pulmonary or liver fibrosis, strictures or premature graying may also be seen, and patients are at increased risk of developing malignancy [89, 90]. Most commonly, symptoms in dyskeratosis congenita do not present until later in life, but severe mutations may present in infancy. Hoyeraal–Hreidarsson syndrome is a severe form of dyskeratosis congenita diagnosed in infancy with findings including cytopenias, intrauterine growth retardation, cerebellar hypoplasia, developmental delay, immunodeficiency, and lacrimal duct stenosis [91–94]. Another severe variant of dyskeratosis congenita that can present in early childhood is Revesz syndrome, characterized by exudative retinopathy and intracranial calcification in addition to the features above, and associated with mutations in TINF2 [89, 95]. The diagnosis of dyskeratosis congenita can be confirmed by the finding of very short telomeres. Mutations in at least 11 genes associated with telomere maintenance are recognized, including DKC1 (MIM #305000), TERT (MIM #613989), and others, though not all causative mutations have been identified [90, 96]. Inheritance varies and can include autosomal dominant, autosomal recessive and X-linked recessive patterns. Children with Hoyeraal–Hreidarsson syndrome are at risk for death in early childhood due to the complications of marrow failure unless they can be successfully transplanted [97].

Paris Trousseau Syndrome (MIM #188025)

Paris Trousseau syndrome (PTS) is a variant of Jacobsen syndrome (MIM 147791) in which thrombocytopenia accompanies congenital cardiac defects such as hypoplastic left heart syndrome and developmental delay [98–101]. Cytogenetic studies show deletion of the terminal portion of chromosome 11q23, encompassing the locus for the megakaryocytic transcription factor FLI1 which is responsible for the platelet phenotype [100, 102,

103]. Bone marrow findings may include micro-megakaryocytes, and ultrastructural studies of platelets may show giant, fused alpha granules and a reduction of dense granules [104]. Consistent with the importance of FLI1 in PTS, isolated mutations in FLI1 have been identified in families with thrombocytopenia and platelet granule abnormalities resembling those seen in patients with PTS [105, 106]. Treatment is generally supportive. Thrombocytopenia tends to improve later in infancy, though platelet function may remain abnormal [107].

Noonan Syndrome

Noonan syndrome is an autosomal dominant disorder associated with abnormal facies, developmental delay, short stature, congenital heart defects, renal anomalies, lymphatic malformations, and bleeding disorders [108]. Its estimated prevalence is between 1:1,000 and 1:2,500 living births. Noonan syndrome is caused by a gain of function mutation in PTPN11, encoding a cytoplasmic protein tyrosine phosphatase called SHP2 that has important regulatory roles in the Ras/MAPK and PI3K pathways [109]. Thrombocytopenia is not usually the dominant symptom in Noonan syndrome, but infants may present with very low platelets [110, 111]. In addition to thrombocytopenia, laboratory abnormalities of hemostasis, including reduced coagulation and platelet function, have been described in the majority of patients [112]. Children with Noonan syndrome are at increased risk for malignancy, such as juvenile myelomonocytic leukemia (JMML) [113, 114] and other cancers [114].

The 22q11.2 Deletion Syndrome

The 22q11.2 deletion syndrome is one of the most commonly diagnosed chromosomal microdeletion syndromes in humans and is associated with a variety of abnormalities including facial abnormalities, palatal abnormalities, cardiac defects and thymic hypoplasia or aplasia [115]. Mild macrothrombocytopenia is commonly associated with the 22q11.2 deletion syndrome, and is thought to be related to heterozygous deletion of the GPIBB gene, located within the deleted portion of chromosome 22 [116, 117]. In the majority of patients, this thrombocytopenia does not result in clinically significant bleeding. Rarely, co-inheritance of a second mutation in GPIBB can lead to true Bernard–Soulier syndrome [118]. Patients with 22q11.2 deletion syndrome are also at increased risk of immune thrombocytopenia (ITP), given their underlying T-cell dysfunction [119], so if thrombocytopenia follows an acquired course, ITP should be considered.

In addition to the congenital disorders described above, thrombocytopenia is common in infants with trisomies 13, 18, and 21. In the first week of life, 83% of infants with trisomy 18 and 75% of those with trisomy 13 were noted to be thrombocytopenic [120]. Several metabolic disorders are associated with thrombocytopenia. Lysosomal storage diseases such as Gaucher disease may present in the newborn period with low platelets [121, 122], and thrombocytopenia may be part of the clinical spectrum in mitochondrial disorders [123]. Sitosterolemia, or Mediterranean macrothrombocytopenia, is caused by mutations in ABCG5 or ABCG8, which encode the sterol efflux transporters sterolin-1 and -2, resulting in accumulation of phytosterols. Affected patients have macrothrombocytopenia and hemolytic anemia, and a review of the smear may show stomatocytes [124–127]. Symptoms may develop in infancy, potentially exacerbated by the use of soy-based formulas or intralipids [128]. While rare, recognition and treatment of an underlying metabolic disorder can avoid important extrahematopoietic complications and may mitigate thrombocytopenia.

Inherited Disorders Associated with Abnormalities of vWF

In some cases, familial thrombocytopenia is associated with increased platelet consumption due to abnormalities of vWF. Examples include type 2B von Willebrand disease (vWD; MIM #613554) and congenital thrombotic thrombocytopenic purpura (TTP; MIM #274150). Thrombocytopenia in these disorders is variable but may be exacerbated in the newborn period given that expression of vWF is increased at birth due to the effects of maternal estrogens, and women may have worsening of their thrombocytopenia during pregnancy for the same reason. Type 2B von Willebrand disease is caused by an activating mutation of VWF that increases its affinity for GPIB on platelets, resulting in increased platelet clearance and loss of high molecular weight vWF multimers. A reciprocal mutation in GPIB that increases its affinity for vWF has a similar phenotype and is called platelet-type vWD. In both disorders, platelet clumps that represent large complexes between platelets and the abnormal vWF may be visible on the peripheral blood smear [129]. The inheritance pattern is autosomal dominant. Bleeding is related primarily to the deficiency of vWF but in severe cases thrombocytopenia may contribute [130]. The diagnosis is suspected if the patient has both low vWF activity and thrombocytopenia; additional laboratory findings may include the loss of high molecular weight vWF multimers. Genetic studies can distinguish between type 2B vWD, and platelet-type vWD. This is most readily achieved by sequencing of vWF exon 28 for the pathogenic variant vWF c.3922C>T, p.Arg1308Cys [130]. Bleeding in patients with type 2B vWD is managed with vWF-containing products and antifibrinolytics [129, 130]. DDAVP is not appropriate in infants due to the risk of hyponatremia and it can exacerbate thrombocytopenia in patients with type 2B disease. In platelet-type vWD, vWF replacement is not effective and platelet transfusion should be used instead [131].

In congenital TTP, deficiency of the von Willebrand cleavage factor ADAMTS13 results in the formation of ultralarge von Willebrand factor multimers and a non-immune, microangiopathic hemolytic anemia. The finding of schistocytes on the peripheral blood smear is the hallmark of this diagnosis. The associated hemolytic anemia may lead to prolonged neonatal jaundice, and renal insufficiency or neuropsychiatric symptoms may also be present [132, 133]. Beyond the newborn period, symptoms may be episodic. Inheritance is autosomal recessive and the diagnosis can be confirmed by the finding of severe deficiency of ADAMTS13 (activity <10%) and identification of homozygous or compound heterozygous mutations. Treatment of congenital TTP includes plasma infusion, to replace the missing ADAMTS13 enzyme activity. Plasma infusions are given daily until clinical stabilization and then prophylactically to control symptoms [134]. The platelet count can be used as a marker of clinical response. Novel approaches to ADAMTS13 replacement, including recombinant products and gene therapy, are in development [135].

Inherited Defects in Platelet Function with Normal Platelet Counts

Glanzmann's Thrombasthenia (MIM #273800)

Glanzmann thrombasthenia (GT) is associated with severe bleeding due to abnormal platelet function, although platelet counts are normal. Symptoms are present at birth. Approximately 500 cases have been reported. GT is caused by autosomal recessive mutations in the gene encoding either platelet glycoprotein alpha-IIb (ITGA2B) or platelet glycoprotein IIIa (ITGB3), with resultant lack of αIIbβ3 integrin expression and deficient platelet aggregation and clot retraction. Patients with GT typically have mucocutaneous bleeding, spontaneous bruising and epistaxis. Intracranial hemorrhage may occur and women typically have excessive menstrual bleeding. Coagulation studies including prothrombin time (PT), activated partial thromboplastin time (aPTT), and fibrinogen are normal and platelet counts and morphology are also normal. Once suspected, the diagnosis can be confirmed by platelet aggregometry showing failure of aggregation to all agonists except for ristocetin [136, 137]; evaluation of platelet glycoprotein receptor expression by flow cytometry can also be performed. Management of bleeding includes use of antifibrinolytics, local measures and recombinant factor VIIA; while platelet transfusions are effective, there is a high rate of alloimmunization and thus they should be reserved for clinically significant bleeding not responding to other therapies [69, 138]. When used, platelets should be leukocyte reduced and, where possible, HLA-matched, to reduce the risks of alloimmunization. Importantly, neonatal alloimmune thrombocytopenia may occur in unaffected infants of mothers with GT, and can cause significant bleeding that is refractory to transfusion [138, 139].

Genetic Testing Strategies

Although genetic testing is now readily available, deciding when to test and what tests to send can be challenging. It is helpful to fully characterize the patient's phenotype and family history prior to initiation of genetic studies, in order to select the appropriate test and interpret the results. It is important to work with a genetics counselor who is familiar with the available tests to choose the appropriate study as well as counsel the family about anticipated or returned results. Several categories of tests are available and have both limitations and benefits.

Single Gene Studies

The advantage of single gene studies is that they are generally the least expensive and, because fewer genes are being examined, the likelihood of finding variants of uncertain significance is lower. In addition, mutations in an unrelated gene, which may not have been intentionally targeted, are not going to be inadvertently discovered. However, if no mutation is found and an inherited condition is strongly suspected, additional genes may need to be examined, which can extend the time and expense required to make a diagnosis. Single gene analyses are particularly well suited for performing family studies when the mutation has already been established.

Next-Generation Sequencing Panels

Next-generation sequencing panels that contain an array of genes associated with a similar phenotype are increasingly popular. These assays are an efficient way to examine multiple candidate genes simultaneously, and, given the amount of information that is returned, they are relatively inexpensive. Panels vary as to which genes they include, and they may not be able to detect copy number variants or certain intronic mutations. Although convenient, by examining a large number of genes there is an increased possibility to find variants of unclear significance, which may be difficult to interpret, or to discover unexpected mutations with potential clinical implications for the patient and family members. For example, *BRCA2* is included in many panels due to its association with Fanconi anemia, and identification of a heterozygous *BRCA2* mutation may lead to new concerns about predisposition to breast cancer without necessarily answering questions about thrombocytopenia. It is important to counsel families about its limitations and the possibility of these unexpected findings prior to sending them for testing.

Whole Exome Sequencing

When suspicion of an inherited disorder is high and more targeted testing approaches have not yielded a diagnosis, whole exome sequencing can be considered. Despite its comprehensive nature, mutations that do not affect coding regions of the genome can still be missed. Genetic counseling is indicated both to ensure the family understands the possible ramifications of this approach, including unexpected findings, and to facilitate obtaining financial clearance.

Even with extensive sequencing for mutations in known genes associated with inherited thrombocytopenia, many patients remain without a diagnosis. A recent study of the use of high throughput next-generation sequencing to diagnose a cohort of patients with suspected inherited thrombocytopenia only yielded a diagnosis in about 35% of patients [140], though others have reported success in establishing a molecular diagnosis in 70% of their cohort [141]. The sensitivity of sequencing assays will vary on the nature of the panel used and the likelihood of an inherited disorder in the patient being tested.

In summary, inherited disorders are a rare but important cause of thrombocytopenia in newborns and infants. A careful evaluation of the peripheral smear, physical findings, and the family history can guide subsequent testing. An accurate diagnosis may have important implications for patient management and family counseling.

References

1. Murray NA. Evaluation and treatment of thrombocytopenia in the neonatal intensive care unit. *Acta Paediatr Suppl* 2002;**91**(438):74–81.

2. Garcia MG, Duenas E, Sola MC, et al. Epidemiologic and outcome studies of patients who received platelet transfusions in the neonatal intensive care unit. *J Perinatol* 2001;**21**(7):415–20.

3. Noris P, Pecci A. Hereditary thrombocytopenias: A growing list of disorders. *Hematology Am Soc Hematol Educ Program* 2017;**2017**(1):385–99.

4. Greinacher A, Pecci A, Kunishima S, et al. Diagnosis of inherited platelet disorders on a blood smear: A tool to facilitate worldwide diagnosis of platelet disorders. *J Thromb Haemost* 2017;**15**(7):1511–21.

5. Noris P, Biino G, Pecci A, et al. Platelet diameters in inherited thrombocytopenias: Analysis of 376

patients with all known disorders. *Blood* 2014;**124** (6):e4-e10.

6. Buchanan GR, Alter BP, Holtkamp CA, Walsh EG. Platelet number and function in Diamond-Blackfan anemia. *Pediatrics* 1981;**68** (2):238–41.

7. Gibson BE, Todd A, Roberts I, et al. Transfusion guidelines for neonates and older children. *Br J Haematol* 2004;**124**(4):433–53.

8. Candotti F. Clinical manifestations and pathophysiological mechanisms of the Wiskott–Aldrich syndrome. *J Clin Immunol* 2018;**38** (1):13–27.

9. Bastida JM, Del Rey M, Revilla N, et al. Wiskott–Aldrich syndrome in a child presenting with macrothrombocytopenia. *Platelets* 2017;**28** (4):417–20.

10. Buchbinder D, Nugent DJ, Fillipovich AH. Wiskott–Aldrich syndrome: Diagnosis, current management, and emerging treatments. *Appl Clin Genet* 2014;7:55–66.

11. Sullivan KE, Mullen CA, Blaese RM, Winkelstein JA. A multi-institutional survey of the Wiskott–Aldrich syndrome. *J Pediatr* 1994;**125**(6 Pt 1):876–85.

12. Alekhina O, Burstein E, Billadeau DD. Cellular functions of WASP family proteins at a glance. *J Cell Sci* 2017;**130**(14):2235–41.

13. Ochs HD. Mutations of the Wiskott–Aldrich syndrome protein affect protein expression and dictate the clinical phenotypes. *Immunol Res* 2009; **44**(1–3):84–8.

14. Notarangelo LD. In Wiskott–Aldrich syndrome, platelet count matters. *Blood* 2013;**121**(9):1484–5.

15. Crispino JD, Horwitz MS. GATA factor mutations in hematologic disease. *Blood* 2017;**129** (15):2103–10.

16. Ochs HD, Slichter SJ, Harker LA, et al. The Wiskott–Aldrich syndrome: Studies of lymphocytes, granulocytes, and platelets. *Blood* 1980;**55**(2):243–52.

17. Mathew P, Conley ME. Effect of intravenous gammaglobulin (IVIG) on the platelet count in patients with Wiskott–Aldrich syndrome. *Pediatr Allergy Immunol* 1995;**6**(2):91–4.

18. Ozsahin H, Cavazzana-Calvo M, Notarangelo LD, et al. Long-term outcome following hematopoietic stem-cell transplantation in Wiskott–Aldrich syndrome: Collaborative study of the European Society for Immunodeficiencies and European Group for Blood and Marrow Transplantation. *Blood* 2008;**111**(1):439–45.

19. Moratto D, Giliani S, Bonfim C, et al. Long-term outcome and lineage-specific chimerism in 194 patients with Wiskott–Aldrich syndrome treated by hematopoietic cell transplantation in the period 1980–2009: An international collaborative study. *Blood* 2011;**118**(6):1675–84.

20. Gabelli M, Marzollo A, Notarangelo LD, Basso G, Putti MC. Eltrombopag use in a patient with Wiskott–Aldrich syndrome. *Pediatr Blood Cancer* 2017;**64**(12).

21. Gerrits AJ, Leven EA, Frelinger AL, et al. Effects of eltrombopag on platelet count and platelet activation in Wiskott–Aldrich syndrome/X-linked thrombocytopenia. *Blood* 2015;**126**(11):1367–78.

22. Alexander WS, Roberts AW, Nicola NA, Li R, Metcalf D. Deficiencies in progenitor cells of multiple hematopoietic lineages and defective megakaryocytopoiesis in mice lacking the thrombopoietic receptor c-Mpl. *Blood* 1996;**87** (6):2162–70.

23. Sitnicka E, Lin N, Priestley GV, et al. The effect of thrombopoietin on the proliferation and differentiation of murine hematopoietic stem cells. *Blood* 1996;**87**(12):4998–5005.

24. Kaushansky K. Thrombopoietin: More than a lineage-specific megakaryocyte growth factor. *Stem Cells* 1997;**15** Suppl 1:97–103; discussion 103.

25. Rose MJ, Nicol KK, Skeens MA, Gross TG, Kerlin BA. Congenital amegakaryocytic thrombocytopenia: The diagnostic importance of combining pathology with molecular genetics. *Pediatr Blood Cancer* 2008;**50** (6):1263–5.

26. Germeshausen M, Ballmaier M, Welte K. Implications of mutations in hematopoietic growth factor receptor genes in congenital cytopenias. *Ann N Y Acad Sci* 2001;**938**:305–20; discussion 20–1.

27. King S, Germeshausen M, Strauss G, Welte K, Ballmaier M. Congenital amegakaryocytic thrombocytopenia: A retrospective clinical analysis of 20 patients. *Br J Haematol* 2005;**131**(5):636–44.

28. Eshuis-Peters E, Versluys AB, Stokman MF, et al. Congenital amegakaryocytic thrombocytopenia Type II presenting with multiple central nervous system anomalies. *Neuropediatrics* 2016;**47** (2):128–31.

29. Martinón-Torres N, Vázquez-Donsión M, Loidi L, Couselo JM. CAMT in a female with developmental delay, facial malformations and central nervous system anomalies. *Pediatr Blood Cancer* 2011;**56**(3):452–3.

30. Bör Ö, Turhan AB, Yarar C. Congenital amegakaryocytic thrombocytopenia with severe neurological findings. *Blood Coagul Fibrinolysis* 2016;**27**(8):936–9.

31. Mukai HY, Kojima H, Todokoro K, et al. Serum thrombopoietin (TPO) levels in patients with amegakaryocytic thrombocytopenia are much higher than those with immune thrombocytopenic purpura. *Thromb Haemost* 1996;**76**(5):675–8.

32. Porcelijn L, Folman CC, Bossers B, et al. The diagnostic value of thrombopoietin level measurements in thrombocytopenia. *Thromb Haemost* 1998;**79**(6):1101–5.

33. Pecci A, Ragab I, Bozzi V, et al. Thrombopoietin mutation in congenital amegakaryocytic thrombocytopenia treatable with romiplostim. *EMBO Mol Med* 2018;**10**(1):63–75.

34. Dasouki MJ, Rafi SK, Olm-Shipman AJ, et al. Exome sequencing reveals a thrombopoietin ligand mutation in a Micronesian family with autosomal recessive aplastic anemia. *Blood* 2013;**122**(20):3440–9.

35. Greenhalgh KL, Howell RT, Bottani A, et al. Thrombocytopenia-absent radius syndrome: A clinical genetic study. *J Med Genet* 2002;**39**(12):876–81.

36. Hall JG. Thrombocytopenia and absent radius (TAR) syndrome. *J Med Genet* 1987;**24**(2):79–83.

37. Hedberg VA, Lipton JM. Thrombocytopenia with absent radii. A review of 100 cases. *Am J Pediatr Hematol Oncol* 1988;**10**(1):51–64.

38. Sultan Y, Scrobohaci ML, Rendu F, Caen JP. Abnormal platelet function, population, and survival-time in a boy with congenital absent radii and thrombocytopenia. *Lancet* 1972;**2**(7778):653.

39. Day HJ, Holmsen H. Platelet adenine nucleotide "storage pool deficiency" in thrombocytopenic absent radii syndrome. *JAMA* 1972;**221**(9):1053–4.

40. Digilio MC, Giannotti A, Marino B, et al. Radial aplasia and chromosome 22q11 deletion. *J Med Genet* 1997;**34**(11):942–4.

41. Klopocki E, Schulze H, Strauss G, et al. Complex inheritance pattern resembling autosomal recessive inheritance involving a microdeletion in thrombocytopenia-absent radius syndrome. *Am J Hum Genet* 2007;**80**(2):232–40.

42. Albers CA, Paul DS, Schulze H, et al. Compound inheritance of a low-frequency regulatory SNP and a rare null mutation in exon-junction complex subunit RBM8A causes TAR syndrome. *Nat Genet* 2012;**44**(4):435–9, S1–2.

43. Albers CA, Newbury-Ecob R, Ouwehand WH, Ghevaert C. New insights into the genetic basis of TAR (thrombocytopenia-absent radii) syndrome. *Curr Opin Genet Dev* 2013;**23**(3):316–23.

44. Fadoo Z, Naqvi SM. Acute myeloid leukemia in a patient with thrombocytopenia with absent radii syndrome. *J Pediatr Hematol Oncol* 2002;**24**(2):134–5.

45. Rao VS, Shenoi UD, Krishnamurthy PN. Acute myeloid leukemia in TAR syndrome. *Indian J Pediatr* 1997;**64**(4):563–5.

46. Kataoka K, Sato T, Yoshimi A, et al. Evi1 is essential for hematopoietic stem cell self-renewal, and its expression marks hematopoietic cells with long-term multilineage repopulating activity. *J Exp Med* 2011;**208**(12):2403–16.

47. Kustikova OS, Schwarzer A, Stahlhut M, et al. Activation of Evi1 inhibits cell cycle progression and differentiation of hematopoietic progenitor cells. *Leukemia* 2013;**27**(5):1127–38.

48. Wieser R. The oncogene and developmental regulator EVI1: Expression, biochemical properties, and biological functions. *Gene* 2007;**396**(2):346–57.

49. Germeshausen M, Ancliff P, Estrada J, et al. MECOM-associated syndrome: A heterogeneous inherited bone marrow failure syndrome with amegakaryocytic thrombocytopenia. *Blood Adv* 2018;**2**(6):586–96.

50. Niihori T, Ouchi-Uchiyama M, Sasahara Y, Kaneko T, Hashii Y, Irie M, et al. Mutations in MECOM, encoding oncoprotein EVI1, cause radioulnar synostosis with amegakaryocytic thrombocytopenia. *Am J Hum Genet* 2015;**97**(6):848–54.

51. Thompson AA, Nguyen LT. Amegakaryocytic thrombocytopenia and radio-ulnar synostosis are associated with HOXA11 mutation. *Nat Genet* 2000;**26**(4):397–8.

52. Walne A, Tummala H, Ellison A, et al. Expanding the phenotypic and genetic spectrum of radioulnar synostosis associated hematological disease. *Haematologica* 2018;**103**(7):e284-e7.

53. Song WJ, Sullivan M G, Legare RD, et al. Haploinsufficiency of CBFA2 causes familial thrombocytopenia with propensity to develop acute myelogenous leukaemia. *Nat Genet* 1999;**23**(2):166–75.

54. Noris P, Favier R, Alessi MC, et al. ANKRD26-related thrombocytopenia and myeloid malignancies. *Blood* 2013;**122**(11):1987–9.

55. Zhang MY, Churpek JE, Keel SB, et al. Germline ETV6 mutations in familial thrombocytopenia and hematologic malignancy. *Nat Genet* 2015;**47**(2):180–5.

56. Noetzli L, Lo RW, Lee-Sherick AB, et al. Germline mutations in ETV6 are associated with thrombocytopenia, red cell macrocytosis and predisposition to lymphoblastic leukemia. *Nat Genet* 2015;**47**(5):535–8.

57. Latger-Cannard V, Philippe C, Bouquet A, et al. Haematological spectrum and genotype-phenotype correlations in nine unrelated families with RUNX1 mutations from the French network on inherited platelet disorders. *Orphanet J Rare Dis* 2016;**11**:49.

58. Feurstein S, Godley LA. Germline ETV6 mutations and predisposition to hematological malignancies. *Int J Hematol* 2017;**106**(2):189–95.

59. Melazzini F, Zaninetti C, Balduini CL. Bleeding is not the main clinical issue in many patients with inherited thrombocytopaenias. *Haemophilia* 2017;**23**(5):673–81.

60. Hock H, Shimamura A. ETV6 in hematopoiesis and leukemia predisposition. *Semin Hematol* 2017;**54**(2):98–104.

61. Godley LA, Shimamura A. Genetic predisposition to hematologic malignancies: Management and surveillance. *Blood* 2017;**130**(4):424–32.

62. Li R, Emsley J. The organizing principle of the platelet glycoprotein Ib-IX-V complex. *J Thromb Haemost* 2013;**11**(4):605–14.

63. Berndt MC, Andrews RK. Bernard–Soulier syndrome. *Haematologica* 2011;**96**(3):355–9.

64. Kunishima S, Naoe T, Kamiya T, Saito H. Novel heterozygous missense mutation in the platelet glycoprotein Ib beta gene associated with isolated giant platelet disorder. *Am J Hematol* 2001;**68**(4):249–55.

65. Ali S, Shetty S, Ghosh K. A novel mutation in GP1 BA gene leads to mono-allelic Bernard–Soulier syndrome form of macrothrombocytopenia. *Blood Coagul Fibrinolysis* 2017;**28**(1):94–5.

66. Poon MC, d'Oiron R. Alloimmunization in congenital deficiencies of platelet surface glycoproteins: Focus on Glanzmann's thrombasthenia and Bernard–Soulier's syndrome. *Semin Thromb Hemost* 2018;**44**(6):604–14.

67. Ozelo MC, Svirin P, Larina L. Use of recombinant factor VIIa in the management of severe bleeding episodes in patients with Bernard-Soulier syndrome. *Ann Hematol* 2005;**84**(12):816–22.

68. Hacihanefioglu A, Tarkun P, Gonullu E. Use of recombinant factor VIIa in the management and prophylaxis of bleeding episodes in two patients with Bernard-Soulier syndrome. *Thromb Res* 2007;**120**(3):455–7.

69. Lee A, Poon MC. Inherited platelet functional disorders: General principles and practical aspects of management. *Transfus Apher Sci* 2018;**57**(4):494–501.

70. Balduini CL, Pecci A, Savoia A. Recent advances in the understanding and management of MYH9-related inherited thrombocytopenias. *Br J Haematol* 2011;**154**(2):161–74.

71. Seri M, Pecci A, Di Bari F, et al. MYH9-related disease: May-Hegglin anomaly, Sebastian syndrome, Fechtner syndrome, and Epstein syndrome are not distinct entities but represent a variable expression of a single illness. *Medicine (Baltimore)* 2003;**82**(3):203–15.

72. Verver E, Pecci A, De Rocco D, et al. R705 H mutation of MYH9 is associated with MYH9-related disease and not only with non-syndromic deafness DFNA17. *Clin Genet* 2015;**88**(1):85–9.

73. Pecci A, Klersy C, Gresele P, et al. MYH9-related disease: A novel prognostic model to predict the clinical evolution of the disease based on genotype-phenotype correlations. *Hum Mutat* 2014;**35**(2):236–47.

74. Harrison P, Cramer EM. Platelet alpha-granules. *Blood Rev* 1993;**7**(1):52–62.

75. Gunay-Aygun M, Falik-Zaccai TC, Vilboux T, et al. NBEAL2 is mutated in gray platelet syndrome and is required for biogenesis of platelet α-granules. *Nat Genet* 2011;**43**(8):732–4.

76. Albers CA, Cvejic A, Favier R, et al. Exome sequencing identifies NBEAL2 as the causative gene for gray platelet syndrome. *Nat Genet* 2011;**43**(8):735–7.

77. Kahr WH, Hinckley J, Li L, et al. Mutations in NBEAL2, encoding a BEACH protein, cause gray platelet syndrome. *Nat Genet* 2011;**43**(8):738–40.

78. Tubman VN, Levine JE, Campagna DR, et al. X-linked gray platelet syndrome due to a GATA1 Arg216Gln mutation. *Blood* 2007;**109**(8):3297–9.

79. Wijgaerts A, Wittevrongel C, Thys C, et al. The transcription factor GATA1 regulates NBEAL2 expression through a long-distance enhancer. *Haematologica* 2017;**102**(4):695–706.

80. Larocca LM, Heller PG, Podda G, et al. Megakaryocytic emperipolesis and platelet function abnormalities in five patients with gray platelet syndrome. *Platelets* 2015;**26**(8):751–7.

81. Nurden AT, Nurden P. The gray platelet syndrome: Clinical spectrum of the disease. *Blood Rev* 2007;**21**(1):21–36.

82. Khincha PP, Savage SA. Neonatal manifestations of inherited bone marrow failure syndromes. *Semin Fetal Neonatal Med* 2016;**21**(1):57–65.

83. Savage SA, Walsh MF. Myelodysplastic syndrome, acute myeloid leukemia, and cancer surveillance in Fanconi anemia. *Hematol Oncol Clin North Am* 2018;**32**(4):657–68.

84. Kutler DI, Auerbach AD. Fanconi anemia in Ashkenazi Jews. *Fam Cancer* 2004;**3**(3–4):241–8.

85. Callén E, Casado JA, Tischkowitz MD, et al. A common founder mutation in FANCA underlies the world's highest prevalence of Fanconi anemia in Gypsy families from Spain. *Blood* 2005;**105**(5):1946–9.

86. Feben C, Kromberg J, Wainwright R, et al. Hematological consequences of a FANCG founder mutation in Black South African patients with Fanconi anemia. *Blood Cells Mol Dis* 2015;**54**(3):270–4.

87. Meetei AR, Levitus M, Xue Y, et al. X-linked inheritance of Fanconi anemia complementation group B. *Nat Genet* 2004;**36**(11):1219–24.

88. Peffault de Latour R, Soulier J. How I treat MDS and AML in Fanconi anemia. *Blood* 2016;**127**(24):2971–9.

89. Savage SA, Alter BP. Dyskeratosis congenita. *Hematol Oncol Clin North Am* 2009;**23**(2):215–31.

90. Agarwal S. Evaluation and management of hematopoietic failure in dyskeratosis congenita. *Hematol Oncol Clin North Am* 2018;**32**(4):669–85.

91. Glousker G, Touzot F, Revy P, Tzfati Y, Savage SA. Unraveling the pathogenesis of Hoyeraal–Hreidarsson syndrome, a complex telomere biology disorder. *Br J Haematol* 2015;**170**(4):457–71.

92. Vogiatzi P, Perdigones N, Mason PJ, Wilson DB, Bessler M. A family with Hoyeraal–Hreidarsson syndrome and four variants in two genes of the telomerase core complex. *Pediatr Blood Cancer* 2013;**60**(6):E4–6.

93. Hreidarsson S, Kristjansson K, Johannesson G, Johannsson JH. A syndrome of progressive pancytopenia with microcephaly, cerebellar hypoplasia and growth failure. *Acta Paediatr Scand* 1988;**77**(5):773–5.

94. Knight SW, Heiss NS, Vulliamy TJ, et al. Unexplained aplastic anaemia, immunodeficiency, and cerebellar hypoplasia (Hoyeraal–Hreidarsson syndrome) due to mutations in the dyskeratosis congenita gene, DKC1. *Br J Haematol* 1999;**107**(2):335–9.

95. Revesz T, Fletcher S, al-Gazali LI, DeBuse P. Bilateral retinopathy, aplastic anaemia, and central nervous system abnormalities: A new syndrome? *J Med Genet* 1992;**29**(9):673–5.

96. Savage SA, Alter BP. The role of telomere biology in bone marrow failure and other disorders. *Mech Ageing Dev* 2008;**129**(1–2):35–47.

97. Ozdemir MA, Karakukcu M, Kose M, Kumandas S, Gumus H. The longest surviving child with Hoyeraal–Hreidarsson syndrome. *Haematologica* 2004;**89**(9):ECR38.

98. Favier R, Douay L, Esteva B, et al. A novel genetic thrombocytopenia (Paris-Trousseau) associated with platelet inclusions, dysmegakaryopoiesis and chromosome deletion AT 11q23. *C R Acad Sci III* 1993;**316**(7):698–701.

99. Breton-Gorius J, Favier R, Guichard J, et al. A new congenital dysmegakaryopoietic thrombocytopenia (Paris-Trousseau) associated with giant platelet alpha-granules and chromosome 11 deletion at 11q23. *Blood* 1995;**85**(7):1805–14.

100. Favier R, Akshoomoff N, Mattson S, Grossfeld P. Jacobsen syndrome: Advances in our knowledge of phenotype and genotype. *Am J Med Genet C Semin Med Genet* 2015;**169**(3):239–50.

101. Grossfeld PD, Mattina T, Lai Z, et al. The 11q terminal deletion disorder: A prospective study of 110 cases. *Am J Med Genet A* 2004;**129A**(1):51–61.

102. Hart A, Melet F, Grossfeld P, et al. Fli-1 is required for murine vascular and megakaryocytic development and is hemizygously deleted in patients with thrombocytopenia. *Immunity* 2000;**13**(2):167–77.

103. Raslóva H, Komura E, Le Couédic JP, et al. FLI1 monoallelic expression combined with its hemizygous loss underlies Paris-Trousseau/Jacobsen thrombopenia. *J Clin Invest* 2004;**114**(1):77–84.

104. Favier R, Jondeau K, Boutard P, et al. Paris-Trousseau syndrome: Clinical, hematological, molecular data of ten new cases. *Thromb Haemost* 2003;**90**(5):893–7.

105. Stockley J, Morgan NV, Bem D, et al. Enrichment of FLI1 and RUNX1 mutations in families with excessive bleeding and platelet dense granule secretion defects. *Blood* 2013;**122**(25):4090–3.

106. Saultier P, Vidal L, Canault M, et al. Macrothrombocytopenia and dense granule deficiency associated with FLI1 variants: Ultrastructural and pathogenic features. *Haematologica* 2017;**102**(6):1006–16.

107. White JG. Platelet storage pool deficiency in Jacobsen syndrome. *Platelets* 2007;**18**(7):522–7.

108. Roberts AE, Allanson JE, Tartaglia M, Gelb BD. Noonan syndrome. *Lancet* 2013;**381**(9863):333–42.

109. Tajan M, de Rocca Serra A, Valet P, Edouard T, Yart A. SHP2 sails from physiology to pathology. *Eur J Med Genet* 2015;**58**(10):509–25.

110. Nunes P, Aguilar S, Prado SN, et al. Severe congenital thrombocytopaenia: First clinical manifestation of Noonan syndrome. *BMJ Case Rep* 2012;**2012**:bcr1020114940.

111. Christensen RD, Yaish HM, Leon EL, Sola-Visner MC, Agrawal PB. A de novo T73I mutation in PTPN11 in a neonate with severe and prolonged congenital thrombocytopenia and Noonan syndrome. *Neonatology* 2013;**104**(1):1–5.

112. Artoni A, Selicorni A, Passamonti SM, et al. Hemostatic abnormalities in Noonan syndrome. *Pediatrics* 2014;**133**(5):e1299–304.

113. Strullu M, Caye A, Lachenaud J, et al. Juvenile myelomonocytic leukaemia and Noonan syndrome. *J Med Genet* 2014;**51**(10):689–97.

114. Kratz CP, Franke L, Peters H, et al. Cancer spectrum and frequency among children with Noonan, Costello, and cardio-facio-cutaneous syndromes. *Br J Cancer* 2015;**112**(8):1392–7.

115. Sullivan KE. Chromosome 22q11.2 deletion syndrome and DiGeorge syndrome. *Immunol Rev* 2019;**287**(1):186–201.

116. Kato T, Kosaka K, Kimura M, et al. Thrombocytopenia in patients with 22q11.2 deletion syndrome and its association with glycoprotein Ib-beta. *Genet Med* 2003;**5**(2):113–19.

117. Liang HP, Morel-Kopp MC, Curtin J, et al. Heterozygous loss of platelet glycoprotein (GP) Ib-V-IX variably affects platelet function in velocardiofacial syndrome (VCFS) patients. *Thromb Haemost* 2007;**98**(6):1298–308.

118. Kunishima S, Imai T, Kobayashi R, et al. Bernard-Soulier syndrome caused by a hemizygous GPIbβ mutation and 22q11.2 deletion. *Pediatr Int* 2013;**55**(4):434–7.

119. DePiero AD, Lourie EM, Berman BW, et al. Recurrent immune cytopenias in two patients with DiGeorge/velocardiofacial syndrome. *J Pediatr* 1997;**131**(3):484–6.

120. Wiedmeier SE, Henry E, Christensen RD. Hematological abnormalities during the first week of life among neonates with trisomy 18 and trisomy 13: Data from a multi-hospital healthcare system. *Am J Med Genet A* 2008;**146A**(3):312–20.

121. Roth P, Sklower Brooks S, Potaznik D, Cooma R, Sahdev S. Neonatal Gaucher disease presenting as persistent thrombocytopenia. *J Perinatol* 2005;**25**(5):356–8.

122. Fairley C, Zimran A, Phillips M, et al. Phenotypic heterogeneity of N370S homozygotes with type I Gaucher disease: An analysis of 798 patients from the ICGG Gaucher Registry. *J Inherit Metab Dis* 2008;**31**(6):738–44.

123. Finsterer J. Hematological manifestations of primary mitochondrial disorders. *Acta Haematol* 2007;**118**(2):88–98.

124. Bastida JM, Benito R, Janusz K, et al. Two novel variants of the ABCG5 gene cause xanthelasmas and macrothrombocytopenia: A brief review of hematologic abnormalities of sitosterolemia. *J Thromb Haemost* 2017;**15**(9):1859–66.

125. Bastida JM, Giros ML, Benito R, et al. Sitosterolemia: Diagnosis, metabolic and hematological abnormalities, cardiovascular disease and management. *Curr Med Chem* 2019;**26**(37):6766–75.

126. Yoo EG. Sitosterolemia: A review and update of pathophysiology, clinical spectrum, diagnosis, and management. *Ann Pediatr Endocrinol Metab* 2016;**21**(1):7–14.

127. Stewart GW, Makris M. Mediterranean macrothrombocytopenia and phytosterolaemia/sitosterolaemia. *Haematologica* 2008;**93**(2):e29.

128. Park JH, Chung IH, Kim DH, et al. Sitosterolemia presenting with severe hypercholesterolemia and intertriginous xanthomas in a breastfed infant: Case report and brief review. *J Clin Endocrinol Metab* 2014;**99**(5):1512–18.

129. Proud L, Ritchey AK. Management of type 2b von Willebrand disease in the neonatal period. *Pediatr Blood Cancer* 2017;**64**(1):103–5.

130. Kruse-Jarres R, Johnsen JM. How I treat type 2B von Willebrand disease. *Blood* 2018;**131**(12):1292–300.

131. Othman M. Platelet-type von Willebrand disease: A rare, often misdiagnosed and underdiagnosed bleeding disorder. *Semin Thromb Hemost* 2011;**37**(5):464–9.

132. Lotta LA, Garagiola I, Palla R, Cairo A, Peyvandi F. ADAMTS13 mutations and polymorphisms in congenital thrombotic thrombocytopenic purpura. *Hum Mutat* 2010;**31**(1):11–19.

133. Krogh AS, Waage A, Quist-Paulsen P. Congenital thrombotic thrombocytopenic purpura. *Tidsskr Nor Laegeforen* 2016;**136**(17):1452–7.

134. Taylor A, Vendramin C, Oosterholt S, Della Pasqua O, Scully M. Pharmacokinetics of plasma infusion in congenital thrombotic thrombocytopenic purpura. *J Thromb Haemost* 2019;**17**:88–98.

135. Plautz WE, Raval JS, Dyer MR, et al. ADAMTS13: Origins, applications, and prospects. *Transfusion* 2018;**58**(10):2453–62.

136. Ferrer M, Tao J, Iruín G, et al. Truncation of glycoprotein (GP) IIIa (616–762) prevents complex formation with GPIIb: Novel mutation in exon 11 of GPIIIa associated with thrombasthenia. *Blood* 1998;**92**(12):4712–20.

137. Poncz M, Rifat S, Coller BS, et al. Glanzmann thrombasthenia secondary to a Gly273–>Asp mutation adjacent to the first calcium-binding domain of platelet glycoprotein IIb. *J Clin Invest* 1994;**93**(1):172–9.

138. Nurden AT. Acquired antibodies to αIIbβ3 in Glanzmann thrombasthenia: From transfusion and pregnancy to bone marrow transplants and beyond. *Transfus Med Rev* 2018;**S0887-7963**(18)30037-3.

139. Barg AA, Hauschner H, Luboshitz J, et al. From thrombasthenia to next generation thrombocytopenia: Neonatal alloimmune thrombocytopenia induced by maternal Glanzmann thrombasthenia. *Pediatr Blood Cancer* 2018;**65**(12):e27376.

140. Wang Q, Cao L, Sheng G, et al. Application of high-throughput sequencing in the diagnosis of inherited thrombocytopenia. *Clin Appl Thromb Hemost* 2018:**24**(9 Suppl):94S–103S.

141. Bastida JM, Lozano ML, Benito R, et al. Introducing high-throughput sequencing into mainstream genetic diagnosis practice in inherited platelet disorders. *Haematologica* 2018;**103**(1):148–62.

Eosinophils and Neutrophils

Kurt R. Schibler and Robert D. Christensen

Eosinophilia and Eosinopenia

Eosinophilia in neonates is identified when the blood concentration of eosinophils exceeds the upper reference range limit. To avoid the potential pitfall of laboratory or technician error, perhaps the definition should be two subsequent eosinophil counts above the upper reference limit. The 95th percentile for blood concentration of eosinophils increases slightly over the first month following birth. Initially a count $\geq 1,200/\mu L$ would exceed the upper range, and by about four weeks a count of above $1,500/\mu L$ would exceed the upper limit [1]. This latter value is similar to that generally used to define eosinophilia in adults [2]. Adults with persistent eosinophilia are well advised to have the situation evaluated, because an association has been seen between persistent eosinophilia and end-organ damage [2]. Some adults with persistent eosinophilia have elevated blood Interkeukin-5 (IL-5) concentrations [3]. Some with hypereosinophilic syndrome have an eosinophilic leukemia involving a translocation in the tyrosine kinase gene [4].

Interleukin-5 (IL-5) probably plays a role as a regulator of eosinophil production. Evidence for this includes the reports of Lee and associates [5] and Dent and coworkers [6] who produced transgenic mice that constitutively over-expressed IL-5. These animals had profound eosinophilia, generally equaling 60% of circulating leukocytes. However, mice with a targeted gene disruption of IL-5 that consequently produce no IL-5, have a reduced number of blood and marrow eosinophils but no other apparent hematologic defects [6]. Further evidence that IL-5 regulates eosinophil production comes from studies of Rennick and colleagues [7] and Sher and associates [8] who used specific neutralizing antibody directed against IL-5 and observed that such inhibits

the eosinophilia otherwise seen in parasitized mice. More evidence that IL-5 stimulates eosinophil production comes from the work of Lu and colleagues [9] who determined that recombinant murine IL-5 had the greatest effect of any factor tested on colony generation of eosinophilic progenitors.

Evidence that IL-5 is a regulator of eosinophil production in humans was provided by Brugnoni and associates, who reported a patient with hypereosinophilia caused by a population of T cells that secreted large amounts of IL-5 [10]. Glucocorticoid administration can result in an abrupt drop in blood eosinophil concentrations, accompanying reduced expression of IL-5 [11]. Interferon-α, which has beneficial effects in many eosinophil-mediated disorders, also inhibits IL-5 gene expression [12]. In a manner reminiscent of the actions of granulocyte colony-stimulating factor on neutrophils, IL-5 stimulates eosinophil function and eosinophil production. Walsh and coworkers observed that IL-5 enhances the adhesion of human eosinophils by a mechanism dependent on CD 11/18 family of adhesions glycoproteins [13]. However, IL-5 does not enhance adhesion of neutrophils. Taken together, this information indicates that IL-5 is a significant physiologic regulator of eosinophil production and function.

Eosinophilia is not a rare finding in the neonatal intensive care unit, but in reports of such, various definitions for eosinophilia have been used. When comparing reports, the definition used for eosinophilia is obviously critical, because the higher the cut-off level used, the lower will be the prevalence of eosinophilia.

The expected range of blood concentrations of eosinophils in neonates has been reported in a few

Neonatal Hematology, Pathogenesis, Diagnosis, and Management of Hematologic Problems, 3rd edition, ed. Pedro A. de Alarcón, Eric J. Werner, Robert D. Christensen, and Martha C. Sola-Visner. Published by Cambridge University Press.

small studies, and more recently in a very larger study including over 80,000 neonates [1]. Medoff and Barbero reported that during the first 12 hours after birth blood eosinophil concentrations range from 20 to 850/μL [14]. On the basis of that report, eosinophilia on the first day of life would be defined as a blood eosinophil count of more than 850/μL. Our large study suggests that a count exceeding 1,200/μL on the day of birth is a more accurate definition of an elevated count [1]. Xanthou reported that by the fifth day after birth eosinophil concentrations had a much greater range than on the first day, with values of 100 to 2,500/μL [15]. Our data suggests that counts as high as 2,500/μL would always be abnormal.

Burell postulated that a complete lack of blood eosinophils in neonates should be considered an abnormality [16]. He found that an absence of eosinophils on the complete blood count (CBC) was common only among infants who fared poorly and subsequently died. He reported that on the day of death there was generally a complete absence of blood eosinophils. Bass reported that blood eosinophil concentrations declined rapidly in the presence of bacterial infection [17]. Our work also suggests that a blood eosinophil count of zero/μL is abnormal, falling below the 5th % reference range [1].

In growing preterm infants, a nonspecific low-grade eosinophilia is so common as to have been given the label "eosinophilia of prematurity." Despite its relatively frequent occurrence, the causes and significance of this condition are uncertain. Defining eosinophilia as blood concentration >700/μL, Gibson and coworkers found that 75% of preterm infants develop eosinophilia [18]. They also observed that this eosinophilia of prematurity generally occurs during a period in which an anabolic state is established. This anabolic state and the accompanying eosinophilia usually are seen in the second or third week of life, and the eosinophilia persists for many days and sometimes for weeks. Portuguez-Molavasi reported that at least one episode of eosinophilia (defined as a count exceeding 1,000/μL) occurred in 35% of all infants admitted to an intensive care nursery [19]. Craver reported that eosinophils can be seen in the cerebrospinal fluid weeks after intraventricular hemorrhage [20], but the significance of this finding is not clear, and this finding did not correlate with blood eosinophil counts.

Although several reports suggest that the eosinophilia of prematurity is benign, the work of Patel and colleagues suggests otherwise [21]. In a retrospective evaluation of 261 admissions to their intensive care unit, eosinophilia (defined as >1,000 eosinophils/μL) was found in 33 patients. When age-matched patients without eosinophilia were compared with these, the development of sepsis was much higher *in* those with eosinophilia. All of 10 neonates born at 26 weeks' gestation or younger who developed eosinophilia also developed at least one nosocomial infection. Twenty of 23 born at >26 weeks' gestation who developed eosinophilia also had sepsis, compared with only 4 of 23 matched infants who did not have eosinophilia. Whether eosinophilia preceded, was concomitant with, or came after the infections is not clear, but these researchers warn of the correlation between eosinophilia and sepsis, particularly with Gram-negative organisms.

The clinical significance of the eosinophilia of prematurity was also addressed by Odelram and associates using the observation that high blood concentrations of eosinophils are often seen in atopic diseases [22]. They attempted to correlate eosinophil counts in neonates with the subsequent development of atopy, determined at the age of 18 months, but little or no correlation was found. Yamamoto and coworkers observed that blood eosinophils counts might be somewhat elevated in neonates who develop chronic lung disease and suggested that eosinophils might become activated in certain patients with hyaline membrane disease and that these cells could subsequently appear in the airways [23]. This postulate accounts for the timing of the eosinophilia of prematurity and the development of chronic lung disease, but not all infants with the eosinophilia of prematurity develop chronic lung disease, and not all neonates with chronic lung disease have antecedent eosinophilia. Others have postulated that medications or constituents of hyperalimentation solutions are responsible for the eosinophilia.

Tissue infiltration with eosinophils has been associated with a variety of pathological conditions in neonates. Most of these conditions are accompanied by blood eosinophilia, and thus eosinophils have been postulated as central to the pathogenesis of these conditions. These include the relatively transient and benign cutaneous eruption within days after birth, termed erythema toxicum neonatorum [24, 25], a similar but much more marked cutaneous eruption termed neonatal eosinophilic pustulosis [26, 27], and infantile eczema [28]. Chronic respiratory inflammation associated with eosinophilic pulmonary infiltrates, sometimes with accompanying blood eosinophilia, include *Chlamydia trachomatis* [29], respiratory syncytial virus [30], and bronchopulmonary dysplasia [23, 31]. Other inflammatory conditions associated with eosinophilic infiltrates and eosinophilia are neonatal eosinophilic esophagitis [32], eosinophilic colitis [33], subcutaneous fat necrosis with eosinophilic granules [34], a variety of infections, necrotizing enterocolitis, and after erythrocyte transfusions [35]. The exact roles of eosinophils in the pathogenesis of these conditions, and whether blood eosinophil counts can be of value in identifying or suspecting these conditions, remain to be determined.

Neutrophilia and Leukemoid Reactions

Reference ranges for blood neutrophil concentrations of neonates are very wide. Neonates born at high altitude (above 4,000 ft) have an even wider range of expected values than do those born at sea level. For instance, blood neutrophil concentrations following birth in Colorado [36] New Mexico [37], and Utah [38] all have a substantially higher 95% reference limit than do those reported in Dallas, Texas [39–41] and Athens, Greece [15, 42]. In these reports, no differences are apparent in the 5% limit, but the 95% limit at high altitude is almost twice that at sea level. The exact mechanism by which high altitude results in considerably higher blood neutrophil counts, over the first days after birth, is unclear. Moreover, it is possible that this difference in upper range limit, ascribed to altitude, is actually the result of differences other than altitude. Large numbers of neutrophil counts from neonates in yet other sites would be helpful in confirming whether there is indeed an important altitude-based difference in blood neutrophil concentration. For instance, data from the neonatal intensive care units (NICUs) at very high altitudes in South America and Asia, and additional data from NICUs at sea level would help resolve this issue.

Bacterial infection is the condition most commonly reported as the cause of neonatal neutrophilia [43, 44]. Chorioamniotitis has been associated with neonatal leukemoid reactions, particularly among extremely low birth weight (ELBW) neonates [45]. Leukemoid reactions were first reported by Krumbhaar in 1926 as an extreme elevation in blood neutrophil concentration [46]. Leukemoid reactions in the NICU have been defined variably as a leukocyte count in excess of $50 \times 10^3/\mu l$, or if more than 2% of the blood leukocytes are immature myeloid cells capable of division (myeloblasts, promyelocytes, or myelocytes). As a consistent approach, at the University of Florida (85 ft above sea level) we defined a neonatal leukemoid reaction as: (1) a blood neutrophil count greater than $30.0 \times 10^3/\mu L$ between birth and 60 hours of life; (2) a count greater than $15.0 \times 10^3 /\mu L$ from 60 hours to 28 days; or (3) greater than 5% blasts, promyelocytes, or myelocytes on a differential blood cell count regardless of the blood neutrophil count [47]. When defined this way, leukemoid reactions were identified in 1.3% of our NICU patients. Evaluating these neonates, even with neutrophil counts as high as 100,000/μL, did not identify any with hyperviscosity and, except for one patient with trisomy 21, all cases of extreme neutrophilia were transient, persisting generally for only a few days. We suspect the responsible kinetic mechanism for this variety of neonatal neutrophilia is increased neutrophil production, not steroid-induced leukocytosis, and is likely from granulocyte colony-stimulating factor (G-CSF) produced during chorioamnionitis or relatively mild to moderately severe neonatal infections [47].

Leukemoid reactions in the NICU, particularly among ELBW and very low birth weight (VLBW) neonates, tend to presage the later development of chronic lung disease. Zanardo et al. suggested that the in utero exposure to proinflammatory cytokines initiating the neonatal leukemoid reaction, conditions the lungs to damage and prolongs the need for supplemental oxygen [48]. Hsiao and Omar also reported this association between early leukemoid reaction, in ELBW neonates, and a higher incidence of bronchopulmonary dysplasia (54% in those with a leukemoid reaction vs. 25% in matched controls that did not have a leukemoid reaction) [49]. However, they found no significant differences in neurodevelopmental outcome between groups at 2 years of age. Zanardo et al. provided further confirmation that histological chorioamnionitis is a risk factor predisposing to leukemoid reaction and subsequently to chronic lung disease [50].

Neonates with Down syndrome have a high prevalence of hematologic abnormalities, including neutrophilia, transient myeloproliferative disorder, congenital leukemia, thrombocytopenia, and polycythemia [51]. Cutaneous vesiculopustular eruptions have been described in those with neonatal myeloproliferative disorders. These lesions contain immature hematopoietic cells similar to blasts, and resolution occurs without specific treatment, concurrent with resolution of the hematologic disorder [52, 53]. Neonates with Down syndrome and a leukemoid reaction have a 20 to 30% probability of developing acute megakaryocyte leukemia, associated with mutations in the N-terminal activation domain of the GATA-1 gene [54, 55].

Case report association have been made between persistent neonatal neutrophilia and persistent severe pulmonary hypertension [56], and between persistent neutrophilia and leukocyte adhesion deficiency [57]. It might be that some of the previous publications on neonatal neutrophilia should be re-examined in light of altitude-appropriate reference ranges [58]. For instance, patients with Down syndrome [51], trisomy 13 [59], and trisomy 18 [59] are all very likely to have neutrophilia in the neonatal period, but the influence of altitude complicates this conclusion. Other considerations discovered by studying very large sample sizes of CBC include that, during the first day following birth, neonates delivered after labor have 20% to 30% higher blood neutrophil counts than do those delivered by cesarean section without labor (38). Also, over the first 3 days, females have higher neutrophil counts than do males, averaging 10% to 20% higher [38].

Neutropenia

Among newborn infants, the CBC is one of the most commonly obtained of all blood tests. Sometimes a CBC is ordered anticipating that neutropenia might be present, as is the case in a neonate with septic shock, or in a small for gestational age (SGA) neonate born after severe preeclampsia. However, most cases where a neonate's CBC reveals neutropenia come as an unexpected puzzle. The neonatologist or pediatrician seeing such a result might

wonder: What conditions should I consider in the differential diagnosis? Will the neutropenia be a significant medical problem or will it be trivial and transient? What steps should I take to evaluate the neutropenia? Should I obtain cultures and initiate antibiotic treatment? Should I order IVIg? Should I order G-CSF?

One reasonable place to start this process is by repeating the CBC, to ensure laboratory error is not responsible for the finding. While the repeat sample is being drawn and run, you might consider the following three issues in order to generate a framework in which to proceed if the repeat test confirms that neutropenia is indeed present. These three questions are: (1) Does the neutropenia appear to be congenital or acquired? (2) Does the baby have signs of illness that could be the result of an infection, or is she/he basically well appearing? (3) Are there additional abnormalities on the CBC?

First, how are you defining neutropenia? Consider the number of neutrophils per microliter of blood, also known as the ANC (absolute neutrophil count) and not just the WBC (white blood cells or leukocytes per microliter). If you find an ANC less than $1,000/\mu L$ twice sequentially, the patient can be said to have neutropenia. If you find two simultaneous ANCs $<500/\mu L$ the patient can be said to have *severe* neutropenia. Counts above $1,000/\mu L$ can technically be neutropenic, if they fall below the 5th percentile reference range. For instance, an ANC of $3,000/\mu L$ 6 hours after birth is indeed an abnormally low ANC. The fact that the ANC is below the reference range signals the presence of pathology. However, it is doubtful that a count as high as $3,000/\mu L$ constitutes a host-defense deficiency or renders the patient at high risk for acquiring an infection. Therefore, we tend to use the diagnosis "neutropenia," or place *neutropenia* on the problem list, only if the ANC is twice, sequentially, less than $1,000/\mu L$.

Table 16.1 shows three questions to consider when evaluating a neonate with neutropenia.

1. **Does the neutropenia appear to be congenital or acquired?** Is this the first CBC obtained on this patient? The common neonatal neutropenias are often seen on the very first CBC. These include the neutropenia of maternal hypertension and the neutropenia associated with early-onset sepsis. Alternatively, has the patient had a normal ANC for days or weeks and now has neutropenia? If so, what else has

Table 16.1 Evaluating a neonate with neutropenia

Three questions to consider when neutropenia is found on a neonate's CBC
1. Does the neutropenia appear to be congenital or acquired?
2. Does the baby have signs of illness that could be the result of an infection, or is she/he basically well appearing?
3. Are there additional abnormalities on the CBC?

changed? Has a significant infectious illness or NEC been acquired? Is this a case of late neutropenia appearing in an otherwise growing preterm neonate, sometimes called "idiopathic neonatal neutropenia"? These late-appearing varieties of neonatal neutropenia cannot be ascribed to maternal hypertension or alloimmune mechanisms.

2. **Does the baby have signs of illness that could be the result of an infection, or is she/he basically well appearing?** Mild infections in neonates tend to result in neutrophilia, while septic shock is more likely to result in neutropenia. Thus, when severe neutropenia if found in a well appearing neonate, the neutropenia is not at all likely to be the neutropenia of sepsis. A well-appearing neonate with neutropenia raises the possibility of immune-mediated neutropenia (alloimmune, maternal autoimmune, or neonatal autoimmune). Similarly, a neonate with any of the varieties of severe congenital neutropenia can appear completely well, unless infection has been acquired. When an otherwise well neonate has syndromic features and neutropenia, it is likely that the neutropenia is part of the syndrome. Other tie-ins with the issue of well versus ill, include hypoglycemia and neutropenia with glycogen storage disease type Ib and pancreatic exocrine insufficiency and neutropenia with Shwachman–Diamond syndrome.

3. **Are there additional abnormalities on the CBC?** Neutropenia resulting from sepsis is generally accompanied by characteristic laboratory features. An increased immature to total (I/T) ratio is common, reflecting the call of neutrophil from the marrow to sites of infection. The hematology laboratory technician sometimes reports morphological changes in the neutrophils, like toxic granulation, Dohle bodies, and vacuolization.

Thrombocytopenia and an elevated MPV sometimes accompany the neutropenia of sepsis. Shock and acidosis are characteristics as well. Contrariwise, the neutropenia of pregnancy-induced hypertension (PIH) should not have a high I/T ratio or the morphological changes of infection.

By considering these three questions, preliminary conclusions can be rapidly reached and these will dictate the next steps. The neutropenia of infection requires appropriate antibiotic coverage and intensive care monitoring and treatment. This is the case in early-onset sepsis and also late onset conditions including NEC and neutropenic late-onset sepsis (most late-onset bacterial infections generate neutrophilia not neutropenia). If the neonate is well but neutropenic, when would antineutrophil antibody tests be helpful and when should the possibility of severe congenital neutropenia be considered?

In general, we suggest waiting until neutropenia has persisted 5 days of more, or until *severe* neutropenia has persisted for 2 days or more, before engaging in further evaluation of the etiology. Transient cases of neutropenia such as the variety related to PIH, will spontaneously remit or at least will significantly improve over this period. When evaluating the possibility of immune-mediated neutropenia the assistance of a specialized neutrophil serology laboratory is needed. The initial evaluation screen can be run on blood drawn from mother and father. If neutropenia persists after a negative immune-neutropenia evaluation, particularly if the ANC remains <500/μL, it is time to consider severe congenital neutropenia.

Given this framework for the initial approach, readers can now consult the following paragraphs, Table 16.2, and the section "Consistent Approaches" for more detail regarding the pathogenesis, evaluation, and treatment of the common and rare varieties of neutropenia among neonates.

The Transient Hyporegenerative Neutropenias Present at Birth

Maternal Hypertension, Donors of Twin–Twin Transfusion Syndrome, Rh Hemolytic Disease

Transient hyporegenerative neutropenia is common among neonates whose mothers had PIH, and in donors of twin–twin transfusions, and in neonates with Rh hemolytic disease. These three

Table 16.2 Classification of varieties of neutropenia in neonates based on timing of presentation and whether they are primarily the result of reduced production vs. accelerated destruction of neutrophils

Categories of neutropenia in neonates
Transient hyporegenerative neutropenias present at birth Maternal hypertension Donors of twin–twin transfusion syndrome Rh hemolytic disease
Neutropenias with accelerated neutrophil destruction generally present in first days Neutropenia of sepsis Immune-mediated
Chronic hyporegenerative neutropenias generally present in first days Severe congenital neutropenia Cyclic Shwachman–Diamond syndrome Syndromic (including reticular dysgenesis)
Neutropenias presenting late in the NICU course Ill neonates (necrotizing enterocolitis, infection) Idiopathic Marrow failure syndromes

varieties of neonatal neutropenia are considered together, because of the many features they have in common. Specifically, they are not accompanied by an elevated I/T ratio or morphological abnormalities of the neutrophils, neutropenia is present at delivery, they have elevated NRBC, reticulocyte counts, and serum erythropoietin concentrations, and the neutropenia generally persists for only a few days [60–66].

Studies of the bone marrow and cultures of the granulocytic progenitors of these patients indicated that the neutropenia is the result of impaired neutrophil production days [60–62, 65, 66]. Zook and coworkers found no association of placental pathology with incidence or severity of neutropenia [67]. Guner et al. found no difference in G-CSF serum levels in neutropenic versus non-neutropenic neonates whose mothers had preeclampsia [68], but Tsao et al. found lower levels of G-CSF in cord blood of infants whose mother had PIH, with the lowest values in those with neutropenia [69].

The issue of whether this variety of transient hyporegenerative neutropenia imparts an antibacterial host-defense defect remains unsettled. Koenig and Christensen [66] and Cadnapaphornchai and Faix [64] observed a significantly larger proportion of late-onset bacterial infection among VLBW neonates who had neutropenia from PIH than among non-neutropenic matched controls. Manzoni et al.

found that *Candida* colonization was significantly increased among those with neutropenia from PIH (62% vs. 35% colonization rate in the first month) [70]. They also found multiple sites of *Candida* colonization to be higher among those with neutropenia (*P*<0.002). In contrast, Teng et al. found no increase in nosocomial infections among VLBW infants with early neutropenia from PIH compared with matched controls who did not have early neutropenia [71].

The administration of G-CSF to neonates with this variety of neutropenia increases the blood neutrophil concentration and increased antibacterial function of neutrophils [72–74], but no evidence indicates fewer infections, or a survival advantage, of the G-CSF recipients. On that basis, we do not recommend G-CSF treatment for neonates with the neutropenia of PIH (see the section on "Consistent Approaches").

Neutropenias Associated with Therapeutic Hypothermia for Hypoxic Ischemic Encephalopathy

Therapeutic hypothermia has become standard of care for term newborn infants diagnosed with hypoxic ischemic encephalopathy in the first few hours after birth [75–78]. In a randomized, controlled, multicenter trial of systemic hypothermia in neonatal hypoxic ischemic encephalopathy, total and leukocyte subsets and serum chemokine levels were measured over time in both hypothermia and normothermia groups as primary outcomes for safety [79]. The hypothermia group had significantly lower median circulating total WBC and leukocyte subclasses than the normothermia group before rewarming. While the absolute neutrophil count rebounded after rewarming in the hypothermia group, chemokines were negatively correlated with their target leukocytes in the hypothermia group, suggesting active chemokine and leukocyte modulation by hypothermia. Relative leukopenia at 60–72 hours correlated with more severe central nervous system injury in the hypothermia group.

The Neutropenias Due to Accelerated Neutrophil Destruction Generally Present at Birth

Neutropenia of Sepsis and the Immune-Mediated Neutropenias

Neonates with overwhelming infection, including septic shock, are very likely to develop neutropenia.

At least two mechanisms can contribute: neutrophil margination and depletion of the marrow neutrophil reserves. Neutrophil margination occurs within hours of intravenous bacterial endotoxin administration and involves a movement of circulating neutrophils to the marginal pool, including sequestration of neutrophils in the pulmonary vasculature [80]. This variety of neutropenia can be sudden and severe, resulting in fewer than 500 neutrophils/μL of blood. If a single bolus of endotoxin is given, the margination neutropenia persists for an hour or so.

Neutropenia accompanying depletion of the neutrophil reserves has a more ominous significance, as it signals few neutrophils in the marrow reserve. Animal studies comparing the hematopoietic response to infection between neonates and adults demonstrate the kinetic differences in the supply and release of neutrophil pools from the bone marrow [81]. These developmental differences increased susceptibility of newborn animals to exhaustion of bone marrow reserves when subjected to experimental infection and ultimately limited their capability to survive these infections [82, 83]. Septic neonates who are neutropenic have a higher mortality than non-neutropenic neonates [84, 85]. Neonates also have an immaturity of neutrophil production. Immaturity of granulopoiesis in preterm neonates is manifest by a low neutrophil cell mass, a reduced capacity for increasing progenitor cell proliferation and frequent occurrence of neutropenia in response to sepsis [86]. This variety of neonatal neutropenia is accompanied by an elevated I/T ratio, morphological findings of neutrophils consistent with infection. Even with excellent NICU care the patient might succumb to the infection, in which case the neutropenia generally persists until death, alternatively if the patient begins to recover from the shock state the neutrophil count generally begins to rise and within a few days might be replaced by neutrophilia.

Isoimmune Neonatal Neutropenia

Isoimmune neonatal neutropenia results from maternal production of IgG directed against antigens on fetal neutrophils [87]. This is analogous to Rh hemolytic disease in that maternal sensitization to fetal neutrophil antigens results in transplacentally acquired IgG antibody destroy the infant's neutrophils [88]. Maternal sensitization may occur during gestation and may occur even in the fetus of a primigravida [89]. The incidence of isoimmune neonatal neutropenia is estimated to be 0.5 to 2 per 1,000 live births [90].

Affected infants frequently develop a fever in the first days of life and are particularly susceptible to cutaneous infections caused by *Staphylococcus aureus*. Beta-hemolytic *Streptococcus* and *Escherichia coli* have also been linked to infections among susceptible infants with this disorder. The onset of infection is usually concurrent with severe neutropenia. In the circulation the concentrations of other myeloid lineages particularly monocytes and eosinophils are typically increased. Characteristic findings on bone marrow evaluation are myeloid hyperplasia with a paucity of mature neutrophils and normal erythropoietic and megakaryocytic elements.

Neutrophil antibodies are detected in the sera of mother and infant. The antibodies react against neutrophils of the patient and of the father, but they do not react against neutrophils from the mother. Several neutrophil-specific antibodies have been implicated, including most commonly human neutrophil alloantigens (HNA)-1, HNA-2, and HNA-3. Other antigenic targets include NC1, SH, SAR, LAN, LEA, CN1, and certain HLA antigens. HNA-1 and NC1 have been identified as isotypes of the FcγIII receptor [87]. HNA-2 is an antigen on glycoprotein (GP)50 and HNA-3 corresponds to an antigen on GP75-90. The infant's neutrophil counts typically normalize over the first 1 to 5 weeks of life as might be expected with the half-life of maternal antibodies.

Treatment for affected infants is supportive. Therapy also includes appropriate antibiotic administration for infections and close follow-up. The use of prophylactic antibiotics has been shown to be ineffective. Intravenous immunoglobulin (IVIg) administration and steroid therapy have not been shown to consistently improve circulating neutrophil counts. For infants with persistence of extremely low neutrophil counts, less than 500 cells per microliter, G-CSF administration might be undertaken. This therapy usually results in a prompt clinical response in circulating neutrophil concentrations.

Maternal Autoimmune Neutropenia

Neonatal autoimmune neutropenia results from transplacental passage of maternal IgG autoantibodies directed against neutrophil antigens. Mothers of these infants can be asymptomatic or have autoimmune neutropenia from systemic lupus erythematosus or idiopathic thrombocytopenic purpura [91, 92].

Neonatal Autoimmune Neutropenia

Autoimmune neutropenia (AIN) is a disorder caused by increased destruction of neutrophils as a result of autoantibodies to the patient's own neutrophils [93]. The incidence is approximately 1 per 100,000 live births [94]. Primary AIN is not associated with other autoimmune disorders such as systemic lupus erythematosus. Reports of associations with parvovirus B19 and β-lactam antibiotics suggest mechanisms such as development of cross-reacting antibodies resulting from molecular mimicry, changes in endogenous antigens, enhanced HLA expression, or loss of suppression of self-reacting lymphocyte clones. HNA-1a (NA-1) autoimmunization has been linked to HLA-DR2, a finding implicating immune response genes [95]. Patients with this immune mediated neutropenia are identified in the first 3 years of life with a variety of infections. In approximately 80% of patients the infections are mild, consisting of abscesses, conjunctivitis, gastroenteritis, otitis media, pyoderma, and upper respiratory infections. In the remaining cases AIN predisposes to serious infections such as meningitis, pneumonia, and sepsis [96]. Diagnosis of AIN is made by detection of neutrophil-specific antibodies [97]. Generally, patients with AIN do not require specific treatment for the neutropenia, however, to increase neutrophil counts in cases of severe infection or before elective surgery, some patients have been treated with corticosteroids, IVIg or G-CSF. Corticosteroids and IVIg increased neutrophil counts in about 50% of individuals, whereas G-CSF increased neutrophil counts in all patients treated [97]. Infections are treated symptomatically with antibiotics. Infants with recurrent infections are often treated with prophylactic antibiotics.

The Chronic Hyporegenerative Neutropenias Generally Present at Birth

Severe Congenital Neutropenia and Cyclic Neutropenia

Severe congenital neutropenia and cyclic neutropenia are rare disorders of myelopoiesis usually caused by heterogeneous mutations in ELANE, the gene that encodes neutrophil elastase [98, 99]. Mutations in CSF3 R, RAS, and

RUNX1 are associated with evolution to myelodysplastic syndrome (MDS) and acute myelogenous leukemia (AML), but the biological basis for the substantial difference in risk of leukemic evolution for cyclic neutropenia versus severe congenital neutropenia is not known [100–102].

Patients with severe congenital neutropenia usually have ANC less than 500 cells/mL without regular cyclic fluctuations and a bone marrow showing maturational arrest of the myeloid lineage. Cyclic neutropenia is characterized neutrophil fluctuations from near 2,000 cells/mL to less than 200 cells/mL at approximately 21 day intervals [103]. The duration of the neutropenic episodes ranges from 3 to 10 days. Other formed elements in the blood with short circulation times such as monocytes, platelets and reticulocytes also cycle. Bone marrow aspirates during periods of neutropenia are noteworthy for cellular hypoplasia or maturational arrest [104]. Individual with cyclic neutropenia have medical histories of repetitive infections occurring in tandem with cyclic episodes of depressed circulating neutrophil concentrations. The severity of infections tends to correlate with the degree of neutropenia. Although cyclic neutropenia is usually benign, death from sepsis occurs in as many as 10% of affected individuals. The disease persists throughout the patients' lifetimes [105].

A recent review of data from the Severe Chronic Neutropenia International Registry (SCNIR) including 307 patients with ELANE mutations was conducted to assess the relationships of mutations and risk for severe outcomes and MDS/AML [106]. The diagnosis was made based on clinical data, and the ELANE mutations were identified later in all cases. The SCNIR population included 40 families with 2 or more affected members (cyclic neutropenia 20 families; severe congenital neutropenia 20 families). The family members with neutropenia had ELANE mutations, and all members with ELANE mutations had neutropenia. Of the 307 patients only 10 were not exposed to G-CSF. For the severe congenital neutropenia patients, there were 15 deaths attributable to MDS/AML and 3 transplant-related deaths in patients who failed to respond to G-CSF, and 4 others of unknown cause. For the cyclic neutropenia patients, there were 8 deaths, none due to MDS/AML. Three deaths were attributable to sepsis; two of these patients were known not to be taking G-CSF as recommended, and one other patient was never treated with G-CSF. One death followed hematopoietic transplantation (not for MDS/ AML). The causes of the other four deaths were: cancer (one), heart failure (one), stroke (one), and unknown (one).

Infections were common in these patients before G-CSF, including mouth ulcers (80%), pneumonia (49%), abscesses (19%), sepsis (17%), cellulitis (12%), and peritonitis (3%). Sixty-one of 97 patients (63%) with mutations unique to SCN reported pneumonia, compared to 31 of 73 patients (42%) with overlapping mutations and 5 of 26 patients (19%) with mutations only seen in cyclic neutropenia. Abscesses occurred in all patient groups: overlapping mutations (4 of 73, 5%), cyclic neutropenia (4 of 26, 15%) or severe congenital neutropenia (19 of 97, 20%) [106].

With longitudinal follow-up, severe events (MDS/AML, stem cell transplant, or death) was far greater in severe congenital neutropenia versus cyclic neutropenia patients (8 of 120 cyclic neutropenia versus 62 of 187 severe congenital neutropenia, $P < 10^{-4}$). The striking excess of severe events over time in severe congenital neutropenia versus cyclic neutropenia and for mutation unique to severe congenital neutropenia versus the overlapping mutations in patients on G-CSF was also highly statistically significant ($P < 10^{-4}$).

The investigators grouped mutations in five principal categories: missense, frameshift, termination, intronic, and deletion or insertion. The missense mutations were most common, and 94% were predicted to have a probable or possible damaging effect on the protein structure by Polyphen 2 analysis. The most striking finding was the association of frameshift mutations in congenital patients with a high risk of abscesses (8/17 evaluable patients, 47%) and evolution to MDS/AML (6/19 patients, 32%). It appears also that a higher proportion of termination mutations are associated with leukemic transformation, but the number of these patients is relatively small. Two mutations C151Y (3/4 patients) and G214 R (3/9 patients) appear to confer a high risk of leukemia. The apparent high risk associated with these mutations may be attributable to major changes in protein structure due to size and charge/polarity differences of exchanged amino acids. Overall, the study demonstrated that

clinically important genotype–phenotype correlations of clinical outcomes and the results of sequencing of ELANE for patients with cyclic and congenital neutropenia. Some mutations appear to be linked to a relatively good prognosis, notably P139 L, IVS4+5 G>A, and S126 L, whereas other mutations, specifically C151Y and G214 R, are associated with a notably poor prognosis. This analysis provides useful information to guide clinical care and to focus research on the cellular and molecular mechanisms for neutropenia and leukemogenesis in these patients [106].

Shwachman–Diamond Syndrome

Shwachman–Diamond syndrome is an autosomal recessive disorder, with an incidence estimated at 1 in 50,000 births, characterized by ineffective hematopoiesis, exocrine pancreatic dysfunction, and metaphyseal dysostosis, and an increased risk of leukemia [107]. Typically, patients with Shwachman–Diamond syndrome present in the first year of life with diarrhea and failure to thrive. In addition to pancreatic insufficiency these patients uniformly develop neutropenia. About 60% of patients are malnourished and short in stature and many also exhibit ichthyotic skin rashes. Shwachman–Diamond syndrome is also associated with other clinical findings including microcephaly, hypertelorism, retinitis pigmentosa, syndactyly, cleft palate, dental dysplasia, skin pigment defects, and myocardial fibrosis [108]. Leukemic transformation has been known to occur. Patients are predisposed to skin infections and pneumonia as a result of the neutropenia. Supportive measures for patients with Shwachman–Diamond syndrome include pancreatic enzymes, antibiotics, transfusions, and granulocyte colony-stimulating factor. The only definitive therapy is bone marrow transplantation.

Boocock and colleagues reported a causal mutation in the SBDS gene (named after Shwachman–Bodian–Diamond syndrome) [109]. Approximately 90% of Shwachman–Diamond syndrome patients have biallelic mutations in the SBDS gene. The structure and function of the SBDS gene has not been determined, but accumulating evidence suggests that the gene plays a role in ribosome biosynthesis and RNA processing [110]. Shwachman–Diamond syndrome cells exhibit abnormal expression of multiple genes involved in ribosome biogenesis and rRNA and mRNA processing and to have decreased expression of several ribosomal protein genes involved in cell growth and survival [111]. Additionally, SBDS has been shown to co-sediment with the 60S ribosomal precursor subunit in sucrose gradients and to associate with the 28S rRNA that is a component of the 60S subunit [110]. Although these findings provide evidence for a role of SBDS in ribosome biogenesis, SBDS is a multifunctional protein and may contribute to non-ribosomal activities that play a role in the clinical phenotype. SBDS genotyping may be used to confirm the definitive diagnosis.

Reticular Dysgenesis

Reticular dysgenesis, also called congenital aleukocytosis, is characterized by severe neutropenia associated with leukopenia, presence of rudimentary thymic lymphoid and splenic tissue, and agammaglobulinemia [112]. Histological examination of the bone marrow, spleen, and lymphoid tissue reveals normal reticular structure with normal erythroid and megakaryocyte elements, but with absent or sparse myeloid cells. Bacterial and viral infections occur early in life and are severe. Aggressive antibiotic therapy and supportive care are necessary for survival. Treatment with G-CSF and granulocyte-macrophage colony-stimulating factor (GM-CSF) has been ineffective. Bone marrow transplantation remains the only long-term treatment option available for infants with this disorder [112, 113].

The Neutropenias Presenting Late in the NICU Course: Necrotizing Enterocolitis and Late-Onset Sepsis, "Idiopathic Neonatal Neutropenia," and Marrow Failure Syndromes

Necrotizing enterocolitis (NEC) can cause neutropenia, and so can severe late-onset infections. An elevated I/T ratio, morphologic changes in neutrophils, and accompanying thrombocytopenia with an elevated MPV suggest that the mechanisms responsible for the neutropenia are those seen in sepsis: margination and accelerated neutrophil utilization. When an NICU patient with a previously normal neutrophil count develop an illness and neutropenia is found, clinical, radiographic, and laboratory features generally indicate whether NEC or sepsis are most likely. We found that NEC was the most common cause of late-onset neutropenia among VLBW infants; accounting for 30% of the late-onset neutropenia and late onset bacterial sepsis accounting for 20% of the late-onset cases [114].

Juul and colleagues described a severe and prolonged but self-resolving variety of neutropenia among preterm neonates [115, 116]. Over 36 months, 2407 neonates were admitted to the NICU of which 429 were VLBW; 14 of which were later diagnosed with "idiopathic neutropenia." In a randomized trial, G-CSF administration resulted in an immediate and marked increase in blood neutrophil concentration (while placebo administration did not), indicating adequate G-CSF-mobilizable marrow neutrophil reserves in this variety of neutropenia. We speculate that this neonatal neutropenia does not constitute a significant deficiency in antibacterial defense, thus no specific treatment is needed. The condition will spontaneously remit in several weeks [116].

Late-onset neutropenia can be a feature of any of the marrow failure syndromes [117]. These disorders typically present with hyporegenerative thrombocytopenia, or anemia, and proceeding to pancytopenia.

Consistent Approaches to Problems and Procedures Related to Neonatal Eosinophilia or Neutropenia

It is important for readers to understand that the following "consistent approaches" were drafted as *general guidelines*, not protocols to be followed with exactness. The approaches given here are rarely the only available rational choices, and readers are urged to consider whether their populations, or their individual patients, would be better served by guidelines different from those provided here. We recognize a lack of evidence on which some of the algorithms and guidelines are based. *Thus, some of what follows, although our best current analysis, is not entirely defensible.* Surely, many of these consistent approaches will change over the next several years as better

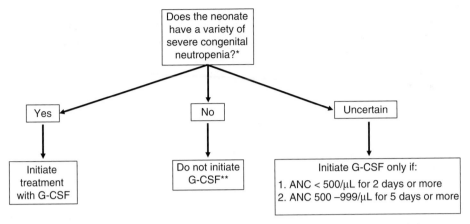

Fig. 16.1 Algorithm to determine administration of G-CSF. *Severe congenital neutropenia includes severe congenital neutropenia, Shwachman–Diamond syndrome, cyclic neutropenia, autoimmune or alloimmune neonatal neutropenia, or any syndrome or condition where severe and chronic neutropenia are a consistent finding. **G-CSF administration is not recommended for neonates with neutropenias of a non-severe, or a non-chronic nature, such as the neutropenia associated with PIH, sepsis, or chronic idiopathic (mild) neutropenia.

information becomes available and improved guidelines can be constructed. The general guidelines are presented under the following headings:

1. A consistent approach to evaluating a neonate with neutropenia
2. A consistent approach to G-CSF administration to a neonate
3. A consistent approach to evaluating eosinophilia in a neonate
4. A consistent approach to bone marrow aspiration/biopsy in a neonate
5. A consistent approach to granulocyte transfusion in the NICU
6. A consistent approach to IVIg administration for neonates with cytopenias

A Consistent Approach to Evaluating a Neonate with Neutropenia

Background

Neutropenia is a relatively common condition in the NICU. As many as 8% of patients admitted to the NICU develop neutropenia at some time during their hospitalization, and among ELBW neonates (<1,000 grams at birth) the prevalence is 35%–40% [118]. Neutropenia can be defined as a blood neutrophil count below the age-appropriate reference range (see Chapter 24). However, it is doubtful that a neutrophil count, if it is above 1,000/μL, conveys a significant risk to the neonate for acquiring

infection, even if such a count is technically in the neutropenic range. We define neonatal neutropenia by the finding of two sequential blood neutrophil counts <1,000/μL, and we define *severe* neonatal neutropenia as two sequential counts <500/μL. We recommend evaluating the cause of the neutropenia only if: (1) the neutropenia is present for at least 5 days, or (2) if *severe* neutropenia is present for at least 2 days.

A Consistent Approach to G-CSF Administration to a Neonate

Background

In the United States, the Food and Drug Administration approve G-CSF for use for use in patients with severe chronic neutropenia, cancer patients receiving myelosuppressive chemotherapy, cancer patients receiving bone marrow transplantation, and patients undergoing peripheral blood hematopoietic stem cell collection. Patients with severe chronic neutropenia generally derive considerable benefit from G-CSF administration. Varieties of neutropenia in neonates for which G-CSF treatment is effective are severe congenital neutropenia, cyclic neutropenia, Shwachman–Diamond syndrome, and alloimmune neutropenia. Almost all patients respond to doses of 5 to 10 μg/kg administered at intervals ranging from every day to once per week to achieve neutrophil

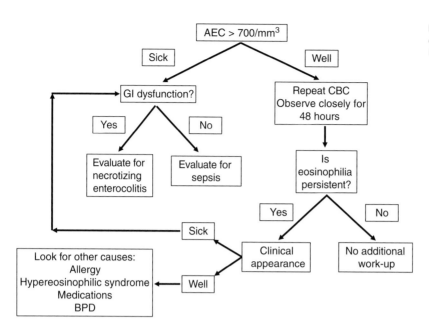

Fig. 16.2 Algorithm to evaluate eosinophilia in the NICU.

concentrations above 500 to 1,000 cells/μL (Fig. 16.1) [119].

A Consistent Approach to Evaluating Eosinophilia in a Neonate

Background

Eosinophilia can be defined as a blood eosinophil count above the age-appropriate 95% reference range. For neonates <3 weeks old, this limit is about 1,200/μL after which it is about 1,500/μL We recommend defining eosinophilia only if two sequential CBCs indicate a blood eosinophil concentration exceeding the 95% reference range [120]. Because the differential diagnosis for eosinophilia in a neonate is extensive, we propose in a simple schemata for evaluating infants with persistent (>48 hours) eosinophilia, see Fig. 16.2.

A consistent Approach to Bone Marrow Aspiration/Biopsy in a Neonate

Background

It is rare that a marrow biopsy or aspirate is needed to determine the cause of a cytopenia in a neonate. Most marrow biopsies are done for the purpose of evaluating cases for congenital marrow failure syndromes because of unexplained severe persistent neutropenia or severe persistent thrombocytopenia. Another reason marrow studies are sometimes done on NICU patients involves treatment registry protocols. Specifically, if a patient is to be entered into a registry for recombinant cytokine treatment, such as G-CSF treatment in a neonate with severe congenital neutropenia, a marrow study will sometimes be required as part of the registry protocol.

Suggested Criteria for Performing a Marrow Biopsy

This study rarely provides the exact cause of the cytopenia, but generally can indicate whether production of the cell type of interest is reduced. Thus, we suggest a marrow biopsy if:

1. Aplastic anemia is suspected.
2. Leukemia is suspected and blood studies are insufficient to confirm the diagnosis.
3. Severe neutropenia or severe thrombocytopenia persist and are unexplained after serological studies (alloimmunization).

A consistent Approach to Granulocyte Transfusion in the NICU

Background and Approach

Granulocyte transfusion have been used very infrequently in neonatology. Animal experiments show granulocyte transfusions can improve the survival rates of septic, neutropenic, neonatal, and adult subjects. However, practical problems with the rapid procurement and administration of neutrophil concentrates severely limit their clinical usefulness. The availability of new generations of effective antibiotics, recombinant hematopoietic growth factors to counter neutropenia, the risk of transmission of infection and the necessity for appropriate technology are some of the factors that have diminished the enthusiasm for use of granulocyte transfusions in neonates. A recent systematic review evaluated the role of granulocyte transfusions as an adjunct to antibiotics in the treatment of neutropenic septic newborns [121]. Authors of this systematic review found that no recent studies of granulocyte transfusion have been conducted in newborn infants. They found no significant difference in mortality of all causes during hospitalization in infants with sepsis and neutropenia who received granulocyte transfusions when compared with placebo or no granulocyte transfusion. We do not recommend the use of granulocyte transfusions in neonates.

A Consistent Approach to IVIg Administration for Neonates with Cytopenias

Background

Intravenous immunoglobulin has been suggested for a variety of neonatal applications. Updates of these putative uses, and the studies testing them, can be found in the Cochrane Neonatal Library.

Prevention of Infection

Nosocomial infections continue to be a significant cause of morbidity and mortality among preterm and/or low birth weight infants. Maternal transport of immunoglobulins to the fetus mainly occurs after 32 weeks' gestation and endogenous synthesis does not begin until several months after birth. Administration of intravenous immunoglobulin provides IgG that can bind to cell surface receptors, provide opsonic activity, activate complement, and promote antibody dependent cytotoxicity. Intravenous immunoglobulin thus has the potential of preventing or altering the course of nosocomial infections.

Ohlsson and Lacy conducted a systematic review to assess the effectiveness and safety of intravenous immunoglobulin (IVIg) administration compared to placebo or no intervention to preterm and/or low birth weight (LBW, less than 2,500 gram birth weight) infants in preventing nosocomial infections [122]. Nineteen studies conducted in many countries were included in this review. The most recent trial was reported in 2000. These included approximately 5,000 preterm and/or LBW infants. Among qualifying studies, the quantity of IVIg per dose varied widely from 120 mg/kg to 1 g/kg. Also, the number of doses varied from a single dose to seven doses. Several different IVIg preparations were used including Gammagard, Sandoglobulin, Gamimmune, Intraglobin; IgVena, Biotransfusion, an unnamed product, Venogamma, and Gammumine-N. When all studies were combined the meta-analysis indicated that IVIg administration resulted in a 3% reduction in sepsis and a 4% reduction in any serious infection, one or more episodes, but was not associated with reductions in other important outcomes: sepsis, necrotizing enterocolitis, intraventricular hemorrhage, or length of hospital stay. Most importantly, IVIg administration did not have any significant effect on mortality from any cause or from infections. Prophylactic use of IVIg was not associated with any short-term serious side effects. From a clinical perspective the small reduction in nosocomial infections without a reduction in mortality or other important clinical outcomes is felt to be of marginal importance. Therefore, we do not recommend IVIg administration as a means of preventing hospital-acquired infections.

Treatment of Infection

Ohlsson and Lacy conducted a systematic review to assess the effectiveness of intravenous immunoglobulin (IVIg) to reduce mortality and morbidity caused by suspected and proven infection in newborn infants [123]. A total of 9 studies evaluating 3973 infants were included in this review. The undisputable results of the largest trial included in this systematic review, INIS trial, which enrolled 3493 infants, and our meta-analyses ($n = 3973$) showed no reduction in mortality during hospital stay, or death or major disability at 2 years of age in infants with suspected or proven infection [124]. Although based on a small sample size ($n = 266$), this update provides additional evidence that IgM-enriched IVIg does not significantly reduce mortality during hospital stay in infants with suspected infection. Routine administration of IVIg or IgM-enriched IVIg to prevent mortality in infants with suspected or proven neonatal infection is not recommended. No further research is recommended.

Immune-Mediated Neutropenia or Thrombocytopenia

For neonates with severe immune-mediated neutropenia we find G-CSF to be more effective in raising the blood neutrophil count, and more conducive to titrating the dosage so as to keep the neutrophil count above 1,000/µL. Therefore, we do not recommend IVIg as a treatment for immune-mediated neutropenia. For immune-mediated thrombocytopenia IVIg can sometimes be helpful. Specifically, IVIg can be used for alloimmune cases where maternal apheresed platelets or typed (usually HPA-lb) platelets are not available for a neonate with severe thrombocytopenia and hemorrhage. Severe thrombocytopenic hemorrhage is rare in neonates whose mothers have autoimmune thrombocytopenia (such as ITP), but in such cases IVIg administration can be useful, along with random donor platelet transfusions.

Immune-Mediated Hemolytic Anemia

IVIg can reduce the rate of hemolysis of antibody-coated erythrocytes. Thus, neonates with immune-mediated hemolytic jaundice might be spared an exchange transfusion, or the number of exchange transfusion might be reduced, if IVIg is administered early during the course of hemolytic jaundice while the serum bilirubin concentration is rising.

Other Potential Uses

We know of no evidence that IVIg is useful for Coombs-negative anemias, non-immune cytopenias including PIH, or chronic benign neutropenia. Therefore, we do not recommend IVIG administration for any of these conditions.

References

1. Christensen RD, Jensen J, Maheshwari A, Henry E. Reference ranges for blood concentrations of eosinophils and monocytes during the neonatal period defined from over 63,000 records in a multihospital health-care system. *J Perinatol* 2010;**30**(8):540–5.

2. McCurley TL, Greer JP. Diagnostic approach to malignant and nonmalignant disorders of the phagocytic and immune systems. In Greer JP, Foerster J, Rodgers GM, et al. eds. *Wintrobe's Clinical Hematology* (Philadelphisa PA: Lippincott/Williams & Wilkins: 2009), pp. 1513–14.

3. Simon HU, Plotz SG, Dummer R, et al. Abnormal clones of T cells producing interleukin-5 in idiopathic eosinophilia. *N Engl J Med* 1999;**341** (15):1112–20.

4. Gotlib J. Molecular classification and pathogenesis of eosinophilic disorders: 2005 update. *Acta Haematol* 2005;**114**(1):7–25.

5. Lee NA, McGarry MP, Larson KA, et al. Expression of IL-5 in thymocytes/T cells leads to the development of a massive eosinophilia, extramedullary eosinophilopoiesis, and unique histopathologies. *J Immunol* 1997;**158**(3):1332–44.

6. Dent LA, Strath M, Mellor AL, Sanderson CJ. Eosinophilia in transgenic mice expressing interleukin 5. *J Exp Med* 1990;**172**(5):1425–31.

7. Rennick DM, Thompson-Snipes L, Coffinan RL, et al. In vivo administration of antibody to interleukin-5 inhibits increased generation of eosinophils and their progenitors in bone marrow of parasitized mice. *Blood* 1990; **76**(2):312–16.

8. Sher A, Coffman RL, Hieny S, et al. Interleukin 5 is required for the blood and tissue eosinophilia but not granuloma formation induced by infection with *Schistosoma mansoni. Proc Natl Acad Sci USA* 1990;**87**(1):61–5.

9. Lu L, Lin ZN, Shen RN, et al. Influence of interleukins 3,5, and 6 on the growth of eosinophil progenitors in highly enriched human bone marrow in the absence of serum. *Exp Hematol* 1990;**18**(11):1180–6.

10. Brugnoni D, Airo R, Rossi G, et al. A case of hypereosinophilic syndrome is associated with the expansion of a CD3-CD4+ T-cell population able to secrete large amounts of interleukin-5. *Blood* 1996;**87**(4):1416–22.

11. Okayama H, Fushimi T, Sllimura S, et al. Glucocorticoids suppressed production and gene expression of interleukin-5 by peripheral blood mononuclear cells in atopic patients and normal subjects. *J Allergy Clin Immunol* 1994;**93** (6):1006–12.

12. Krishnaswamy G, Smith J, Srikandl S, et al. Lymphoblastoid interferon-alpha inhibits T cell proliferation and expression of eosinophil-activating cytokines. *J Interferon Cytokine Res* 1996;**16**(10): 819–27.

13. Walsh GM, Hartnell A, Wardlaw AJ, et al. IL-5 enhances the in vitro adhesion of human eosinophils, but not neutrophils, in a leucocyte integrin (CD11/18)-dependent manner. *Immunology* 1990;**71** (2):258–65.

14. Medoff HS, Barbero GJ. Total blood eosinophil counts in the newborn period. *Pediatrics* 1950;**6**(5):737–42.

15. Xanthou M. Leucocyte blood picture in ill newborn babies. *Arch Dis Child* 1972;**47**(255):741–6.

16. Burrell JM. A comparative study of the circulating eosinophil level in babies. *Part I. Premature infants. Arch Dis Child* 1952;**27**(134):337–40.

17. Bass DA. Behavior of eosinophil leukocytes in acute inflammation. II. Eosinophil dynamics during acute inflammation. *J Clin Invest* 1975;**56**(4):870–9.

18. Gibson, EL, Y Vaucher, Corrigan JJ Jr. Eosinophilia in premature infants: Relationship to weight gain. *J Pediatr* 1979;**95**(1):99–101.

19. Portuguezmalavasi A, Coteboileau T, Aranda JV. Eosinophilia in the newborn, possible role in adverse drug-reactions. *Pediatrc Res* 1980;**14**(4):537–8.

20. Craver RD. The cytology of cerebrospinal fluid associated with neonatal intraventricular hemorrhage. *Pediatr Pathol Lab Med* 1996;**16**(5):713–19.

21. Patel L, Garvey B, Arnon S, Roberts IA. Eosinophilia in newborn infants. *Acta Paediatr* 1994;**83**(8):797–801.

22. Odelram H, Bjorksten B, Leander E, Kjellman NI. Predictors of atopy in newborn babies. *Allergy* 1995;**50**(7):585–92.

23. Yamamoto C, Kojima T, Hatrori K, et al. Eosinophilia in premature infants: Correlation with chronic lung disease. *Acta Paediatrica* 1996;**85**(10):1232–5.

24. Morgan AJ, Steen CJ, Schwartz RA, Janniger CK. Erythema toxicum neonatorum revisited. *Cutis* 2009;**83**(1):13–16.

25. Matsumoto K, Shimanouchi Y, Kawakubo K, et al. Infantile eczema at one month of age is associated with cord blood eosinophilia and subsequent development of atopic dermatitis and wheezing illness until two years of age. *Int Arch Allergy Immunol* 2005;**137** Suppl 1:69–76.

26. Marchini, G, Ulfgren AK, Loré K, et al. Erythema toxicum neonatorum: An immunohistochemical analysis. *Pediatr Dermatol* 2001;**18**(3):177–87.

27. Ladrigan MK, LeBoit PE, Frieden IJ. Neonatal eosinophilic pustulosis in a 2-month old. *Pediatr Dermatol* 2008;**25**(1):52–5.

28. Asgari M, Leiferman KM, Piepkorn M, Kuechle MK. Neonatal eosinophilic pustulosis. *Int J Dermatol* 2006;**45**(2):131–4.

29. Chiang YC, Shyur SD, Huang LH, et al. Chlamydia trachomatis pneumonia: Experience in a medical center. *Acta Paediatr Taiwan* 2005;**46**(5):284–8.

30. Lindemans, CA, Kimpen JL, Luijk B, et al. Systemic eosinophil response induced by respiratory syncytial virus. *Clin Exp Immunol* 2006;**144**(3):409–17.

31. Brostrom EB, Katz-Salamon M, Lundahl J, Halldén G, Winbladh B. Eosinophil activation in preterm infants with lung disease. *Acta Paediatr*, 2007;**96**(1):23–8.

32. Pentiuk SP, Miller CK, Kaul A. Eosinophilic esophagitis in infants and toddlers. *Dysphagia* 2007;**22**(1):44–8.

33. Ohtsuka, Y, Shimizu T, Shoji H, et al. Neonatal transient eosinophilic colitis causes lower gastrointestinal bleeding in early infancy. *J Pediatr Gastroenterol Nutr* 2007;**44**(4):501–5.

34. Tajirian A, Ross R, Zeikus P, Robinson -Bostom L. Subcutaneous fat necrosis of the newborn with eosinophilic granules. *J Cutan Pathol* 2007;**34**(7):588–90.

35. Juul SE, Haynes JW, McPherson RJ. Evaluation of eosinophilia in hospitalized preterm infants. *J Perinatol* 2005;**25**(3):182–8.

36. Carballo C, Foucar K, Swanson P, Papile LA, Watterberg KL. Effect of high altitude on neutrophil counts in newborn infants. *J Pediatr* 1991;**119**(3):464–6.

37. Maynard EC, Reed C, Kircher T. Neutrophil counts in newborn infants at high altitude. *J Pediatr* 1993;**122**(6):990–1.

38. Schmutz N, Henry E, Jopling J, Christensen RD. Expected ranges for blood neutrophil concentrations of neonates: The Manroe and Mouzinho charts revisited. *J Perinatol* 2008;**28**(4):275–81.

39. Manroe BL, Weinberg AG, Rosenfeld CR, Browne R. The neonatal blood count in health and disease. I. Reference values for neutrophilic cells. *J Pediatr* 1979;**95**(1):89–98.

40. Mouzinho A, Rosenfeld CR, Sanchez PJ, Risser R. Revised reference ranges for circulating neutrophils in very-low-birth-weight neonates. *Pediatrics* 1994;**94**(1):76–82.

41. Manroe BL. Neutrophil values in infants born at high altitudes. *J Pediatr* 1992;**120**(2 Pt 1):334–5.

42. Xanthou M. Leucocyte blood picture in healthy full-term and premature babies during neonatal period. *Arch Dis Child* 1970;**45**(240):242–9.

43. Newman TB, Puopolo KM, Wi S, Draper D, Escobar GJ. Interpreting complete blood counts soon after birth in newborns at risk for sepsis. *Pediatrics* 2010; **126**(5):903–9.

44. Hornik CP, Benjamin DK, Becker KC, et al. Use of the complete blood cell count in late-onset neonatal sepsis. *Pediatr Infect Dis J* 2012;**31**(8):803–7.

45. Rastogi S, Rastogi D, Sundaram R, Kulpa J, Parekh AJ. Leukemoid reaction in extremely low-birth-weight infants. *Am J Perinatol* 1999;**16**(2):93–7 .

46. Krumbhaar EB. Leukemoid blood pictures in various clinical conditions. *Am J Med Sci* 1926;**172**(4):519–32.

47. Calhoun DA, Kirk JF, Christensen RD. Incidence, significance, and kinetic mechanism responsible for leukemoid reactions in patients in the neonatal intensive care unit: a prospective evaluation. *J Pediatr* 1996;**129**(3):403–9.

48. Zanardo V, Savio V, Giacomin C, et al. Relationship between neonatal leukemoid reaction and bronchopulmonary dysplasia in low-birth-weight infants: a cross-sectional study. *Am J Perinatol* 2002;**19**(7):379–86.

49. Hsiao R, Omar SA. Outcome of extremely low birth weight infants with leukemoid reaction. *Pediatrics* 2005;**116**(1):e43-e51.

50. Zanardo V, Vedovato S, Trevisanuto DD, et al. Histological chorioamnionitis and neonatal leukemoid reaction in low-birth-weight infants. *Hum Pathol* 2006;**37**(1):87–91.

51. Henry E, Walker D, Wiedmeier SE, Christensen RD. Hematological abnormalities during the first week of life among neonates with Down syndrome: Data from a multihospital healthcare system. *Am J Med Genet A* 2007;**143A**(1):42–50.

52. Nijhawan A, Baselga E, Gonzalez-Ensenat MA, et al. Vesiculopustular eruptions in Down syndrome neonates with myeloproliferative disorders. *Arch Dermatol* 2001;**137**(6):760–3.

53. Burch JM, Weston WL, Rogers M, Morelli JG. Cutaneous pustular leukemoid reactions in trisomy 21. *Pediatr Dermatol* 2003;**20**(3):232–7.

54. Xu G, Nagano M, Kanezaki R, et al. Frequent mutations in the GATA-1 gene in the transient myeloproliferative disorder of Down syndrome. *Blood* 2003;**102**(8):2960–8.

55. Crispino JD. GATA1 in normal and malignant hematopoiesis. *Semin Cell Dev Biol* 2005;**16**(1):137–47.

56. Engmann C, Donn SM. Severe neutrophilia in an infant with persistent pulmonary hypertension of the newborn. *Am J Perinatol* 2003;**20**(7):347–51.

57. Alizadeh P, Rahbarimanesh AA, Bahram MG, Salmasian H. Leukocyte adhesion deficiency type 1 presenting as leukemoid reaction. *Indian J Pediatr* 2007;**74**(12):1121–3.

58. Lambert RM, Baer VL, Wiedmeier SE, et al. Isolated elevated blood neutrophil concentration at altitude does not require NICU admission if appropriate reference ranges are used. *J Perinatol* 2009;**29**(12):822–5.

59. Wiedmeier SE, Henry E, Christensen RD. Hematological abnormalities during the first week of life among neonates with trisomy 18 and trisomy 13: Data from a multi-hospital healthcare system. *Am J Med Genet A* 2008;**146A**(3):312–20.

60. Brazy JE, Grimm JK, Little VA. Neonatal manifestations of severe maternal hypertension occurring before the thirty-sixth week of pregnancy. *J Pediatr* 1982;**100**(2):265–71

61. Koenig JM, Christensen RD. Incidence, neutrophil kinetics, and natural history of neonatal neutropenia associated with maternal hypertension. *N Engl J Med* 1989;**321**(9):557–62.

62. Koenig JM, Christensen RD. The mechanism responsible for diminished neutrophil production in neonates delivered of women with pregnancy-induced hypertension. *Am J Obstet Gynecol* 1991;**165**(2):467–73.

63. Doron MW, Makhlouf RA, Katz VL, et al. Increased incidence of sepsis at birth in neutropenic infants of mothers with preeclampsia. *J Pediatr* 1994;**125**(3):452–8.

64. Cadnapaphornchai M, Faix RG. Increased nosocomial infection in neutropenic low birth weight (2000 grams or less) infants of hypertensive mothers. *J Pediatr* 1992;**121**(6): 956–61.

65. Koenig JM, Hunter DD, Christensen RD. Neutropenia in donor (anemic) twins involved in the twin-twin transfusion syndrome. *J Perinatol* 1991;**11**(4):355–8.

66. Koenig JM, Christensen RD. Neutropenia and thrombocytopenia in infants with Rh hemolytic disease. *J Pediatr* 1989;**114**(4 Pt 1):625–31.

67. Zook KJ, Mackley AB, Kern J, Paul DA. Hematologic effects of placental pathology on very low birthweight infants born to mothers with preeclampsia. *J Perinatol* 2009;**29**(1):8–12.

68. Guner S, Yigit S, Cetin M, et al. Evaluation of serum granulocyte colony stimulating factor levels in infants of preeclamptic mothers. *Turk J Pediatr* 2007;**49**(1):55–60.

69. Tsao PN, Teng R-J, Tang J-R, Yau K-I T. Granulocyte colony-stimulating factor in the cord blood of premature neonates born to mothers with pregnancy-induced hypertension. *J Pediatr* 1999;**135**(1):56–9.

70. Manzoni P, Farina D, Monetti C, et al. Early-onset neutropenia is a risk factor for *Candida* colonization in very low-birth-weight neonates. *Diagn Microbiol Infect Dis* 2007;**57**(1):77–83.

71. Teng RJ, Wu TJ, Garrison RD, Sharma R, Huday ML. Early neutropenia is not associated with an increased rate of nosocomial infection in very low-birth-weight infants. *J Perinatol* 2009;**29**(3):219–24.

72. Ahmad M, Fleit HB, Golightly MG, LaGamma EF. In vivo effect of recombinant human granulocyte colony-stimulating factor on phagocytic function and oxidative burst activity in septic neutropenic neonates. *Biol Neonate* 2004;**86**(1):48–54.

73. Zuppa AA, Girlando P, Florio MG, et al. Influence of maternal preeclampsia on recombinant human granulocyte colony-stimulating factor effect in neutropenic neonates with suspected sepsis. *Eur J Obstet Gynecol Reprod Biol* 2002;**102**(2):131–6.

74. Kocherlakota P, La Gamma EF. Preliminary report: rhG-CSF may reduce the incidence of neonatal sepsis in prolonged preeclampsia-associated neutropenia. *Pediatrics* 1998;**102**(5):1107–11.

75. Shankaran S, Pappas A, Laptook AR, et al. Outcomes of safety and effectiveness in a multicenter randomized, controlled trial of whole-body hypothermia for neonatal hypoxic-ischemic encephalopathy. *Pediatrics* 2008;**122**(4):e791–8.

76. Azzopardi DV, Strohm B, Edwards AD, et al. Moderate hypothermia to treat perinatal asphyxial encephalopathy. *N Engl J Med* 2009;**361**(14):1349–58.

77. Jacobs SE, Morley CJ, Inder TE, et al. Whole-body hypothermia for term and near-term newborns with hypoxic-ischemic encephalopathy: A randomized controlled trial. *Arch Pediatr Adolesc Med* 2011;**165**(8):692–700.

78. Simbruner G, Mittal RA, Rohlmann F, et al. Systemic hypothermia after neonatal encephalopathy: Outcomes of neo.nEURO.network RCT. *Pediatrics* 2010;**126**(4):e771–8.

79. Jenkins DD, Lee T, Chiuzan C, et al. Altered circulating leukocytes and their chemokines in a clinical trial of therapeutic hypothermia for neonatal hypoxic ischemic encephalopathy*. *Pediatr Crit Care Med* 2013;**14**(8):786–95

80. Cybulsky MI, Movat HZ. Experimental bacterial pneumonia in rabbits: Polymorphonuclear leukocyte margination and sequestration in rabbit lungs and quantitation and kinetics of 51Cr-labeled polymorphonuclear leukocytes in *E. coli*-induced lung lesions. *Exp Lung Res* 1982;**4**(1):47–66.

81. Erdman SH, Christensen RD, Bradley PP, Rothstein G. Supply and release of storage neutrophils. A developmental study. *Biol Neonate* 1982;**41**(3–4):132–7

82. Christensen RD, Rothstein G. Exhaustion of mature marrow neutrophils in neonates with sepsis. *J Pediatr* 1980;**96**(2):316–18.

83. Christensen RD. Neutrophil kinetics in the fetus and neonate. *Am J Pediatr Hematol Oncol* 1989;**11**(2):215–23.

84. al-Mulla ZS, Christensen RD. Neutropenia in the neonate. *Clin Perinatol* 1995;**22**(3):711–39.

85. Rodwell, RL, Taylor K, Tudehope D, Gray P. Hematologic scoring system in early diagnosis of sepsis in neutropenic newborns. *Pediatr Infect Dis J* 1993;**12**(5):372–6.

86. Carr R. Neutrophil production and function in newborn infants. *Br J Haematol* 2000;**110**(1):18–28.

87. Maheshwari A, Christensen RD. Developmental granulopoiesis. In Polin RA, Fox WW, Abman SH, eds. *Fetal and Neonatal Physiology* (Philadelphia, PA: Saunders, 2004).

88. Boxer LA, Yokoyama M, Lalezari P. Isoimmune neonatal neutropenia. *J Pediatr* 1972;**80**(5):783–7.

89. Lalezari P, Radel E. Neutrophil-specific antigens: Immunology and clinical significance. *Semin Hematol* 1974;**11**(3):281–90.

90. Levine DH, Madyastha PR. Isoimmune neonatal neutropenia. *Am J Perinatol* 1986;**3**(3):231–3.

91. Conway LT, Clay ME, Kline WE, et al. Natural history of primary autoimmune neutropenia in infancy. *Pediatrics* 1987;**79**(5):728–33.

92. Lalezari P, Khorshidi M, Petrosova M. Autoimmune neutropenia of infancy. *J Pediatr* 1986;**109**(5):764–9.

93. Veldhuisen B, Porcelijn L, Ellen van der Schoot C, de Haas M. Molecular typing of human platelet and neutrophil antigens (HPA and HNA). *Transfus Apher Sci* 2014;**50**(2):189–99.

94. Boxer LA, Greenberg MS, Boxer GJ, Stossel TP. Autoimmune neutropenia. *N Engl J Med* 1975;**293**(15):748–53.

95. Lyall EG, Lucas GF, Eden OB. Autoimmune neutropenia of infancy. *J Clin Pathol* 1992;**45**(5):431–4.

96. Bux J. Molecular nature of granulocyte antigens. *Transfus Clin Biol* 2001;**8**(3):242–7.

97. Farruggia P. Immune neutropenias of infancy and childhood. *World J Pediatr* 2016;**12**(2):142–8.

98. Horwitz M, Benson K, Person R, et al. Mutations in ELA2, encoding neutrophil elastase, define a 21-day biological clock in cyclic haematopoiesis. *Nat Genet* 1999;**23**(4): 433–6.

99. Dale DC, Person RE, Bolyard AA, et al. Mutations in the gene encoding neutrophil elastase in congenital and cyclic neutropenia. *Blood* 2000;**96**(7):2317–22.

100. Beekman R, Touw IP. G-CSF and its receptor in myeloid malignancy. *Blood* 2010;**115**(25):5131–6.

101. Link DC, Kunter G, Kasai Y, et al. Distinct patterns of mutations occurring in de novo AML versus AML arising in the setting of severe congenital neutropenia. *Blood* 2007;**110**(5):1648–55.

102. Skokowa J, Steinemann D, Katsman-Kuipers JE, et al. Cooperativity of RUNX1 and CSF3 R mutations in severe congenital neutropenia: A unique pathway in myeloid leukemogenesis. *Blood* 2014;**123**(14): 2229–37.

103. Kostmann R. Infantile genetic agranulocytosis; agranulocytosis infantilis hereditaria. *Acta Paediatr Suppl* 1956;**45**(Suppl 105):1–78.

104. Bonilla MA, Gillio AP, Ruggeiro M, et al. Effects of recombinant human granulocyte colony-stimulating factor on neutropenia in patients with congenital agranulocytosis. *N Engl J Med* 1989;**320**(24):1574–80.

105. Dale DC, Bolyard AA, Hammond WP. Cyclic neutropenia: Natural history and effects of long-term treatment with recombinant human granulocyte colony-stimulating factor. *Cancer Invest* 1993;**11**(2):219–23.

106. Makaryan V, Zeidler C, Bolyard AA, et al. The diversity of mutations and clinical outcomes for ELANE-associated neutropenia. *Curr Opin Hematol* 2015;**22**(1):3–11.

107. Shwachman H, Diamond LK, Oski FA, Khaw KT. The syndrome of pancreatic insufficiency and bone marrow dysfunction. *J Pediatr* 1964;**65**:645–63.

108. Burroughs L, Woolfrey A, Shimamura A. Shwachman–Diamond syndrome: A review of the clinical presentation, molecular pathogenesis, diagnosis, and treatment. *Hematol Oncol Clin North Am* 2009;**23**(2):233–48.

109. Boocock GR, Morrison JA, Popovic M, et al. Mutations in SBDS are associated with Shwachman-Diamond syndrome. *Nat Genet* 2003;**33**(1):97–101.

110. Ganapathi KA, Austin KM, Lee CS, et al. The human Shwachman–Diamond syndrome protein, SBDS, associates with ribosomal RNA. *Blood* 2007;**110**(5):1458–65.

111. Rujkijyanont P, Adams S-L, Beyene J, Dror Y. Bone marrow cells from patients with Shwachman–Diamond syndrome abnormally express genes involved in ribosome biogenesis and RNA processing. *Br J Haematol* 2009;**145**(6):806–15.

112. Roper M, Parmley RT, Crist WM, Kelly DR, Cooper MD. Severe congenital leukopenia (reticular dysgenesis).Immunologic and morphologic characterizations of leukocytes. *Am J Dis Child* 1985;**139**(8):832–5.

113. Bertrand Y, Müller S, Casanova J, et al. Reticular dysgenesis: HLA non-identical bone marrow transplants in a series of 10 patients. *Bone Marrow Transplant* 2002;**29**(9):759–62.

114. Christensen RD, Henry E, Wiedmeier SE, Stoddard RA, Lambert DK. Low blood neutrophil concentrations among extremely low birth weight neonates: data from a multihospital health-care system. *J Perinatol* 2006;**26**(11):682–7.

115. Juul SE, Calhoun DA, Christensen RD. "Idiopathic neutropenia" in very low birthweight infants. *Acta Paediatr* 1998;**87**(9):963–8.

116. Juul SE, Christensen RD. Effect of recombinant granulocyte colony-stimulating factor on blood neutrophil concentrations among patients with "idiopathic neonatal neutropenia": A randomized, placebo-controlled trial. *J Perinatol* 2003;**23**(6):493–7.

117. Rivers A, Slayton WB. Congenital cytopenias and bone marrow failure syndromes. *Semin Perinatol* 2009;**33**(1):20–8.

118. Nittala S, Subbarao GC, Maheshwari A. Evaluation of neutropenia and neutrophilia in preterm infants. *J Matern Fetal Neonatal Med* 2012;**25**(Suppl 5):100–3.

119. Corey SJ, Wollman MR, Deshpande RV. Granulocyte colony-stimulating factor and congenital neutropenia–risk of leukemia? *J Pediatr* 1996;**129**(1):187–8.

120. Sullivan SE, Calhoun DA. Eosinophilia in the neonatal intensive care unit. *Clin Perinatol* 2000;**27**(3): 603–22, vi.

121. Pammi M, Brocklehurst P. Granulocyte transfusions for neonates with confirmed or suspected sepsis and neutropenia. *Cochrane Database Syst Rev* 2011;**10**:CD003956.

122. Ohlsson A, Lacy JB. Intravenous immunoglobulin for preventing infection in preterm and/or low-birth-weight infants. *Cochrane Database Syst Rev*, 2004;**1**:CD000361.

123. Ohlsson A, Lacy JB. Intravenous immunoglobulin for suspected or proven infection in neonates. *Cochrane Database Syst Rev*, 2015;**3**:CD001239.

124. Inis Collaborative Group, Brocklehurst P, Farrell B, et al. Treatment of neonatal sepsis with intravenous immune globulin. *N Engl J Med* 2011;**365**(13):1201–11.

Functional Phagocyte Disorders in the Neonate

Thomas F. Michniacki and Kelly Walkovich

Introduction

In addition to quantitative neutrophil abnormalities, innate immunity, and thus risk of infection in a neonate, may be negatively impacted by qualitative phagocyte defects. The term phagocyte stems from the Greek "phagein" meaning "to eat or devour" and "cyte" meaning "cell" and refers to hematopoietic derived cells, namely monocytes, macrophages and neutrophils capable of engulfing and digesting microorganisms, foreign particles, and cellular debris. Neutrophils are also classified as granulocytes, given the characteristic presence of granules in their cytoplasm that play a key role in neutrophil function.

Term and preterm infants have age-appropriate inherent limitations in the functional capabilities of their neutrophils but may also present with additional pathologic phagocytic disorders. It is imperative that clinicians who care for neonates understand the normal immunological dysfunction of the newborn neutrophil and are able to recognize and care for neonates suspected of having a functional phagocyte disorder.

Neutrophil Development in the Neonate

Leukocytes within the mononuclear-phagocyte system, including neutrophils, monocytes, macrophages, eosinophils, and basophils, are derived from a common progenitor cell located within the bone marrow, the colony-forming unit granulocyte-monocyte (CFU-GM). The proliferation and differentiation of these early progenitor cells depends on numerous cytokines with granulocyte-macrophage colony-stimulating factor (GM-CSF) and granulocyte colony-stimulating factor (G-CSF) being the most prominent. Neutrophil development proceeds from the most immature cells capable of mitotic division, i.e., myeloblast to promyelocyte to myelocyte, to immature cells undergoing maturation, i.e., metamyelocyte to band to mature neutrophils. It is these immature neutrophil progenitors that create a reserve pool within the bone marrow capable of cellular division and neutrophil mobilization at times of need [1, 2]. Term neonates have a vastly reduced proliferative pool with estimates at about 10% of adult values. This diminished pool results in a depressed ability to mount an appropriate response to infectious organisms, with newborns often exhausting their neutrophil reserves during active infections and having an elevated risk of mortality and morbidity secondary to sepsis. It is not until approximately 4 weeks of age that neutrophil pool quantities reach those of adults. Small for gestational age, preterm and extremely low birth rate neonates have further diminished proliferative pools and additionally may manifest neutropenia regardless of infection status, secondary to reduced neutrophil production. Reduced phagocytic cell production may be a result of decreased G-CSF and GM-CSF levels in these infants [2–4].

Granulopoiesis, the formation of granules within a cell, is an imperative developmental step during neutrophil maturation, with additional creation of secretory vesicles within the mature neutrophil to assist with cellular migration and adherence. Azurophilic, specific, and gelatinase granules contribute substantially to the extracellular/intracellular antimicrobial and migratory/extravasation properties of neutrophils. Certain neonatal granule protein levels, including lactoferrin and bactericidal permeability-increasing proteins, do appear to be reduced compared to adults with preterm infants also showing decreased degranulation capabilities [2, 3, 5]

Neonatal Hematology, Pathogenesis, Diagnosis, and Management of Hematologic Problems, 3rd edition, ed. Pedro A. de Alarcón, Eric J. Werner, Robert D. Christensen, and Martha C. Sola-Visner. Published by Cambridge University Press.

Neutrophil Function in the Neonate

See Table 17.1 for a summary of neonatal neutrophil function characteristics and defects.

Migration and Adherence

Once released from the bone marrow storage pool, neutrophils are capable of migrating from the circulatory system into extravascular sites of inflammation. This process involves multiple steps, all of which show altered ability within the neonate. Following entry into the bloodstream, adherence to the vascular endothelial cells with subsequent leukocyte rolling and adherence is facilitated by cellular membrane molecules. As neutrophils transiently interact and roll along vascular cell surfaces they adhere to sites of inflammation through an interaction between L-selectin on neutrophils and P- and E-selectins on endothelial cells [1]. A firm attachment to the vascular surface is formed by shedding of L-selectin and increased expression of beta2-integrins on the neutrophil with ensuing binding of the beta2-integrins to intercellular endothelial adhesions molecules 1 and 2 (ICAM-1 and ICAM-2) on endothelial cells. Neonatal neutrophils, especially those found in preterm infants, appear to have decreased rolling and adhesion capabilities due to reduced L-selectin expression,

L-selectin shedding, and beta2-integrin protein upregulation. An immature vascular endothelium with suboptimal P-selectin may also contribute to poor neutrophil rolling and adhesion [2, 3, 6].

Diapedesis and Basement Membrane Passage

Diapedesis, in which neutrophils migrate between endothelial cells and into the extravascular space, requires a cytoskeleton capable of deformability in addition to the beta2-integrin and ICAM interactions noted above. Furthermore, successful movement through the endothelial basement membrane is facilitated by neutrophil release of digestive enzymes, including elastase and collagenase [1, 2]. Neutrophils from newborns exhibit increased rigidity likely secondary to altered F-actin levels and abnormal membrane fluidity with resultant inability to modify cellular shape upon stimulation. Reduced elastase degranulation capabilities in preterm infants likely also affects passage through the endothelial basement membrane [2–4, 6].

Chemotaxis

The movement of neutrophils within the extravascular space across a gradient of chemotactic factors is termed chemotaxis. This cellular

Table 17.1 Neonatal neutrophil function characteristics

Neutrophil function	Neonatal defect
Migration and adherence	Neonatal neutrophils, particularly preterm infants, have reduced L-selectin expression, L-selectin shedding and beta2-integrin protein upregulation Immature vascular endothelium with suboptimal P-selectin
Diapedesis and basement membrane passage	All newborns exhibit increased neutrophil rigidity secondary to altered F-actin levels and abnormal membrane fluidity Reduced elastase degranulation capabilities in preterm infants affects passage through the endothelial basement membrane
Chemotaxis	Reduced expression and function of chemotactic sensory receptors in newborns Suboptimal intracellular free calcium levels following activation Preterm infants may not show significant improvement in chemotaxis until 2 months of age Sepsis, indomethacin, and magnesium sulfate may negatively affect chemotactic abilities
Phagocytosis	Impaired ability to upregulate CR3 in both preterm and term infants Preterm neonates show significantly less expression of Fc gamma receptors Preterm neonates have greatly reduced phagocytosis, but nearly normal phagocytic abilities are restored if focus of phagocytosis is opsonized appropriately
Respiratory burst	Ill term and preterm neonates exhibit suppressed respiratory burst Healthy preterm newborns show decreased capacity to upregulate oxidative burst following bacterial stimulation Respiratory burst deficiencies appear to persist throughout times of infection and until 2 months of age
Neutrophil extracellular traps (NETs)	NETs creation impaired in both term and preterm infants

propulsion requires sensory receptors for various chemotactic peptide molecules. Impaired kinesis of newborn neutrophils results from not only reduced expression but decreased function of these receptors. Intracellular calcium plays an important role in chemotaxis following receptor stimulation and neutrophils within neonates appear to have suboptimal intracellular free calcium levels following activation [1, 2]. Term infants reach adult chemotactic abilities by approximately 2 weeks of age but preterm infants may not show significant improvement in chemotaxis until 2 months of age [6]. Sepsis, indomethacin administration, and intrapartum exposure to magnesium sulfate may further negatively affect chemotactic abilities [3, 7].

Phagocytosis

Upon entry into areas of inflammation neutrophils may encounter pathogens necessitating phagocytosis to aid in microbial clearance. Successful phagocytosis by neutrophils is aided by complement receptors, particularly the CR3 receptor, and Fc gamma receptors, which bind immunoglobulins as both complement and immunoglobulin are key contributors to opsonization. The ability to upregulate CR3 is decreased in both preterm and term infants. The expression of Fc gamma receptors in term infants appears to be comparable to adults but preterm neonates show significantly less expression of these receptors [6]. Interestingly, measurement of the phagocytic ability of neutrophils from term newborns was similar to adult controls but preterm neonates manifested greatly reduced phagocytosis when whole blood assays were used. The phagocytic defect observed in preterm infants can be improved by exposing the neutrophils to serum from adults or therapeutic immunoglobulin. Thus it appears that preterm and term neonates can show nearly normal phagocytic abilities if the focus of phagocytosis is opsonized appropriately [3].

Respiratory Burst

Following ingestion by phagocytosis, microorganisms are internalized into phagosomes, which then fuse with lysosomes and granules that contain proteolytic enzymes. These enzymes are next activated in the phagolysosome and digest the microorganism via generation of reactive oxygen species (using NADPH oxidase) and nitric oxide (using nitric oxide synthetase). Myeloperoxidase may additionally use the reactive oxygen species to create hypochlorous acid, which further assists in destruction in pathogens [1,3]. Under nonstressed conditions neutrophils from healthy newborns appear to show an intense respiratory burst response with increased reactive oxygen species generation. This elevated response is not sustained though at times of stress, including pulmonary or infectious insult, with neutrophils from ill neonates exhibiting suppressed respiratory burst. Healthy preterm newborns additionally show a reduced capacity to upregulate oxidative burst following bacterial stimulation. These neonatal respiratory burst deficiencies appear to persist throughout times of infection but will often normalize by 2 months of age in healthy infants [2–4].

Neutrophil Extracellular Traps (NETs)

Neutrophils also participate in a non-phagocytosis method of killing through the creation of neutrophil extracellular traps (NETs). NETs consist of DNA fragments and granule proteins extruded from neutrophils that form an extracellular scaffold of fibers with a high concentration of antimicrobial components with the ability to capture and destroy microbes. NET formation results from a cellular process that is separate from necrosis or apoptosis. The creation of NETs by both term and preterm infants is impaired and appears to further potentially increase their risk of infections [3, 4, 8].

Therapies to Overcome Neonatal Neutrophil Functional Deficiencies

The administration of G-CSF and GM-CSF can increase mobilization of neutrophils from the bone marrow, increase beta2-integrins expression on neutrophils (although they reduce L-selectin levels), and improve the phagocytic and respiratory burst properties of neutrophils [4, 7]. Studies show conflicting results on whether treatment with colony-stimulating factor reduces mortality in neonates with confirmed or presumed sepsis, although absolute neutrophil counts do increase in these patients following the administration of G-CSF [9–11].

Further large randomized studies are necessary to clarify any potential benefit of colony-stimulating factors in ill neonates. It has been found, however, that early postnatal prophylactic GM-CSF in extremely preterm infants (below 31 weeks' gestation) improves neutropenia but does not decrease rates of sepsis or improve survival [12].

It has been theorized that treatment with intravenous immunoglobulin may improve opsonic and phagocytic activity in septic neonates and potentially lead to improved survival rates but trials exploring this have had diverging results with no definitive conclusion being reached as to whether administration of immune globulin is beneficial in neonates with sepsis or not [4, 13–16]. Studies do show that there is not sufficient benefit to premature infants to routinely recommend prophylactic treatment with immune globulins [4, 16–18].

Functional Phagocyte Disorders in the Neonate

Table 17.2 summarizes disorders of the neutrophil, clinical manifestations, testing and treatments. Further details can be found in the sections that follow.

CARD9 Deficiency

CARD9 deficiency is an autosomal recessive disorder due to mutations in caspase recruitment domain-containing protein 9 (CARD9), an intracellular myeloid signaling molecule downstream of C-type lectin and Toll-like receptors [19]. Mutations in *CARD9* render the neutrophil defective against *Candida* and other serious fungal infections. Patients with CARD9 deficiency not unexpectedly present with a heightened susceptibility to fungal diseases including central nervous system and gastrointestinal tract infections with *Candida*, invasive *Exophiala* infections, and persistent mucocutaneous candidiasis. The invasiveness of the fungal disease is likely secondary to the killing defect of neutrophils and separates CARD9 deficiency from other disorders with chronic mucocutaneous candidiasis.

The deficit in fungal immunity is a result of the breakdown of the normal host defense. Normal host defense against *Candida* relies on opsonins, especially complement, and importantly the interaction of β-glucan and mannan residues on the surface of *Candida* with the C-type lectins expressed on the plasma membrane of myeloid cells to trigger an inflammatory response [20]. Activation of the C-type lectin or Toll-like receptors via recognition of fungal cell wall components results in phosphorylation of CARD9 and formation of a trimeric complex with B-cell lymphoma 10 (BCL10) and mucosa-associated lymphoid tissue lymphoma translocation gene 1 (MALT1). Formation of this trimeric CARD9-BCL10-MALT1 complex subsequently activates NF-κB and generates a pro-inflammatory response with IL-6 and IL-1β production that enhances antifungal, particularly anti-*Candida*, neutrophil function. CARD9 is also induces T-helper cells to produce interleukin-17 (IL-17), which plays a major role in the clearance of *Candida* [20]. Treatment of CARD9 deficiency relies on aggressive anti-fungal therapy in combination of with G-CSF and/or GM-CSF.

Chédiak–Higashi Syndrome

Chédiak–Higashi syndrome (CHS) is an autosomal recessive disorder that manifests with oculocutaneous albinism, neurologic dysfunction, abnormal coagulation, an elevated risk of hemophagocytic lymphohistiocytosis (HLH), and frequent infections with bacterial pathogens. A defect in the *CHS1/LYST* gene leads to abnormalities in lysosomal/vesicular transport and granulopoiesis. Giant azurophilic granules develop within patient neutrophils and other granulocytes and their appearance can assist in the diagnosis of patients [1]. Additionally, CHS neutrophils are deficient in granule proteases, suffer from delayed/incomplete degranulation and display faulty chemotaxis. [1, 21]. These functional neutrophil defects lead to recurrent and potentially serious cutaneous, respiratory tract, and mucous membrane bacterial infections. The lysosome and granule dysfunctions of the disorder lead to the clinical manifestations of albinism and coagulopathy as a result of improper transportation of melanosomes within melanocytes and reduction in platelet-dense bodies creating a platelet storage pool deficiency. Further hematological manifestations of the syndrome include neutropenia and a risk of development of hemophagocytic lymphohistiocytosis as the patient ages and enters the "accelerated phase" of the disorder. Patients

Table 17.2 Congenital disorders of the neutrophil

Disorder	Gene mutation	Inheritance pattern	Clinical manifestations	Specific diagnostic testing	Treatment
CARD9 deficiency	CARD9	AR	Invasive fungal infections, meningoencephalitis with Candida, chronic mucocutaneous candidiasis, deep and disseminated dermatophytosis	Skin biopsy with granulomatous dermatitis, extensive fungal evaluation	Anti-fungal prophylaxis, GM-CSF, consider HSCT
Chédiak–Higashi syndrome	LYST	AR	Oculocutaneous albinism, progressive neurologic dysfunction, giant granules within granulocytes, recurrent infections, bleeding diathesis, risk of hemophagocytic lymphohistiocytosis (HLH)	Platelet aggregation study, neuroimaging, EMG/EEG, peripheral smear evaluation, light microscopy of hair shafts, HLH evaluation studies, genetic testing	Antimicrobial prophylaxis, G-CSF, +/– interferon gamma, HLH targeted therapies, HSCT
Chronic granulomatous disease	CYBB CYBA NCF1 NCF2 NCF4	XL AR AR AR AR	Recurrent bacterial infections particularly with catalase-positive organisms, colitis, granuloma formation, risk of fungal disease and mulch pneumonitis	Neutrophil functional testing (DHR and NBT), ESR/CRP trending, imaging to rule out infections with inflammatory marker rises, genetic testing	Prophylaxis with TMP-SMX and itraconazole, +/– interferon-gamma, aggressive infection management with broad spectrum antimicrobials, glucocorticoids for liver abscess/mulch pneumonitis/Nocardia pneumonia, immunosuppression for severe inflammation, bone marrow transplantation
Glycogen storage disease type 1b	SLC37A4 or G6PC	AR	Hypoglycemia, seizures, lactic acidosis, hyperuricemia and hyperlipedimia. Neutropenia with defective chemotaxis, perioral and perianal infections, protracted diarrhea and colitis	Biallelic pathogenic variants in G6PC or SLC37A4 genes on molecular genetic testing or hepatic enzyme activity of glucose 6 phosphatase	Metabolic support by expert metabolic team to provide nutrition and particularly to control hypoglycemia, hyperuricemia and renal and hepatic complications. G-CSF therapy for neutropenia and recurrent infections
Hyperimmunoglobulin E syndromes (STAT3 LOF)	STAT3	AD	Recurrent "cold" skin abscesses (esp. S. aureus), eczema, retained primary teeth, coarse facial features, vascular anomalies, elevated IgE, eosinophilia, fractures, allergies	Serum IgE and eosinophils, vaccine response studies, dental radiology imaging, Th17 cell count, usage of diagnostic scoring system, annual PFTs/CXRs, genetic testing	Aggressive eczema management, TMP-SMX prophylaxis, +/– interferon-gamma
IRAK4 deficiency	IRAK4	AR	Lack of fever, unexpectedly low C-reactive protein (CRP) in setting of infection, recurrent invasive bacterial infections, inadequate polysaccharide vaccine response	Vaccine response studies, absence of toll-like receptor induced cytokine production, genetic testing	Antimicrobial prophylaxis, intravenous immunoglobulin (IVIg), antipneumococcal vaccination

Table 17.2 (cont.)

Disorder	Gene mutation	Inheritance pattern	Clinical manifestations	Specific diagnostic testing	Treatment
MyD88 deficiency	MYD88	AR	Recurrent infections, especially pneumococcal	Vaccine response studies, absence of toll-like receptor induced cytokine production, genetic testing	Quality skin care, antimicrobial prophylaxis, IVIg, antipneumococcal vaccination
Leukocyte adhesion deficiency (LAD)	ITGB2	AR	Leukocytosis, delayed umbilical cord separation, impaired wound healing, severe periodontitis, gingivitis, ulcerative skin lesions, colitis, HPV infections	CD18 and CD11 evaluation via flow cytometry, genetic testing	Excellent oral hygiene, antimicrobial prophylaxis, GM-CSF not useful, HSCT with severe disease
	SLC35C1	AR	Leukocytosis, recurrent infections, intellectual disability, depressed nasal bridge, Bombay blood phenotype	Analysis of blood phenotype, absence of CD15a on flow cytometry, genetic testing	Antimicrobial prophylaxis, excellent oral hygiene, fucose supplementation
	FERMT3	AR	Leukocytosis, recurrent infections, bleeding, osteoporosis-like bone abnormalities	Analysis of integrin activation and expression, genetic testing Functional assays for neutrophils and platelet adhesion, genetic testing	Antimicrobial prophylaxis, platelet transfusions with bleeding, HSCT
Mendelian susceptibility to mycobacterial diseases (IRF8 deficiency)	IRF8	AR	Severe monocytopenia and lack of dendritic cells, disseminated BCG infection, intellectual delay	Mendelian susceptibility to mycobacterial diseases flow cytometry	Mycobacterial prophylaxis, consideration for HSCT in severe disease
Myeloperoxidase deficiency	MPO	Mixed	Often asymptomatic, Candida infections in the setting of diabetes	Histochemical staining for MPO	Antimicrobial prophylaxis in those with recurrent infections
NF-κB essential modifier (NEMO) deficiency	IKBKG	XL	Immunodeficiency, mycobacterial susceptibility, ectodermal dysplasia, inflammatory/autoimmunity	Immunoglobulin levels, vaccination responses, genetic testing	IVIg, azithromycin, and TMP-SMX prophylaxis, HSCT
Neutrophil-specific granule deficiency	CEBPE SMARCD2	AR	Increased pyogenic infections, absence of specific granules, frequent bi-lobed neutrophils, risk of MDS/AML	Light and electron microscopy evaluation of neutrophils, biochemical measurements of granule proteins	Antimicrobial prophylaxis, aggressive management of infections, GM-CSF with severe infections, HSCT in those with risk of malignant transformation
Shwachman–Diamond syndrome	SDBS DNAJC21 EFL1 SRP54	AR AR AR AD	Pancreatic exocrine insufficiency, steatorrhea, skeletal abnormalities, short stature, elevated transaminases, bone marrow failure, risk for MDS/AML	Bone marrow evaluation, ultrasound of pancreas, serum trypsinogen (<3yo) or isoamylase (>3yo), genetic screening	G-CSF, annual bone marrow evaluations with FISH for MDS genetic alterations, pancreatic enzyme replacement, HSCT in those with severe disease
Wiskott–Aldrich syndrome	WAS	XL	Bleeding, immunodeficiency, eczema, malignancy	WAS protein analysis via flow cytometry, mean platelet value, genetic testing	Prophylactic antimicrobials, irradiated platelets, IVIG, rituximab in those with autoimmune cytopenias, HSCT

are additionally at risk of developing progressive neurologic abnormalities, including ataxia, peripheral neuropathy, seizures, motor/sensory deficits, and cognitive decline [1, 22].

Diagnosis should be considered in those caring for neonates exhibiting albinism and frequent pyogenic infections. Examination of the infant's blood smear may reveal absolute neutropenia and the presence of the classic large granules within all granulocytes, including neutrophils. Examination of fetal hair may reveal giant melanin granules. Definitive diagnosis is made via mutational testing for the CHS1/LYST gene. In those with a family history of the syndrome, prenatal diagnosis is additionally possible via analysis of chorionic villus or amniotic cells [1, 22].

Therapy is aimed at prophylactic administration of antibiotics, often trimethoprim-sulfamethoxazole, and aggressive treatment with antimicrobial therapy in those with proven or suspected infection. G-CSF administration may improve neutropenia. Patients often are referred to undergo hematopoietic stem cell transplantation (HSCT) prior to the development of hemophagocytic lymphohistiocytosis or devastating infections, but HSCT does not correct the neurologic deficits [1]. Treatment with ascorbic acid at high doses may improve the function of neutrophils in those with CHS and is reasonable to trial in patients [1, 23–25]

Chronic Granulomatous Disease

Chronic granulomatous disease (CGD) occurs with an estimated frequency of 1:200,000 live births and is due to mutations that disrupt the oxidative burst capacity of the nicotinamide adenine dinucleotide phosphate (NAPDH) oxidative complex in phagocytes [26]. Mutations in any of the genes (CYBB, CYBA, NFC1, NFC2, NFC4) that encode the five subunits (gp91phox, p22phox, p47phox, p67phox, p40phox, respectively) of NAPDH oxidase result in CGD. Defective oxidative burst results in the inability of neutrophils, monocytes and macrophages to kill many organisms, particularly catalase-positive bacteria such as Staphylococcus aureus, Burkholderia cepacia, Serratia marcescens, Nocardia, Samonella, and fungi such as Aspergillus.

Patients with CGD frequently present in infancy with the majority of patients presenting by childhood with severe or recurrent catalase-positive bacterial or fungal infections affecting the skin, lungs, liver, and lymph nodes. Fungal infections are the most common cause of death and carry a higher mortality risk than bacterial infections, although infections in CGD patients may be clinically underwhelming even with extensive disease [27]. Besides infections, patients with CGD are prone to inflammatory complications including granuloma formation and inflammatory bowel disease [28]. The dihydrorhodamine 123 (DHR) oxidation test can functionally assess the oxidative burst in clinically concerning patients. Gene sequencing can further confirm the disorder. Of note, patients with the X-linked form of CGD, due to mutations in CYBB, generally present with more severe disease as do patients with completely absent or extremely low residual superoxide production [29].

Treatment of CGD relies on aggressive treatment of active infections as well as prophylactic antimicrobials, e.g., trimethoprim-sulfamethoxazole, and antifungals, e.g., itraconazole [30]. Many patients also benefit from the use of interferon-gamma, although treatment with interferon-gamma is not universal [31]. Patients can be cured with hematopoietic stem cell transplant but the decision to proceed to transplant is based on the degree of disease severity and the quality of the donor match [32]. A limited number of patients have also been treated with gene therapy.

Glycogen Storage Disease Type 1b

Glycogen storage disease type 1b, also known as glucose-6-phosphatase deficiency or von Gierke disease, is an autosomal recessive condition most prominently associated with hypoglycemia and renal/hepatic abnormalities, but the disorder may also manifest neutropenia with dysfunctional neutrophil chemotaxis and respiratory burst capabilities [33, 34]. The majority of patients present with neutropenia prior to 1 year of age, although the neutropenia may be intermittent. The clinical impact of the neutropenia and neutrophil dysfunction is often clinically apparent in patients with the presence of perioral and perirectal infections as well as protracted diarrhea/colitis frequently reported [33]. A definitive diagnosis is made via genetic testing and G-CSF administration may reduce the frequency and severity of infections.

Hyperimmunoglobulin E Syndromes

Patients with autosomal dominant hyperimmunoglobulin E (hyper-IgE) syndrome most often have a mutation in the signal transducer and activator of transcription 3 (*STAT3*) gene causing defects in the JAK-STAT pathway with clinical manifestations of severe eczema and frequent sinopulmonary infections and staphylococcal abscesses. Facial features of patients are often coarse with a broad nasal base and bridge. Skeletal abnormalities include retention of primary teeth and scoliosis. Laboratory analysis reveals the presence of eosinophilia and IgE levels frequently >2,000 IU/mL. The majority of patients, 81%, present with an erythematous papulopustular in the newborn period [1, 35]. Various immune abnormalities are associated with this disorder disorder. These include failure of Th17 CD4 cell differentiation and reduced memory B cells. Although patients with hyper-IgE syndrome do not present with neutropenia they appear to have deficits in the chemotactic abilities of their neutrophils. Reduced IL-17 levels additionally appear to negatively affect the recruitment and expansion of neutrophils needed at times of inflammation [1, 36–38]. Of note, patients with DOCK8 deficiency present with hyperimmunoglobulin E with elevated IgE, recurrent infections, and eczema but do not have the neutrophil chemotactic defects, nor retained teeth. DOCK8 deficiency patients are often distinguishable from STAT3 LOF patients due to their propensity for food allergies and cutaneous viral infections. Similarly, phosphoglucomutase 3 (PGM 3) deficiency leads to a hyperimmunoglobulin E-like syndrome with elevations in IgE, recurrent sinopulmonary infections, and eczema but without the characteristic facial features or neutrophil chemotactic defects seen in autosomal dominant hyper-IgE syndrome [39, 40].

Hyper-IgE secondary to STAT3 dysfunction should be suspected in neonates with the distinct eczematous rash and a family history of the syndrome. Numerous scoring systems have been created to assist in the diagnosis of patients although confirmation of the diagnosis is made through genetic testing. Management involves meticulous skin care and antimicrobial prophylaxis with trimethoprim-sulfamethoxazole to reduce the frequency of cutaneous and sinopulmonary infections. There is currently no defined role for bone marrow transplantation and its usage is controversial [35, 41, 42].

IRAK4 Deficiency/MyD88 Deficiency

Toll-like receptors (TLRs) are surface molecules found predominantly on leukocytes that function as critical components of innate immunity via recognition of microbial antigens and subsequent activation of intracellular pathways to trigger antimicrobial and inflammatory cellular processes. Deficiency of the cytoplasmic signaling molecules IRAK4 and MyD88 that interact with TLRs can lead to an elevated risk of invasive pyogenic bacterial infections, most notably *Pseudomonas aeruginosa*, *Staphylococcus aureus*, and *Streptococcus pneumoniae* [43]. In addition to inadequate cytokine production (particularly tumor necrosis factor-alpha, IL-1, and IL-6) and hypogammaglobulinemia, dysfunctional neutrophil migration, recruitment and phagocytosis appear to play a role in the increased infection susceptibility observed in children with IRAK4 or MyD88 deficiency [44, 45]. Those afflicted with either condition often show a lack of fever and unexpectedly low markers of inflammation in setting of infection. An inadequate response to polysaccharide vaccines may also be observed. Aggressive treatment of bacterial infections with additional consideration for prophylactic antibiotics and immunoglobulin replacement are the preferred treatment modalities [43].

Leukocyte Adhesion Deficiency

Leukocyte adhesion deficiency (LAD) is a rare autosomal recessive immunodeficiency with dysfunctional immune cell migration wherein phagocytes cannot leave the vasculature to migrate normally into tissues under infection or inflammation. The disorder is clinically characterized by neutrophilia, infections with the notable absence of pus, impaired wound healing and in some cases delayed umbilical cord detachment. Three different subtypes of LAD exist.

LAD-1 is estimated to occur in 1:1 million live births and is due to bi-allelic mutations in *ITGB2*, the gene encoding the beta2 (β2) integrin CD18, that lead to impairment in β2 integrin expression, heterodimer formation with an α-integrin subunit and/or function [46]. Normal integrin expression is essential for an appropriate inflammatory response. Thus, phagocytes with little-to-no or defective CD18 have impaired binding to intercellular adhesion molecules (ICAMs and iC3b) on activated endothelial cells, rendering the leukocytes incapable of egressing from the vasculature to sites of microbial entry and injury [47]. Significant periodontal disease and colitis are seen in LAD-1 patients likely as a result of the absence of tissue neutrophils in the oropharynx and gastrointestinal tract and subsequent lack of inhibition of the IL-23/IL-17 axis, precipitating an upregulated chronic hyperinflammatory response [48]. Patients with LAD-1 can be diagnosed via flow cytometry to detect the absence of CD18 expression. Severely affected patients can be cured with hematopoietic stem cell transplant, while all patients should receive aggressive antimicrobial management of infections and regular preventative oral hygiene.

Patients with LAD-2 have a defect in fucosylation of macromolecules, especially selectins. Without properly fucosylated selectins, circulating neutrophils are not able to tether to the vascular endothelium during the "rolling" phase of tissue migration. Additional manifestations of LAD-2, which help clinically distinguish the disorder from LAD-1, are the high frequency of neurologic manifestations, craniofacial anomalies, and the presence of the rare Bombay erythrocyte phenotype.

LAD-3 is exquisitely rare and is due to a defect in integrin activation associated with mutations in kindlin 3. The defect affects both neutrophils and platelets, thus a bleeding diathesis is seen in association with the LAD phenotype.

Mendelian Susceptibility to Mycobacterial Diseases (IRF8 Deficiency)

Mendelian susceptibility to mycobacterial disease (MSMD) disorders are caused by various genetic defects that affect the mononuclear phagocyte/T helper cell type 1 (Th1) and interleukin-12/interferon-gamma pathways leading to an increased risk of not only mycobacterial infections but additionally *Salmonella*, *Listeria*, fungi, and various viruses [1, 49]. Patients with mutations in the interferon regulatory factor 8 (*IRF8*) gene appear to have reduced neutrophil oxidative respiratory burst capabilities along with potential abnormalities in granulopoiesis [50]. Fascinatingly, there has been a recent discovery of additional X-linked mutations in *CYBB* that cause similar

infectious predispositions as MSMD rather than the types of infections classically observed in those diagnosed with chronic granulomatous disease who may also present with *CYBB* gene alterations. Patients with these mutations showed defective oxidative burst in macrophages only, rather than all phagocytes, and thus presents with a different clinical phenotype than those with CGD [49].

Myeloperoxidase Deficiency

Myeloperoxidase (MPO) deficiency is the most common phagocyte functional disorder with 1 in 4,000 people of European descent having a complete deficiency, although it is rarely symptomatic. MPO is synthesized in both neutrophils and monocytes and is primarily located within azurophilic granules. The MPO-rich azurophilic granules are either fused to the phagosome or released into the extracellular space to assist in bactericidal activity by catalyzing the conversion of hydrogen peroxide into cytotoxic hypochlorous acid [1, 51]. In symptomatic individuals, disseminated fungal infections, particularly *Candida* species, may cause significant morbidity and is most often seen in the context of poorly controlled diabetes mellitus [52, 53]. A diagnosis can be secured through histochemical staining of neutrophils for myeloperoxidase, although a complete enzymatic deficiency can lead to abnormal DHR oxidative testing and a misdiagnosis of chronic granulomatous disease. Aggressive treatment of acute fungal infections in those with a history of clinical manifestations is the preferred treatment along with tight glucose control [1].

NF-κB Essential Modifier (NEMO) Deficiency

The transcription factor, nuclear factor kappa B (NF-κB), is a crucial regulator of various genes that play an important role in human inflammation and immunity. Mutations in the gene *IKBKG* leads to alterations in the protein NF-κB essential modifier (NEMO), which results in decreased activity of NF-κB and subsequent X-linked clinical manifestations of increased risk of mycobacterial and viral infections, hypogammaglobulinemia, and a condition known as ectodermal dysplasia [54]. Sparse hair, conical teeth, hypohidrosis with associated heat intolerance, and various skin rashes are commonly found in those presenting with ectodermal dysplasia. Autoinflammation with colitis and oral ulcers may also be observed in NEMO deficiency [1, 55]. The infectious and inflammatory manifestations of the disorder appear to be primarily driven by dysfunctions of B-cell isotype-class switching and T-/NK-cell impairment but neutrophils additionally seem to be affected through modified responses to lipopolysaccharides, alterations in GM-CSF/G-CSF release, and diminished activation of NADPH oxidase [54, 56, 57]. Immunoglobulin levels, antibody responses to vaccinations and an analysis of toll-like receptor function may aid in the diagnosis although a definitive diagnosis is obtained through genetic screening. Immunoglobulin replacement with antimicrobial prophylaxis against mycobacterial species and *Pneumocystis jiroveci* is crucial in the treatment of the disorder. In those severely affected there may also be a role for hematopoietic stem cell transplantation [55, 58, 59].

Neutrophil-Specific Granule Deficiency

The rare autosomal-recessive condition, neutrophil-specific granule deficiency, is characterized by a lack of specific and gelatinase neutrophilic granules with additional abnormalities observed in azurophilic granules and the ability of neutrophils to properly mobilize, undergo chemotaxis, and mount an optimal oxidative response [60]. The condition occurs secondary to an alteration in the myeloid-specific transcription factor, CEBPE, which results in inadequate progression of promyelocytes into myelocytes. Mutations in the *SMARCD2* gene, which interacts with CEBPE, may additionally cause the disorder While azurophilic granules are produced in promyelocytes and myeloblasts, specific and gelatinase granules are primarily synthesized in the later stages of neutrophil development. Specific granule defect patients thus have deficits with numerous neutrophilic granule subtypes. Those with the condition suffer from persistent cutaneous and pulmonary bacterial infections. Diagnosis may be made through light and electron microscopy analysis showing absent or empty granules within neutrophils. Biochemical measurements of granule proteins may also be used [1, 61]. Treatment is aimed at administration of prophylactic antimicrobials in those with frequent infections and successful bone marrow transplantation has been reported [62].

Shwachman–Diamond Syndrome

Shwachman–Diamond syndrome (SDS) is a condition that most often presents during infancy with clinical manifestations consisting of neutrophil dysfunction, neutropenia with possible progression to bone marrow failure, skeletal abnormalities, and pancreatic exocrine dysfunction. The condition is most commonly due to alterations in the *SBDS* gene, which appears to affect ribosomal formation and assembly, but recent studies have shown that mutations in *DNAJC21*, *EFL1*, and *SRP54* may also lead to a presentation similar to SDS [63–65]. Exocrine pancreatic insufficiency causes steatorrhea, poor weight gain, and fatty-infiltration of the pancreas on ultrasound evaluation. Short stature, axial skeleton dystrophies, metaphyseal dyplasia, and abnormal thumbs are the most common skeletal anomalies observed. In those with bone marrow failure progression to myelodysplasia and/or acute myeloid leukemia may occur. Recurrent infections with bacterial pathogens occur due to neutropenia with additional impairment of monocyte and neutrophil chemotactic abilities, although neutrophil respiratory burst activity seems to remain intact in those with SDS [66, 67].

Diagnosis of the syndrome is aided by discovery of neutropenia or pancytopenia on complete blood cell count analysis. Bone marrow evaluation can be used to demonstrate marrow hypocellularity and to rule out progression to dysplasia or malignancy. Pancreatic function can be assessed through obtainment of serum trypsinogen, pancreatic isoamylase, or fecal elastase. Abdominal ultrasound of the pancreas may also be helpful. A positive genetic evaluation secures a diagnosis. Those with the disorder should have annual bone marrow evaluations and be provided pancreatic enzyme replacement. G-CSF administration may improve neutropenia and hematopoietic stem cell transplantation can be curative for the immunologic and hematologic manifestations of the disease [1, 66, 68].

Wiskott–Aldrich Syndrome

The X-linked condition Wiskott–Aldrich syndrome (WAS) is characterized by immunodeficiency, eczema, and thrombocytopenia. Mutations in the *WAS* gene lead to altered production of the WAS protein (WASP). Thrombocytopenia is often present at birth and is associated with a reduced mean platelet volume with concurrent elevated platelet clearance and platelet functional defects. Autoimmunity with hemolytic anemia, inflammatory bowel disease, and vasculitic processes can occur. Severity of eczema varies and usually presents prior to 1 year of age [1]. Patients with WAS manifest numerous immunologic abnormalities including dysfunctional T lymphocytes, hypogammaglobulinemia, poor antibody response to vaccinations, and reduced natural killer cell cytotoxicity. Additionally, neutrophils exhibit decreased phagocytosis and chemotaxis likely due in part to abnormal podosome production. There is also evidence that beta2-integrins are affected in those with WAS mutations leading to neutrophil migration, adhesion, and respiratory burst defects [69, 70]. Immune dysfunction leads to recurrent sinopulmonary, otitis media, and cutaneous infections. Of note, females heterozygous for the WAS mutation may exhibit clinical signs and symptoms if significant skewed X-chromosome inactivation is present [1].

Identification of the WAS gene verifies the diagnosis in those manifesting a clinical picture consistent with the syndrome. Western blotting or flow cytometry of WASP expression may also aid in the diagnosis. Supportive care is provided through prophylactic trimethoprim-sulfamethoxazole to help prevent bacterial and *P. jirovecii* infections. Acyclovir prophylaxis is considered in those with frequent herpes simplex virus infections and regular intravenous immunoglobulin administration shows benefit in those with antibody deficiency. Platelet transfusions must be irradiated and free of cytomegalovirus. Rituximab therapy has been utilized in those with severe cytopenias secondary to autoimmunity. Bone marrow transplantation is currently the only curative option for *WAS* but gene therapy may become readily available in the future [1, 71].

Summary

It is clear that an elevated infectious risk is found in term and preterm infants due to numerous inherent defects in the various functional capabilities of their neutrophils and relatively immature phagocytic system. These abnormalities resolve over time as the child ages but clinicians caring for newborns should be aware of the presence of suboptimal neonate neutrophil functionality. Various disorders, ranging from those with subtle phagocyte defects to overwhelming neutrophil dysfunction, can further increase immunodeficiency in a neonate leading to a significant morbidity and mortality risk. Proper identification and initial management of newborns afflicted with these conditions is imperative to improving their outcomes.

References

1. Orkin SH, Fisher DE, Ginsburg D, et al. eds. *Nathan and Oski's Hematology and Oncology of Infancy and Childhood*. 8th ed. (Philadelphia PA: Saunders/Elsevier, 2015).

2. Urlichs F, Speer CP. Neutrophil function in preterm and term infants. *NeoReviews* 2004;**5**(10): e417–e430.

3. Lawrence SM, Corriden R, Nizet V. Age-appropriate functions and dysfunctions of the neonatal neutrophil. *Front Pediatr* 2017;**5**:23.

4. Melvan JN, Bagby GJ, Welsh DA, Nelson S, Zhang P. Neonatal sepsis and neutrophil insufficiencies. *Int Rev Immunol* 2010;**29**(3):315–48.

5. Levy O. Innate immunity of the newborn: Basic mechanisms and clinical correlates. *Nat Rev Immunol* 2007;**7**(5):379–90.

6. Carr R. Neutrophil production and function in newborn infants. *BJHaem* 2000;**110**(1):18–28.

7. Chandra S, Haines H, Michie C, Maheshwari A. Developmental defects in neutrophils from preterm infants. *NeoReviews* 2007;**8**(9):e368–76.

8. Lipp P, Ruhnau J, Lange A, et al. Less neutrophil extracellular trap formation in term newborns than in adults. *Neonatology* 2017;**111**(2):182–8.

9. Chaudhuri J, Mitra S, Mukhopadhyay D, Chakraborty S, Chatterjee S. Granulocyte colony-stimulating factor for preterms with sepsis and neutropenia: A randomized controlled trial. *J Clin Neonatol* 2012;**1**(4):202–6.

10. Aktaş D, Demirel B, Gürsoy T, Ovalı F. A randomized case-controlled study of recombinant human granulocyte colony stimulating factor for the treatment of sepsis in preterm neutropenic infants. *Pediatr Neonatol* 2015;**56**(3):171–5.

11. Carr R, Modi N, Doré C. G-CSF and GM-CSF for treating or preventing neonatal infections. *Cochrane Database Syst Rev* 2003;**3**: CD003066.

12. Carr R, Brocklehurst P, Doré CJ, Modi N. Granulocyte-macrophage colony stimulating factor administered as prophylaxis for reduction of sepsis in extremely preterm, small for gestational age neonates (the PROGRAMS trial): a single-blind, multicentre,

randomised controlled trial. *Lancet* 2009;**373** (9659):226–33.

13. Capasso L, Borrelli A, Cerullo J, et al. Role of immunoglobulins in neonatal sepsis. *Transl Med UniSa* 2015;**11**:28–33.

14. Franco ACBF, Torrico AC, Moreira FT, et al. Adjuvant use of intravenous immunoglobulin in the treatment of neonatal sepsis: A systematic review with a meta-analysis. *J Pediatr (Rio J)* 2012;**88**(5):377–83.

15. INIS Collaborative Group, Brocklehurst P, Farrell B, et al. Treatment of neonatal sepsis with intravenous immune globulin. *N Engl J Med* 2011;**365**(13):1201–11.

16. Jenson HB, Pollock BH. Meta-analyses of the effectiveness of intravenous immune globulin for prevention and treatment of neonatal sepsis. *Pediatrics* 1997;**99**(2):E2.

17. Jenson HB, Pollock BH. The role of intravenous immunoglobulin for the prevention and treatment of neonatal sepsis. *Semin Perinatol* 1998;**22** (1):50–63.

18. Ohlsson A, Lacy JB. Intravenous immunoglobulin for preventing infection in preterm and/or low birth weight infants. *Cochrane Database Syst Rev* 2013;**2**(7):CD000361.

19. Glocker E-O, Hennigs A, Nabavi M, et al. A homozygous CARD9 mutation in a family with susceptibility to fungal infections. *N Engl J Med* 2009;**361**(18):1727–35.

20. Netea MG, Maródi L. Innate immune mechanisms for recognition and uptake of Candida species. *Trends Immunol* 2010;**31**(9):346–53.

21. Clark RA, Kimball HR. Defective granulocyte chemotaxis in the Chediak–Higashi syndrome. *J Clin Invest* 1971;**50**(12):2645–52.

22. Kaplan J, De Domenico I, Ward DM. Chediak–Higashi syndrome. *Curr Opin Hematol* 2008;**15** (1):22–9.

23. Gallin JI, Elin RJ, Hubert RT, et al. Efficacy of ascorbic acid in Chediak–Higashi syndrome (CHS): Studies in humans and mice. *Blood.* 1979;**53**(2):226–34.

24. Boxer LA, Watanabe AM, Rister M, et al. Correction of leukocyte function in Chediak–Higashi syndrome by ascorbate. *N Engl J Med* 1976;**295**(19):1041–5.

25. Boxer LA, Albertini DF, Baehner RL, Oliver JM. Impaired microtubule assembly and polymorphonuclear leucocyte function in the Chediak–Higashi syndrome correctable by ascorbic acid. *Br J Haematol* 1979;**43**(2):207–13.

26. Winkelstein JA, Marino MC, Johnston RB, et al. Chronic granulomatous disease. Report on

a national registry of 368 patients. *Medicine (Baltimore)* 2000;**79**(3):155–69.

27. Marciano BE, Spalding C, Fitzgerald A, et al. Common severe infections in chronic granulomatous disease. *Clin Infect Dis* 201515;**60** (8):1176–83.

28. Marciano BE, Rosenzweig SD, Kleiner DE, et al. Gastrointestinal involvement in chronic granulomatous disease. *Pediatrics* 2004;**114** (2):462–8.

29. Kuhns DB, Alvord WG, Heller T, et al. Residual NADPH oxidase and survival in chronic granulomatous disease. *N Engl J Med* 2010;**363** (27):2600–10.

30. Gallin JI, Alling DW, Malech HL, et al. Itraconazole to prevent fungal infections in chronic granulomatous disease. *N Engl J Med* 2003;**348**(24):2416–22.

31. The International Chronic Granulomatous Disease Cooperative Study Group. A controlled trial of interferon gamma to prevent infection in chronic granulomatous disease. *N Engl J Med* 1991;**324**(8):509–16.

32. Güngör T, Teira P, Slatter M, et al. Reduced-intensity conditioning and HLA-matched haemopoietic stem-cell transplantation in patients with chronic granulomatous disease: a prospective multicentre study. *Lancet* 2014;**383**(9915):436–48.

33. Visser G, Rake JP, Fernandes J, et al. Neutropenia, neutrophil dysfunction, and inflammatory bowel disease in glycogen storage disease type Ib: Results of the European study on glycogen storage disease type I. *J Pediatr* 2000;**137**(2):187–91.

34. Melis D, Fulceri R, Parenti G, et al. Genotype/phenotype correlation in glycogen storage disease type 1b: A multicentre study and review of the literature. *Eur J Pediatr* 2005;**164**(8):501–8.

35. Sowerwine KJ, Holland SM, Freeman AF. Hyper-IgE syndrome update. *Ann N Y Acad Sci* 2012;**1250**:25–32.

36. Hill HR, Ochs HD, Quie PG, et al. Defect in neutrophil granulocyte chemotaxis in Job's syndrome of recurrent "cold" staphylococcal abscesses. *Lancet* 1974;**2**(7881):617–19.

37. Dinauer MC. Disorders of neutrophil function: An overview. *Methods Mol Biol* 2007;**412**:489–504.

38. Szczawinska-Poplonyk A, Kycler Z, Pietrucha B, et al. The hyperimmunoglobulin E syndrome: Clinical manifestation diversity in primary immune deficiency. *Orphanet J Rare Dis* 2011;**6** (1):76.

39. Sassi A, Lazaroski S, Wu G, et al. Hypomorphic homozygous mutations in phosphoglucomutase 3 (PGM3) impair immunity and increase serum IgE

levels. *J Allergy Clin Immunol.* 2014;**133** (5):1410–19.E13.

40. Zhang Y, Yu X, Ichikawa M, et al. Autosomal recessive phosphoglucomutase 3 (PGM3) mutations link glycosylation defects to atopy, immune deficiency, autoimmunity, and neurocognitive impairment. *J Allergy Clin Immunol* 2014;**133**(5):1400–9, e14095.

41. Mogensen TH. STAT3 and the Hyper-IgE syndrome: Clinical presentation, genetic origin, pathogenesis, novel findings and remaining uncertainties. *JAKSTAT.* 2013;**2**(2):e23435.

42. Davies EG, Thrasher AJ. Update on the hyper immunoglobulin M syndromes. *Br J Haematol* 2010;**149**(2):167–80.

43. Picard C, von Bernuth H, Ghandil P, et al. Clinical Features and Outcome of Patients With IRAK-4 and MyD88 Deficiency. *Medicine (Baltimore)* 2010;**89**(6):403–25.

44. Bouma G, Doffinger R, Patel SY, et al. Impaired neutrophil migration and phagocytosis in IRAK-4 deficiency. *Br J Haematol* 2009;**147**(1):153–6.

45. Jarchum I, Liu M, Shi C, Equinda M, Pamer EG. Critical role for MyD88-mediated neutrophil recruitment during *Clostridium difficile* colitis. *Infect Immun* 2012;**80**(9):2989–96.

46. Harris ES, Weyrich AS, Zimmerman GA. Lessons from rare maladies: Leukocyte adhesion deficiency syndromes. *Curr Opin Hematol* 2013;**20**(1):16–25.

47. Rotrosen D, Gallin JI. Disorders of phagocyte function. *Annu Rev Immunol* 1987;**5**:127–50.

48. Moutsopoulos NM, Konkel J, Sarmadi M, et al. Defective neutrophil recruitment in leukocyte adhesion deficiency type I disease causes local IL-17-driven inflammatory bone loss. *Sci Transl Med* 2014;**6**(229):229ra40.

49. Bustamante J, Boisson-Dupuis S, Abel L, Casanova J-L. Mendelian susceptibility to mycobacterial disease: Genetic, immunological, and clinical features of inborn errors of IFN-γ immunity. *Semin Immunol* 2014;**26**(6):454–70.

50. Bigley V, Maisuria S, Cytlak U, et al. Biallelic interferon regulatory factor 8 mutation: A complex immunodeficiency syndrome with dendritic cell deficiency, monocytopenia, and immune dysregulation. *Journal of Allergy and Clinical Immunology* 2018;**141**(6):2234–48.

51. Klebanoff SJ, Kettle AJ, Rosen H, Winterbourn CC, Nauseef WM. Myeloperoxidase: A front-line defender against phagocytosed microorganisms. *J Leukoc Biol* 2013;**93**(2):185–98.

52. Chiang AK, Chan GC, Ma SK, et al. Disseminated fungal infection associated with myeloperoxidase deficiency in a premature neonate. *Pediatr Infect Dis J* 2000;**19**(10):1027–9.

53. Ludviksson BR, Thorarensen O, Gudnason T, Halldorsson S. *Candida albicans* meningitis in a child with myeloperoxidase deficiency. *Pediatr Infect Dis J* 1993;**12**(2):162–4.

54. Uzel G. The range of defects associated with nuclear factor kappaB essential modulator. *Curr Opin Allergy Clin Immunol* 2005;**5**(6):513–18.

55. Kawai T, Nishikomori R, Heike T. Diagnosis and treatment in anhidrotic ectodermal dysplasia with immunodeficiency. *Allergol Int* 2012;**61** (2):207–17.

56. Choi M, Rolle S, Wellner M, et al. Inhibition of NF-kappaB by a TAT-NEMO-binding domain peptide accelerates constitutive apoptosis and abrogates LPS-delayed neutrophil apoptosis. *Blood* 2003;**102**(6):2259–67.

57. Singh A, Zarember KA, Kuhns DB, Gallin JI. Impaired priming and activation of the neutrophil NADPH oxidase in patients with IRAK4 or NEMO deficiency. *J Immunol* 2009;**182**(10):6410–17.

58. Pai S-Y, Levy O, Jabara HH, et al. Allogeneic transplantation successfully corrects immune defects, but not susceptibility to colitis, in a patient with nuclear factor-kappaB essential modulator deficiency. *J Allergy Clin Immunol* 2008;**122** (6):1113–1118.e1.

59. Dupuis-Girod S, Cancrini C, Le Deist F, et al. Successful allogeneic hemopoietic stem cell transplantation in a child who had anhidrotic ectodermal dysplasia with immunodeficiency. *Pediatrics* 2006;**118**(1):e205–211.

60. Gallin JI, Fletcher MP, Seligmann BE, et al. Human neutrophil-specific granule deficiency: a model to assess the role of neutrophil-specific granules in the evolution of the inflammatory response. *Blood* 1982;**59**(6):1317–29.

61. McIlwaine L, Parker A, Sandilands G, Gallipoli P, Leach M. Neutrophil-specific granule deficiency. *Br J Haematol* 2013;**160**(6):735.

62. Wynn RF, Sood M, Theilgaard-Mönch K, et al. Intractable diarrhoea of infancy caused by neutrophil specific granule deficiency and cured by stem cell transplantation. *Gut* 2006;**55** (2):292–3.

63. Dhanraj S, Matveev A, Li H, et al. Biallelic mutations in DNAJC21 cause Shwachman–Diamond syndrome. *Blood* 2017;**129**(11):1557–62.

64. Stepensky P, Chacón-Flores M, Kim KH, et al. Mutations in EFL1, an SBDS partner, are associated with infantile pancytopenia, exocrine pancreatic insufficiency and skeletal anomalies in a

Shwachman-Diamond like syndrome. *J Med Genet* 201754(8):558–66.

65. Carapito R, Konantz M, Paillard C, et al. Mutations in signal recognition particle SRP54 cause syndromic neutropenia with Shwachman–Diamond-like features. *J Clin Invest* 2017;**127**(11):4090–103.

66. Bezzerri V, Cipolli M. Shwachman–Diamond syndrome: Molecular mechanisms and current perspectives. *Mol Diagn Ther* 2019;**23**(2):281–90.

67. Rochowski A, Sun C, Glogauer M, Alter BP. Neutrophil functions in patients with inherited bone marrow failure syndromes. *Pediatr Blood Cancer* 2011;**57**(2):306–9.

68. Nelson AS, Myers KC. Diagnosis, treatment, and molecular pathology of Shwachman–Diamond syndrome. *Hematol Oncol Clin North Am* 2018;**32**(4):687–700.

69. Thrasher AJ, Burns SO. WASP: a key immunological multitasker. *Nat Rev Immunol* 2010;**10**(3):182–92.

70. Ochs HD, Slichter SJ, Harker LA, et al. The Wiskott–Aldrich syndrome: studies of lymphocytes, granulocytes, and platelets. *Blood* 1980;**55**(2):243–52.

71. Massaad MJ, Ramesh N, Geha RS. Wiskott–Aldrich syndrome: A comprehensive review. *Ann N Y Acad Sci* 2013;**1285**:26–43.

Chapter

18

Bleeding Disorders

Manuela Albisetti and Paul Monagle

Introduction

Bleeding symptoms presenting in the neonatal period usually present a diagnostic and therapeutic challenge for treating physicians. Bleeding disorders may be due to either congenital or acquired coagulation disorders, and may be related to mortality or long-term morbidity when not appropriately and timely diagnosed. While severe congenital coagulation defects usually present in the first hours to days of life with distinct symptoms in otherwise well newborns, acquired coagulation disorders usually present in sick newborns with a variety of presentations and distinct etiologies that differ from older children and adults. In newborns, the diagnosis of coagulation abnormalities based upon plasma concentrations of components of the hemostatic system requires age-appropriate reference ranges because plasma concentrations of several procoagulant and inhibitor proteins are physiologically decreased at birth. The aim of this chapter is to discuss clinical presentation, diagnosis, and management of the most common congenital and acquired bleeding disorders in newborns, excluding platelet disorders.

General Information

Developmental Hemostasis

Components of the hemostatic system are already synthetized by the fetus starting at 10 weeks' gestational age. At birth, all factors of the coagulation and fibrinolytic system are present and measurable. However, the concentration of several factors differs significantly from older children and adults. In the coagulation system, plasma concentrations of the vitamin K-dependent factors (F), contact factors, and the capacity to generate thrombin are decreased in newborns as compared to adults, while other factors such as fibrinogen, FV, FVIII, and FXIII are similar or increased at birth [1–5]. Plasma concentrations of the inhibitors antithrombin, heparin cofactor II, protein C, and protein S are decreased at birth up to 50% of older children and adult values. By contrast, the plasma concentration of α_2-macroglobulin in newborns is increased approximately twice compared to adult values. In the fibrinolytic system, plasma concentrations of plasminogen, tissue-plasminogen activator, α_2-antiplasmin (α_2-AP) and plasminogen activator inhibitor-1 (PAI-1) are also significantly decreased in newborns compared to adults [1–3]. All these specific age-dependent features of the hemostatic system are considered physiological and do not predispose newborns to an increased risk of hemorrhage. However, these differences may hamper the diagnosis of a bleeding disorder in newborns or even lead to misclassification of coagulation defects when reference ranges of coagulation established for adults are used to interpret laboratory results of newborns with bleeding disorders. For this reason, accurate interpretation of coagulation tests in newborns can only be performed using age-dependent reference ranges, keeping in mind that these reference ranges may vary depending on the reagent and analyzer used in the laboratory [4, 6].

Clinical Presentation

Unexplained bleeding symptoms in otherwise healthy full-term newborns should be carefully investigated because it may reflect the presence of a severe congenital factor deficiency. Bleeding

Neonatal Hematology, Pathogenesis, Diagnosis, and Management of Hematologic Problems, 3rd edition, ed. Pedro A. de Alarcón, Eric J. Werner, Robert D. Christensen, and Martha C. Sola-Visner. Published by Cambridge University Press. © Cambridge University Press 2021.

manifestations include persistent oozing from the umbilical stump, bleeding into the scalp resulting in large cephalohematomas, subdural hemorrhage, bruising, soft-tissue hemorrhage, bleeding following circumcision, persistent bleeding from puncture sites or, more rarely, gastrointestinal bleeding. Bleeding into joints, which is typical for older infants with severe hemophilia A or B, rarely occurs in newborns.

A small but important proportion of newborns present with an intracranial hemorrhage (ICH) as the first manifestation of their bleeding tendency, and a major cause of morbidity such as neurological impairment and developmental delay [7]. Intracranial hemorrhage can occur in both full-term and premature newborns and in a variety of locations. Intracranial hemorrhage in full-term newborns is rare and usually occurs either spontaneously or secondary to a variety of insults such as birth asphyxia, trauma, vitamin K (VK) deficiency, disseminated intravascular coagulation (DIC), and several congenital factor deficiencies [8–9]. The reported incidence of ICH in newborns with severe hemophilia A or B ranges between 3% and 4%. This incidence is significantly increased compared to the one reported in non-hemophiliac newborns ranging from 0.03% after elective caesarean to 0.1% after vacuum extraction [10–12]. Other rarer inherited factor deficiencies possibly causing ICH include FV, FVII, FX, FXI, and FXIII. Non-hematological causes such as arteriovenous malformations also need to be considered in neonates who have spontaneous ICH.

The characteristic form of ICH in premature newborns is an intraventricular hemorrhage (IVH) which is characterized by bleeding from the fragile microvasculature of the subependymal germinal matrix that may extend into the lateral ventricles and/or brain parenchyma [13–17]. Approximately 20% to 40% of premature infants born before 32 weeks' gestational age or with a birth weight less than 1,500 grams develop an ICH [14]. Most IVHs occur in the first 24 hours, with almost all developing by 72 hours of life [14, 18]. The pathophysiologic mechanism of IVH in premature infants is incompletely understood and likely multifactorial [19]. Abnormalities of cerebral blood flow resulting in ischemia, and subsequent reperfusion of brain tissue are the most likely causes. Other potential contributing mechanisms include the fragility of the germinal matrix capillaries, oxidative damage to the endothelium, and concurrent impairment of the coagulation system including decreased plasma concentrations of some coagulant proteins, thrombocytopenia, and enhanced local fibrinolytic activity [20–21]. Factors such as vaginal delivery, labor, intrapartum asphyxia, respiratory distress syndrome, increased mean diastolic and systolic blood pressure, and decreased superior vena cava flow due to an immature myocardium have been associated with IVH in premature newborns [22–23]. The role of VK deficiency in the development of IVH has been assessed in three randomized controlled trials evaluating the role of VK administration to mothers during pregnancy in preventing IVH in newborns. Two demonstrated benefit and one did not [24–26].

Laboratory Investigations

Bleeding symptoms in newborns require prompt and accurate laboratory investigations to ensure appropriate treatment and possibly avoid long-term morbidity. A stepwise approach including coagulation screening tests (prothrombin time (PT), activated partial thromboplastin time (aPTT), and fibrinogen) followed by specific coagulation protein assays as indicated by the screening test results is recommended. Depending on the clinical circumstances, if screening tests are normal, factor XIII deficiency must still be excluded. This approach of stepwise evaluation of otherwise healthy newborns with bleeding symptoms and abnormal coagulation screening tests is depicted in Table 18.1.

In newborns, the diagnosis of many congenital factor deficiencies based upon plasma concentrations can be difficult because plasma concentrations of several coagulation proteins are physiologically decreased at birth (see Table 18.2) [1–5]. Mild to moderate congenital deficiencies of prothrombin, FV, FVIII, FIX, FX, and FXI result in plasma concentrations that may overlap with neonatal physiological values. By contrast, plasma concentrations resulting from either mild to moderate FVII deficiency or severe deficiency of FV, FVII, FVIII, FIX, FX, and FXIII can be easily distinguished from physiologic values (see Table 18.2).

Prenatal diagnosis of most congenital factor deficiencies is performed by amniocentesis or chorionic villus biopsy. The prenatal diagnosis of congenital deficiencies of specific coagulation

Table 18.1 Evaluation of otherwise healthy newborns with bleeding symptoms and abnormal coagulation screening tests

Type or location of bleeding	Abnormal tests				No abnormal tests
	PT	aPTT	PT + aPTT	PT + aPTT + fibrinogen	
Umbilical stump		FVIII, FIX, (vWF)	FV, FX	Fibrinogen	FXIII, α2-AP
After circumcision		FVIII, FIX, FXI		Fibrinogen	
Bruising	VK deficiency		FX		
Soft-tissue		(vWF)	FV	Fibrinogen	FXIII
Gastrointestinal	VK deficiency	FVIII, FIX	FII, FV, FX		
Puncture sites	VK deficiency	FVII, FIX, (vWF)	FX	Fibrinogen	
Cephalhematoma		FVIII, FIX			
Intracranial	FVII, VK deficiency	FVIII, FIX, FXI, (vWF)	FII, FV, FX		FXIII

Abbreviations: PT, prothrombin time; aPTT, activated partial thromboplastin time; F, factor; vWF, von Willebrand factor; VK, vitamin K.

Table 18.2 Plasma concentrations of coagulation proteins in full-term healthy newborns and in congenital factor deficiencies

Factor	Plasma concentration (U/ml)		
	At birth	By factor deficiency	
		Severe	Mild–moderate
II	0.27–0.64	–	<0.01–0.20
V	0.34–1.45	<0.01	0.02–0.20
VII	0.28–1.43	<0.01	0.01–0.15
VIII	0.50–1.78	<0.01	0.01–0.50
IX	0.15–0.91	<0.01	0.01–0.50
X	0.12–0.87	<0.01	0.01–0.15
XI	0.10–0.87	–	<0.01–0.70
XIII	0.11–0.93	<0.01	–

Abbreviations: units per milliliter (U/ml)

proteins is largely confined to severe hemophilia A and B although deficiencies of FV, FVII, FXIII, and vWF (von Willebrand factor) have also been diagnosed prenatally [27]. Prenatal diagnosis of vWF deficiency is only indicated for type 3 or severe von Willebrand disease (vWD) [28–29]. Recently, droplet digital PCR and targeted massively parallel sequencing for maternal plasma DNA analysis was developed to noninvasively determine fetal mutational status in pregnancies at risk for hemophilia A and B [30]. Early diagnosis

permits either termination of the pregnancy or early intervention when indicated.

Congenital Hemorrhagic Disorders

Hemostatic Proteins

For congenital deficiencies of components of the hemostatic system, both a severe and a milder form occur. Severe congenital deficiencies of prothrombin, factor (F)V, FVII, FVIII, FIX, FX, FXI, fibrinogen, FXIII, and α2AP can all present with bleeding in the first days of life [31–33]. Mild congenital deficiencies of these proteins usually do not cause bleeding at birth in otherwise healthy full-term newborns. Although von Willebrand disease (vWD) is the most common bleeding disorder during childhood, only rare severe forms of vWF deficiency present with bleeding in newborns. Deficiencies of FXII, high molecular weight kininogen, and prekallikrein do not cause bleeding and are not discussed further.

Inheritance

Congenital deficiencies of prothrombin, FV, FVII, FX, FXI, FXIII, fibrinogen, and α2AP are inherited as autosomal recessive traits with consanguinity present in many families [34]. Deficiencies of FVIII (hemophilia A) and FIX (hemophilia B), the most common congenital bleeding disorders to present in newborns, are inherited as sex-linked recessive traits. Although vWF deficiency is predominantly inherited as an autosomal dominant pattern, cases of autosomal recessive inheritance have been reported [35–36]. Rarely, combined deficiencies of prothrombin, FVII, FIX, and FX, or FV and FVIII present in newborns [37–38].

Congenital Factor Deficiencies

The following provides specific information on the presentation and management of congenital factor deficiencies with an emphasis on severe forms.

Factor VIII Deficiency

Factor VIII is a heterodimer with a molecular weight of 330,000 consisting of a COOH-terminal-derived light-chain in a metal ion-dependent association with an NH_2-terminal heavy-chain fragment. The gene for FVIII is located on the long arm of the human X chromosome in the most distal band Xq28 (see Table 18.3). Following activation by FXa or thrombin, FVIIIa acts as a cofactor for the FIXa-mediated activation of FX, which subsequently converts prothrombin to thrombin in the presence of FVa, negatively charged phospholipids, and calcium.

Severe FVIII deficiency (FVIII <1%) is the most common congenital coagulation disorder to present in newborns. A small percentage of newborns with moderate (FVIII 1%–5%) or mild (FVIII 5%–50%) FVIII deficiency may also present following an acquired hemostatic challenge [39]. Based upon

recent cohort studies, 40% to 60% of children with severe hemophilia A are clinically symptomatic as newborns. A further 40% present by 1 year of age, and 50% have had a major bleed by 1.5 years [40–42]. Common presentations are ICH, muscle and mouth bleeding, cephalic hematoma, bleeding from the umbilical stump, and following circumcision [11, 43–46]. Rarer reported clinical presentations include bleeding in the adrenal gland, hematoma of the liver, splenic rupture, and radial artery pseudoaneurysm following radial artery puncture [47–49]. Although rare, severe hemophilia A may occur in females and present at birth. The plasma concentrations of FVIII in these female newborns is, in general, less than <0.01 U/ml.

Treatment

Currently, FVIII concentrates (plasma derived or recombinant) are the treatment of choice [50]. Recently, data from a randomized trial have shown that previous untreated children receiving plasma-derived factor VIII had a lower incidence of inhibitors than those treated with recombinant factor VIII [51]. From these data, newborns with hemophilia A requiring FVIII substitution should preferably receive plasma-derived factor VIII as first-line therapy. No data are available so far on the incidence of inhibitors in previous untreated patients treated with the new half-life extended FVIII concentrates. Alternative therapy to FVIII replacement has been used in newborns undergoing circumcision. In one study of 10 patients

Table 18.3 Properties of coagulation proteins

Factor	Chromosome	Molecular weight	Plasma concentration (µg/ml)	Half-life (hours)	Minimal hemostatic level
I	4q26-q28	330,000	3,000	120	0.5–1.0 g/L
II	11p11.2	72,000	100	72	0.15–0.40 U/ml
V	1q21-q25	330,000	10	12–36	0.10–0.25 U/ml
VII	13q34	50,000	0.5	4–6	0.05–0.10 U/ml
VIII	Xq28	330,000	0.1	12–15	0.30–0.50 U/ml
IX	Xq27	56,000	5	18–30	0.20–0.50 U/ml
X	13q34	58,800	10	65	0.10–0.20 U/ml
XI	4q32-q35	160,000	5	65	0.10–0.30 U/ml
XIII	a: 6p24p25 b: 1q31-q32	320,000	60	72–240	0.10–0.50 U/ml
vWF	12pter-p12	309,000	5–10	12	0.30–0.50 U/ml

Abbreviations: micrograms per milliliter (µg/ml); grams per liter (g/L); units per milliliter (U/ml); factor (F); a subunit of FXIII (a); b subunit of FXIII (b); von Willebrand factor (vWF)

with severe hemophilia A, local fibrin glue was used instead of infusion of FVIII concentrate. Only two of three patients who bled postoperatively required FVIII concentrate [52]. Insufficient data are available to support the benefit of prophylactic doses of FVIII intrauterine or shortly after birth in newborns suspected or confirmed to have hemophilia in order to offset the trauma of labor and reduce the risk of ICH. The role of the new non-FVIII treatment options (Emicizumab, Fitusiran, Concizumab) as first line therapy in newborns with hemophilia A is still under debate.

Factor IX Deficiency

Human FIX is a vitamin K (VK)-dependent single-chain glycoprotein with a molecular weight of 56,000. The gene for FIX is located on the tip of the long arm of the X chromosome at position Xq27 (see Table 18.3). Following activation by FXIa or FVIIa complexed with tissue factor, FIXa complexed with FVIIIa on membrane surfaces activates FX, which subsequently converts prothrombin to thrombin.

Bleeding due to severe FIX deficiency (FIX <1%) in newborns occurs at the same sites as for FVIII deficiency [11, 41–46]. The diagnosis of mild FIX deficiency (FIX 5%–40%) in newborns may be difficult because of physiologically decreased FIX levels as low as 0.15 U/ml and the potential for concurrent VK deficiency in these patients (see Table 18.1).

Treatment

Plasma-derived and recombinant FIX concentrates are the replacement products of choice and preferable to prothrombin complex concentrates (PCC). No data are available so far on the incidence of inhibitors in previous untreated patients treated with the new half-life extended FIX concentrates.

Afibrinogenemia and Hypofibrinogenemia

The fibrinogen molecule is a dimer with a molecular weight of 330,000 consisting of three pairs of polypeptide chains named Aα-, Bβ, and γ-chain. These three chains are encoded by three separate genes located on chromosome 4 (see Table 18.3). Following enzymatic cleavage of fibrinopeptides by

thrombin, fibrinogen is converted into insoluble fibrin inducing clot formation.

Fibrinogen deficiency is rare. Bleeding due to afibrinogenemia has been reported in newborns following circumcision, or as umbilical stump bleeding and soft tissue hemorrhage, and bleeding from puncture sites [52–56].

Treatment

Although fresh frozen plasma (FFP) can be used as initial therapy, cryoprecipitate or fibrinogen concentrates are preferable. Fresh frozen plasma at a dose of 10–20 ml/kg or cryoprecipitate at a dose of 1 U/5 kg of body weight will usually raise the plasma fibrinogen level 50 to 100 mg/dl and last for 4–5 days, reflecting the long plasma half-life of fibrinogen (see Table 18.3). One fibrinogen concentrate is available in Europe (Haemocomplettan HS, CSL Behring) and North America (Riastap, CSL Behring). The dose required for children depends on the type of bleeding and on the weight of the patient [52–56].

Prothrombin Deficiency

Prothrombin is a VK-dependent plasma glycoprotein with a molecular weight of 72,000. The gene for prothrombin is located on chromosome 11 at position 11p11.2 (see Table 18.3). Prothrombin is converted to thrombin by FXa in the presence of FVa, phospholipids and calcium.

Deficiency of prothrombin is very rare. Knockout mouse models demonstrated that life expectancy in unchallenged adults genetically depleted of prothrombin was about 5 to 7 days. The loss of viability was associated with the development of severe hemorrhagic events within multiple tissues, particularly in the heart and brain. These models suggested that the conditional loss of prothrombin is uniformly not compatible with maintenance of hemostasis or long-term survival [57]. Patients with prothrombin levels below 30%–40% may present with prolonged postinjury bleeding, mucosal bleeding, hematomas, and hemarthroses [58]. Bleeding complications due to prothrombin deficiency are reported in two newborns and consisted of gastrointestinal bleeding and ICH [59–61].

Treatment

Bleeding secondary to prothombin deficiency can be treated with FFP at a loading dose of 10–20 ml/

kg followed by 3 ml/kg every 12–24 hours. Although PCC contains significant amount of prothrombin, administration of PCC should be carefully monitored because the presence of other VK-dependent factors in PCC may activate the coagulation cascade leading to thrombotic complications [34, 62].

Factor V Deficiency

Factor V is a single-chain glycoprotein with a molecular weight of 330,000. The gene for FV is located on chromosome 1 at position 1q21-25 (see Table 18.3). Following activation by thrombin or FXa, FVa acts as a cofactor for the FXa-mediated activation of prothrombin.

Bleeding due to severe FV deficiency has been reported in newborns. The clinical presentations include ICH, subdural hematoma, bleeding from the umbilical stump, gastric hemorrhage, and soft tissue hemorrhage [63–64]. Antenatal intraventricular hemorrhage (IVH) was reported in three newborns [65–67].

Treatment

Currently, only FFP is available as a replacement source for FV. When bleeding occurs infusions of FFP at an initial dose of 10–20 ml/kg, followed by infusions of 3 to 6 ml/kg can correct the bleeding defect (see Table 18.3). Platelet transfusion may provide an alternative source of FV and a valuable treatment in concomitant to FFP [34, 68]. While the administration of recombinant FVIIa (rFVIIa) (NovoNordisk) has been successfully used in patients with FV deficiency not responding to FFP, there have been no reports on the use of rFVIIa in neonatal hemorrhage so far.

Factor VII Deficiency

Factor VII is a VK-dependent single-chain zymogen with a molecular weight of 50,000. The gene for FVII is located on the long arm of chromosome 13 at position 13q34 (see Table 18.3). Factor VII is a component of the extrinsic pathway of blood coagulation. Following activation by binding to its cofactor, tissue factor, FVIIa catalyzes activation of additional FVII and activates both FX and FIX.

Severe FVII deficiency (FVII <1%) usually causes significant bleeding equivalent to that seen in patients with severe hemophilia, that manifests within the first 6 months of life. Patients with FVII levels of greater than 5% generally have mild hemorrhagic episodes. The most common reported bleeding complication in newborns with congenital FVII deficiency is ICH [69–71]. In a review of 75 patients with FVII deficiency, ICH was observed in 12 (16%) patients. In 5 (41%) out of these 12 patients, ICH occurred in the first week of life with fatal outcome [72]. Recently, a newborn with a severe ICH due to congenital FVII deficiency having a novel homozygous mutation of NM_000131.4 c.272_277 delins CCTCTC on 13th chromosome was reported [73]. Congenital FVII deficiency may occur in infants with Dubin–Johnson syndrome or Gilbert syndrome [74–76].

Treatment

Bleeding episodes due to FVII deficiency can be treated with FFP, PCC or FVII concentrates, either plasma-derived factor VII or recombinant factor VIIa depending upon availability. For severe hemorrhage, FFP should be administered at an initial dose of 20 ml/kg followed by a dose of 3 to 6 ml/kg repeated every 8 to 12 hours until healing occurs. Although FFP or PCC can be used as initial therapy, FVII concentrate has become the replacement product of choice. However, careful monitoring is required because of the risk of thromboembolisms (TEs) [34, 69, 77]. A recovery study of rFVIIa has been reported for a newborn with severe FVII deficiency and ICH. The drug was administered intravenously every 4 hours at doses of 15, 22, and 30 μg/kg. Factor VII:C was >100% between 30 and 180 minutes after each infusion with mean trough levels over 25% for all three doses. Infusions were well tolerated and maintained effective hemostasis with a good clinical outcome [79]. The successful treatment of intracranial hemorrhage in newborns with severe FVII deficiency using rFVIIa at doses ranging from 20 to 150 μg/kg every 4 to 6 hours has been described in several case reports [80–82]. In 1988, Daffos et al. used fetal blood sampling to diagnose FVII deficiency at 24 weeks' gestational age and the fetus was transfused in utero at 37 weeks' gestational age with 200 U of FVIIa concentrate. Subsequently the baby was born without hemorrhagic complications and did not bleed as a newborn [83].

von Willebrand Factor Deficiency

The von Willebrand factor is an adhesive multimeric glycoprotein with a molecular weight of

309,000. The gene for vWF is located on the short arm of chromosome 12 at position 12pter-p12 (see Table 18.3). Following simultaneous binding of vWF to the glycoprotein Ib receptor on platelet surfaces and to collagen in the subendothelium, vWF mediates the adhesion of platelets to the injured vascular wall. Platelet adhesion is mediated by the highest molecular weight multimers of vWF. In addition, vWF acts as a plasma carrier and stabilizing protein for FVIII.

von Willebrand disease includes partial or complete deficiency of vWF (type 1, and 3), qualitative variants with decreased platelet-dependent function (type 2A, and 2 M), qualitative variants with increased affinity for platelet glycoprotein Ib (type 2B), and qualitative variants with markedly decreased affinity for FVIII (type 2 N). Although vWD is the most common congenital bleeding disorder, patients rarely present as newborns because plasma concentrations of vWF are increased at birth with an increased proportion of high molecular weight multimers [84–85]. Bleeding due to vWF deficiency are rarely reported in newborns. Two infants with type 2B vWD presented with bleeding at blood sampling and soft tissue sites. Repeated platelet counts were less than 50×10^9/L, and the bleeding time and aPTT were prolonged. The vWF multimeric structure was characterized by the absence of the high molecular weight forms, and the patient's platelets aggregated at much lower ristocetin concentrations than did controls [86]. One infant with type 2A vWD presented with bleeding from the umbilical stump and later with life threatening epistaxis [87]. Two newborns with type 3 vWD presented at the age of 5 and 7 days respectively, with ICH and subdural hemorrhage [88–89].

Treatment

The goal of the therapy for vWD is to normalize platelet adhesion and increase plasma concentrations of FVIII. Although partially purified FVIII concentrates contain large amounts of vWF, not all of them are able to normalize platelet adhesion because they only contain low- and mid-molecular weight multimers [91]. Several partially purified FVIII concentrates containing some of the high-molecular weight vWF multimers that have been successfully used to treat bleeding in patients with vWD are available (Bayer, CSL Behring, Octapharma, Takeda). Both type 2 and type 3 vWD can present in newborns and may require treatment with FVIII-vW concentrates at a dose varying from 5 to 40 U/ml initially administered every 12 to 24 hours.

Factor X Deficiency

Factor X is a VK-dependent two-polypeptide-chain molecule with a molecular weight of 58,800. The gene for FX is located on the long arm of chromosome 13 at position 13q34 (see Table 18.3). Following activation by the FVIIa-tissue factor complex or the FIXa-FVIIIa complex, FXa converts prothrombin to thrombin in the presence of FVa, phospholipids, and calcium.

Bleeding complications due to severe FX deficiency have been reported in newborns. The most common clinical presentation was ICH, but other sites of bleeding were also reported including bleeding from the umbilical stump or from heel prick sites, gastrointestinal bleeding, scrotal hemorrhage, and spontaneous bruising [92–94]. Subdural hemorrhage was diagnosed antenatally in one newborn [95].

Treatment

Uncomplicated bleeding episodes can be treated with FFP at an initial dose of 20 ml/kg followed by a dose of 5–10 ml/kg every 24 hours until hemostasis occurs. For severe bleeding episodes, PCC can also be used at doses which depend upon the concentration of FX contained in the concentrate. However, repeated administration of PCC should be avoided because of the risk of TEs and disseminated intravascular coagulation (DIC). For similar reasons, high doses of PCC that increase FX levels by more than 50% of normal should also be avoided. Successful primary prophylaxis with PCC in four newborns presenting with bleeding within 24–72 hours of birth has been described by McMahon et al [96]. In all children, early prophylaxis prevented development of arthropathy and improved quality of life [34, 97]. A new human plasma-derived FX concentrate (Coagadex; BioProducts Laboratory, Elstree, UK) for the treatment of hereditary FX deficiency was approved in 2016 in the United States and Europe. Clinical studies have shown that administration of this concentrate at a dose of 25 IU/kg is safe and efficacious for on-demand treatment and short-term prophylaxis in patients with moderate-to-severe hereditary FX deficiency [98].

Factor XI Deficiency

Factor XI is a homodimer composed of two identical chains bound together by disulfide bonds, and with a molecular weight of 160,000. The gene for FXI is located on chromosome 4 at position 4q32-35 (see Table 18.3). Following activation by FXIIa, FXIa mediates the activation of FIX in the presence of calcium.

Deficiency of FXI is rare, and is different from other coagulation protein deficiencies in that bleeding symptoms do not necessarily correlate with plasma concentrations of FXI nor do all patients bleed [99]. Bleeding complications due to severe FXI deficiency are reported in two newborns. One newborn bled after circumcision at the age of 3 days, while another newborn was diagnosed prenatally with bilateral subdural hemorrhage [100–101].

Treatment

Bleeding episodes requiring treatment can be controlled with either FFP at a dose of 10 to 20 ml/kg followed by a dose of 3 to 6 ml/kg every 24 hours until hemostasis is achieved or FXI concentrates (Bio Products, LFB) [34, 99].

Factor XIII Deficiency

Factor XIII is a tetramer consisting of two A subunits and two B subunits with a molecular weight of 320,000. The gene for the A subunit of FXIII is located on chromosome 6 at 6p24-25, while the gene for the B subunit is located on chromosome 1 at position 1q31-32 (see Table 18.3). The catalytic activity of FXIII resides in the A subunit. After binding to calcium, FXIII is converted to its activated form by thrombin during fibrin formation. Activated FXIII catalyzes the formation of peptide bonds between adjacent molecules of fibrin monomers, leading to a mechanical and chemical stability of the fibrin clot.

Severe FXIII deficiency typically manifests at birth with bleeding from the umbilical stump or ICH [102–105]. Other clinical presentations of homozygous FXIII deficiency include delayed wound healing, abnormal scar formation, and recurrent soft tissue hemorrhage with tendency to form hemorrhagic cysts. Intracranial hemorrhage occurs even in the absence of a trauma in approximately one-third of all affected patients [106]. Heterozygous newborns are not clinically affected.

Treatment

Fresh frozen plasma, cryoprecipitate as well as plasma derived (CSL Behring) or recombinant (NovoNordisk) FXIII concentrates can be used for the treatment of FXIII deficient patients. Newborns with FXIII deficiency should be placed on a prophylactic regimen of FXIII because of the high incidence of ICH. Plasma concentrations of FXIII over 1% are effective and the very long half-life of FXIII permits once a month therapy. Therefore, prophylactic replacement therapy is achieved either with little doses of FFP (2–3 ml/kg) administered every 4 to 6 weeks, cryoprecipitate at a dose of 1 bag/10–20 kg every 3 to 6 weeks or, preferably, with plasma-derived FXIII concentrate at a dose of 10 to 20 U/kg every 4 to 6 weeks depending on the clinical situation and the pre-infusion plasma concentration of FXIII [34, 106–107]. In the phase 3 trial evaluating the recombinant FXIII in patients older than 6 years with congenital FXIII-A subunit deficiency, a dose of 35 U/kg of rFXIII was safe and effective in preventing bleeding episodes [108].

Familial Multiple Factor Deficiencies

Congenital deficiencies of two or more coagulation proteins have been reported for 16 different combinations of coagulation factors [109–110]. Bleeding in the neonatal period has only been reported for two infants with combined factor deficiencies. One infant with FII, FVII, FIX, and FX deficiency presented with spontaneous bruising and bleeding from the umbilical stump which persisted until 3 months of age when the infant was treated with FFP [111]. A second infant with FV and FVIII deficiency presented with serious bleeding (undescribed) in the first week of life [112]. Multiple factor deficiencies, including combined FXI and FXII, FXI and FVIII, and FVIII, FXI, FXII and FXIII deficiencies, have been observed in patients with Noonan's syndrome [113].

Treatment

Initial therapy is usually with FFP. Subsequent treatment will vary depending upon the specific factors affected.

Alpha$_2$-Antiplasmin Deficiency

Alpha$_2$-antiplasmin is a single-chain glycoprotein with a molecular weight of 63,000 and a plasma half-life of approximately 60 hours. The gene for α$_2$-AP is located on chromosome 18 at position p11.1-q11.2. Alpha$_2$-antiplasmin is a major inhibitor of the fibrinolytic cascade by forming an irreversible inactive complex with plasmin.

Alpha$_2$-antiplasmin deficiency is a rare congenital disorder that presents with normal coagulation screening tests. A common presentation is bleeding from the umbilical stump [114]. Reports of older children and adults describe bleeding in the central nervous system, epistaxis, hemarthrosis, spontaneous intramedullary hematoma, and excessive bleeding during surgery or following minor trauma [115–117].

Treatment

Successful administration of antifibrinolytic agents including tranexamic acid and epsilon-aminocaproic acid have been reported to treat bleeding episodes or as prophylaxis during surgical procedures in adult patients with α$_2$-AP deficiency [118]. Tranexamic acid was administered by continuous infusion or either hourly infusion or orally during 14 days by procedures [119]. No data on dose requirements of antifibrinolytic agents in newborns and children with α$_2$-AP deficiency are available.

Acquired Hemorrhagic Disorders

The most common causes of acquired hemorrhagic disorders in newborns are VK deficiency, DIC, and liver disease.

Vitamin K Deficiency

Mechanism of Action of Vitamin K

Vitamin K is a cofactor essential for the γ-carboxylation process of the VK-dependent factors, FII, FVII, FIX, FX, and inhibitor proteins C and S. These proteins bind calcium through the gamma carboxyl groups permitting subsequent concentration on negatively charged phospholipid surfaces. The lack of functional activity for VK-dependent coagulation proteins causes bleeding which is reversible with VK therapy.

Sources of Vitamin K

Sources of VK in humans are the diet that provides VK$_1$ (phytonadione) which is particularly present in leafy green vegetables and intestinal bacteria, which synthesize VK$_2$ (menaquinone). Newborns are at increased risk of VK deficiency due to poor placental transfer of VK (10%) during pregnancy, insufficient bacterial colonization of the colon at birth, and inadequate dietary intake of VK in breast-fed babies [120–122]. Finally, drugs including oral anticoagulants, anticonvulsants, rifampicin, or isoniazid administered to mothers during pregnancy can interfere with either VK storage pool or VK function in fetus and newborns [123–125].

Clinical Presentation of Vitamin K Deficiency

Bleeding due to VK deficiency can be classified into three patterns based on the timing and type of complications [126]. A first, early pattern of VK deficiency bleeding (VKDB) is rare and presents in the first 24 hours of life with serious bleeding including ICH, intrathoracic or intra-abdominal bleeding. This early pattern usually manifests in newborns whose mothers have been taken VK antagonists, certain anticonvulsants, or antituberculous drugs. Cases of fetal extensive intracranial hemorrhage due to latent maternal vitamin K deficiency due to severe eating disorder and recurrent vomiting since early pregnancy were reported [127–128]. A second, classic pattern of VKDB presents on days 1 to 7 of life in breast-fed infants, with nose or gastrointestinal bleeding, bruising, bleeding from puncture sites or umbilical stump, or following circumcision. The third, late pattern of VKDB presents beyond the first week of life in breast-fed infants and is usually associated with a variety of diseases that compromise the supply of VK such as diarrhea, cystic fibrosis, α$_1$-antitrypsin deficiency, hepatitis, coeliac disease. and other rare disorders. The late pattern can also occur when recommended prophylactic vitamin K is not administered [129]. This late pattern is characterized by bruising, gastrointestinal bleeding or ICH.

Laboratory Evaluation of Suspected Vitamin K Deficiency

The laboratory tests for detecting the presence of VK deficiency include screening tests (PT and aPTT), and specific factor assays (FII, FVII, FIX, FX) (see Table 18.1). Patients with VK deficiency produce decarboxylated forms of the VK dependent factors (PIVKA) which can be measured directly, or as a discrepancy between coagulant activity and immunological concentration [130–131].

Treatment of Vitamin K Deficiency

Any patient suspected to have VK deficiency should be treated immediately with VK while awaiting laboratory confirmation. The route and specific type of therapy is dictated by the urgency of the clinical situation and potential side effects of therapy.

Bleeding due to VK deficiency should be treated with intravenous or subcutaneous VK at doses appropriate for age. Depending on the severity of bleeding, 10 to 20 ml/kg of stored plasma or FFP should be given. Fresh frozen plasma is particularly useful when the precise nature of the coagulopathy is unknown. Prothrombin complex concentrates can be administered to newborns with life threatening bleeding or ICH in alternative to FFP. However, administration of PCCs requires careful monitoring because of the risk of thromboembolic complications. The amount of plasma required to totally correct a severe VK deficiency is so large that it may result in volume overload. The successful administration of rFVIIa has been reported in five newborns with ICH due to VK deficiency. In all patients, rapid correction of coagulopathy allowed early neurosurgical intervention, and no bleeding extension was observed after infusion of rFVIIa at doses ranging between 90 and 200 µg/kg (see Table 18.4) [128, 132–134].

Prophylactic Vitamin K Administration

Two major randomized controlled trials assessed the benefits of VK prophylaxis using clinical bleeding as the outcome measure [135–136]. In the first study, 3338 full-term infants were randomized to receive either placebo, or menadione (100 µg or 5 mg) intramuscularly. Healthcare personnel, who were unaware of the type of therapy, assessed minor and major bleeding outcomes. The incidence of ICH as well as minor bleeding was significantly increased in the placebo group compared to both treatment arms. This clinical result was supported by laboratory tests showing that the PT was prolonged in infants with hemorrhagic complications and corrected when VK was given. In the second study, 470 infants were randomized to receive VK or nothing. The study population consisted of male infants who were undergoing circumcision. Bleeding following circumcision was observed in 32 out of 230 infants not receiving VK compared to 6 out of 240 infants treated with VK. The same investigators reproduced these results in a subsequent, smaller, non-blinded trial [137].

The benefit of prophylactic VK in neonates has also been demonstrated by several epidemiological trials conducted in different countries. Independently of the administration route and dosing regimen used, VK prophylaxis at birth clearly protects newborns against classical VKDB [138]. However, for the prevention of late VKBD, some controversy still exists with regard to the mode of application and dosing. While oral administration of a single dose of 1 mg VK at birth protects against early and classical VKDB, it seems indeed not effective in preventing late VKDB [138–139]. Repeated or continuous oral VK supplementation was shown to be as effective as intramuscular prophylaxis but requires appropriate compliance, and may not fully protect infants with cholestatic disease from late VKDB [139–140]. The efficacy of oral VK prophylaxis may be improved by the use of a new mixed-

Table 18.4 Newborns with vitamin K deficiency bleeding treated with rFVIIa

Publication	Age (weight)	Clinical presentation	Dose of rFVIIa (µg/kg)	Outcome
Brady et al. [132]	7 weeks (4 kg) 7 weeks (3.9 kg)	ICH ICH	100 100	No intraoperative bleeding. No bleeding extension No bleeding extension
Flood et al. [134]	5 weeks	Subdural hemorrhage	200	Rapid correction of coagulopathy. No bleeding extension
Hubbard et al. [129]	5 weeks (4 kg) 5 weeks	ICH ICH	100 90	Rapid correction of coagulopathy. No bleeding extension Rapid correction of coagulopathy. No bleeding extension

Table 18.5 Current recommendations for vitamin K prophylaxis in healthy newborns in different countries

Country	Recommended vitamin K prophylaxis
Australia	All newborns: 1 mg IM on day 1 For parents who decline injection, healthcare providers should recommend an oral dose of 2.0 mg vitamin K at the time of the first feeding, a second dose given 72–120 hours after birth and a third dose given at 4 weeks
Canada	Newborns with birth weight ≤1,500 g: 0.5 mg IM within first 6 hours of birth Newborns with birth weight >1,500 g: 1.0 mg IM within first 6 hours of birth For parents who decline injection, health care providers should recommend an oral dose of 2.0 mg vitamin K at the time of the first feeding, to be repeated at 2 to 4 and 6 to 8 weeks of age
Germany	All newborns: 2 mg oral on day 1, day 4 to 10, and day 28 to 42
Switzerland	All newborns: 2 mg* oral at 4 hours, 4 days, and 4 weeks
USA	All newborns: 1–2 mg IM on day 1

Note: * Mixed-micellar VK preparation.

Abbreviations: milligram (mg); gram (g); intramuscular (IM); United States of America (USA).

micellar, water-soluble VK formulation [141–142]. Current recommendations for VK prophylaxis in healthy newborns in different countries are listed in Table 18.5. In 2016, the ESPGHAN Committee on Nutrition published a position paper to provide recommendations for setting up local guidelines for the prevention of VKDB in newborns and infants [143]. The group recommends that healthy newborn infants should either receive 1 mg of vitamin K1 by intramuscular injection at birth; or 3 × 2 mg vitamin K1 orally at birth, at 4 to 6 days and at 4 to 6 weeks; or 2 mg vitamin K1 orally at birth, and a weekly dose of 1 mg orally for 3 months. Intramuscular application is the preferred route for efficiency and reliability of administration. The oral route is not appropriate for preterm infants and for newborns who have cholestasis or impaired intestinal absorption or are too unwell to take oral vitamin K1, or those whose mothers have taken medications that interfere with vitamin K metabolism [143].

Pregnant women receiving oral anticonvulsant therapy should receive VK in the third trimester to prevent overt VK deficiency in their infants at birth.

The frequency of VKDB is on the increase again in many westernized countries predominantly due to refusal of VK injections at birth. This practice is strongly linked to vaccine refusal. Appropriate education of parents, and/or documentation of reasons for refusal of VK is important. Parents who refuse VK for their infant should be given clear instructions about when to present urgently for medical attention as approximately

50% of children who present with late VKDB will have a signal bleed that gives an opportunity for early intervention [144–146].

Disseminated Intravascular Coagulation

Etiology

Disseminated intravascular coagulation (DIC) is not a disorder in itself but a process that is secondary to a variety of age-specific underlying diseases [147]. In premature newborns, DIC usually develops secondary to respiratory distress syndrome, congenital viral infections, serious bacterial infections, hypothermia, and meconium or amniotic fluid aspiration syndromes. In full-term infants, DIC usually occurs in association with adverse events affecting the feto-placental unit resulting in asphyxia, shock and release of tissue thromboplastin at the time of birth [148–149].

Pathogenetic Mechanism

The pathogenetic mechanism of DIC is a systemic activation of coagulation mediated by several cytokines, particularly interleukin-6. This process leads to a tissue factor-mediated increased generation of thrombin and a decreased generation of natural anticoagulants including antithrombin, protein C, and tissue factor–pathway inhibitor, and consequently to extensive intravascular deposition of fibrin. The simultaneous inhibition of the fibrinolytic pathway, due to increased plasma concentration of plasminogen activator inhibitor-1 (PAI-1), prevents an adequate removal of fibrin from small vessels resulting in extensive thrombosis and organ failure. The process also leads to consumption of platelets and coagulation factors, which may cause severe hemorrhage [147].

Clinical Presentation and Diagnosis

Clinically affected infants usually present with bleeding complications which include diffuse oozing from mucous membranes or sites of invasive procedures, hematuria, hemoptysis, bruising, hematomas, and, in some cases, ICH. The diagnosis of DIC is based upon compatible clinical features in conjunction with abnormalities of specific coagulation tests. The classic laboratory abnormalities which reflect clinically significant DIC include prolongation of screening tests (PT, aPTT), thrombocytopenia, decreased plasma concentrations of specific coagulation factors (fibrinogen, FV, and FVIII) and inhibitors (antithrombin (AT), heparin cofactor (HC)II, protein C), and increased concentrations of fibrinogen degradation products (FDP). The diagnosis of DIC can be facilitated by very sensitive tests that measure the in vivo effects of thrombin and/or plasmin generation. These tests include prothrombin activation fragment 1 and 2, and thrombin-antithrombin (TAT) complexes. However, abnormalities in these tests alone do not necessarily signify the presence of DIC nor the need to treat. For example, increased plasma concentrations of TAT complexes are present in cord plasma from healthy infants and likely reflect activation of the coagulation system during the normal birth process [150–152].

Treatment

The cornerstone of treatment of DIC in all patients remains the successful treatment of the underlying disease [153]. Treatment of the secondary hemostatic disorder may be helpful, but has to be considered as an adjuvant therapy. Since decreased concentrations of platelets and coagulation factors may cause serious bleeding, replacement therapy with platelet concentrates and plasma in the form of FPP or cryoprecipitate may be beneficial in clinically symptomatic newborns. Transfusion of factor concentrates is generally not recommended because of contamination with activated coagulation factors, which could, at least theoretically, augment the already activated coagulation system. Clinically practical goals when treating newborns that are bleeding from DIC are to maintain the

platelet count above 50×10^9/L, fibrinogen concentrations above 1.0 g/L, and PT and aPTT values near normal values for age. Although replacement of natural inhibitors of coagulation including AT and protein C may be an appropriate therapy in patients with DIC, the lack of large clinical trials cannot support a general recommendation to use them [154–155]. Another attractive therapy option in patients with DIC is to inhibit the activation of the coagulation system by using heparin. However, heparin may increase the risk of bleeding and there are no trials showing that it is helpful. The use of heparin is usually limited to patients with large vessel thrombosis [156–158]. Several uncontrolled and two randomized clinical trials in newborns with DIC have been published. Gobel et al. randomized 36 infants to either unfractionated heparin (UFH) or placebo [159], while Gross et al. randomized 33 newborns to either exchange transfusion, administration of FFP and platelets, or no specific therapy [160]. Although no beneficial effect of therapy was shown, both trials were not conclusive because the sample sizes were insufficient to detect a 50% reduction in mortality.

Liver Disease

Etiology

The causes of liver disease associated with an increased risk of bleeding in the neonatal period includes congenital heart disease with severe cardiac low output, hypoxia, extra-hepatic biliary atresia, inherited metabolic disorders, and viral hepatitis.

Pathogenetic Mechanism

The mechanisms responsible for hemostatic impairment in liver disease include decreased synthesis of coagulation factors, activation of both the coagulation and fibrinolytic systems, poor clearance of activated hemostatic components, loss of coagulation proteins into ascitic fluid, thrombocytopenia, platelet dysfunction, and concomitant VK deficiency. The pathogenesis may change with the underlying cause of the liver disease [161]. Frequently this condition presents in association with DIC.

Clinical Presentation

The clinical presentation is variable and usually dependent on the underlying disorder. Symptoms include ecchymoses and petechiae, mucous membrane bleeding, hemorrhage from gastrointestinal varices or into the abdomen, and ICH.

Laboratory Evaluation

Laboratory abnormalities include prolongation of screening tests (PT, aPTT), thrombocytopenia, and prolonged bleeding time. Plasma concentrations of FVII, FV, fibrinogen, and plasminogen are decreased, while FDP and D-dimer are frequently increased. A normal concentration of FVIII, reflecting significant extra-hepatic synthesis, can help distinguish severe liver disease from DIC.

Treatment

Treatment modalities include factor replacement in the form of FFP and cryoprecipitate, platelet transfusions, and VK administration. A conceptual approach to treatment of hemostatic problems due to liver disease in children has recently been suggested [153]. In recent years, rFVIIa has been increasingly used in infants with liver disease [162–169]. Brown et al. treated 10 infants with bleeding complications and coagulopathy due to liver failure [164]. Recombinant FVIIa administered at a dose of 80 µg/kg quickly normalized the PT and maintained improved hemostasis even when coagulopathy had been refractory to FFP. Therapy with rFVIIa subjectively reduced clinical bleeding and also improved fluid balance [164]. A pediatric case series by Pettersson et al., including four infants, suggests that rFVIIa may be of benefit in the short-term management of life-threatening bleeding in children with severe liver disease [165]. In this study, prophylactic administration of rFVIIa was also useful to prevent bleeding during diagnostic and therapeutic procedures in these children [165]. A successful treatment of an iatrogenic liver injury in a 1,200 g infant using rFVIIa administered on three doses each of 100 µg/kg has also been reported [170].

References

1. Andrew M, Paes B, Milner R, et al. Development of the human coagulation system in the full-term infant. *Blood* 1987;**70**:165–72.

2. Andrew M, Paes B, Milner R, et al. Development of the human coagulation system in the healthy premature infant. *Blood* 1988;**72**:1651–7.

3. Andrew M, Paes B, Johnston M. Development of the hemostatic system in the neonate and young infant. *Am J Pediatr Hematol Oncol* 1990;**12**:95–104.

4. Appel IM, Grimminck B, Geerts J, et al. Age dependency of coagulation parameters during childhood and puberty. *J Thromb Haemost* 2012;**10**:2254–63.

5. Toulon P, Berruyer M, Brionne-Francois M, et al. Age dependency for coagulation parameters in paediatric populations. Results of a multicentre study aimed at defining the age-specific reference ranges. *J Thromb Haemost* 2016;**116**:9–16.

6. Monagle P, Barnes C, Ignjatovic V, et al. Developmental haemostasis. Impact for clinical haemostasis laboratories. *Thromb Haemost* 2006;**95**:362–72.

7. Gupta SN, Kechli AM, Kanamalla US. Intracranial hemorrhage in term newborns: Management and outcomes. *Pediatr Neurol* 2009;**40**:1–12.

8. Abbondanzo SL, Gootenberg JE, Lofts RS, et al. Intracranial hemorrhage in congenital deficiency of factor XIII. *Am J Pediatr Hematol Oncol* 1988;**10**:65–8.

9. Struwe F. Intracranial hemorrhage and occlusive hydrocephalus in hereditary bleeding disorders. *Dev Med Child Neurol* 1970;**12**:165–9.

10. Smith AR, Leonard N, Heisel Kurth M. Intracranial hemorrhage in newborns with hemophilia: The role of screening radiologic studies in the first 7 days of life. *J Pediatr Hemato Oncol* 2008;**30** :81–4.

11. Ljung RC. Intracranial hemorrhage in haemophilia A and B. *Br J Haematol* 2008;**140**:378–84.

12. Tarantino MD, Gupta SL, Brusky RM. The incidence and outcome of intracranial hemorrhage in newborns with haemophilia: Analysis of the Nationwide Inpatient Sample database. *Haemophilia* 2007;**13**:380–2.

13. McCrea HJ, Ment LR. The diagnosis, management, and postnatal prevention of intraventricular hemorrhage in the preterm neonate. *Clin Perinatol* 2008;**35**:777–92.

14. Owens R. Intraventricular hemorrhage in the premature neonate. *Neonatal Netw* 2005;**24**:55–71.

15. Hayden CK, Shattuck KE, Richardson CJ, et al. Subependymal germinal matrix hemorrhage in fullterm neonates. *Pediatrics* 1985;**75** :714–18.

16. Mack LA, Wright K, Hirsch JH, et al. Intracranial hemorrhage in premature infants: Accuracy in sonographic evaluation. *Am J Roentgenol* 1981;**137**:245–50.

17. Antoniuk S, da Silva RV. Periventricular and intraventricular hemorrhage in the premature infants. *Rev Neurol* 2000;**31**:238–43.

18. Dolfin T, Skidmore MB, Fong KW, et al. Incidence, severity and timing of subependymal

and intraventricular hemorrhages in preterm infants born in a perinatal unit as detected by serial real-time ultrasound. *Pediatrics* 1983;**71**:541–6.

19. Ment LR, Duncan CC, Ehrenkranz RA. Intraventricular hemorrhage of the preterm neonate. *Semin Perinatol* 1987;**11** :132–41.

20. Clark CE, Clyman RI, Roth RS, et al. Risk factor analysis of intraventricular hemorrhage in low-birth-weight infants. *J Pediatr* 1981;**99**:625–8.

21. Cooke RW. Factors associated with periventricular hemorrhage in very low birthweight infants. *Arch Dis Child* 1981;**56**:425–31.

22. Gronlund JU, Korvenranta H, Kero P, et al. Elevated arterial blood pressure is associated with peri-intraventricular hemorrhage. *Eur J Pediatr* 1994;**153**:836–41.

23. Kluckow M, Evans N. Low superior vena cava flow and intraventricular hemorrhage in preterm infants. *Arch Dis Child Fetal Neonatal Ed* 2000;**82**: F188–94.

24. Morales WJ, Angel JL, O'Brien WF, et al. The use of antenatal vitamin K in the prevention of early neonatal intraventricular hemorrhage. *Am J Obstet Gynecol* 1988;**159**:774–9.

25. Pomerance JJ, Teal JG, Gogdok JF, et al. Maternally administered antenatal vitamin K_1: Effect on neonatal prothrombin activity, partial thromboplastin time, and intraventricular hemorrhage. *Obstet Gynecol* 1987;**70**:235–41.

26. Kazzi NJ, Ilagen MB, Liang KC. Maternal administration of vitamin K does not improve the coagulation profile of preterm infants. *Pediatrics* 1989;**84**:1045–50.

27. Peyvandi F, Jayandharan G, Chandy M, et al. Genetic diagnosis of hemophilia and other inherited bleeding disorders. *Haemophilia* 2006;**12** (Suppl 3):82–9.

28. Peake IR, Bowen D, Bignell P, et al. Family studies and prenatal diagnosis in severe von Willebrand disease by polymerase chain reaction amplification of a variable number tandem repeat region of the von Willebrand factor gene. *Blood* 1990;**76**:555–61.

29. Federici AB. Diagnosis of inherited von Wiillebrand disease: A clinical perspective. *Semin Thromb Hemost* 2006;**32**:555–65.

30. Hudecova I, Jiang P, Davies J, et al. Noninvasive detection of F8 int22h–related inversions and sequence variants in maternal plasma of hemophilia carriers. *Blood* 2017;**130**(3):340–7.

31. Buchanan GR. Coagulation disorders in the neonate. *Pediatr Clin North Am* 1986;**33**:203–20.

32. Montgomery RR, Marlar RA, Gill JC. Newborn haemostasis. *Clin Hematol* 1985;**14**:443–60.

33. Gibson B. Neonatal haemostasis. *Arch Dis Child* 1989;**64**:503–6.

34. Bolton–Maggs PH, Perry DJ, Chalmers EA, et al. The rare coagulation disorders: Review with guidelines for management from the United Kingdom Haemophilia Centre Doctors' Organisation. *Haemophilia* 2004;**10**:593–628.

35. Lopez–Fernandez MF, Blanco–Lopez MJ, Castineira MP, et al. Further evidence for recessive inheritance of von Willebrand disease with abnormal binding of von Willebrand factor to factor VIII. *Am J Hematol* 1992;**40**:20–7.

36. Eikenboom JC, Reitsma PH, Peerlinck KM, et al. Recessive inheritance of von Willebrand's disease type I. *Lancet* 1993;**341**:982–6.

37. Spreafico M, Peyvandi F. Combined FV and FVIII deficiency. *Haemophilia* 2008;**14**:1201–08.

38. Girolami A, Ruzzon E, Tezza F, et al. Congenital FX deficiency combined with other clotting defects or with other abnormalities: A critical evaluation of the literature. *Haemophilia* 2008;**14**:323–8.

39. Chalmers EA. Neonatal coagulation problems. *Arch Dis Child Fetal Neonatal Ed* 2004;**89**:F475–8.

40. Chalmers EA. Haemophilia and the newborn. *Blood Rev* 2004;**18**:85–92.

41. Baehner RL, Strauss H. Hemophilia in the first year of life. *N Engl J Med* 1966;**275**:524–8.

42. Conway JH, Hiltgartner MW. Initial presentation of paediatric hemophiliacs. *Arch Pediatr Adolesc Med* 1994;**148**:589–94.

43. Ljung R, Chambost H, Stain AM, et al. Haemophilia in the first years of life. *Haemophilia* 2008;**14**(Suppl 3):188–95.

44. Pollman H, Richter H, Ringkamp H, et al. When are children diagnosed as having severe haemophilia and when do they start to bleed? A 10 year single centre PUP study. *Eur J Pediatr* 1999;**158**:S166–70.

45. Klinge J, Auberger K, Auerswald G, et al. Prevalence and outcome of intracranial hemorrhage in haemophiliacs: A survey of the paediatric group of the German Society of Thrombosis and Haemostasis (GTH). *Eur J Pediatr* 1999;**158**:S162–5.

46. Kulkarni R, Lusher JM. Intracranial and extracranial hemorrhages in newborns with hemophilia: A review of the literature. *J Pediatr Hematol Oncol* 1999;**21**:289–95.

47. Le Pommelet C, Durand P, Laurian Y, et al. Haemophilia A: Two cases showing unusual features at birth. *Haemophilia* 1998;**4**:122–5.

48. Johnson–Robbins LA, Porter JC, Horgan MJ. Splenic rupture in a newborn with hemophilia A:

Case report and review of the literature. *Clin Pediatr (Phila)* 1999;**38**:117–19.

49. Fields JM, Saluja S, Schwartz DS, et al. Hemophilia presenting in an infant as a radial artery pseudoaneurysm following arterial puncture. *Pediatr Radiol* 1997;**27**:763–4.

50. DiMichele D, Neufeld EJ. Hemophilia. A new approach to an old disease. *Hematol Oncol Clin North Am* 1998;**12**:1315–44.

51. Peyvandi F, Mannucci PM, Garagiola I, et al. A randomized trial of factor VIII and neutralizing antibodies in hemophilia A. *N Engl J Med* 2016;**374**:2054–64.

52. Martinowitz U, Varon D, Jonas P, et al. Circumcision in hemophilia: The use of fibrin glue for local hemostasis. *J Urol* 1992;**148**:855–7.

53. de Moerloose P, Neerman–Arbez M. Congenital fibrinogen disorders. *Semin Thromb Hemost* 2009;**35**:356–66.

54. Manios S, Schenck W, Kunzer W. Congenital fibrinogen deficiency. *Acta Pediatr Scand* 1968;**57**:145–80.

55. Fried K, Kaufman S. Congenital afibrinogenemia in 10 offspring of uncle–niece marriages. *Clin Genet* 1980;**17**:223–7.

56. Toledano A, Lachassinne E, Roumegoux C, et al. Treatment of congenital afibrinogenemia in a premature neonate. *Ann Pharmacother* 2008;**42**:1145–6.

57. Mullins ES, Kombrinck KW, Talmage KE, et al. Genetic elimination of prothrombin in adult mice is not compatible with survival and results in spontaneous hemorrhagic events in both heart and brain. *Blood* 2009;**15** (113):696–704.

58. Menegatti M, Peyvandi F. Treatment of rare factor deficiencies other than hemophilia. *Blood* 2019;**133**, 415–24.

59. Gill F, Shapiro S, Schwartz E. Severe congenital hypoprothrombinemia. *J Pediatr* 1978;**93**:264–6.

60. Viola L, Chiaretti A, Lazzareschi I, et al. Intracranial hemorrhage in congenital factor II deficiency. *Pediatr Med Chir* 1995;**17**:593–4.

61. Strijks E, Poort SR, Renier WO, et al. Hereditary prothrombin deficiency presenting as intracranial haematoma in infancy. *Neuropediatrics* 1999;**30**:320–4.

62. Meeks SL, Abshire TC. Abnormalities of prothrombin: A review of the pathophysiology, diagnosis, and treatment. *Haemophilia* 2008;**14**:1159–63.

63. Salooja N, Martin P, Khair K, et al. Severe factor V deficiency and neonatal intracranial

hemorrhage :a case report. *Haemophilia* 2000, **6**:44–6.

64. Ehrenforth S, Klarmann D, Zabel B, et al. Severe factor V deficiency presenting as subdural haematoma in the newborn. *Eur J Pediatr* 1998;**157**:1032.

65. Whitelaw A, Haines M, Bolsover W, et al. Factor V deficiency and antenatal ventricular hemorrhage. *Arch Dis Child* 1984;**59**:997–9.

66. Bonvini G, Cotta–Ramusino A, Ricciardi G. Congenital factor V deficiency and intraventricular hemorrhage of prenatal origin. *Pediatr Med Chir* 1994;**16**:93–4.

67. Ellestad SC, Zimmerman SA, Thornburg C, et al. Severe factor V deficiency presenting with intracranial hemorrhage during gestation. *Haemophilia.* 2007;**13**:4 32–4.

68. Huang JN, Koerper MA. Factor V deficiency: A concise review. *Haemophilia* 2008;**14**:1164–69.

69. Lapecorella M, Mariani G, International Registry on Congenital Factor VII Deficiency. Factor VII deficiency: Defining the clinical picture and optimizing therapeutic options. *Haemophilia.* 2008;**14**:1170–5.

70. Rabiner S, Winick M, Smith C. Congenital deficiency of factor VII associated with hemorrhagic disease of the newborn. *Pediatrics* 1960;**25**:101–5.

71. Matthay K, Koerper M, Ablin AR. Intracranial hemorrhage in congenital factor VII deficiency. *J Pediatr* 1979;**94**:413–15.

72. Ragni M, Lewis J, Spero J, et al. Factor VII deficiency. *Am J Hematol* 1981;**10**:79–88.

73. Kader S, Mutlu M, Acar FA, et al. Homozygous congenital factor VII deficiency with a novel mutation, associated with severe spontaneous intracranial bleeding in a neonate. *Blood Coagul Fibrinolysis* 2018;**29**:476–80.

74. Seligsohn U, Shani M, Ramot B. Gilbert syndrome and factor-VII deficiency. *Lancet* 1970;**1**:1398.

75. Levanon M, Rimon S, Shani M, et al. Active and inactive factor VII in Dubin–Johnson syndrome with factor-VII deficiency, hereditary factor-VII deficiency and on coumadin administration. *Br J Haematol* 1972;**23**:669–77.

76. Seligsohn U, Shani M, Ramot B. Dubin–Johnston syndrome in Israel: Association with factor VII deficiency. *Quart J Med* 1970;**39**:569–84.

77. Mathew P, Young G. Recombinant factor VIIa in paediatric bleeding disorders: A 2006 review. *Haemophilia* 2006;**12**:457–2.

78. Worth LL, Hoots WK. Development of a subdural vein thrombosis following aggressive factor VII

replacement for postnatal intracranial hemorrhage in a homozygous factor VII–deficient infant. *Haemophilia*1998;4:757–61.

79. Wong WY, Huang WC, Miller R, et al. Clinical efficacy and recovery levels of recombinant FVIIa (NovoSeven) in the treatment of intracranial hemorrhage in severe neonatal FVII deficiency. *Haemophilia* 2000;6:50–4.

80. Chuansumrit A, Visanuyothin N, Puapunwattana S, et al. Outcome of intracranial hemorrhage in infants with congenital factor VII deficiency. *J Med Assoc Thai* 2002;85(Suppl 4): S1059–64.

81. Karimi M. Successful control of central nervous system bleeding in two newborns with severe factor Vii deficiency using rFVIIa administered via Port-a-Cath. *Semin Hematol* 2008;45 Suppl 1:S74.

82. Farah RA, Hamod D, Melick N, et al. Successful prophylaxis against intracranial hemorrhage using weekly administration of activated recombinant factor VII in a newborn with severe factor VII deficiency. *J Thromb Haemost* 2007;5:433–4.

83. Daffos F, Forestier F, Kaplan C, et al. Prenatal diagnosis and management of bleeding disorders with fetal blood sampling. *Am J Obstet Gynecol* 1988;158:939–46.

84. Katz JA, Moake JL, McPherson PD, et al. Relationship between human development and disappearance of unusually large von Willebrand factor multimers from plasma. *Blood* 1989;73:1851–8.

85. Weinstein MJ, Blanchard R, Moake JL, et al. Fetal and neonatal von Willebrand factor (vWF) is unusually large and similar to the vWF in patients with thrombotic thrombocytopenic purpura. *Br J Haematol* 1989;72:68–72.

86. Donner M, Holmberg L, Nilsson IM. Type IIB von Willebrand's disease with probable autosomal recessive inheritance and presenting as thrombocytopenia in infancy. *Br J Haematol* 1987;66:349–54.

87. Bignall P, Standen G, Bowen DJ, et al. Rapid neonatal diagnosis of von Willebrand's disease by use of the polymerase chain reaction (Letter). *Lancet* 1990;336:638–9.

88. Gazengel C, Fischer A, Schlegel N, et al. Treatment of type III von Willebrand's disease with solvent/detergent–treated factor VIII concentrates. *Nouv Rev Fr Hematol* 1988;30:225–7.

89. Wetzstein V, Budde U, Oyen F, et al. Intracranial hemorrhage in a term newborn with severe von Willebrand disease type 3 associated with sinus venous thrombosis. *Haematologica* 2006;9(Suppl):ECR60.

90. Lopez–Fernandez MF, Lopez–Berges C, Corral M, et al. Assessment of multimeric structure and ristocetin-induced binding to platelets of von Willebrand factor present in cryoprecipitate and different factor VIII concentrates. *Vox Sang* 1987;52:15–19.

91. Mannucci PM. Treatment of von Willebrand's disease. *N Engl J Med* 2004;351:683–94.

92. Machin S, Winter M, Davies S, et al. Factor X deficiency in the neonatal period. *Arch Dis Child* 1980;55:406–8.

93. Ruane B, McCord F. Factor X deficiency: A rare cause of scrotal hemorrhage. *Irish Med J* 1990;83:163.

94. el Kalla S, Menon NS. Neonatal congenital Factor X deficiency. *Pediatr Hematol Oncol* 1991;8:347–54.

95. De Sousa C, Clark T, Bradshaw A. Antenatally diagnosed subdural hemorrhage in congenital factor X deficiency. *Arch Dis Child* 1988;63:1168–74.

96. McMahon C, Smith J, Goonan C, Byrne M, Smith OP. The role of primary prophylactic factor replacement therapy in children with severe factor X deficiency. *Br J Haematol* 2002;119(3):789–91.

97. Brown DL, Kouides PA. Diagnosis and treatment of inherited factor X deficiency. *Haemophilia* 2008;14:1176–82.

98. Shapiro E. Plasma-derived human factor X concentrate for on–demand and perioperative treatment in factor X–deficient patients: Pharmacology, pharmacokinetics, efficacy, and safety. *Expert Opin Drug Metab Toxicol* 2017;13, 97–104.

99. Gomez K, Bolton–Maggs P. Factor XI deficiency. *Haemophilia* 2008;14:1183–9.

100. Kitchens C. Factor XI. A review of its biochemistry and deficiency. *Semin Thromb Haemostas* 1991;17:55–72.

101. Barozzino T, Sgro M, Toi A, et al. Fetal bilateral subdural hemorrhage s. Prenatal diagnosis and spontaneous resolution by time of delivery. *Prenat Diagn* 1998;18:496–503.

102. Diehl R, Thouvenin S, Reynaud J, et al. Factor XIII deficiency in a newborn. *Arch Pediatr* 2007;14:890–2.

103. Ozsoylu S, Altay C, Hi Csonmez G. Congenital factor XIII deficiency: Observation of two cases in the newborn period. *Am J Dis Child* 1971;122:541–3.

104. Francis J, Todd P. Congenital factor XIII deficiency in a neonate. *Br Med J* 1978;2:1532.

105. Solves P, Altes A, Ginovart G, et al. Late hemorrhagic disease of the newborn as a cause of intracerebral bleeding. *Ann Hematol* 1997;**75**:65–6.

106. Hsieh L, Nugent D. Factor XIII deficiency. *Haemophilia* 2008;**14**:1190–200.

107. Gootenberg JE. Factor concentrates for the treatment of factor XIII deficiency. *Curr Opin Hematol* 1998;**5**:372–5.

108. Inbal A, Oldenburg J, Carcao M, et al. Recombinant factor XIII: A safe and novel treatment for congenital factor XIII deficiency. *Blood* 2012;**119**:5111–17.

109. Mammen E, Murano G, Bick RL. Combined congenital clotting factor abnormalities. *Semin Thromb Haemostas* 1983;**9**:55–6.

110. Spreafico M, Peyvandi F. Combined FV and FVIII deficiency. *Haemophilia* 2008;**14**:1201–8.

111. McMillan C, Roberts H. Congenital combined deficiency of coagulation factors II, VII, IX and X. *N Engl J Med* 1966;**274**:1313–15.

112. Mazzone D, Fichera A, Pratico G, et al. Combined congenital deficiency of factor V and factor VIII. *Acta Haemat* 1982;**68**:337–8.

113. Sharland M, Patton MA, Talbot S, et al. Coagulation-factor deficiencies and abnormal bleeding in Noonan's syndrome. *Lancet* 1992;**339**:19–21.

114. Yoshioka A, Kamitsuji H, Takase T, et al. Congenital deficiency of alpha-2-plasmin inhibitor in three sisters. *Haemostasis* 1982;**11**:176–84.

115. Leebeek FW, Stibbe J, Knot EA, et al. Mild haemostatic problems associated with congenital heterozygous alpha 2-antiplasmin deficiency. *Thromb Haemost* 1988;**59**:96–100.

116. Kettle P, Mayne EE. A bleeding disorder due to deficiency of alpha-2-antiplasmin. *J Clin Pathol* 1985;**38**:428–9.

117. Devaussuzenet VMP, Ducou–le–Pointe HA, Doco AM, et al. A case of intramedullary hematoma associated with congenital alpha2-plasmin inhibitor deficiency. *Pediatr Radiol* 1998;**28**:978–80.

118. Schwartz BS, Williams EC, Conlan MG, et al. Epsilon-aminocaproic acid in the treatment of patients with acute promyelocytic leukemia and acquired alpha-2-plasmin inhibitor deficiency. *Ann Intern Med* 1986;**105**:873–7.

119. Zarnovicanova M, Mocikova K. A homozygous quantitative defect of alpha 2-antiplasmin in a family from central Slovakia. *Bratisl Lek Listy* 2000;**101**:28–30.

120. Mandelbrot L, Guillaumont M, Forestier F, et al. Placental transfer of vitamin K$_1$ and its implications in fetal hemostasis. *Thromb Haemost* 1988;**60**:39–43.

121. Greer FR, Mummah–Schendel LL, Marshall S, et al. Vitamin K$_1$ (phylloquinone) and Vitamin K$_2$ (menaquinone) status in newborns during the first week of life. *Pediatrics* 1988;**81**:137–40.

122. Hiraike H, Kimura M, Itokawa Y. Distribution of K vitamins (phylloquinone and menaquinones) in human placenta and maternal and umbilical cord plasma. *Am J Obstet Gynecol* 1988;**158**:564–9.

123. Srinivasan G, Seeler RA, Tiruvury A, et al. Maternal anticonvulsant therapy and hemorrhagic disease of the newborn. *Obstet Gynecol* 1982;**59**:250–2.

124. Laosombat V. Hemorrhagic disease of the newborn after maternal anticonvulsant therapy: A case report and literature review. *J Med Assoc Thailand* 1988;**71**:643–8.

125. Eggermont E, Logghe N, Van De Casseye W, et al. Haemorrhagic disease of the newborn in the offspring of rifampicin and isoniazid treated mothers. *Acta Paediatr Belg* 1976;**29**:87–90.

126. Shearer MJ. Vitamin K deficiency bleeding (VKDB) in early infancy. *Blood Rev* 2009;**23**:49–59.

127. Goto T, Kakita H, Takasu M, et al. A rare case of fetal extensive intracranial hemorrhage and whole-cerebral hypoplasia due to latent maternal vitamin K deficiency. *J Neonatal Perinatal Med* 2018;**11**:191–4.

128. Sotodate G, Matsumoto A, Konishi Y, et al. Fetal intracranial hemorrhage due to maternal subclinical vitamin K deficiency associated with long–term eating disorder. *J Obstet Gynaecol Res* 2019;**45**:461–5.

129. Hubbard D, Tobias JD. Intracerebral hemorrhage due to hemorrhagic disease of the newborn and failure to administer vitamin K at birth. *South Med J* 2006;**99**:1216–20.

130. Widdershoven J, Lambert W, Motohara K, et al. Plasma concentrations of vitamin K$_1$ and PIVKA-II in bottle-fed and breast-fed infants with and without vitamin K prophylaxis at birth. *Eur J Pediatr* 1988;**148**:139–42.

131. Motohara K, Endo F, Matsuda I. Screening for late neonatal vitamin K deficiency by acarboxyprothrombin in dried blood spots. *Arch Dis Child* 1987;**62**:370–5.

132. Brady KM, Easley RB, Tobias JD. Recombinant activated factor VII (rFVIIa) treatment in infants

with hemorrhage. *Pediatr Anesth* 2006;**16**:1042–6.

133. Clarke P, Shearer MJ. Vitamin K deficiency bleeding after missed prophylaxis: Rapid synergist effect of vitamin K therapy on hemostasis. *South Med J* 2007;**100**:612–13.

134. Flood VH, Galderisi FC, Lowas SR, et al. Hemorrhagic disease of the newborn despite vitamin K prophylaxis at birth. *Pediatr Blood Cancer* 2008;**50**:1075–7.

135. Vietti TJ, Murphy TP, James JA, Pritchard JA. Observation on the prophylactic use of vitamin K in the newborn. *J Pediatr* 1960;**56**:343–6.

136. Sutherland JM, Glueck HI. Hemorrhagic disease of the newborn: Breast feeding as a necessary factor in the pathogenesis. *Am J Dis Child* 1967;**113**:524–33.

137. Vietti TJ, Stephens JC, Bennett KR. Vitamin K-1 prophylaxis in the newborn. *JAMA* 1961;**176**:791–3.

138. Puckett RM, Offringa M. Prophylactic vitamin K for vitamin K deficiency bleeding in neonates. *Cochrane Database Syst Rev* 2000;**2000**(4): CD002776.

139. Van Winckel M, De Bruyne R, Van De Velde S, et al. Vitamin K, an update for the pediatrician. *Eur J Pediatr* 2009;**168**:127–34.

140. Cornelissen M, Von Kries R, Loughnan P, et al. Prevention of vitamin K deficiency bleeding: Efficacy of different multiple oral dose schedules of vitamin K. *Eur J Pediatr* 1997;**156**:126–30.

141. Greer FR, Marshall SP, Severson RR, et al. A new mixed micellar preparation for oral vitamin K prophylaxis: Randomized controlled comparison with an intramuscular formulation in breast fed infants. *Arch Dis Child* 1998;**79**:300–5.

142. Schubiger G, Stocker C, Banziger O, et al. Oral vitamin K1 prophylaxis for newborns with a new mixed-micellar preparation of phylloquinone: 3 years' experience in Switzerland. *Eur J Pediatr* 1999;**158**:599–602.

143. Mihatsch WA., Braegger C, Bronsky J, et al. Prevention of vitamin K deficiency bleeding in newborn infants: A position paper by the ESPGHAN committee on nutrition. *JPGN* 2016;**63**:123–9.

144. Busfield A, Samuel R, McNinch A, et al. Vitamin K deficiency bleeding after NICE guidance and withdrawal of Konakion neonatal: British Paediatric Surveillance Unit Study, 2006–2008. *Arch Dis Child* 2013;**98**:41–7.

145. McNinch A, Busfield A, Tripp J. Vitamin K deficiency bleeding in Great Britain and Ireland: British Paediatric Surveillance Unit surveys, 1993–94 and 2001–02. *Arch Dis Child* 2007;**92**:759–66.

146. Darlow BA, Phillips AA, Dickson NP. New Zealand surveillance of neonatal vitamin K deficiency bleeding (VKDB): 1998–2008. *J Paediatr Child Health* 2011;**47**:460–64.

147. Levi M, ten Cate H. Disseminated intravascular coagulation. *N Engl J Med* 1999;**341**:586–92.

148. Anderson J, Brown JK, Cockburn F. On the role of disseminated intravascular coagulation on the pathology of birth asphyxia. *Dev Med Child Neurol* 1974;**16**:581–91.

149. Chessells J, Wigglesworth J. Coagulation studies in severe birth asphyxia. *Arch Dis Child* 1971;**46**:253–6.

150. Suarez CR, Menendez CE, Walenga JM, et al. Neonatal and maternal hemostasis: Value of molecular markers in the assessment of hemostatic status. *Semin Thromb Hemostas* 1984;**10**:280–4.

151. Yuen PM, Yin JA, Lao TT. Fibrinopeptide A levels in maternal and newborn plasma. *Eur J Obstet Gynecol Reprod Biol* 1989;**30**:239–44.

152. Suarez CR, Walenga J, Mangogna LC, et al. Neonatal and maternal fibrinolysis: Activation at time of birth. *Am J Hematol* 1985;**19**:365–72.

153. Magnusson M, Ignjatovic V, Hardikar W, Monagle P. A conceptual and practical approach to haemostasis in paediatric liver disease. *P Arch Dis Child* 2016;**101**:854–9.

154. Ettingshausen CE, Veldmann A, Beeg T, et al. Replacement therapy with protein C concentrate in infants and adolescents with meningococcal sepsis and purpura fulminans. *Semin Thromb Hemostas* 1999;**25**:537–41.

155. Rintala E, Kauppila M, Seppala OP, et al. Protein C substitution in sepsis–associated purpura fulminans. *Crit Care Med* 2000;**28**:2373–8.

156. Haneberg B, Gutteberg TJ, Moe PJ, et al. Heparin for infants and children with meningococcal septicemia. Results of a randomized therapeutic trial. *NIPH Ann* 1983;**6**:43–7.

157. Blum D, Fondu P, Denolin–Reubens R, et al. Early heparin therapy in 60 children with acute meningococcemia: Relationship between clinical manifestations and coagulation abnormalities. *Acta Chir Belgica* 1973;**4**:288–97.

158. Hathaway WE. Heparin therapy in acute meningococcemia. *J Pediatr* 1991;**82**:900–1.

159. Gobel U, von Voss H, Jurgens H, et al. Efficiency of heparin in the treatment of newborn infants with respiratory distress syndrome and

disseminated intravascular coagulation. *Eur J Pediatr* 1980;**133**:47–9.

160. Gross S, Filston H, Anderson JC. Controlled study of treatment for disseminated intravascular coagulation in the neonate. *J Pediatr* 1982;**100**:445–8.

161. Beattie W, Magnusson M, Hardikar W, et al. Characterization of the coagulation profile in children with liver disease and extrahepatic portal vein obstruction or shunt. *Pediatr Hematol Oncol.* 2017;**34**:107–19.

162. Kawada Y, Shiiki M, Miyagawa T, et al. Successful treatment of an infant with fulminant hepatitis by factor VII concentrate. *Rinsho Ketsueki* 1989;**30**:1982–6.

163. Hedner U, Glazer S, Falch J. Recombinant activated factor VII in the treatment of bleeding episodes in patients with inherited and acquired bleeding disorders. *Transfus Med Rev* 1993;**7**:78–83.

164. Brown JB, Emerick KM, Brown DL, et al. Recombinant factor VIIa improves coagulopathy caused by liver failure. *J Pediatr Gastroenterol Nutr* 2003;**37**:268–72.

165. Pettersson M, Fischler B, Petrini P, et al. Recombinant FVIIa in children with liver disease. *Thromb Res* 2005;**116**:185–97.

166. Leblebisatan G, Sasmaz I, Antmen B, et al. Management of life–threatening hemorrhages and unsafe interventions in nonhemophiliac children by recombinant factor VIIa. *Clin Appl Thromb Hemost* 2010;**16**:77–82.

167. McQuilten ZK, Barnes C, Zatta A, et al. Haemostasis Registry Steering Committee. Off-label use of recombinant factor VIIa in pediatric patients. *Pediatrics* 2012;**129**: e1533–e40.

168. Chuansumrit A, Teeraratkul S, Wanichkul S, et al. rFVIIa Study Group: Recombinant-activated factor VII for control and prevention of hemorrhage in nonhemophilic pediatric patients. *Blood Coagul Fibrinolysis* 2010;**21**:354–62.

169. Al–Said K, Anderson R, Wong A, Le D. Recombinant factor VIIa for intraoperative bleeding in a child with hepatoblastoma and review of recombinant activated factor VIIa use in children undergoing surgery. *J Pediatr Surg* 2008;**43**:e15–e9.

170. Abdullaha F, Hunterb C, Hargrove C, et al. Recombinant factor VIIa for treatment of massive liver fracture in a premature infant. *J Pediatr Surg* 2006;**41**:1764–7.

Neonatal Thrombosis

Gary Woods and Matthew A. Saxonhouse

Introduction

Thromboembolism (TE) in pediatrics is relatively rare compared with adults, with an estimated venous thromboembolism (VTE) incidence of 0.07–0.14/10,000 children [1, 2]. A bimodal age distribution has been well demonstrated in the pediatric VTE population and children less than 1 year of age, especially those less than 1 month of age, are most commonly affected [1, 2]. The incidence of VTE in this very young population, particularly when hospitalized, is increasing [3–6]. Between 1997 and 2018, up to a 13-fold increase in neonatal TE incidence has been described in all live births and a greater than six-fold increase in neonatal TE incidence has been described for neonatal intensive care unit (NICU) admissions [4–7]. This increase has been attributed to improving survival rates in critically ill and/or premature neonates, the increased utilization of central venous catheters (CVC), and a much greater awareness of VTE and the associated risk factors in this population [3, 6, 8, 9]. The aim of this chapter is to review the congenital and acquired risk factors associated with neonatal TE and to discuss the clinical presentation, diagnosis, and management of this rare complication that has been shown to significantly impact the morbidity and mortality rates of those afflicted [1–3, 8].

Risk Factors

Developmental Hemostasis

Developmental hemostasis is a term used to describe the physiologic changes in the dynamic hemostatic system evolving from intrauterine life, through the neonatal and pediatric time periods, into its maturation in adulthood [10]. The variations in procoagulant and anticoagulant activities in neonates compared with adults has been well described and is even more pronounced in premature infants [11, 12]. At birth, the plasma concentration of procoagulants factor (F) V, FVIII, FXIII, and von Willebrand have been shown to have similar, if not increased, activities compared to adult levels [10, 13]. All vitamin K dependent factors, including procoagulant FII, FVII, FIX, and FX and anticoagulant proteins C and S, are decreased and can take months to even years to reach adult normal values [13]. Procoagulants FXI and FXII, have also been shown to be decreased compared to adult norms, and anticoagulants antithrombin and plasminogen have also been shown to have significantly less activity in neonates [10, 13].

Although these differences seem to infer a prothrombotic state, other factors, including a decreased ability to generate thrombin, provide a balance that prevents spontaneous TE in otherwise well neonates [14]. However, if other acquired or congenital risk factors are present (see Table 19.1), this balance can be disrupted, predisposing certain neonates to TE [15].

Clinical Risk Factors

Studies have shown that male gender, extreme prematurity (<25–27 weeks' gestational age), extremely low birth weight (<1,000 g), and prolonged NICU stay all increase the risk for neonatal TE [2–4, 16]. Most pediatric VTE are associated with at least one if not more clinical risk factors, and neonatal VTE are no different, with over 80% of symptomatic neonatal TE being associated with the presence of acquired risk factors (see Table 19.I) [1, 2, 4–6]. The primary risk factor associated with

Neonatal Hematology, Pathogenesis, Diagnosis, and Management of Hematologic Problems, 3rd edition, ed. Pedro A. de Alarcón, Eric J. Werner, Robert D. Christensen, and Martha C. Sola-Visner. Published by Cambridge University Press. © Cambridge University Press 2021.

Table 19.1 Risk factors for the development of neonatal TE

Maternal risk factors	Delivery risk factors	Neonatal risk factors
Infertility	Emergent cesarean section	Central venous/arterial catheters*
Oligohydramnios	Fetal heart rate abnormalities	Congenital heart disease
Inherited thrombophilia	Instrumentation	Sepsis
Preeclampsia	Meconium stained fluid	Meningitis
Diabetes		Birth asphyxia
Fetal growth restriction		Respiratory distress syndrome
Chorioamnionitis		Dehydration
Prolonged rupture of membranes		Congenital nephritic/nephrotic syndrome
Autoimmune disorders		Necrotizing enterocolitis
Fetal thrombotic vasculopathy		Inherited thrombophilia
		Polycythemia
		Pulmonary hypertension
		Surgery
		Extracorporeal membrane oxygenation
		Medications (steroids)

Notes: *Greatest risk factor for thrombosis.

From Saxonhouse and Manco-Johnson. The evaluation and management of neonatal coagulation disorders. *Semin Perinatol* 2009;33:52–65, 56, with permission [14]; and data from[4, 17, 101, 105, 131–138].

the vast majority of neonatal TE development is the presence of a CVC or arterial catheter, with a reported symptomatic CVC-associated VTE incidence of 2.2%–33.6% [2, 4, 5, 17–20]. The greatest VTE risk factor in premature infants is the presence of an umbilical venous catheter (UVC) [21]. Sepsis and any congenital heart disease have also been shown to carry significant risk in neonatal TE [7, 9].

Along with neonatal risk factors, there are maternal factors that directly affect the risk of neonatal TE. Maternal diabetes, hypertension, fetal thrombotic vasculopathy, preeclampsia, prolonged rupture of membranes, and chorioamnionitis have all been reported as risk factors, but the reports vary [7, 14, 22]. Maternal autoimmune conditions can also influence neonatal TE development. Maternal antiphospholipid antibodies, including anticardiolipin, β2-glycoprotein, and lupus anticoagulant, seem to confer a significant risk of neonatal TE, especially perinatal arterial ischemic stroke (PAIS). These antibodies can cause placental thromboses or may cross the placenta and directly influence TE development in the neonate [23–25].

Inherited Thrombophilia

The role of inherited thrombophilia (IT) in neonatal TE is poorly defined [26]. The literature is scarce, but between 20% and 33% of neonatal TE has been associated with IT [4, 6]. A recent systematic review of the literature found that

while thrombophilic conditions may play a role in neonatal TE, clinical risk factors have more influence on the development of TE [27]. This seems to be particularly true regarding CVC related neonatal TE, where only few cases have an associated IT [28, 29]. More recent evidence has suggested that multiple IT or a combination of an IT and a clinical risk factor influence neonatal TE development [14]. Clinical risk factors seem to more heavily influence neonatal TE development, but IT evaluation may be appropriate in certain situations, especially in unprovoked TE or if there is a family history of TE, depending on the thrombosis severity, location, as well as the number of acquired risk factors present [30]. Due to the large volume of blood typically needed to perform the investigations, a step-wise approach can be used with only certain studies required during the acute event and others obtained around 3–6 months of life (see Table 19.2).

Activated protein C is a vitamin K dependent anticoagulant that inactivates the activated forms of FV (FVa) and FVIII (FVIIIa). A mutation in FV, most commonly FV Leiden (FVL), can lead to a resistance in activated protein C, resulting in a thrombophilic state. It is the most common IT, with heterozygous mutations affecting about 5% of the white European population, and it confers about a 5-fold increased TE risk and 80-fold increased TE risk in adults with heterozygous and homozygous mutations, respectively [31–34]. Although most

Table 19.2 Laboratory evaluation for inherited thrombophilia

Laboratory testing if other acquired risk factors present	Laboratory testing if other acquired risk factors *not* present
Antiphospholipid antibody panel, Anticardiolipin and lupus anticoagulant (IgG, IgM)*	Antiphospholipid antibody panel, anticardiolipin and lupus anticoagulant (IgG, IgM)*
Protein C activity**	Protein C activity**
Protein S activity**	Protein S activity**
Lipoprotein(a)**	Antithrombin (activity assay)**
Plasminogen level **(if considering thrombolytic therapy)	Factor V Leiden***
Antithrombin III (AT-III) (activity assay)**	Prothrombin G***
Factor V Leiden***	PAI-1 4G/5G mutation***
Factor II G20210A (prothrombin G)***	Homocysteine** (if elevated, screen for methylenetetrahydrofolate reductase gene mutation)
	Lipoprotein a**
	FVIII activity**
	FXII activity**
	Plasminogen activity**
	Heparin cofactor II**

Notes: *May be performed from maternal serum during first few months of life.

** Protein-based assays are affected by the acute thrombosis and must be repeated at 3–6 months of life, before a definitive diagnosis may be made. Therefore, recommend that complete evaluation (excluding DNA-based assays) be performed at 3–6 months of life [107, 136]. If anticoagulation is being administered, then these assays should be obtained 14–30 days after discontinuing the anticoagulant. Lipoprotein(a) levels may need to be repeated at 8–12 months of life.

***DNA-based assays.

Adapted from Saxonhouse and Manco-Johnson. The evaluation and management of neonatal coagulation disorders. *Semin Perinatol* 2009;33:52–65, 59, with permission [14]. Refs: [131, 132, 136, 139, 140].

individuals with a FVL mutation will not have their first TE event until later in life, there have been meta-analyses that have shown a significant association with FVL mutations and neonatal cerebral sinus venous thrombosis (CSVT) [35].

Prothrombin gene 2021A (PTG) mutation is the second most common IT, as 1%–2% of the white European population is affected. This mutation increases circulating prothrombin, the precursor to thrombin, concentrations by 15%–30%, which increases the TE risk about two- to three-fold in the adult population [36, 37]. There have been reports of PTG mutations in neonatal TE, but these are rare, and other studies have shown no significant neonatal TE risk with this mutation [15, 35].

Protein C deficiency is a rare condition resulting in the inability to inactivate FVa and FVIIIa, which results in an approximate 10-fold increased risk of TE in the general population in those heterozygous for the mutation [38]. Although there are case reports and case series suggesting heterozygous protein C deficiency may increase arterial and venous TE in neonates, especially CSVT, numerous studies report that the risk of neonatal TE is relatively low [27, 39–41].

Homozygous protein C deficiency is rare, but manifests hours after birth with cerebral damage noted in utero, large vessel thrombosis, and most commonly purpura fulminans, a dermal vascular necrosis that causes a progressive hemorrhagic necrosis of the skin [42, 43]. Newborns will have a diffuse disseminated intravascular coagulation with resulting hemorrhagic complications with large bullae lesions primarily on the extremities, buttock, abdomen, scrotum, and other sites of pressure [44]. Treatment would include either fresh frozen plasma (FFP) at 10–20 ml/kg every 12 hours or the use of protein C concentrates until there is resolution of the skin lesions [45, 46]. After the initial treatment, protein C concentrates are safe, efficient, and available for prophylactic use in severe congenital protein C deficiency [47].

Protein S is a vitamin K-dependent endogenous anticoagulant that acts as a cofactor for the activated protein C inactivation of FVa and FVIIIa [48]. It usually circulates as an active free form and a complement 4B (C4B) bound inactive form, but, due to a deficiency of C4B, it circulates predominantly in the free form in neonates [49, 50]. A recent systematic review of the literature showed that very few neonatal and pediatric TE are due to heterozygous protein S deficiency [27]. Compound heterozygous and homozygous protein S deficiencies are rare and usually present at birth with purpura fulminans [51–53]. There are no isolated protein S concentrates available, so treatment involves FFP at 10–20 ml/kg every 12 hours until lesions resolve, with potential long-term pharmacologic anticoagulation to follow [54].

Antithrombin is a serine protease inhibitor that inactivates FIIa (thrombin), FIXa, FXa, FXIa, and FXIIa [55]. It may be acquired, especially in congenital nephrotic syndrome, or inherited. Heterozygous antithrombin deficiency has been reported in neonatal arterial and venous TE but is not associated with purpura fulminans. It is, however, associated with TE in unusual sites like the coronary arteries, the aorta, and the central nervous system [56–61]. Homozygous antithrombin deficiency is quite rare but has been implicated in severe spontaneous venous and arterial TE in neonates. Neonatal pulmonary artery TE, IVC/abdominal vein, and extremity venous TE have all been reported [62–64]. Treatment would require anticoagulation, but heparin may not be effective as it relies on antithrombin as a substrate so substitution of antithrombin with a plasma derived concentrate is usually required and has been shown to be effective [65].

Lipoprotein(a) (Lp(a)) is composed of a polypeptide chain and low-density lipid particle and is structurally similar to plasminogen. Due to the resemblance, it competes with plasminogen in binding to fibrin, which reduces fibrinolytic activity. Elevated levels of Lp(a) can reduce fibrinolytic activity significantly enough that TE risk is increased. Although pediatric venous and arterial TE have both been described, the true risk associated with neonatal TE and elevated Lp(a) is not well defined, but it seems that elevated Lp(a) may play a role in neonatal PAIS [66, 67].

Clinical Presentations and Locations of Neonatal TE

Locations for the variety of neonatal TE and the proper imaging modalities to diagnose them are presented below. Many of the gold standard imaging techniques used in adults are unable to be utilized in neonates, thus Doppler ultrasonography (US) is the most widely and safely used modality [20].

Arterial TE

Perinatal Arterial Ischemic Stroke (PAIS)

Perinatal arterial ischemic stroke refers to insults, ischemic or hemorrhagic, occurring from 20 weeks' gestational age to 28 days postnatally. PAIS is defined as a condition with acute encephalopathy, seizures, or neurologic deficits presenting in the term or preterm infant before the 29th postnatal day with brain imaging confirming a parenchymal infarct in the appropriate arterial region [68, 69]. Most abnormalities occur in the left hemisphere within the distribution of the middle cerebral artery with the origin of the left carotid artery from the aorta allowing for a more direct vascular route to the brain as a corridor for cardiac emboli [23, 70]. Multi-focal cerebral infarctions may occur, but these tend to be embolic in origin. Many potential risk factors have been implicated in the etiology of PAIS (see Table 19.1). Between 22 and 70% of congenital hemiplegic cerebral palsy in neonates has been attributed to PAIS [23, 71, 72]. Other neurological comorbidities include seizure disorders, delayed language development, and behavioral disorders [25].

Placental pathology is a major risk factor for PAIS. Maternal/fetal conditions including fetal thrombotic vasculopathy and antiphospholipid antibody syndrome may result in emboli that break off the placental circulation and enter the fetal circulation [73, 74]. Studies have identified prothrombotic risk factors, especially elevated lipoprotein (a) and protein C deficiency, in as much as 68% of neonates with PAIS [66].

Screening for neonates with suspected PAIS can be done with cranial ultrasound (CUS) as it is the least invasive method. However, studies have found that 75% of cases of PAIS were missed using this modality alone [75]. Therefore, all cases of suspected PAIS should have MRI with diffusion-weighted imaging (DW MRI) performed [76]. This technique allows the detection of cerebral edema, which is an early sign of cerebral ischemic damage [77, 78]. Angiography can also be performed and allows for the detection of thromboses if there is a history of instrumentation/difficult delivery [79].

Iatrogenic/Spontaneous Arterial TE

Umbilical arterial catheters (UACs) and peripheral arterial catheters (PAL) are frequently used in the NICU (10%–64% of neonates) as means for continuous monitoring of arterial blood pressure and blood gases [15]. Femoral arterial catheters are used more frequently in neonates with congenital heart disease or those requiring extensive surgery. Despite their value, they can have devastating complications such as infection, limb loss, renal failure, and even death [80–82]. High UAC positioning (T6-9) has been found to have fewer clinical complication, while low dose continuous heparin infusion at 1 u/ml prolongs catheter patency but does not reduce the risk of TE [83, 84]. Catheter material, duration of placement, and solutions infused influence the risk for catheter related TE. Suspicion of an arterial TE should be confirmed by Doppler US but contrast angiography may be required for complicated cases [18].

Venous TE

Catheter-Related TE

Although vital to the improvement in care to the most critical of neonates, the presence of a central venous catheter (CVC) represents the greatest risk for TE. Additional risk factors further increase this risk. Providers must evaluate the risks and benefits every day that a CVC remains in place and prompt removal should occur whenever the risks of a CVC outweigh its benefits. Damage to blood vessel walls during insertion, disrupted blood flow, infusion of substances that damage endothelium, and thrombogenic catheter materials are the main reasons that TE develop [85, 86]. The exact incidence of CVC-related TE varies but recent reports have ranged from 0.7% to 67% [19, 87, 88].

The majority of CVCs placed in neonates include umbilical venous catheters (UVCs) and peripherally inserted central venous catheters (PICCs) [85]. Autopsy studies have estimated that 20%–65% of infants who die with a UVC in situ have microscopic evidence of TE [16, 89, 90]. Intracardiac TE from UVC placement ranges from 1.8% to 5.3% [85].

Persistent infection and/or thrombocytopenia, line dysfunction, and bilateral lower limb edema should alert the clinician of a possible UVC-related TE [91]. Most centers remove UVCs within 7 days of placement, but they should always be removed by 14 days [92]. PICCs or surgically placed CVCs tend to remain in place

for weeks until antibiotic treatment is completed, or an infant has reached adequate enteral feedings. Signs of either PICC or CVC-related TE include unilateral limb swelling/pain/discoloration, superior vena cava syndrome, chylothorax, chylopericardium, intracardiac thrombosis, persistently positive blood cultures, thrombocytopenia, and cardiac failure [21, 93, 94].

Evaluation for CVC-related TE should start with Doppler US but false negative results can occur due to obstruction of the distal subclavian veins by the clavicles [18].

Intracardiac TE and TE in Infants with Complex Congenital Heart Disease

A major complication of a CVC in neonates is the development of a right atrial TE. This type of TE has been associated with endocarditis, pulmonary arterial obstruction, ventricular dysfunction, and death [5, 95–97]. Right atrial and other types of intracardiac thrombi have also been reported commonly in neonates undergoing repair for complex congenital heart disease [98]. Reviews of neonates who underwent palliative repair found evidence of thrombi in 23%–33%, whereas a more recent case-control study performed at a high-level referral NICU demonstrated an incidence of intracardiac TE of 22.5 cases per 1,000 admissions [99] [95].

Echocardiography is the preferred modality for diagnosing either right atrial TE formation, intracardiac vegetations, or TE formation in infants with single ventricle physiology. Signs suggestive of an atrial TE include new onset murmur, sepsis, persistent thrombocytopenia, and cardiac failure.

Renal Vein Thrombosis (RVT)

The most prevalent noncatheter-related TE during the neonatal period, RVT has an incidence of about 0.5 per 1,000 NICU admissions [5]. Recent reviews have demonstrated that about 70% of cases are unilateral, with 64% of these involving the left kidney and a male predominance [100–102]. The cardinal signs suggesting RVT are macroscopic hematuria, a palpable abdominal mass, and thrombocytopenia. Other symptoms include oliguria, proteinuria, acute renal failure, and hypertension. Risk factors are frequently found in RVT cases, with prematurity and perinatal asphyxia being the most common [100].

Because of the potential association of an IT and RVT, an evaluation for an IT is warranted. Doppler US is the modality of choice for diagnosing RVT in neonates with radiographic criteria including presence of echogenic clot, venous distension secondary to presence of a thrombus, or absence of flow [100].

Complications of RVT include adrenal hemorrhage, extension of the clot into the IVC, renal failure, hypertension, and death [101]. Survival is currently at around 85%, however, renal atrophy did not seem to change whether supportive care or anticoagulation/fibrinolysis were used, suggesting that many of these events may be in utero and chronic in nature [100].

Portal Vein Thrombosis (PVT)

Sepsis/omphalitis and UVC use represent the two major risk factors for PVT [103]. Diagnosis may be difficult since most cases are clinically silent. Doppler US is the preferred modality for evaluation. Cavernous transformation of the portal vein with subsequent splenomegaly and reversal of portal flow are used to document severity [103]. Although spontaneous resolution of asymptomatic PVT in neonates is common, detection of PVT warrants close observation to follow for signs of portal hypertension. This complication may manifest itself up to 10 years after the neonatal period [103].

Cerebral Sinovenous Thrombosis (CSVT)

A subcategory of perinatal stroke, CSVT symptoms are similar to PAIS [104, 105]. Other clinical findings may include anemia and/or thrombocytopenia. Predisposing risk factors are common, with infection, perinatal complications, and IT being the most frequently reported [105]. The superficial and lateral sinuses are the most frequently involved vessels, and up to 30% of cases have reported venous infarction with subsequent hemorrhage [23, 106]. Intraventricular hemorrhages (especially in term neonates) and hemorrhages within the caudate nucleus and thalamus are associated with thrombosis of the deep cerebral venous sinuses. Therefore, the presence of an intraventricular hemorrhage or thalamic hemorrhage in a term or late preterm infant warrants evaluation for CSVT [106]. Diagnosis of CSVT is best made through diffusion MRI with venography [21, 30, 91, 107]. Mortality rates for neonatal CSVT range from 2% to 24%, with long-term complications consisting of

cerebral palsy, epilepsy, and cognitive impairments in 10%–80% of infants [108–110].

Management
General Information

When possible, neonates with TE should be managed under the care of an experienced pediatric hematologist or neonatologist with pediatric hematology consultation at tertiary care centers with appropriate radiologic, pharmacologic, surgical, and laboratory support [111]. Management is based on the type of TE, location, severity, and risk factors. Most neonatal TE are managed with therapeutic anticoagulation, but there are situations where active monitoring for thrombus extension without anticoagulation therapy is appropriate, as studies have demonstrated spontaneous resolution of TE in up to 50% of asymptomatic neonates with UVCs [88, 112–114]. In addition, the smaller the thrombus, the more likely it will spontaneously resolve [114]. Therefore, certain neonatal TE can be monitored closely with serial US investigations, with the intent to initiate anticoagulation should the TE increase in size or become symptomatic. The duration and type of therapy depends on the location and size of the TE. The complexity in the decision of when and how long to treat neonatal TE reinforces the notion that the care should be managed under the guidance of experienced providers [111]. Long-term complications such as post-thrombotic syndrome may develop as a result of a catheter-related thrombosis from 1 month to up to 10 years following the event [115].

Arterial TE

Current guidelines recommend anticoagulation for PAIS if there is an ongoing cardioembolic source or evidence of recurrent PAIS [91, 116]. Arterial catheters should be immediately removed whenever there is suspicion or confirmation of a TE [91]. If vascular spasm occurs, removal of the catheter may alleviate symptoms. If spasm persists, warming of the contralateral extremity for 15 minutes may resolve symptoms. However, persistent symptoms may require the local application of 2% nitroglycerin ointment at 4 mm/kg with close monitoring of blood pressure [117]. Management options for neonates with arterial

317

Table 19.3 Management of neonatal arterial TE

Type	Severity	Treatment
Femoral arterial catheter related	Non-limb threatening	Anticoagulation
	Limb or organ threatening	Anticoagulation but change to thrombolytic therapy if clot does not improve or symptoms worsen within 24–48 hours
PAL related	Non-limb threatening	Anticoagulation
	Limb threatening	Thrombolytic therapy followed by anticoagulation
Spontaneous or UAC related	Non-limb or organ threatening	Anticoagulation
	Limb or organ threatening	Thrombolytic therapy followed by anticoagulation

Notes: See Tables 19.7 and 19.10 for dosing guidelines.
Reference: [91].

TE include therapeutic anticoagulation or potentially thrombolytic therapy (see Table 19.3).

Venous TE

Many neonatal TE will be found in association with a CVC. Prior to removing any CVC, including UVCs, that has an associated VTE, it is recommended that 3–5 days of therapeutic anticoagulation be administered to prevent emboli [111]. Currently, most neonatal CVC-associated VTE are treated with therapeutic anticoagulation with thrombolysis reserved for life or limb threatening VTE. Current management strategies are extrapolated from adult data, but the optimal management neonatal CVC-associated VTE is currently being evaluated in the Netherlands [87]. Depending on risk categories, CVC-associated VTE will be managed with either thrombolysis followed by therapeutic anticoagulation, therapeutic anticoagulation alone, or close observation. This will be one of the first studies evaluating treatment options specifically in this population and it will provide a unified, national approach to neonatal thromboses as all NICUs in the Netherlands will follow this protocol [87]. Thrombolytics and/or anticoagulation should also be used for neonates with infective endocarditis that is resistant to antibiotic therapy alone and should be based on the size and symptoms of the TE [118].

Treatment guidelines for RVT (Table 19.4) and PVT (Table 19.5) are provided. There are currently no evidence-based neonatal PVT treatment guidelines due to insufficient data, thus treatment for each neonate should be individualized [103]. Also, there is no evidence to suggest that anticoagulation would improve outcomes, primarily reducing rate of portal hypertension. Due to the lack of evidence, avoidance of anticoagulation if possible is the guiding principle, but if anticoagulation in initiated, duration of therapy should be as short as possible [103].

A systematic review of anticoagulation for CSVT in neonates demonstrated that anticoagulation did reduce the risk of thrombus propagation, but did not have a significant effect on mortality before discharge either in the presence or absence of pre-existing intracranial hemorrhage (ICH) [111, 119]. Current recommendations are to initiate anticoagulation in the presence of CSVT. Risk vs. benefit must be taken into account if acute hemorrhage is present. Anticoagulation should be continued for 6 weeks with repeat imaging at that time. Surgery is reserved for those with hydrocephalus or large intracerebral hematomas with mass effect.

Anticoagulation Therapy with Heparins

Treatment guidelines for anticoagulant dosing regimens for neonates are extrapolated from adult and pediatric data since there are no randomized controlled trials, which at this point will likely never be completed due to the risk of withholding this therapy [111, 117]. This is disappointing as the significant differences in the coagulation system of neonates make it difficult to assess the true risk for serious complications, specifically intracranial hemorrhage (ICH), which is potentially increased even more in premature infants. The presence of certain clinical factors, including recent central nervous system surgery, active bleeding, recent seizure activity, or significant coagulopathy, need to be considered in this especially at risk population as they can affect the initiation of anticoagulant therapy as well as the type of therapy selected [15]. Family discussions

Table 19.4 Management of neonatal renal vein thrombosis (RVT)

	Unilateral RVT	Bilateral RVT
Absence of renal impairment and/or no extension into the inferior vena cava	May consider supportive care with monitoring of the RVT for extension or initiate anticoagulation. If extension occurs, initiate anticoagulation	Anticoagulation
Extension into the inferior vena cava or presence of renal impairment	Anticoagulation*	Anticoagulation*
Renal failure	N/A	Initial thrombolytic therapy with rt-TPA*, followed by anticoagulation

Notes: Adapted from Saxonhouse MA. Management of neonatal thrombosis. *Clin Perinatol* 2012;39:195, with permission [117].
*For dosing options, please see Tables 19.7–19.10.
Data from references [91, 101, 102, 111, 134, 141].

Table 19.5 Management of neonatal portal venous thrombosis

Treatment plan	Description	Recommended ultrasound (US) follow-up
Observation	Non-occlusive thrombus and no evidence of portal hypertension	2–3 days
Anticoagulation*	Occlusive thrombus or idiopathic	10 days. If thrombus resolved, may stop therapy. If still present, treat for 6 weeks to 3 months depending on US follow up
Thrombolysis*	End-organ compromise with extension of the thrombosis into the IVC, RA, and/or RV	Daily. May stop thrombolysis when symptoms improve but would transition to anticoagulation for 6 weeks to 3 months

Notes: IVC, inferior vena cava; RA, right atrium; RV, right ventricle
*For dosing options, please see Tables 19.7–19.10.
Data from Ref. [111].
Adapted from Williams S, Chan AK. Neonatal portal vein thrombosis: Diagnosis and management. *Semin Fetal Neonatal Med* 2011;16:337; with permission.

highlighting the risks and goals for treatment must be documented prior to initiating any therapy. Before initiating any treatment, absolute and relative contraindications to antithrombotic therapy should be reviewed (Table 19.6).

Heparin anticoagulants require antithrombin (AT) to achieve their therapeutic effect. Antithrombin baseline levels are lower in neonates compared with children and adults and neonates clear heparin at an increased rate, thus neonatal dosing may be at higher levels than adult recommended dosing in order to attain therapeutic levels [15]. In rare cases, significant difficulty obtaining therapeutic heparin levels may occur and monitoring AT activity may be recommended with administration of AT concentrate. If AT is administered, close monitoring of heparin levels

is required as supratherapeutic anticoagulant levels can be obtained which would increase the risk of bleeding complications. This is not frequently recommended and should only take place with pediatric hematology assistance.

Low molecular weight heparin (LMWH) is a commonly used anticoagulant in infants and children that selectively inhibits activated factor X (FXa), with enoxaparin utilized most frequently [3, 120–122]. Clinical trials have shown that LMWH generally has fewer bleeding complications than unfractionated heparin (UFH), has a longer half-life, and has a consistent pharmacokinetic and pharmacodynamic profile [123, 124]. LMWH therapy has been effective in the NICU with centers reporting either partial or complete resolution of TE events in 59%–100% of neonates

Table 19.6 Contraindications for anticoagulation/thrombolysis

	Absolute	Relative
Medical conditions	1. CNS surgery or ischemia (including birth asphyxia) within 10 days 2. Active bleeding 3. Invasive procedures within 3 days 4. Seizures within 48 hours	1. Platelet count < 50 × 104/microliter (100 × 104/microliter for ill neonates) 2. Fibrinogen concentration <100 mg/dL 3. INR > 2 4. Severe coagulation deficiency 5. Hypertension

Notes: CNS, central nervous system; INR, international normalized ratio.

Adapted from Manco-Johnson. Controversies in neonatal thrombotic disorders. In Ohls RY, ed. *Hematology, Immunology and Infectious Disease: Neonatology Questions and Controversies* (Philadelphia, PA: Saunders Elsevier, 2008), p. 68; with permission [24].
Data from refs. [17, 18, 91, 107, 142]

Table 19.7 Recommended dosing for anticoagulant therapy in neonates

Gestational age*	UFH	LMWH
≤32 weeks >32 weeks	15 units/kg per hour 28 units/kg per hour	1.5 mg/kg SQ q 12 hours 1.5–1.7 mg/kg SQ q 12 hours
		Prophylactic dosing 0.75 mg/kg SQ q 12 hours Goal for anti-factor Xa level of 0.1–0.3 U/ml

Notes: * Dosing applies also to post-conceptional age (GA + weeks of life)

Monitoring for UFH: Maintain anti-Xa UFH assay level of 0.3–0.7 U/ml. Levels should be checked 4–6 hours after initiating therapy. If loading dose provided, check level 4–6 hours after loading dose provided. If need to make changes in dosing, check levels 4–6 hours after each change in infusion rate.

Monitoring for LMWH: Maintain anti-Xa LMWH assay level of 0.5 to 1.0 U/ml. Check level 4 hours after the 2nd or 3rd dose. If therapeutic, repeat within 24–48 hours. If remain therapeutic, then may check weekly [143].

Complete blood count, platelet count, and coagulation screening (including activated partial thromboplastin time, prothrombin time, PT, and fibrinogen) should be performed prior to starting anticoagulation.

Bolus dosing for UFH should be performed only if there is a significant risk or evidence of thrombus progression [127]. Otherwise, avoid bolus dosing in neonates. If bolus dosing is recommended: ≤32 weeks 25 units/kg IV over 10 minutes; >32 weeks 50 units/kg IV over 10 minutes.

If infant with renal dysfunction, dosing should be discussed with pharmacist.
Data from references [91, 107, 144]

treated [125, 126]. Initial dosing guidelines are based on gestational age (Table 19.7), followed by close monitoring with adjustments as needed to maintain a therapeutic LMWH anti-Xa assay level of 0.5–1 units/mL (Table 19.8). Maintaining therapeutic levels in neonates may be a challenge [111]. A recent review evaluating enoxaparin use in 240 neonates found that the mean maintenance dose of enoxaparin ranged from 1.48 to 2.27 mg/kg q 12 h for all infants, but was higher for preterm neonates at 1.9 to 2.27 mg/kg q 12 h [125, 126]. These findings have influenced the current recommended dosing (Table 19.7).

Although UFH has been largely replaced by LMWH in the treatment of neonatal TE, there are still situations where it would be an appropriate anticoagulant treatment choice. UFH has similar activity against both FXa and FIIa. UFH has a much shorter half-life than LMWH and can be easily reversed with protamine [15]. Thus, in critically ill children where the risk for bleeding is higher, UFH may be a more appropriate choice. Initial dosing recommendations are dependent on gestational age (see Table 19.7) with adjustments as needed to obtain a target anti-Xa UFH assay level of 0.35–0.7 U/ml (Table 19.9). The most recent review of UFH dosing in neonates does not recommend a loading dose due to an increased bleeding risk and lack of evidence suggesting that recurrent thromboses are due to sub-therapeutic anti-factor Xa

Table 19.8 Neonatal LMWH dose titration guideline

Anti-Xa low molecular weight heparin assay (U/ml)	Dose adjustment	Next anti-Xa low molecular weight heparin assay
<0.1	Increase dose by 25%	4 hours after next dose following adjustment*
0.11–0.34	Increase dose by 25%	4 hours after 2nd dose following adjustment
0.35–0.49	Increase dose by 10%	4 hours after 2nd dose following adjustment
0.5–1.0	No change	24–48 hours then weekly. If weekly levels are within therapeutic range three consecutive times, can space to monthly. If change in renal function or signs of bleeding, check level 4 hours after next dose.
1.1–1.5	Decrease dose by 20%	4 hours after 2nd dose following adjustment
1.6–2.0	Hold dose until anti-Xa <1.0 units/ml, then decrease dose by 30%	Check level every 6 hours until <1.0 units/ml; then 4 hours after next dose following adjustment
>2.0	Hold dose until anti-Xa <0.5 units/ml, then decrease dose by 40%	Check level every 12 hours until <0.5 units/ml; then 4 hours after next dose following adjustment

Notes: *Consider waiting until after 2nd dose following adjustment if dose >2.5mg/kg.

Important information: Goal anti-Xa: 0.5–1.0U/ml; anti-Xa level to be checked, 4 hours after 2nd or 3rd dose of initial regimen

Table 19.9 Neonatal UFH dose titration guidelines

Infant ≤32 weeks corrected GA		Infant >32 weeks corrected GA	
Anti-Xa UFH assay level (U/ml)	Round to the nearest 10th unit	Anti-Xa UFH assay level (U/ml)	Round to the nearest 10th unit
Less than 0.2	Bolus 25 units/kg once Increase drip by 1.5 units/kg per hour	Less than 0.2	Bolus 50 units/kg IV once Increase drip by 2.8 units/kg per hour
0.2–0.29	Increase drip by 1.5 units/kg per hour	0.2–0.29	Increase drip by 2.8 units/kg per hour
0.3–0.7	No change	0.3–0.7	No change
0.71–0.8	Decrease drip by 1.5 units/kg per hour	0.71–0.8	Decrease drip by 2.8 units/kg per hour
0.81–0.99	Hold drip for 1 hour then decrease drip by 1.5 units/kg per hour	0.81–0.99	Hold drip for 1 hour then decrease drip by 2.8 units/kg per hour
1 or greater	Hold drip for 1 hour then decrease drip by 3 units/kg per hour	1 or greater	Hold drip for 1 hour then decrease drip by 4.2 units/kg per hour

UFH assay levels during the first 24 hours of anticoagulation [127]. Loading doses should be reserved for neonates with significant risk or evidence of thrombus progression. UFH therapy should be limited for short-term use and attempts to convert to LMWH should occur if longer therapy is required. Therapy is usually limited to 2–14 days, but data to support this recommendation are lacking [91].

Thrombolysis

Thrombolytic therapy utilizing recombinant tissue plasminogen activator (rTPA) is generally reserved for neonates with life or limb threatening TE. The safety and efficacy of rTPA treatment in neonates has been reported in case series and cohort studies demonstrating complete or partial clot lysis in 84%–94% of cases with no significant bleeding complications reported [128].

Plasminogen levels in neonates are at about 50% of adult levels and thus, due to the mechanism of action of rTPA, it is recommended that plasminogen supplementation be utilized prior to initiating this therapy [11, 111]. Dosing recommendations for rTPA (Table 19.10) are based on limited data, and careful laboratory monitoring of

Table 19.10 Neonatal rTPA dosing guidelines

Clinical situation	Recommended dosing	Appropriate monitoring
Limb/life threatening thrombus	0.03 mg/kg per hour Infuse unfractionated heparin (UFH) at 10 units/kg per hour	Dose escalation up to 0.3 mg/kg per hour can be considered, but must be done slowly with continuing monitoring of the patient* Supplementation with plasminogen (FFP at 10 ml/kg) prior to commencing therapy is recommended to ensure adequate thrombolysis [13]

Follow up and dose adjustments

For arterial thrombi, reimage at 6–8 hour intervals, for venous thrombi, reimage at 12–24 hour intervals.

If repeat imaging reveals clot lysis <50%, INCREASE infusion to next dosing level and repeat imaging in 12–24 hours.

If repeat imaging reveals clot lysis 51–94%, continue same dose of infusion and repeat imaging in 12–24 hours.

If repeat imaging reveals clot lysis >95%, stop infusion, and initiate anticoagulation protocol.

If no clot dissolution is evident 12–24 hours after starting infusion and/or d-dimers are not increasing, may also give additional 10 ml/kg of FFP to provide plasminogen to increase efficacy of rTPA.

Attempt to maintain fibrinogen levels >100 mg/dl (provide cryo if <100) and platelet counts >50,000.

rTPA infusion should not be used for >96 hours unless deemed appropriate by neonatology and hematology.

Notes: * Dose titrations can be made every 12–24 hours and are as follows: 0.06 mg/kg per hour → 0.1 mg/kg per hour → 0.2 mg/kg per hour → 0.3 mg/kg per hour. Max dose is 0.3 mg/kg per hour.

fibrinogen levels, platelet counts, and plasminogen (if able) are recommended with replacement as needed to help reduce the risk of severe bleeding [15]. Simultaneous infusion of UFH at a dose of 10 U/kg per hour is recommended to inhibit clot propagation [107, 129]. Once the blood clot is adequately lysed, rTPA therapy should be discontinued with initiation of therapeutic anticoagulation, preferably LMWH.

The main risk associated with rTPA is significant bleeding, specifically ICH. Although some reports suggest preterm infants in particular may be at risk for developing ICH with thrombolytic therapy, others suggest that the risk is similar to more mature neonates [130]. Due to these concerns, ensuring that other clinical bleeding risk factors, including hypertension, thrombocytopenia, and vitamin K deficiency, are corrected prior to initiating thrombolytic therapy is recommended.

Conclusion

Neonatal TE represents an increasing problem of neonates admitted to a NICU. The lack of randomized clinical trials and limited data guiding management of TE emergencies forces neonatologists and hematologists to base their treatment decisions on case series, expert opinion, and published guidelines. Current studies are attempting to determine optimal protocols and care for neonates with symptomatic TE. At this point, the ultimate goal of anyone caring

for neonates with symptomatic TE is to treat effectively without causing additional harm. As care continues to improve for the smallest preterm neonates, so will the risks of CVC-associated VTE. The importance of future studies and improved data registries investigating treatment options for neonatal TE will enhance the care provided to these neonates.

References

1. Andrew M, David M, Adams M, et al. Venous thromboembolic complications (VTE) in children: First analyses of the Canadian Registry of VTE. *Blood* 1994;**83**(5):1251–7.

2. van Ommen CH, Heijboer H, Büller HR, et al. Venous thromboembolism in childhood: A prospective two-year registry in The Netherlands. *J Pediatr* 2001;**139**(5):676–81.

3. Raffini L, Huang YS, Witmer C, Feudtner C. Dramatic increase in venous thromboembolism in children's hospitals in the United States from 2001 to 2007. *Pediatrics* 2009;**124**(4):1001–8.

4. Nowak-Gottl U, von Kries R, Gobel U. Neonatal symptomatic thromboembolism in Germany: Two-year survey. *Arch Dis Child Fetal Neonatal Ed*, 1997;**76**(3):F163–7.

5. Schmidt B, Andrew M. Neonatal thrombosis: Report of a prospective Canadian and international registry. *Pediatrics* 1995. **96**(5 Pt 1):939–43.

6. Saracco P, Bagna R, Gentilomo C, et al. Clinical data of neonatal systemic thrombosis. *J Pediatr* 2016;**171**:60–6 e1.

7. Bhat R, Kumar R, Kwon S, Murthy K, Liem RI. Risk factors for neonatal venous and arterial thromboembolism in the neonatal intensive care unit: A case control study. *J Pediatr* 2018;**195**:28–32.

8. Setty BA, O'Brien SH, Kerlin BA. Pediatric venous thromboembolism in the United States: A tertiary care complication of chronic diseases. *Pediatr Blood Cancer* 2012;**59**(2):258–64.

9. Nag U, Greenberg R, Leraas HJ, et al. Risk factors for thrombosis in the neonatal intensive care unit: Analysis of a large national database. *Blood* 2017;**130** (Supplement 1): 3351.

10. Monagle P, Barnes C, Ignjatovic V, et al. Developmental haemostasis: Impact for clinical haemostasis laboratories. *Thromb Haemost* 2006;**95**(2):362–72.

11. Andrew M, Paes B, Milner R, et al. Development of the human coagulation system in the full-term infant. *Blood* 1987;**70**(1):165–72.

12. Andrew M, Paes B, Milner R, et al. Development of the human coagulation system in the healthy premature infant. *Blood* 1988;**72**(5):1651–7.

13. Attard C, van der Straaten T, Karlaftis V, Monagle P, Ignjatovic V. Developmental hemostasis: Age-specific differences in the levels of hemostatic proteins. *J Thromb Haemost* 2013;**11** (10):1850–4.

14. Saxonhouse MA, Manco-Johnson MJ. The evaluation and management of neonatal coagulation disorders. *Semin Perinatol* 2009;**33** (1):52–65.

15. Saxonhouse MA, Thrombosis in the neonatal intensive care unit. *Clin Perinatol* 2015;**42** (3):651–73.

16. Schmidt B, Zipursky A. Thrombotic disease in newborn infants. *Clin Perinatol* 1984;**11** (2):461–88.

17. Beardsley DS. Venous thromboembolism in the neonatal period. *Semin Perinatol* 2007;**31** (4):250–3.

18. Greenway A, Massicotte MP, Monagle P. Neonatal thrombosis and its treatment. *Blood Rev* 2004;**18** (2):75–84.

19. Park CK, Paes BA, Nagel K, et al. Neonatal central venous catheter thrombosis: Diagnosis, management and outcome. *Blood Coagul Fibrinolysis* 2014;**25**(2):97–106.

20. Pettit J. Assessment of infants with peripherally inserted central catheters: Part 1. Detecting the most frequently occurring complications. *Adv Neonatal Care* 2002;**2**(6):304–15.

21. Rajagopal R, Cheah FC, Monagle P. Thromboembolism and anticoagulation management in the preterm infant. *Semin Fetal Neonatal Med* 2016;**21**(1):50–6.

22. Narang S, Roy J, Stevens TP, et al. Risk factors for umbilical venous catheter-associated thrombosis in very low birth weight infants. *Pediatr Blood Cancer* 2009;**52**(1):75–9.

23. Chalmers EA. Perinatal stroke: Risk factors and management. *Br J Haematol* 2005;**130**(3):333–43.

24. Manco-Johnson M. Controversies in neonatal thrombotic disorders. In Ohls R YM, ed. *Hematology, Immunology and Infections Disease: Neonatology Questions and Controversies* (Philadelphia, PA: Saunders Elsevier, 2008), pp. 58–74.

25. Nelson KB, Causative factors in cerebral palsy. *Clin Obstet Gynecol* 2008;**51**(4):749–62.

26. Saracco P, Parodi C, Fabris V, et al. Management and investigation of neonatal thromboembolic events: genetic and acquired risk factors. *Thromb Res* 2009; **123**(6):805–9.

27. Klaassen IL, van Ommen CH, Middeldorp S. Manifestations and clinical impact of pediatric inherited thrombophilia. *Blood* 2015;**125** (7):1073–7.

28. Demirel N, Aydin M, Zenciroglu A, et al. Neonatal thrombo-embolism: Risk factors, clinical features and outcome. *Ann Trop Paediatr* 2009;**29** (4):271–9.

29. Salonvaara M, Riikonen P, Kekomäki R, Heinonen, K. Clinically symptomatic central venous catheter-related deep venous thrombosis in newborns. *Acta Paediatr* 1999;**88**(6):642–6.

30. O'Brien SH. Perinatal thrombosis: Implications for mothers and neonates. *Hematology Am Soc Hematol Educ Program* 2015;**2015**:48–52.

31. Dahlback B. The protein C anticoagulant system: Inherited defects as basis for venous thrombosis. *Thromb Res* 1995;**77**(1):1–43.

32. Dahlback B. Inherited thrombophilia: Resistance to activated protein C as a pathogenic factor of venous thromboembolism. *Blood* 1995;**85** (3):607–14.

33. van der Meer FJ, Koster T, Vandenbroucke JP, Briët E, Rosendaal FR. The Leiden Thrombophilia Study (LETS). *Thromb Haemost* 1997;**78**(1):631–5.

34. Price DT, Ridker PM. Factor V Leiden mutation and the risks for thromboembolic disease: A clinical perspective. *Ann Intern Med* 1997;**127** (10):895–903.

35. Laugesaar R, Kahre T, Kolk A, et al. Factor V Leiden and prothrombin 20210G>A mutation and paediatric ischaemic stroke: A case-control study and two meta-analyses. *Acta Paediatr* 2010;**99**(8):1168–74.

36. Poort SR, Rosendaal FR, Reitsma PH, Bertina RM. A common genetic variation in the 3'-untranslated region of the prothrombin gene is associated with elevated plasma prothrombin levels and an increase in venous thrombosis. *Blood* 1996;**88**(10):3698–703.

37. Junker R, Koch HG, Auberger K, et al. Prothrombin G20210A gene mutation and further prothrombotic risk factors in childhood thrombophilia. *Arterioscler Thromb Vasc Biol* 1999;**19**(10):2568–72.

38. Allaart CF, Poort SR, Rosendaal FR, et al. Increased risk of venous thrombosis in carriers of hereditary protein C deficiency defect. *Lancet* 1993;**341**(8838):134–8.

39. Tridapalli E, Stella M, Capretti MG, Faldella G. Neonatal arterial iliac thrombosis in type-I protein C deficiency: a case report. *Ital J Pediatr* 2010;**36**:23.

40. De Stefano V, Leone G, Mastrangelo S, et al. Clinical manifestations and management of inherited thrombophilia: retrospective analysis and follow-up after diagnosis of 238 patients with congenital deficiency of antithrombin III, protein C, protein S. *Thromb Haemost* 1994;**72**(3):352–8.

41. De Stefano V, Finazzi G, Mannucci PM. Inherited thrombophilia: Pathogenesis, clinical syndromes, and management. *Blood* 1996;**87**(9):3531–44.

42. Auletta MJ, Headington JT. Purpura fulminans. A cutaneous manifestation of severe protein C deficiency. *Arch Dermato*, 1988;**124**(9):1387–91.

43. Adcock DM, Brozna J, Marlar RA. Proposed classification and pathologic mechanisms of purpura fulminans and skin necrosis. *Semin Thromb Hemost* 1990;**16**(4):333–40.

44. Alessi MC, Aillaud MF, Paut O, et al. Purpura fulminans in a patient homozygous for a mutation in the protein C gene–prenatal diagnosis in a subsequent pregnancy. *Thromb Haemost* 1996;**75**(3):525–6.

45. Marlar RA, Montgomery RR, Broekmans AW. Report on the diagnosis and treatment of homozygous protein C deficiency. Report of the Working Party on Homozygous Protein C Deficiency of the ICTH-Subcommittee on Protein C and Protein S. *Thromb Haemost* 1989;**61**(3):529–31.

46. Dreyfus M, Magny JF, Bridey F, et al. Treatment of homozygous protein C deficiency and neonatal purpura fulminans with a purified protein C concentrate. *N Engl J Med* 1991;**325**(22):1565–8.

47. Kroiss S, Albisetti M. Use of human protein C concentrates in the treatment of patients with severe congenital protein C deficiency. *Biologics* 2010;**4**:51–60.

48. Walker FJ. Regulation of activated protein C by a new protein. A possible function for bovine protein S. *J Biol Chem* 1980;**255**(12):5521–4.

49. Moalic P, Gruel Y, Body G, et al. Levels and plasma distribution of free and C4b-BP-bound protein S in human fetuses and full-term newborns. *Thromb Res* 1988;**49**(5):471–80.

50. Schwarz HP, Muntean W, Watzke H, Richter B, Griffin JH. Low total protein S antigen but high protein S activity due to decreased C4b-binding protein in neonates. *Blood* 1988;**71**(3):562–5.

51. Pegelow CH, Ledford M, Young J, Zilleruelo G. Severe protein S deficiency in a newborn. *Pediatrics* 1992;**89**(4 Pt 1):674–6.

52. Hui CH, Lam CC, Sze CS. A family of protein S deficiency including two adults with homozygous deficiency. *Thromb Haemost* 1997;**78**(3):1158–9.

53. Pung-amritt P, Poort SR, Vos HL, et al. Compound heterozygosity for one novel and one recurrent mutation in a Thai patient with severe protein S deficiency. *Thromb Haemost* 1999;**81**(2):189–92.

54. Mahasandana C, Suvatte V, Chuansumrit A, et al. Homozygous protein S deficiency in an infant with purpura fulminans. *J Pediatr* 1990;**117**(5):750–3.

55. Lane DA, Caso R. Antithrombin: structure, genomic organization, function and inherited deficiency. *Baillieres Clin Haematol* 1989;**2**(4):961–98.

56. Bjarke B, Herin P, Blomback M. Neonatal aortic thrombosis. A possible clinical manifestation of congenital antithrombin 3 deficiency. *Acta Paediatr Scand* 1974;**63**(2):297–301.

57. Winter JH, Fenech A, Ridley W, et al. Familial antithrombin III deficiency. *Q J Med* 1982;**51**(204):373–95.

58. Brenner B, Fishman A, Goldsher D, Schreibman, D. Cerebral thrombosis in a newborn with a congenital deficiency of antithrombin III. *Am J Hematol* 1988;**27**(3):209–11.

59. Peeters S, Vandenplas Y, Jochmans K, et al. Myocardial infarction in a neonate with hereditary antithrombin III deficiency. *Acta Paediatr* 1993;**82**(6–7):610–13.

60. Jochmans K., Lissens W, Vervoort R, et al. Antithrombin-Gly 424 Arg: A novel point mutation responsible for type 1 antithrombin deficiency and neonatal thrombosis. *Blood* 1994;**83**(1):146–51.

61. Newman RS, Spear GS, Kirschbaum N. Postmortem DNA diagnosis of factor V Leiden in

a neonate with systemic thrombosis and probable antithrombin deficiency. *Obstet Gynecol* 1998;**92**(4 Pt 2):702–5.

62. Swoboda V, Zervan K, Thom K, et al. Homozygous antithrombin deficiency type II causing neonatal thrombosis. *Thromb Res* 2017;**158**:134–7.

63. Chowdhury V, Lane DA, Mille B, et al. Homozygous antithrombin deficiency: Report of two new cases (99 Leu to Phe) associated with arterial and venous thrombosis. *Thromb Haemost* 1994;**72**(2):198–202.

64. Roman K, Rosenthal E, Razavi R. Pulmonary arterial thrombosis in a neonate with homozygous deficiency of antithrombin III: Successful outcome following pulmonary thrombectomy and infusions of antithrombin III concentrate. *Cardiol Young* 2000;**10**(3):275–8.

65. Shiozaki A, Arai T, Izumi R, Niiya K, Sakuragawa N. Congenital antithrombin III deficient neonate treated with antithrombin III concentrates. *Thromb Res* 1993;**70**(3):211–16.

66. Gunther G, Junker R, Sträter R, et al. Symptomatic ischemic stroke in full-term neonates: Role of acquired and genetic prothrombotic risk factors. *Stroke* 2000;**31**(10):2437–41.

67. Nowak-Gottl U, Junker R, Hartmeier M, et al. Increased lipoprotein(a) is an important risk factor for venous thromboembolism in childhood. *Circulation* 1999;**100**(7):743–8.

68. Gacio S, Munoz Giacomelli F, Klein F. Presumed perinatal ischemic stroke: A review. *Arch Argent Pediatr* 2015;**113**(5):449–55.

69. Fernandez-Lopez D, Natarajan N, Ashwal S, Vexler ZS. Mechanisms of perinatal arterial ischemic stroke. *J Cereb Blood Flow Metab* 2014;**34**(6):921–32.

70. Hunt RW, Inder TE. Perinatal and neonatal ischaemic stroke: A review. *Thromb Res* 2006;**118**(1):39–48.

71. Lynch JK, Nelson KB. Epidemiology of perinatal stroke. *Curr Opin Pediatr* 2001;**13**(6):499–505.

72. Lynch JK, Nelson KB, Curry CJ, Grether JK. Cerebrovascular disorders in children with the factor V Leiden mutation. *J Child Neurol* 2001;**16**(10):735–44.

73. Elbers J, Viero S, MacGregor D, DeVeber G, Moore AM. Placental pathology in neonatal stroke. *Pediatrics* 2011;**127**(3):e722–9.

74. Giacchetti L, De Gaudenzi M, Leoncini A, et al. Neonatal renal and inferior vena cava thrombosis associated with fetal thrombotic vasculopathy: A case report. *J Med Case Rep* 2017;**11**(1):248.

75. Estan J, Hope P. Unilateral neonatal cerebral infarction in full term infants. *Arch Dis Child Fetal Neonatal Ed* 1997;**76**(2):F88–93.

76. Venkataraman A, Kingsley PB, Kalina P, et al. Newborn brain infarction: Clinical aspects and magnetic resonance imaging. *CNS Spectr* 2004;**9**(6):436–44.

77. Lövblad KO, el-Koussy M, Guzman R, et al. Diffusion-weighted and perfusion-weighted MR of cerebral vasospasm. *Acta Neurochir Suppl* 2001;**77**:121–6.

78. Mader I, Schöning M, Klose U, Küker W. Neonatal cerebral infarction diagnosed by diffusion-weighted MRI: Pseudonormalization occurs early. *Stroke* 2002;**33**(4):1142–5.

79. Mercuri, E., Cowan F, Gupte G, et al. Prothrombotic disorders and abnormal neurodevelopmental outcome in infants with neonatal cerebral infarction. *Pediatrics* 2001;**107**(6):1400–4.

80. Greenberg R, Waldman D, Brooks C, et al. Endovascular treatment of renal artery thrombosis caused by umbilical artery catheterization. *J Vasc Surg* 1998;**28**(5):949–53.

81. Nouri S, Mahdhaoui N, Beizig S, et al. Thrombose aortique néonatale majeure: à propos d'une observation [Major neonatal aortic thrombosis: A case report]. *Arch Pediatr* 2007;**14**(9):1097–100.

82. Seibert JJ, Northington FJ, Miers JF, Taylor BJ. Aortic thrombosis after umbilical artery catheterization in neonates: prevalence of complications on long-term follow-up. *AJR Am J Roentgenol* 1991;**156**(3):567–9.

83. Barrington KJ. Umbilical artery catheters in the newborn: Effects of position of the catheter tip. *Cochrane Database Syst Rev* 2000;**2**:CD000505.

84. Barrington KJ. Umbilical artery catheters in the newborn: Effects of heparin. *Cochrane Database Syst Rev* 2000;**2**:CD000507.

85. Bhat R, Monagle P. The preterm infant with thrombosis. *Arch Dis Child Fetal Neonatal Ed* 2012;**97**(6):F423–8.

86. Sellitto M, Messina F. Central venous catheterization and thrombosis in newborns: Update on diagnosis and management. *J Matern Fetal Neonatal Med* 2012;**25**(Suppl 4):26–8.

87. Sol JJ, van de Loo M, Boerma M, et al. NEOnatal Central-venous Line Observational study on Thrombosis (NEOCLOT): Evaluation of a national guideline on management of neonatal catheter-related thrombosis. *BMC Pediatr* 2018;**18**(1):84.

88. van Elteren HA, Veldt HS, Te Pas AB, et al. Management and outcome in 32 neonates with thrombotic events. *Int J Pediatr* 2011;**2011**:217564.

89. Khilnani P, Goldstein B, Todres ID. Double lumen umbilical venous catheters in critically ill neonates: a randomized prospective study. *Crit Care Med* 1991;**19**(11):1348–51.

90. Tanke RB, van Megen R, Daniels O. Thrombus detection on central venous catheters in the neonatal intensive care unit. *Angiology* 1994;**45**(6):477–80.

91. Monagle P, Chan AKC, Goldenberg NA, et al. Antithrombotic therapy in neonates and children: Antithrombotic Therapy and Prevention of Thrombosis, 9th ed: American College of Chest Physicians Evidence-Based Clinical Practice Guidelines. *Chest* 2012;**141**(2 Suppl):e737S–801S.

92. O'Grady NP, Alexander M, Burns LA, et al. Guidelines for the prevention of intravascular catheter-related infections. *Infect Control Hosp Epidemiol* 2002;**23**(12):759–69.

93. Saxonhouse MA, Burchfield DJ. The evaluation and management of postnatal thromboses. *J Perinatol* 2009;**29**(7):467–78.

94. Andrew ME, Monagle P, deVeber G, Chan AK. Thromboembolic disease and antithrombotic therapy in newborns. *Hematology Am Soc Hematol Educ Program* 2001;358–74.

95. Ulloa-Ricardez A, Romero-Espinoza L, Estrada-Loza Mde J, González-Cabello HJ, Núñez-Enríquez JC. Risk factors for intracardiac thrombosis in the right atrium and superior vena cava in critically ill neonates who required the installation of a central venous catheter. *Pediatr Neonatol* 2016;**57**(4):288–94.

96. Hermansen MC, Hermansen MG. Intravascular catheter complications in the neonatal intensive care unit. *Clin Perinatol* 2005;**32**(1):141–56, vii.

97. Torres-Valdivieso MJ, Cobas J, Barrio C, et al. Successful use of tissue plasminogen activator in catheter-related intracardiac thrombus of a premature infant. *Am J Perinatol* 2003;**20**(2):91–6.

98. Cholette JM, Rubenstein JS, Alfieris GM, et al. Elevated risk of thrombosis in neonates undergoing initial palliative cardiac surgery. *Ann Thorac Surg* 2007;**84**(4):1320–5.

99. Fenton KN, Siewers RD, Rebovich B, Pigula FA. Interim mortality in infants with systemic-to-pulmonary artery shunts. *Ann Thorac Surg* 2003;**76**(1):152–6; discussion 156–7.

100. Bidadi B, Nageswara Rao AA, Kaur D, Khan SP, Rodriguez V. Neonatal renal vein thrombosis: Role of anticoagulation and thrombolysis. An institutional review. *Pediatr Hematol Oncol* 2016;**33**(1):59–66.

101. Lau KK, Stoffman JM, Williams S, et al. Neonatal renal vein thrombosis: Review of the English-language literature between 1992 and 2006. *Pediatrics* 2007;**120**(5):e1278–84.

102. Messinger Y, Sheaffer JW, Mrozek J, Smith CM, Sinaiko AR. Renal outcome of neonatal renal venous thrombosis: Review of 28 patients and effectiveness of fibrinolytics and heparin in 10 patients. *Pediatrics* 2006;**118**(5):e1478–84.

103. Williams S, Chan AK. Neonatal portal vein thrombosis: Diagnosis and management. *Semin Fetal Neonatal Med* 2011;**16**(6):329–39.

104. deVeber G, Andrew M, Adams C, et al. Cerebral sinovenous thrombosis in children. *N Engl J Med* 2001;**345**(6):417–23.

105. Wasay M, Dai AI, Ansari M, Shaikh Z, Roach ES. Cerebral venous sinus thrombosis in children: A multicenter cohort from the United States. *J Child Neurol* 2008;**23**(1):26–31.

106. Wu YW, Hamrick SE, Miller SP, et al. Intraventricular hemorrhage in term neonates caused by sinovenous thrombosis. *Ann Neurol* 2003;**54**(1):123–6.

107. Manco-Johnson MJ. How I treat venous thrombosis in children. *Blood* 2006;**107**(1):21–9.

108. Berfelo FJ, Kersbergen KJ, van Ommen CH, et al. Neonatal cerebral sinovenous thrombosis from symptom to outcome. *Stroke* 2010;**41**(7):1382–8.

109. Kersbergen KJ, Groenendaal F, Benders MJ, et al. The spectrum of associated brain lesions in cerebral sinovenous thrombosis: relation to gestational age and outcome. *Arch Dis Child Fetal Neonatal Ed* 2011;**96**(6):F404–9.

110. Moharir MD, Shroff M, Pontigon AM, et al. A prospective outcome study of neonatal cerebral sinovenous thrombosis. *J Child Neurol* 2011;**26**(9):1137–44.

111. Monagle P, Cuello CA, Augustine C, et al. American Society of Hematology 2018 Guidelines for management of venous thromboembolism: Treatment of pediatric venous thromboembolism. *Blood Advances* 2018;**2**(22):3291–316.

112. Bendaly EA, Batra AS, Ebenroth ES, Hurwitz RA. Outcome of cardiac thrombi in infants. *Pediatr Cardiol* 2008;**29**(1):95–101.

113. Butler-O'Hara M, Buzzard CJ, Reubens L, et al. A randomized trial comparing long-term and short-term use of umbilical venous catheters in premature infants with birth weights of less than 1251 grams. *Pediatrics* 2006;**118**(1):e25–35.

114. Kim JH, Lee YS, Kim SH, et al. Does umbilical vein catheterization lead to portal venous

thrombosis? Prospective US evaluation in 100 neonates. *Radiology* 2001;**219**(3):645–50.

115. Bacciedoni V Attie M, Donato H, Comité Nacional de Hematología, Oncología y Medicina Transfusional. Thrombosis in newborn infants. *Arch Argent Pediatr* 2016;**114**(2):159–66.

116. van der Aa NE, Benders MJ, Groenendaal F, de Vries LS. Neonatal stroke: A review of the current evidence on epidemiology, pathogenesis, diagnostics and therapeutic options. *Acta Paediatr* 2014;**103**(4):356–64.

117. Saxonhouse MA. Management of neonatal thrombosis. *Clin Perinatol* 2012;**39**(1):191–208.

118. Marks KA, Zucker N, Kapelushnik J, Karplus M, Levitas A. Infective endocarditis successfully treated in extremely low birth weight infants with recombinant tissue plasminogen activator. *Pediatrics* 2002;**109**(1):153–8.

119. Rossor T, Arichi T, Bhate S, Hart AR, Raman Singh R. Anticoagulation in the management of neonatal cerebral sinovenous thrombosis: A systematic review and meta-analysis. *Dev Med Child Neurol* 2018;**60**(9):884–891.

120. Kerlin BA, Blatt NB, Fuh B, et al. Epidemiology and risk factors for thromboembolic complications of childhood nephrotic syndrome: A Midwest Pediatric Nephrology Consortium (MWPNC) study. *J Pediatr* 2009;**155**(1):105–10, 110 e1.

121. Young G. Old and new antithrombotic drugs in neonates and infants. *Semin Fetal Neonatal Med* 2011;**16**(6):349–54.

122. Chan AK, Monagle P. Updates in thrombosis in pediatrics: Where are we after 20 years? *Hematology Am Soc Hematol Educ Program* 2012;**2012**:439–43.

123. Bounameaux H. Unfractionated versus low-molecular-weight heparin in the treatment of venous thromboembolism. *Vasc Med* 1998;**3**(1):41–6.

124. Samama MM, Gerotziafas GT. Comparative pharmacokinetics of LMWHs. *Semin Thromb Hemost* 2000;**26**(Suppl 1):31–8.

125. Malowany JI, Knoppert DC, Chan AK, Pepelassis D, Lee DS. Enoxaparin use in the neonatal intensive care unit: Experience over 8 years. *Pharmacotherapy* 2007;**27**(9):1263–71.

126. Malowany JI, Monagle P, Knoppert DC, et al. Enoxaparin for neonatal thrombosis: A call for a higher dose for neonates. *Thromb Res* 2008;**122**(6):826–30.

127. Bhatt MD, Paes BA, Chan AK. How to use unfractionated heparin to treat neonatal thrombosis in clinical practice. *Blood Coagul Fibrinolysis* 2016;**27**(6):605–14.

128. Hartmann J, Hussein A, Trowitzsch E, Becker J, Hennecke KH. Treatment of neonatal thrombus formation with recombinant tissue plasminogen activator: six years' experience and review of the literature. *Arch Dis Child Fetal Neonatal Ed* 2001;**85**(1):F18–22.

129. Wang M, Hays T, Balasa V, et al. Low-dose tissue plasminogen activator thrombolysis in children. *J Pediatr Hematol Oncol* 2003;**25**(5):379–86.

130. Zenz W, Arlt F, Sodia S, Berghold A. Intracerebral hemorrhage during fibrinolytic therapy in children: a review of the literature of the last thirty years. *Semin Thromb Hemost* 1997;**23**(3):321–32.

131. Alioglu B, Ozyurek E, Tarcan A, et al. Heterozygous methylenetetrahydrofolate reductase 677C-T gene mutation with mild hyperhomocysteinemia associated with intrauterine iliofemoral artery thrombosis. *Blood Coagul Fibrinolysis* 2006;**17**(6):495–8.

132. Boffa MC, Lachassinne E. Infant perinatal thrombosis and antiphospholipid antibodies: a review. *Lupus* 2007;**16**(8):634–41.

133. Kenet G, Nowak-Gottl U. Fetal and neonatal thrombophilia. *Obstet Gynecol Clin North Am* 2006;**33**(3):457–66.

134. Kosch A, Kuwertz-Bröking E, Heller C, et al. Renal venous thrombosis in neonates: Prothrombotic risk factors and long-term follow-up. *Blood* 2004;**104**(5):1356–60.

135. Lee J, Croen LA, Backstrand KH, et al. Maternal and infant characteristics associated with perinatal arterial stroke in the infant. *JAMA* 2005;**293**(6):723–9.

136. Nowak-Göttl U, Duering C, Kempf-Bielack B, Sträter R. Thromboembolic diseases in neonates and children. *Pathophysiol Haemost Thromb* 2003;**33**(5–6):269–74.

137. Raju TN, Nelson KB, Ferriero D, Lynch JK, NICHD-NINDS Perinatal Stroke Workshop Participants. Ischemic perinatal stroke: Summary of a workshop sponsored by the National Institute of Child Health and Human Development and the National Institute of Neurological Disorders and Stroke. *Pediatrics* 2007;**120**(3):609–16.

138. Wu YW, Lynch JK, Nelson KB. Perinatal arterial stroke: understanding mechanisms and outcomes. *Semin Neurol* 2005;**25**(4):424–34.

139. Kenet G, Lütkhoff LK, Albisetti M, et al. Impact of thrombophilia on risk of arterial ischemic stroke or cerebral sinovenous thrombosis in neonates and children: A systematic review and meta-analysis of observational studies. *Circulation* 2010;**121**(16):1838–47.

140. Rosendaal FR. Venous thrombosis: The role of genes, environment, and behavior. *Hematology Am Soc Hematol Educ Program*, 2005:1–12.

141. Marks SD, Massicotte MP, Steele BT, et al. Neonatal renal venous thrombosis: Clinical outcomes and prevalence of prothrombotic disorders. *J Pediatr* 2005;**146**(6):811–16.

142. Thornburg C, Pipe S. Neonatal thromboembolic emergencies. *Semin Fetal Neonatal Med* 2006;**11**(3):198–206.

143. Molinari AC, Banov L, Bertamino M, et al. A practical approach to the use of low molecular weight heparins in VTE treatment and prophylaxis in children and newborns. *Pediatr Hematol Oncol*, 2015;**32**(1):1–10.

144. Armstrong-Wells JM, Manco-Johnson MJ. Neonatal thrombosis. In De Alarcón PW, Werner EJ, Christensen RD, eds. *Neonatal Hematology* (New York: Cambridge University Press, 2013), p. 282.

Chapter

20

Transfusion Practices

Cyril Jacquot, Yunchuan D. Mo, and Naomi L. C. Luban

Neonatal transfusion therapy requires an understanding of the dynamic interactions of the feto-maternal unit, the physiologic changes that accompany the transition from fetus to neonate to infant, and the underlying pathophysiology of different hematologic disorders. Guidelines for neonatal transfusions remain controversial, since most have been extrapolated from evidence in adults or based on small studies in neonates with marginal statistical validity. Compared to older children and adults, neonates have small total blood volumes but high blood volume per body weight. Because of the limited capacity to expand their blood volume to compensate for their rapid growth, many sick and/or premature infants require significant blood component support, especially within the first weeks of life. Immaturity of many organ systems predisposes them to metabolic derangements from blood products and their additive solutions, and to the infectious and immunomodulatory hazards of transfusion, such as transfusion-acquired CMV (TA-CMV) infection and transfusion-associated graft versus host disease (TA-GVHD). Therefore, component modifications are often required to compensate for the infant's small blood volume, immunologic immaturity, and/or compromised organ function, and constitute the uniqueness of neonatal transfusion therapy.

Pretransfusion Testing

A sample of cord blood is often collected in all newborn infants at the time of delivery, but routine testing of cord blood for ABO group and Rh type is not necessary for healthy newborn infants unless the mother is Rh-negative and/or has a positive antibody screen [1]. For sick infants,

ABO and Rh type should be determined on samples obtained from both mother and baby. Cord blood may be used for initial testing, but should be confirmed with an infant's sample. The infant's blood group is determined from the red blood cells (RBCs) alone, since the corresponding iso-agglutinins anti-A and anti-B in the serum/plasma are usually weak or absent. Screening for atypical antibodies may be performed on maternal blood if available, or in the neonatal serum/plasma. A conventional cross-match is unnecessary if atypical antibodies are not demonstrable. Further compatibility testing during any one hospital course up to 4 months of age can be omitted for repeated small-volume transfusions since the formation of alloantibodies in the first 4 months of life is extremely rare [1]. However, this requires that the initial antibody screen is negative and all transfused RBCs are group O, Rh-negative, or ABO- and Rh-compatible. If the infant is supported with plasma and platelets, then passive acquisition of antibody may occur, and cross-matching is indicated, particularly for major surgical procedures, where large volumes of blood may be transfused [2]. If the antibody screen is positive, then serological investigation to identify the antibody is necessary. Full compatibility testing should be performed with appropriately selected blood, negative for the antigen(s) to which the antibody is directed.

Red Blood Cell Transfusions

Anemia in the neonatal period may be secondary to blood loss, hemolysis, or impaired production of RBCs. The usual postnatal decline in RBC mass that occurs in all newborns is more pronounced in preterm infants, resulting in hemoglobin levels

Neonatal Hematology, Pathogenesis, Diagnosis, and Management of Hematologic Problems, 3rd edition, ed. Pedro A. de Alarcón, Eric J. Werner, Robert D. Christensen, and Martha C. Sola-Visner. Published by Cambridge University Press. © Cambridge University Press 2021.

that drop to 8 g/dL in VLBW infants (very low birth weight, 1,000–1,500 g), and to 7 g/dl in ELBW infants (extremely low birth weight, <1,000 g), by 4 to 8 weeks of age [3]. This phenomenon, termed anemia of prematurity (AOP), is primarily due to lower hemoglobin concentrations at birth, frequent blood sampling, low total blood volume to blood sampling ratio, increased risk for other comorbidities, and a diminished erythropoietic response [4]. In sick infants requiring intensive care, frequent blood sampling for laboratory tests and blood gas monitoring results in significant iatrogenic anemia and have been correlated directly to transfusion requirements [5]. Approximately 65%–90% of VLBW infants require multiple small volume RBC transfusions [6]. Controlling for the degree of prematurity and severity of illness, there is considerable variation in transfusion practice in different centers, which significantly impacts the number and volume of RBCs transfused. This indicates a large discretionary element in the utilization of RBC transfusions, and is not surprising given the paucity of convincing evidence based data to guide clinicians [7, 8].

The definition of "nonphysiologic" versus "physiologic" anemia in preterm neonates, and the hemoglobin levels at which to transfuse, is fraught with controversy. Tissue oxygen delivery is determined not only by the hemoglobin concentration but also by the proportion of fetal to adult hemoglobin, level of RBC 2,3-diphosphoglycerate (2,3-DPG), cardiac output, and arterial oxygen tension [3, 9]. Tachypnea, periodic breathing or apnea, tachycardia, poor feeding, poor growth, decreased activity, and anaerobic metabolism resulting in lactic acidosis all are considered to be indicators of significant anemia. However, many of these symptoms, signs, and tests are nonspecific and do not correlate well to hemoglobin levels or respond consistently to RBC transfusions [10]. Attempts to identify accurate indicators of peripheral oxygen delivery through the use of nonradioactive measures of circulating blood volume, and near-infrared spectroscopy to measure fractional oxygen extraction have had variable results. Neither method has proven to be an accurate predictor of transfusion, based at least in part on study design and technical aspects of the devices used [11, 12].

Risks of Transfusion Therapy

Advances in donor recruitment, blood screening, and processing have decreased the risks associated with blood transfusion. As part of patient blood management, current transfusion considerations and guidelines focus on reducing both transfusion number and donor exposures. Nevertheless, hematologic, immunologic, infectious, cardiovascular, and metabolic complications can occur. Many of these risks exist for transfusion recipients of any age, whereas others pose a greater threat to the neonatal recipient. These potential risks affect the choice and processing of blood products. Parents must be advised of the risks, benefits, and alternatives to transfusion, and informed consent should be documented in the medical record along with the indications for, and results of, the prescribed transfusion.

Indications

Many guidelines have been published regarding indications for RBC transfusion based on expert opinion from clinical experience rather than on actual statistically powered randomized controlled trials. Therefore, transfusion thresholds remain controversial because there are few studies which address the appropriateness of these transfusion triggers in neonates. Current guidelines for replacement transfusion therapy in neonates are given in Table 20.1 [2, 4]. Infants with significant cardiopulmonary disease generally require more aggressive RBC transfusion support, whereas infants receiving minimal cardiopulmonary

Table 20.1 Guidelines for red blood cell replacement for neonates

Clinical status	Target hematocrit
For severe cardiopulmonary disease (requiring mechanical ventilation with FiO2 >0.35)	>40%–45%
For moderate cardiopulmonary disease	>30%–35%
For major surgery	>30%–35%
For infants with stable anemia with unexplained apnea/bradycardia, tachycardia, or poor growth	>20%–25%

Notes: Modified from: references [6, 13]. Definitions for level of severity of cardiopulmonary disease may be defined individually by institution.

support, with acceptable weight gain, and with minimal episodes of apnea and bradycardia, require less aggressive support [4, 6, 13]. Some have advocated the use of absolute reticulocyte counts in stable, growing infants with anemia of prematurity, proposing that an absolute reticulocyte count of $>75–100 \times 10^3/\mu L$ is a reliable predictor of a future rise in hemoglobin (Hb), and that RBC transfusion can be avoided in the absence of clinical signs of anemia and significant iatrogenic blood loss [6].

Restrictive versus Liberal RBC Transfusion Thresholds

Two studies attempted to address high versus low threshold transfusion guidelines based on level of respiratory support in ELBW and VLBW infants. Although very different in design and outcome, neither study clearly established an appropriate hemoglobin target. While the multi-institutional Canadian Premature Infants in Need of Transfusion (PINT) study demonstrated no advantage for liberal transfusion practices [14], the Bell study from Iowa suggested that restrictive transfusion was associated with more apneic episodes, intraparenchymal brain hemorrhage, and periventricular leukomalacia [15]. The discrepant results may be due to a greater Hb difference in restrictive/liberal transfusion groups (2.7 gm/dL versus 1.1 gm/dL), and a higher overall Hb value in the liberal transfusion group in the Bell study compared to the PINT study.

In contrast to short-term effects, long-term (average 12 years of age) neurodevelopmental measurements in the Bell study cohort showed reduced brain volumes for neonates transfused using liberal guidelines [16]. Meanwhile, previously enrolled ELBW infants from the PINT study were followed up at 18 to 21 months' corrected age. Although liberal transfusion practices did not result in a statistically significant difference in death or the presence of cerebral palsy, severe cognitive delay (mental development index score [MDIC] <70), or severe visual or hearing impairment, post-hoc analysis with cognitive delay redefined (MDIC <85) showed a significant difference favoring the liberal threshold group [17].

More recently, a meta-analysis published in 2016 did not identify statistically significant differences in a range of harmful outcomes between neonates exposed to restrictive and liberal RBC transfusion practice [18]. It has been argued that a more liberal approach to RBC transfusion may be warranted, due to the decreasing infectious risks of RBC transfusions, the ability to decrease donor exposures using repeat RBC transfusions from the same donor, and the possible neuroprotective advantage of more liberal RBC transfusion practices. Further studies are needed to guide decisions for RBC transfusion support, given the unclear short- and long-term benefits and risks of liberal transfusion practices. The NICHD sponsored Transfusion of Premature (TOP) trial (NCT01702805) will determine whether higher hemoglobin thresholds for ELBW patients will result in improved neurodevelopmental outcomes.

RBC Preparations

RBCs are stored in one of several anticoagulant-preservative (AP) solutions to improve red cell viability and to extend storage time. All AP solutions contain citrate, phosphate, and dextrose (CPD), which function as an anticoagulant, a buffer and a source of RBC metabolic energy, respectively. The addition of mannitol and adenine to existing additive solutions has increased the shelf life of RBCs from 21 days (CPD) to 35 days (CPDA-1) and to 42 days for extended-storage AP solutions (Adsol® [AS-1], Nutricel® [AS-3], Optisol® [AS-5]) by stabilizing the RBC membrane and maintaining 2,3-DPG and adenosine triphoshate (ATP) within erythrocytes. RBC units collected in citrate–phosphate–dextrose-adenine (CPDA-1) usually have a hematocrit (Hct) of approximately 70%, whereas RBCs in newer extended-storage AP solutions have a Hct of 60% or less. Studies have shown that extended-storage preservative solutions are safe, and as efficacious as CPDA-1 RBCs in increasing the Hct in neonates receiving small-volume transfusions (10–15 mL/kg) [19–21]. However, there are no clinical studies that have confirmed or refuted the effect of an AP on metabolic abnormalities in massive transfusion (>20 mL/kg) for the neonate. Of particular concern is the potential for adenine-induced nephrotoxicity [20] and intolerable fluid shifts secondary to the diuretic effects of mannitol (present in AS-1, AS-5, and AS-7 but not AS-3) [19] in neonatal patients with limited blood volumes [2]. Therefore, some experts recommend avoiding RBCs stored in extended-storage media

(AS-1, AS-3, AS-5) for large-volume transfusions until such data have been published.

All blood components must be filtered before transfusion. The standard 120–170 μm pore-size filter is adequate for red cells, plasma, and platelets. Microaggregate filters (10–20 μm pore size) can screen out 20–120 μm particles, which include clumped platelets, fibrin, and nonviable granulocytes that accumulate during storage. These filters are unnecessary when components undergo prestorage leukodepletion, which is recommended for recipients at risk for transfusion transmitted cytomegalovirus (TT-CMV) (see the subsection Cytomegalovirus under the section on Transfusion-Transmitted Infections on p. XXX). In addition to reducing the risk of TT-CMV, leukoreduction has dramatically decreased the incidence of febrile non-hemolytic transfusion reactions (FNHTRs) in RBC and PLT transfusions since being implemented, from 10% to approximately 0.1%–3% (0.2% for prestorage leukoreduction) [22, 23]. Leukocyte reduction has also been proven to reduce the incidence of HLA alloimmunization in adults [24].

Dose and Administration

There is little information on the optimal volume of RBCs to be transfused to correct anemia; however, most infants are transfused 10–15 mL/kg, depending upon their cardiovascular status. One small study indicated that transfusion of 20 mL/kg of packed red blood cells (PRBCs) results in a significantly greater rise in hematocrit in VLBW infants, as compared with transfusion of 10 ml/kg, without detrimental effects on pulmonary function, vital signs, or serum potassium; however, all infants in this study received furosemide immediately following transfusion [25]. Conclusions on the safety of transfusing 20 mL/kg RBCs has not yet been established. Formulae used to calculate volumes for transfusions are provided in Table 20.2.

Warming small-volume RBC aliquots before transfusion is not necessary, particularly if the transfusion is given slowly over 2 to 3 hours. However, hypothermia can develop after massive transfusion unless the RBCs are first warmed. Controlled blood warming devices should be used for large-volume transfusions, particularly exchange and intra-operative transfusions. Blood components dispensed in syringes cannot be warmed in water baths because of the risk of contamination, but they may be warmed adequately when placed in warm-air incubators for 30 minutes before transfusion [2, 26]. Overheating, with resultant hemolysis, may occur when syringe aliquots are placed under radiant warmers or phototherapy lights [26].

Table 20.2 Formulae for transfusion of red cell products

I. Estimated blood volumes
- Fetus ≈ 140 mL/kg (or 0.14 mL/g)
- Preterm ≈ 100–120 mL/kg
- Full-term ≈ 80–85 mL/kg
- Adult ≈ 70–75 mL/kg

II. Calculation of volume of packed RBC transfusion
- PRBC volume $= EBV \times \frac{(\text{Hct desired} - \text{Hct observed})}{\text{Hct of packed red cell unit}}$.

III. Calculation for exchange transfusion
- 2-volume exchange volume (preterm) = 100 mL/kg × 2, or 200 mL/kg
- 2-volume exchange volume (term) = 85 mL/kg × 2, or 170 mL/kg

III. Calculations for partial exchange transfusion
Polycythemia
- Exchange volume (mL) $= EBV \times \frac{(\text{Observed Hct} - \text{Desired Hct})}{\text{Observed Hct}}$.

  Example: 1 kg preterm infant with Hct 68%, desired post partial exchange Hct 55%:
  Volume of exchange (mL) = 100 × (68 − 55)/68 = ~20 ml of crystalloid exchanged with WB.

Severe anemia
- Exchange volume (mL) $= EBV \times \frac{(\text{desired Hct} - \text{observed Hct})}{(\text{Hct of unit} * - \text{observed Hct})}$.

  Example: 1 kg preterm infant with Hct 21%, desired post-Hct 45%:
  Volume of exchange (mL) = 100 × (45 − 21)/(70* − 21) = ~49 mL of CPDA RBCs exchanged with WB.

*(CPDA-1RBCs Hct ~70%: whole blood withdrawn is replaced with packed RBCs.)

When phototherapy is in progress, the blood component and tubing should be shielded from the UV light by using aluminum foil to prevent overheating and hemolysis. At the other extreme, freezing and lysis may occur if RBC products are stored in unmonitored refrigerators or freezers.

Whole-Blood Transfusion

A whole-blood (WB) unit contains approximately 450–500 mL of blood and 70 mL of AP solution. The shelf life of WB depends on the AP solution in which it is stored (i.e., 35 days in CPDA-1; 42 days in extended-storage media). Whole blood stored longer than 48 hours does not contain functional platelets or granulocytes, and coagulation factors (especially V and VIII) decrease throughout storage. Many blood centers rarely collect WB for allogeneic use because reconstituted WB, prepared by combining a unit of RBCs with an appropriate volume of compatible fresh frozen plasma (FFP), can be used for the same clinical effect. Whole blood or reconstituted WB is the product of choice in the setting of massive transfusion or acute blood loss, where restoration of oxygen-carrying capacity and blood volume are needed simultaneously. Primary indications for WB or reconstituted RB use in neonates include resuscitation of patients with acute blood loss in excess of 25% of their total blood volume (TBV) (i.e., ruptured vasa previa) [27], exchange transfusions, cardiopulmonary bypass, extracorporeal membrane oxygenation (ECMO), and continuous hemofiltration [28]. There is little advantage of WB in the emergency setting for the acute resuscitation of the neonate over packed RBCs and crystalloid or colloid solutions since other blood components replete in hemostatic elements may need to be subsequently transfused. When reconstituted WB is needed for large volume transfusion procedures, the neonate may be given plasma that is ABO compatible with the neonate's RBCs, but RBCs that are compatible with maternal serum. This may mean that the ABO group of the RBC and plasma units may be different. An alternative used by some transfusion centers entails the use of low isohemagglutinin titer, group-O, Rh compatible WB, if available [4]. This decreases the risk of hemolysis in non-O patients transfused with the WB. The most recent AABB Standards set guidelines on the use of such low-titer WB [1].

The use of fresh WB (<48 hours old) to either prime the cardiopulmonary bypass (CPB) circuit and/or meet postoperative transfusion requirements have had conflicting results reported in randomized controlled trials. Transfusion of fresh WB has previously been associated with significantly less postoperative blood loss compared with the transfusion of multiple blood components separately following bypass surgery for complex congenital heart disease in children less than 2 years of age. This has been attributed to better platelet function in fresh WB, as measured by 30 minute and 3 hour postoperative platelet aggregation responses to ADP and epinephrine [29]. Friesen et al. also showed that the collection of fresh autologous WB (replacing with 5% albumin) prior to heparinization and reinfusion following CPB was associated with greater improvement of coagulation status after CPB in infants (>1 month old) with non-cyanotic heart disease undergoing non-complex open heart surgery [30]. It is difficult to generalize the benefit in all infants because the CPB circuit was primed with a crystalloid solution, and cyanotic or complex patients may not tolerate the anemia and potential hemodynamic changes prior to CPB caused by this technique [30]. A subsequent prospective trial compared fresh WB to reconstituted WB for priming the CPB circuit in children <1 year of age ($n = 200$) undergoing open-heart surgery and found contrasting results. Infants who received reconstituted WB had a shorter stay in the intensive care unit than those who received fresh WB. There was no difference between the two groups in: early postoperative chest-tube output, transfusion requirements, levels of serum mediators of inflammation, or cardiac troponin I levels [31]. Unfortunately, there was no report of the age of the RBCs reported for the group who received reconstituted WB, making it difficult to attribute their findings to the age of RBCs used. Most recently, Gruenwald et al. prospectively compared the use of reconstituted *fresh* WB (RFWB), defined as <48 hours, versus standard blood component therapy (*stored* components used for reconstitution) both during CPB and within the first 24 hours postoperatively ($n = 64$) [32]. Lower chest tube loss in the first 24 hours postoperatively, shorter ventilation times, shorter hospital stay, and lower inotropic scores were reported for those neonates receiving RFWB versus those receiving standard blood component therapy [32].

Nonetheless, there currently exists no consensus within the United States on the use of fresh WB or RFWB for CPB pump priming or postoperative transfusion support in neonates with congenital heart disease. Decisions are often made by individual institutions based on inventory, the overall activity of cardiothoracic service, and the complexity of the patients treated. It should be noted that fresh WB (<48 hours old) is not universally available.

Donor Exposure

In the 1980s, 80%–90% of VLBW infants received multiple transfusions, often from different donors [33, 34]. Over the past two decades, a concerted effort to minimize the potential risks of transfusions by reducing the number of transfusions and donor exposures has been made through improvements in clinical care, decrease in laboratory blood draw volumes, noninvasive monitoring techniques, and the adoption of conservative transfusion guidelines. Using these methods, one tertiary-level nursery reported decreases in both the percentage of VLBW infants transfused, and number of RBC transfusions/VLBW infant from 88% to 65% and from 7.0 to 4.9 respectively [6].

Several studies have documented the safety of using RBCs stored in extended storage AP solutions until the expiration date of 35–42 days [35–37]. One or two preterm infants for whom multiple RBC transfusions are anticipated are assigned to dedicated units of freshly collected RBCs. Small aliquots are obtained repeatedly from the dedicated unit(s), using sterile connecting devices to transfer the RBCs into a separate bag, without compromising the integrity of the primary storage bag [38]. A closed-system filter-syringe set may alternatively be used in place of a transfer bag [39]. Previous studies have shown a 64% reduction in donor exposures in VLBW infants who received RBCs through a dedicated single-donor system [35]. Furthermore, multiple prospective studies have also shown that CPDA-1 and AS-3-preserved single-donor split RBC packs are safe for use in neonatal small-volume transfusions after 35 days and 42 days of storage respectively. No clinically significant changes in post-transfusion pH, ionized calcium, and potassium levels, and comparable hematocrit increments to fresh and or washed RBC products were demonstrated [35, 40, 41]. Many limited-donor

programs report the reduction of donor exposures to approximately 2.0 per VLBW infant, with those neonates born before 28 weeks' gestation and those between 28 and 31 weeks with IUGR at highest risk of needing more than one donor [42]. To minimize blood waste without compromising the goal of limiting donor exposure, many have devised models to predict each infant's transfusion requirements, whereby those infants predicted to have high transfusion requirements are assigned to receive blood from a dedicated RBC unit, while other infants are assigned to receive blood from a unit that is shared among as many as four similar infants [43].

One prospective study has been conducted in premature infants to evaluate whether fresh RBCs (≤7 days) decreased morbidity and mortality in VLBW infants compared with standard RBCs. In the Age of Red Blood Cells in Premature Infants (ARIPI) trial conducted in Canada, 188 infants provided with fresh RBC transfusions (mean age of transfused RBCs 5.1 days, SD 2.0 days) did not demonstrate an improvement in a composite outcome measure of major neonatal morbidities (necrotizing enterocolitis [NEC], intraventricular hemorrhage [IVH], bronchopulmonary dysplasia [BPD], and retinopathy of prematurity [ROP]) or death at 30 and 90 days compared with the 189 infants who received standard RBC products (mean age of transfused RBCs 14.6 days, SD 8.3 days) despite having 60% more donor exposures [44]. Although an unblinded randomized control trial suggested an advantage in clinical outcomes in neonates with congenital heart disease receiving reconstituted fresh WB defined as less than 48 hours old when dispensed for cardiopulmonary bypass pump priming and postoperative transfusion support [32], the role of fresh RBCs for routine transfusion support in premature infants has not shown a clear benefit. ARIPI has subsequently been criticized for insufficient separation of mean RBC storage time between its two cohorts (<2 weeks) and for inadequately addressing the issue of storage lesion in the oldest additive solution units (35–42 days). The use of a relatively liberal transfusion strategy may also have contributed to better clinical outcomes than would be expected with restrictive practices [45]. Although the saline–adenine–glucose–mannitol (SAGM) additive solution used in the study is widely available in Canada and Europe, its restricted distribution in other regions may limit the relevance of its conclusions in countries like the United States where other types of additive solutions are utilized. However, based on the results of this and other recent randomized clinical trials in older children and adults such as ABLE [46], RECESS [47], TOTAL [48], and INFORM [49], recent guidelines for neonatal transfusion do not recommend limiting the age of transfused RBCs to <10 days [50, 51].

Directed (Including Parental) Donor Transfusions

Directed donations from first- and second-degree relatives rather than from voluntary blood donors are perceived by the lay public to have a lower risk of transmitting viral infections, although there are no scientific data to support this contention. One study showed that although biological parents were interested in donating for their infants, many were found to be ineligible for serological and medical reasons. However, those eligible were able to supply all small-volume RBC transfusions for their infants using a single-donor system in which RBCs were stored in AS-3 for 42 days or less [52, 53]. A retrospective review at a pediatric institution found that parental donors had higher rates of infectious disease testing positivity than community donors [54].

The transfusion of blood from biologic parents poses unique immunologic and serologic risks to the neonate. TA-GVHD is a well-recognized complication of the use of familial blood, therefore all blood components obtained from blood relatives should be irradiated before transfusion. Maternal plasma may contain antibodies directed against paternal red cell, leukocyte, and platelet antigens that are also expressed on neonatal cells. Anti-leukocyte and anti-platelet antibodies have been found in 16% and 12% of mothers, respectively [55]. Exposing the infant to these antibodies within maternal blood components can potentially result in hemolysis, thrombocytopenia, or transfusion-related acute lung injury (TRALI). Therefore, maternal RBCs and platelets should be washed or plasma-reduced prior to transfusion. Conversely, paternal blood products are a poor choice in neonates with immune mediated hemolysis (hemolytic disease of the fetus and newborn, or HDFN) or neonatal alloimmune thrombocytopenia (NAIT) because the transfused paternal cells express the antigens to which the neonate has passively acquired antibodies from the mother. Therefore, fathers and paternal blood relatives should not serve as donors for blood components containing cellular elements unless maternal serum is shown to lack lymphocytotoxic antibodies [4, 52].

Given these concerns, when parental-directed donation is considered for an infant, the following recommendation should be reviewed with families and the provider [56]:

- All parental cellular blood components must be irradiated before transfusion to the neonate to prevent TA-GVHD.
- If maternal RBCs or platelets are transfused, they should be given as washed cells or should be plasma reduced and irradiated.
- Fathers are not recommended as RBC donors for their newborns.
- Fathers should not donate granulocytes or platelets to their infants unless maternal serum is shown to lack lymphocytotoxic antibodies.

Recombinant Erythropoietin

Despite the fact that over 30 clinical studies have been performed to evaluate the efficacy and safety of recombinant human erythropoietin (rHuEpo) in neonates, there currently exists no clear consensus as to whether its use minimizes the need for blood transfusions without risk to the neonate. Reasons for the lack of consensus are multifactorial, including limitations in study designs; variation in infant demographics, transfusion practices, supportive care, and blood sampling techniques between studies, and the difficulty assessing the clinical impact of results [57].

Early randomized controlled trials demonstrated that most VLBW infants given rHuEPO received fewer and lower-volume RBC transfusion during the study period, with maximum benefit being seen in larger, more stable preterm infants [58–60]; however, conflicting results were reported for rHuEPO benefit in ELBW infants [61, 62]. Early (<8 days of age) and late (≥8 days of age) rHuEPO treatment protocols subsequently were designed to prevent and treat AOP respectively, by decreasing RBC transfusions. Although both regimens have been shown to reduce RBC transfusion, it remains uncertain whether the absolute reduction in transfusion volume achieved is clinically significant without preventing or decreasing donor exposures, in an era of single-donor, dedicated RBC unit transfusion practices [63].

The Cochrane Collaboration carried out three systematic reviews on the use of rHuEPO in neonates [64–66]. Their meta-analyses of both early and late rHuEPO use showed no clear benefit in terms of significantly decreasing donor exposures, nor was there any effect on incidence of comorbidities. Although the number and volume of RBC transfusions per infant were decreased, the clinical impact of these results was trivial (i.e., <1 transfusion/infant, 7 mL/kg of RBCs respectively in late rHuEPO-exposed infants) [64]. RBC transfusion was not avoided in early or late rHuEPO-exposed infants, when RBCs transfused prior to study entry were considered. Furthermore, a statistically significant increased risk of ROP (> grade 3) was noted in neonates who received early rHuEPO therapy [66]. rHuEPO alone exerts only modest effects on transfusion burden, and so therefore should be used cautiously in light of the risk of ROP. Its role for reducing transfusions in preterm infants in conjunction with methods to reduce iatrogenic blood loss, conservative transfusion practices, and autologous transfusion, remains to be determined. The role of rHuEPO as a neuroprotectant has been investigated by several groups; secondary analyses of these studies for transfusion may prove the additional information that will support its use in infant patient blood management [67].

Autologous Transfusion

Autologous transfusion in an infant can occur by collection, storage, and re-infusion of autologous cord blood (ACB) or by delaying cord clamping [68]. The placenta contains 75–125 ml of blood at birth depending on the gestational age of the infant. This serves as a substantial volume of fetal blood, and could be an ideal source for autologous RBCs for the neonate, eliminating the potential risks of transfusion transmitted diseases and TA-GVHD. However, high rates of bacterial contamination (15.8%) [69] and small collection volumes from infants less than 1,000 g have raised concerns as to whether such preparations are beneficial in ensuring safe care to neonates.

More recently, lower rates of bacterial contamination in stored ACB units (no contamination from ACB units derived from cesarean deliveries), acceptable volume yields, equivalent efficacy/safety of ACB-derived RBCs to allogeneic RBCs, and significant reduction of neonates with birth weight between 1,000 g and 2,500 g requiring allogeneic RBCs have increased interest in this blood product [70, 71]. Nonetheless, protocols for ensuring proper collection without bacterial contamination and adequate anticoagulation are still being refined; additional large, randomized controlled trials are needed to validate the safety, efficacy, and usefulness of this process [72, 73].

Delayed umbilical cord clamping (30 to 120 seconds) of premature infants has been reported as a successful variation on autologous transfusion. This simple maneuver has been shown to significantly increase RBC mass and circulating blood volume during the first 24 hours of life, while decreasing the immediate need of blood transfusions and the incidence of intraventricular hemorrhage in the preterm infant [74–76].

One limitation with delayed cord clamping is the required delay of 30 seconds or more in neonatal resuscitation during a VLBW delivery. As an alternative, "milking" or "stripping" the cord has been proposed. This is done by holding the placental end of the umbilical cord, and gently moving blood within the umbilical vessels toward the neonate. This "stripping" is performed one to four times prior to clamping and cutting the cord. In a randomized controlled trial of 40 VLBW infants (stripping versus immediate clamping), Hosono et al. reported that those infants in the stripped group had higher hemoglobin values and blood pressures at NICU admission, shorter duration of ventilation, lower odds of requiring a RBC transfusion, and lower odds of developing an IVH [77]. Subsequently, Rabe et al. compared delayed cord clamping versus cord stripping in a randomized trial ($n = 58$) and found no differences between the two groups in hemoglobin values, number of RBC transfusions, or morbidities [78]. A Cochrane review in 2012 showed that delayed cord clamping up to 180 seconds or umbilical cord milking versus immediate cord clamping resulted in 39% fewer transfusions for anemia, 41% fewer patients with IVH and 38% fewer patients with NEC [79, 80]. Similarly, a randomized clinical trial in 2017 found that delayed cord clamping reduced anemia at 8 and 12 months in infants at high risk for iron deficiency [81]. The American College of Obstetricians and Gynecologists currently recommends a delay in umbilical cord clamping in vigorous term and preterm infants for at least 30–60 seconds after birth [82].

Exchange Transfusion

Neonatal exchange transfusion is the replacement of the majority of RBC mass and plasma with compatible RBCs and plasma from one or more donors. The amount of blood exchanged generally is expressed in relation to the recipient's blood volume (e.g., as a single or double-volume exchange, or a partial exchange).

Indications

The majority of exchange transfusions are performed for the treatment of hemolytic disease of the fetus and newborn (HDFN). Exchange transfusion procedures are frequently used in newborns with severe hyperbilirubinemia from other causes in order to prevent kernicterus and other toxicity [2]. Although not tested in RCTs, the procedure has also been used successfully, albeit infrequently, to remove exogenous (drugs) or endogenous (metabolic) toxins [83, 84], treat severe autoimmune hemolytic anemia [85, 86], correct life-threatening hyperkalemia [87, 88], and to treat neonatal sepsis unresponsive to other therapy [89].

When performed for HDFN, exchange transfusions correct anemia, replace the infant's antibody coated RBCs with antigen-negative RBCs, remove free maternal antibody in the plasma, and decrease bilirubin levels. The American Academy of Pediatrics has established exchange therapy criteria for infants of ≥35 weeks' gestation based on a nomogram incorporating post-natal age and total serum bilirubin (TSB) levels. Prematurity, hypoxemia, acidosis, hypothermia, and sepsis predispose to kernicterus at lower levels of bilirubin, and prompt earlier intervention.

A number of studies have been published on the use of intravenous immunoglobulin (IVIg, 0.5–1 gm/kg) as adjuvant treatment for Rhesus and ABO HDFN, and have demonstrated a reduction in the duration of phototherapy and the need for exchange transfusion [90–92]. The most recent Cochrane Collaboration meta-analysis, which included 658 infants in 9 studies, affirmed that IVIg administration can significantly reduce the need for exchange transfusion in term infants with Rhesus and ABO HDFN, although the authors could not provide even a weak recommendation for the use of IVIg based on the lack of demonstrable benefit in the least biased studies and overall low quality of the evidence [93]. However, in light of the potential for serious adverse outcomes in 5% of infants following exchange therapy, IVIg may be considered when serum bilirubin levels continue to rise despite aggressive phototherapy or when the bilirubin level is within 2–3 mg/dL of the exchange level [94].

The efficiency of exchange transfusion diminishes exponentially as the procedure continues. For this reason, a double-volume exchange is preferred for most procedures, as little is gained by exceeding two blood volumes. The kinetics of exchange are very similar, regardless of whether a continuous (simultaneous withdrawal and replacement) or discontinuous technique (alternating withdrawal and replacement) is used. The effectiveness of exchange transfusion varies with the component being removed, and is highest for RBCs. A double-volume exchange transfusion results in removal of approximately 85% of the neonate's RBCs but only 25%–45% of bilirubin and/or maternal alloantibody. This is because of a slowly equilibrating tissue-bound pool for bilirubin, antibody, and similar substances. Repeat exchange transfusions are often needed in infants with severe HDFN because of rebound of bilirubin following the initial procedure, resulting from persistent maternal antibody destruction of sensitized infant RBCs and equilibration of extravascular and intravascular bilirubin. The use of albumin before exchange transfusion in an effort to mobilize tissue bilirubin has not been definitively demonstrated to improve efficiency of bilirubin removal [95].

Component Preparation

Either stored WB if available or reconstituted WB can be used for neonatal exchange transfusions. RBCs chosen for the exchange should be fresh (preferably < 7 days). If available, CPDA-1 units may be preferentially selected over additive solution units because the safety of extended storage media has not been amply studied for neonatal large-volume transfusions. If only older CPDA units or additive solution units are available, the RBC units may be volume reduced or washed. All components should be CMV risk reduced, irradiated, and sickle-negative, with final hematocrit of 40%–50% [4]. If the delivery of an infant with severe HDFN is anticipated, then group O Rh-negative blood cross-matched against the mother's plasma may be prepared prior to birth. Blood prepared after delivery should be negative for the implicated antigen(s) and may be cross-matched against a maternal or neonatal sample. In ABO HDFN, the blood must be group O and Rh-compatible between mother and infant. If group O whole blood is selected, the products should have a low isoagglutinin titer. Group O RBCs are often reconstituted with AB plasma to ensure that no isoagglutinins are present, although this practice results in two donor exposures per exchange transfusion. Blood prepared for exchange transfusion for nonimmune indications such as nonimmune hyperbilirubinemia, drug overdose, and sepsis, are cross-matched against the infant only.

Administration

The volume needed for administering a double-volume exchange can be calculated using the formula in Table 20.2. The blood is warmed through a temperature-controlled in-line blood warmer, and the exchange transfusion is either performed by the traditional push–pull method using a single vascular access (typically the umbilical vein), or by isovolumetric techniques utilizing two access sites for simultaneous removal of the infant's blood and administration of replacement blood products [96]. Aliquots of 5–20 mL with a maximum of 5 mL/kg are withdrawn or infused in the discontinuous method, at a rate not exceeding 5 mL/kg every 3 minutes to avoid rapid fluctuations in intracranial pressure [97]. When an isovolumetric exchange is being done, volumes to be removed/reinfused should not exceed 2 mL/kg per minute. The duration of the exchange is usually 1 to 2 hours.

Complications

Potential complications of exchange transfusion include hypocalcemia, hyper- and hypoglycemia, hyperkalemia, dilutional thrombocytopenia and coagulopathy, umbilical vein/artery thrombosis, NEC, and infection. Previous estimates on the risk of death or permanent serious sequelae were relatively high for neonates, particularly those who were premature and/or those with underlying illnesses. In a retrospective study examining adverse events among 106 neonates undergoing 140 exchange transfusions performed between 1980 and 1995, overall mortality was 2%, and 8% in those infants classified as "ill." Death or serious complications were noted in 12% of sick neonates, but less than 1% for healthy infants (defined as only having hyperbilirubinemia) [89].

More recent reviews show fewer serious complications. A recent retrospective review of 55 neonates undergoing 66 exchange transfusions between 1992 and 2002, reported the majority of adverse events were asymptomatic laboratory abnormalities, including thrombocytopenia (44%), hypocalcemia (29%), and metabolic acidosis (24%) [98]. Adverse events were more frequent in exchanges performed on preterm infants with gestational age < 32 weeks or infants with other significant comorbidities, and when umbilical catheters were used versus other methods of central venous access. There was a single death reported in a severely ill infant; however, it was unclear if this was directly related to exchange transfusion [98]. These improved rates of serious adverse events have been confirmed in other reports [99]. Considering the declining rate of exchange transfusions in the 21st century, current mortality rates range from 0.3% in term neonates up to 10% in preterm neonates [100, 101]. Regardless, the potential risk of adverse events from exchange transfusion needs to be balanced against the risk of bilirubin encephalopathy in ill infants.

Partial Exchange Transfusion

Partial exchange transfusion (PET) is used to correct severe anemia without the risk of fluid overload and heart failure in critically ill hydropic infants, but is more commonly used to decrease the Hct in neonates with polycythemia-hyperviscosity syndrome. This syndrome is diagnosed in infants with a Hct above 65%–70% and with symptoms attributed to polycythemia, which include hypoglycemia, tachypnea, congestive heart failure, hypotonia, tremors, seizures, renal insufficiency, and/or NEC [102]. Reducing the Hct to approximately 55% causes rapid amelioration of the clinical manifestations of polycythemia and is associated with reversal of cerebral blood-flow abnormalities in symptomatic infants. The long-term benefit of early PET for neonatal poly-cythemia is questionable. In a long-term follow up study of 93 polycythemic infants randomized to receive either PET or supportive care, fewer neu-rologic abnormalities and fine-motor delays were noted at 2 years, but only limited benefits were seen at 7 years for the infants who received PET [103, 104]. Common indications include a Hct ≥70%, or a Hct between 65% and 70% in a symptomatic infant. Use of isotonic crystalloid replacement solutions through peripheral vessels rather than the umbilical vein is preferred in most instances because it has been found to be as effec-tive as 5% albumin and plasma for replacement [105]. The technique of partial exchange transfu-sion is similar to that used in larger volume exchange [106]. Exchange volume calculations are listed in Table 20.2. More recent publications have focused on continuous exchange as an alter-native to the traditional push–pull methods [107].

Intrauterine Fetal Transfusion

Intrauterine transfusion (IUT) has been used for the correction of critical anemia resulting from HDFN, fetal parvovirus B19 infection, twin-to-twin transfusion, fetomaternal hemorrhage, and homozygous alpha-thalassemia. Fetal transfu-sions may be administered by intraperitoneal, or intravascular via cordocentesis or intrahepatic venous puncture [108, 109]. Intraperitoneal trans-fusion (IPT) has been largely replaced by direct intravascular transfusion (IVT), since IVT cir-cumvents the problem of poor absorption of RBCs from the peritoneal cavity of severely hydropic fetuses, and also allows precise diagnos-tic evaluation of the fetal status by means of fetal blood sampling. IPT may be necessary when intravascular access is difficult, due to narrow umbilical vessels (gestational age, GA <20 weeks) or increased fetal size. Furthermore, IPT can also be used in conjunction with IVT to prolong the interval between procedures and produce a more stable fetal Hct [108, 109]. A recent study indi-cates that IVIg may be an effective non-invasive alternative to IUT prior to 20 weeks' gestation [110].

Intrauterine transfusions are generally per-formed when the fetal middle cerebral artery peak systolic velocity (MCA-PSV) exceeds 1.5 multiples of the median (MoM) for gestational age or there is evidence of hydrops suggestive of moderate to severe anemia [111]. The usual trans-fusion goal is a fetal Hct of 40%–45%, not to exceed a fourfold increase in Hct so as to avoid acute changes in blood viscosity [4]. Hct levels fall by approximately 1% per day, but can decrease more rapidly in fetuses with severe HDFN. This necessitates repeat transfusion every 21–28 days or more frequently (i.e., 7–14 days) for fetuses with more brisk hemolysis until suppression of fetal erythropoiesis occurs [112]. Overall survival for hydropic fetuses undergoing IUTs is approxi-mately 78%–90%, with more severely hydropic fetuses having lower survival rates (55%) [113]. The perinatal loss rate is approximately 1%–3%. Risk factors associated with procedure-related fetal death include very low pretransfusion fetal Hct, large increases in post-transfusion Hct (> fourfold), increases in umbilical venous pres-sure during IUT, umbilical arterial puncture, and transamniotic cord needling [113–115]. Fresh (<7 days) CPD(A), CMV risk-reduced, irradiated blood is recommended for all IUTs. Older CPD(A) units or extended storage RBC units may be volume reduced or washed prior to use. The blood should be cross-match compatible with maternal serum, and antigen-negative for the offending antibody (or antibodies) in cases of HDFN, warmed to physiologic body temperature, and packed to a Hct of 75%–85% in the appropriate volume as calculated using formulas in Table 20.2.

Intrauterine transfusions are usually initiated at 20 weeks' gestation and continued until 34–35 weeks' gestation with delivery at 37–38 weeks, depending on disease severity. Infants with severe HDFN, who receive multiple IUTs often require less phototherapy and fewer exchange transfu-sions in the neonatal period [116]. After several IUTs, suppression of erythropoiesis is common, rendering these infants virtually devoid of reticu-locytes, with their red cell mass derived almost entirely from donor RBCs [108]. This results in a more dramatic nadir period in which the major-ity of transfused infants may need several RBC transfusions within the first 3 months of life [117]. Meticulous communication between the NICU and transfusion center is imperative as misleading initial blood grouping and false-negative DAT may occur in the heavily intrauterine transfused infant.

Intrauterine platelet transfusions have been used to treat severely thrombocytopenic fetuses with neonatal alloimmune thrombocytopenia

(NAIT) to prevent antenatal intracranial hemorrhage [118, 119]. Predictors of disease severity include a maternal history of prior affected pregnancies and fetal/neonatal intracranial hemorrhage occurring at an early gestational age. Mothers may be treated with steroids and IVIg based on risk stratification. Repeated transfusions at weekly intervals often are necessary because of the short survival time of transfused platelets. Irradiated washed maternal platelets may be used for single transfusions, but for repeated transfusions, a panel of selected platelet antigen-negative donors should be recruited. All products should be CMV risk-reduced and irradiated.

Platelet Transfusions

Neonatal thrombocytopenia, defined as a platelet count <150 × 10^9/L, complicates 22%–35% of all NICU admissions [120], and results from decreased platelet production, increased peripheral destruction, or a combination of these two processes, as typically seen in sick infants. Neonates have different risks of bleeding given an equivalent degree of thrombocytopenia. For example, thrombocytopenic neonates with IUGR have a relatively low risk of major hemorrhage whereas those with sepsis or NEC have an intermediate risk, and those with neonatal alloimmune thrombocytopenia (NAIT) have a high risk as demonstrated by a 10%–20% incidence of intracranial hemorrhage (ICH). Differences in platelet function, concurrent coagulopathy, and immunological factors are likely causes for these discrepancies.

Indications and Transfusion Thresholds

Quantitative and qualitative platelet disorders may cause significant bleeding with resulting morbidity, the most serious being ICH. One randomized controlled trial addressing whether platelet transfusions reduce major bleeding in neonates showed no difference in the incidence of new ICHs or extension of existing hemorrhages between infants given prophylactic platelet transfusions to maintain platelet counts of at least 150 × 10^9/L or to control infants who were transfused to maintain platelet counts greater than 50 × 10^9/L without evidence of bleeding [121]. However, this study did not address bleeding risk or transfusion benefit for neonates with platelet counts below 50 × 10^9/L.

In a cross-sectional observational study of neonatal outcomes with severe thrombocytopenia, Stanworth et al. failed to show a clear relationship between nadir platelet count/degree of thrombocytopenia and major hemorrhage (IVH, pulmonary, intra-abdominal, hematuria) [122]. In the 169 neonates studied with severe thrombocytopenia (platelet count nadir <60,000/µL), 154 (91%) did not experience major hemorrhage. Of the 15 (9%) that experienced major hemorrhage, 12 patients (80%) had a platelet count nadir before the hemorrhage of greater than 20,000/µL [122], and follow-up analysis revealed that thrombocytopenia alone was not a strong indicator of bleeding risk, whereas gestational age (<34 weeks), early onset of postnatal thrombocytopenia (<10 days after birth), and coexistence of NEC were strong clinical risk factors for bleeding in this population [123]. Retrospective studies have also failed to establish a link between the severity of thrombocytopenia and risk of IVH [124] across both liberal and restrictive transfusion practices [125, 126]. A recent retrospective study of VLBW infants demonstrated that a restrictive platelet transfusion protocol using platelet count thresholds of 25,000/µL in clinically stable neonates and 50,000/µL in clinically unstable neonates, extremely premature neonates within the first week of life, or neonates at high risk of major bleeding was not associated with an increased risk for IVH compared with a more aggressive transfusion protocol [125].

Platelets for Neonatal Transfusion Study 2 (PlaNet 2) (ISRCTN 87736839), an RCT in the UK, Ireland, and the Netherlands comparing prophylactic platelet transfusion thresholds of 25,000/µL and 50,000/µL in terms of mortality and major bleeding complications in 660 premature infants (less than 34 weeks), reported results in 2019 [127]. Infants randomized to the higher transfusion threshold had higher occurrence of a new major bleeding episode or death than infants randomized to the lower threshold (26% versus 19%, $p = 0.02$) [127]. The authors are unsure of the etiology but suggest that cytokines, inflammatory mediators, fluid shifts or adult donor platelets interacting with the neonatal coagulation milieu may play a role. Of note, the neonates studied had few, if any, risk factors for bleeding, and represented a small percent (660 of 3731) of infants assessed for eligibility.

Nevertheless, in their recent retrospective review, Sparger and colleagues found that a majority of neonatal platelet transfusions in the US continue to be administered for pre-transfusion platelet counts of ≥50,000/μL in VLBW infants despite evidence that platelet transfusion has little appreciable impact on the risk of IVH after adjustment for underlying clinical variables [128].

Antibody-mediated perinatal thrombocytopenia may be secondary to transplacentally transmitted maternal antibodies directed against both maternal and neonatal platelet antigens (neonatal ITP), or against paternally inherited fetal/neonatal platelet antigen (NAIT). Each etiology carries a distinct degree of thrombocytopenia and distinct bleeding risk. Incidences of severe thrombocytopenia (platelet count $<20 \times 10^9$/L) and ICH in infants born with neonatal ITP occurs in approximately 1%–5% and 1% respectively, with the majority of ICH occurring in infants having platelet count nadirs below 10×10^9/L [129, 130]. Platelet transfusions of any antigen type and/or maternal platelets are relatively ineffective in infants with neonatal ITP [131], and are advocated only in life-threatening bleeding emergencies, although thrombocytopenia usually responds to IVIg and/or corticosteroids [129, 132]. In contrast to neonatal ITP, NAIT carries a substantial risk of ICH, half occurring in utero before 28 weeks' gestation [132, 133]. A 7 year prospective study reported an overall incidence of ICH in neonates with NAIT of 14%, and indicated that individuals with fetomaternal incompatibility at human platelet antigen-5b (HPA-5b) may bleed at higher platelet counts [134]. For this reason, the threshold for platelet transfusion for neonates with NAIT remains unclear. A generally accepted standard platelet threshold of $25–30 \times 10^9$/L for neonates without other bleeding risk factors, and a higher trigger ($50–100 \times 10^9$/L) for preterm neonates,

clinically unstable neonates, and neonates with NAIT [132, 135]. Hemorrhage associated with acquired (i.e., ECMO, CPB, antiplatelet medications, uremia) or congenital qualitative platelet abnormalities (i.e., Bernard–Soulier syndrome) are treated with platelet transfusions even if the platelet count is within normal range.

Preparations

A standard platelet unit from a single whole blood donation contains 5.5×10^{10} platelets in 50–70 mL of plasma. Apheresis platelets, also called single-donor platelets (SDPs), contain a minimum of 3.0×10^{11} platelets in approximately 250 mL of plasma (range: 200 to 400 mL). Apheresis platelets can be split into multiple small aliquots by means of a sterile connecting device in the same fashion as RBCs, offering the advantage of limiting donor exposures. Each whole blood unit (or whole blood equivalent of an apheresis unit) may be volume reduced to 15–20 mL for patients with significant fluid restrictions, but this process is associated with significant platelet loss of 15%–35% and may affect platelet function adversely. The shelf life of WB-derived and apheresis platelets ranges from 5 to 7 days, depending on additional testing for bacterial contamination; volume-reduced platelets expire 4 hours after manipulation. Table 20.3 lists various indications for irradiation of cellular blood products (RBCs, platelets, granulocytes) in the neonatal population, although many institutions elect to provide universally irradiated cellular blood components to all infants under the age of 12 months (or older) due to delayed presentation/diagnosis of congenital immunodeficiency syndromes.

Platelets express intrinsic ABO antigens, but not Rh antigens. Whenever possible, the platelets should be ABO- and Rh- compatible because intravascular hemolysis following transfusion of

Table 20.3 Indications for administering irradiated blood components to neonates*

- Transfusion to a premature infant with birthweight <1,200 g
- Neonatal exchange transfusion
- Intrauterine transfusion, or postnatal transfusion in neonate who had received intrauterine transfusion
- Known or suspected congenital cellular immunodeficiency
- Significant immunosuppression related to chemotherapy or radiation treatment
- Transfusion of a cellular blood component obtained from a blood relative
- Transfusion of an HLA-matched or crossmatched platelet product

Notes: Modified from references [2, 4].

*Irradiation of cellular blood components. FFP, TP, and cryoprecipitate do not require irradiation.

ABO-incompatible platelets has been reported in infants [136]. Although Rh matching does not affect post-transfusion platelet increment, small amounts of RBCs (up to 0.2 to 0.3 mL) are present in WB-derived platelets and can cause Rh sensitization in an Rh-negative recipient. Compared to WB-derived concentrates, apheresis platelets contain much less RBC volume (0.0004–0.0005 mL), which is below the minimal volume (0.03 mL) reported to cause Rh alloimmunization [137]. Overall, the frequency of RhD alloimmunization from transfusion of D+ platelets (both apheresis and WB-derived) to both immunocompetent and immunocompromised Rh negative patients has been demonstrated to be low (<1.5%) in recent studies [138]. Nevertheless, administration of Rh immune globulin (RhIg intramuscular dose: 100 IU/mL RBCs transfused, intravenous dose: 90 IU RhIG/mL RBCs) may be considered for Rh-negative neonates, especially females, within 72 hours of exposure to Rh-positive RBCs through platelet transfusion [139].

Dose and Administration

Platelet dosing in neonates may be calculated based on mL/kg or Equivalent Units/kg. An Equivalent Unit (EU) is the volume of a platelet aliquot that contains a minimum of 5.5×10^{10} platelets. Since one apheresis unit contains at least 3×10^{11} platelets, an apheresis platelet unit is equivalent to approximately 6 units of WB-derived platelets. The standard dose based on this method is 1 EU/5–10 kg with a minimum dose of one EU. EU-based dosing offers the advantage of reducing platelet content variability in the transfused product since a minimum dose of platelets will be administered regardless of its volume. This may be clinically significant in sick neonates with thrombocytopenia. A dose of 5–10 mL/kg of WB-derived platelets is expected to yield a platelet increment of $50–100 \times 10^9$/L. However, in neonates with increased platelet destruction (as seen in sepsis, DIC, and NAIT), actual post-transfusion increments may be significantly lower.

With NAIT, fetomaternal incompatibility for the HPA-1a and HPA-5b antigens is responsible for 80% and 15% of cases in white Europeans respectively, whereas other antigens may be responsible in other racial groups. If the HPA incompatibility is unknown, then the mother is likely to be the most readily available source of antigen-negative platelets.

Maternal platelets should be washed free of antibody-containing plasma and irradiated before transfusion [4]. In the event that maternal platelets are unavailable and laboratory confirmation of the offending antigen is pending, then transfusion of platelets negative for both HPA-1a and HPA-5b is likely to be successful in 95% of white European infants. A retrospective analysis of neonates with severe NAIT demonstrated an increase above a threshold of 40×10^9/L in 24/27 newborns and an increase above a threshold of 80×10^9/L in 16/27 newborns. Therefore, platelet transfusions from random donors are an appropriate strategy in the management of severe NAIT when antigen-negative platelets are unavailable [140, 141]. Platelets should never be warmed or infused through umbilical arterial lines.

Plasma and Cryoprecipitate Transfusions

Plasma can be prepared by either WB separation or by apheresis. When the plasma product is frozen to −18 °C or colder within 8 or 24 hours of collection it is labeled as fresh frozen plasma (FFP) or plasma frozen within 24 hours after phlebotomy (PF24), respectively, and can be stored at this temperature for up to 1 year [4]. Both products are considered to be functionally equivalent for coagulation factor replacement and are used interchangeably in most transfusion practices. Plasma is available in volumes of approximately 250–300 mL if collected from whole-blood donations; or up to 600 mL if derived from apheresis; however, plasma can be separated into a system of multiple satellite bags, and frozen as aliquots for infants who receive only fractions of a plasma unit. Furthermore, plasma can be further subdivided into aliquots via sterile connecting devices after being thawed for multiple neonates, stored at 1–6 °C for up to 5 days, and transfused as thawed plasma (TP) [2]. Although TP has approximately 40% activity of heat labile factors (Factor V and VIII), effective hemostasis is retained at this level, making TP clinically similar to FFP [142].

Crossmatching is not performed, since type-specific or AB-negative product is typically issued. Because the freezing process renders the frozen-thawed plasma component free of viable leukocytes, leukoreduction and irradiation are unnecessary. Plasma is not screened for CMV IgG; therefore, passive transfer of CMV antibody in plasma may result in positive CMV IgG testing in the transfused neonate. This does not represent CMV infection, and the antibody disappears in a time course consistent with the 21 day half-life of gamma globulin [143]

Solvent/detergent-treated plasma serves as an alternative to standard plasma products with decreased risk of transmission of enveloped viruses [144]. Octaplas™ (genesis Biopharma) received Health Canada approval in 2005 and FDA approval in January 2013. It has been available in Europe since 1992 and several countries (e.g., Norway, Republic of Ireland, and Finland) have entirely converted their plasma supply from FFP to Octaplas™. Each lot is prepared from a pool of 630 to 1520 units of FFP, which provides a more consistent level of coagulation factors. The risk of allergic reactions and TRALI appears reduced due to the process of filtration to remove cellular debris as well as the dilution of individual donor plasma proteins. The product is available in 200 mL aliquots, but these cannot be divided into smaller portions, limiting their use in smaller patients. Octaplas™ preparation includes affinity ligand chromatography (to remove prions), several filtration steps, and S/D treatment with trinitrobutyl phosphate and Triton X-100. Through such preparation processes, Octaplas™ is associated with reduced risk of bacterial contamination [145]. In the United States, the shelf-life is 3 years when stored below −18 °C (compared to 1 year for FFP or PF24).

Plasma is used primarily to treat acquired coagulation factor deficiencies as a result of disseminated intravascular coagulation (DIC), dilutional coagulopathy, liver failure, or vitamin K deficiency from malabsorption, biliary disease, warfarin effect, or maternal anticonvulsant therapy. Plasma should be used for specific factor replacement in congenital factor deficiencies only when specific viral-inactivated plasma-derived or recombinant factor concentrates are unavailable [2]. FDA-approved commercial factor concentrates are now available for FVIIa, FVIII, FIX, FXIII, von Willebrand factor (vWF); prothrombin complex, protein C, antithrombin, and fibrinogen. Plasma is not indicated for volume expansion, enhancement of wound healing, or first-line treatment for congenital factor deficiencies when commercial factor concentrates are

available. Although earlier studies demonstrated that the incidence of IVH was reduced by prophylactic plasma transfusion, recent evidence has disproved any effect of prophylactic transfusion on rates of death or disability in preterm infants [146]. The use of plasma as a source of immunoglobulins for the treatment of neonatal sepsis, or for the treatment of immunodeficiency states is also unwarranted [147]. There is also no evidence that prophylactic plasma transfusion in neonates undergoing CPB either prevents excessive bleeding or decreases transfusion requirements despite the universal reduction in components of the coagulation and fibrinolytic systems [148]. Bleeding in this situation is often related to platelet dysfunction with or without thrombocytopenia and responds better to platelet administration.

The typical dose of plasma administered is 10–15 mL/kg as this will replace approximately 10%–30% of most factors immediately following transfusion [149]. Further doses are determined by the clinical situation, underlying disease process, and the half-life of the factor(s) being replaced. Furthermore, both the prothrombin time (PT) and activated partial thromboplastin time (aPTT) are prolonged in the neonate as a result of depressed vitamin K dependent factors in neonates, requiring correlation of lab values to clinical status of the infant when assessing plasma component needs in the sick neonate. It is essential to obtain appropriately collected, non-heparinized specimens for evaluation of coagulation factor deficiencies prior to plasma transfusion.

Cryoprecipitate is the protein fraction derived from FFP thawed at 1–6 °C, which is then resuspended in approximately 10–15 mL of plasma and refrozen to −18 °C for storage up to 1 year. Each unit of cryoprecipitate is derived from a single WB donation, and contains a minimum of 80 units of factor VIII activity and 150 mg of fibrinogen [1]. Although there are no standards for the quantity of the other factors, cryoprecipitate also contains vWF, factor XIII, and fibronectin [27]. Cryoprecipitate is the treatment of choice for severe acquired hypofibrinogenemia (<150 mg/dL) associated with bleeding. In general, an infant should receive 1 unit of cryoprecipitate per 5 kg, which increases the total fibrinogen by about 100 mg/dL [143]. Bleeding associated with von Willebrand disease, hemophilia A, and congenital fibrinogen deficiency (including afibrinogenemia and hypofibrinogenemia) should be treated with FDA-licensed recombinant factor concentrates and/or viral inactivated pooled plasma-derived factor concentrates whenever possible.

Granulocyte Transfusions

Despite effective antimicrobial therapy, sepsis-related mortality in preterm infants remains high (up to 15%), as a result of the underlying incompetence of the preterm infant's immune system. A small neutrophil storage pool and sepsis-related defects in neutrophil deformability, chemotaxis, phagocytosis, and oxidative killing, lead to significant neutropenia and qualitative neutrophil deficiencies in the presence of bacterial infection. Furthermore, placental transfer of IgG is low prior to 32 weeks' gestation, resulting in hypogammaglobulinemia [150, 151].

The Resolving Infection in Neutropenia with Granulocytes (RING) randomized clinical trial [152] compared standard antimicrobial therapy alone against daily granulocyte transfusion from donors stimulated with granulocyte colony-stimulating factor (G-CSF) and dexamethasone in addition to standard therapy and found no difference in survival or microbial response in the granulocyte arm, although secondary analyses indicated that higher doses of granulocytes achieved through G-CSF stimulation were associated with better outcomes than lower doses [153]. Although children (defined as <18 years of age) were included in this study, they comprised only a minority of the total number of subjects (6/49 in control arm, 4/48 in granulocyte arm) [152]. Studies of the efficacy of granulocyte transfusions for the treatment of life-threatening infections in neonatal patients are difficult to evaluate because of small numbers of patients with varying degrees of illness and supportive care regimens, differing methods of harvesting neutrophils, and different transfusion protocols. Meta-analysis of the safety and efficacy of granulocyte infusion adjunctive to antimicrobial therapy in the treatment of septic neutropenic neonates failed to show that granulocyte infusions reduce mortality or morbidity, although a reduction in the latter approached statistical significance [154]. In spite of the conflicting evidence, granulocyte transfusion may rarely be considered in neonates with qualitative neutrophil defects with severe (or progressive) bacterial or fungal infection who

have not responded to appropriate aggressive antimicrobial treatment [135].

Granulocyte concentrates (GCs) for neonatal use are prepared by automated leukapheresis of healthy stimulated donors, and should contain 1.0–2.0×10^9 PMNs/kg in 10–15 mL/kg volume. As discussed above, there is evidence that granulocyte yield may be increased by co-stimulating donors with dexamethasone and G-CSF [153]. Once initiated, daily granulocyte transfusions are recommended until there is clinical improvement and evidence of neutrophil count recovery (ANC + bands >3 $\times 10^9$/L in the first week of life; >1.5 $\times 10^9$/L thereafter). The component must be ABO- and Rh-compatible and cross-matched with the recipient, since the product contains a large number of RBCs (Hct: 15%–20%). All GCs should be gamma irradiated but NOT leukodepleted and infused as soon as possible after collection using standard 170 μm filters. Cytomegalovirus-negative donors may be preferentially selected when the recipient is known to be CMV negative because of the risk of CMV transmission, although it may be difficult to consistently provide granulocytes from seronegative donors in areas with high CMV prevalence. It is essential that the medical team and the infant's parents be aware and consent to the fact that FDA-mandated infectious disease testing will not be completed before the product is released for transfusion because of the product's 24-hour outdate. This ensures that the risks and benefits of transfusing an untested blood product are considered by all parties.

Intravenous immunoglobulin and growth factors (G-CSF and GM-CSF) have also been attempted to augment traditional antimicrobial therapy to support septic neonates, but the efficacy of such agents requires further investigation. In meta-analysis, the addition of G-CSF or GM-CSF to antibiotic therapy in preterm infants with suspected systemic infection did not reduce immediate mortality, although a significant reduction in mortality was seen in septic neonates with neutropenia [155]. Prophylactic administration of IVIg has not been shown to confer any significant reduction in mortality in infants with suspected infections [156]. Furthermore, IVIg was shown to be inferior in terms of overall survival to granulocyte transfusions when used in conjunction with antimicrobials in neonates with presumed bacterial infection and neutropenia [157].

Granulocyte transfusions have unique risks, and include varying degrees of pulmonary reactions which range from mild transient respiratory distress in 25%–50%, to severe pulmonary edema, hypoxia, and ARDS in about 1% of all transfusions in adults. They are also associated with a high incidence of febrile reactions. Pulmonary complications have been reported in 4% of transfused infants [158], and severe pulmonary reactions resembling TRALI have been reported [159, 160]. Amphotericin B administered within 6 hours of GCs has been suspected to potentiate severe pulmonary reactions, but has not been confirmed in RCTs [161].

Extracorporeal Membrane Oxygenation

Extracorporeal membrane oxygenation (ECMO) is the use of prolonged extracorporeal circulation and gas exchange through a membrane oxygenator to provide temporary life support in patients with profound cardiorespiratory failure who fail to respond to conventional therapy. The transfusion service plays a vital role in supporting the needs of infants on ECMO by providing blood products for the initiation of ECMO as well as ongoing transfusion support throughout the course of ECMO, which may be quite extensive. Under ideal circumstances, fresh, ABO, and Rh compatible RBCs along with type-specific plasma are used to prime the ECMO circuit. However, in cases where ECMO deployment occurs emergently, there may be insufficient time for preparation of blood products meeting all of the above criteria. Provisions for urgent use (i.e., ECMO circuit disruption) often require an inventory of group O-negative RBCs. Blood products used for ECMO should be fresh (<5–10 days), CMV risk-reduced, gamma irradiated, and sickle-negative. Although there is mounting anecdotal evidence that RBCs preserved in extended storage media are safe for ECMO, many ECMO centers use CPDA-stored RBC products or reduce the amount of additive solution prior to use [2].

Hemostatic complications during ECMO are multifactorial and include the following: systemic heparinization to prevent clot formation in the circuit, qualitative and quantitative platelet deficiencies resulting from activation and consumption within the circuit, activation of the coagulation cascade and simultaneous fibrinolysis

from continuous contact of plasma proteins with the prosthetic surfaces, and underlying predisposing factors to coagulopathy (i.e., acidosis, DIC, hypoxia). For these reasons, bleeding is common in ECMO patients. Despite aggressive blood component support, the Extracorporeal Life Support Organization (ELSO) registry reports a 15% incidence of ICH and 7% incidence of other major bleeding throughout an ECMO course [162, 163].

Ongoing blood product support throughout ECMO varies based on transfusion triggers and the indication for ECMO [164]. Platelet counts decrease by a mean of 26% from baseline counts within 15 minutes of initiating ECMO and continue to decline further thereafter, while platelet function is reduced considerably. Sepsis while on ECMO increases platelet requirements. Consequently, platelet counts generally are maintained between 100 and 200 $\times$ 10^9/L, depending on the assessed risk of hemorrhage in the individual infant [165]. Maintaining a platelet count $\geq 150 \times 10^9$/L is recommended for high risk infants, and $\geq 200 \times 10^9$/L is often recommended postoperative in diaphragmatic hernia repair cases and/or for active bleeding. Cryoprecipitate is administered to maintain fibrinogen ≥ 100 mg/dL, and Hct is maintained at 40%–45%, to optimize oxygen delivery [166].

In the past, blood usage for neonates on ECMO resulted in a mean of 30 donor exposures per ECMO course; however, this been reduced to 7–10 donor exposures in many centers by employing donor exposure-limiting strategies (i.e., use of single-donor split products) [167].

Management of ECMO Patients Using Factor Concentrates such as Antithrombin III

Although on-demand dosing of antithrombin concentrates (Thrombate, ATryn) for pediatric patients on ECMO increases antithrombin levels and decreases heparin requirements for at least 12 hours after dosing, no statistical differences in the number of circuit changes, in vivo clots or hemorrhages, transfusion requirements, hospital or ICU length of stay, or in-hospital mortality were identified compared to controls [168, 169]. Similarly, studies of antithrombin supplementation in children on cardiopulmonary bypass have demonstrated decreased heparin doses without significant impact on clinical outcomes [170].

Adverse Reactions to Blood Transfusion

The physiological immaturity of various organ systems in the newborn gives rise to significant differences in the incidence and types of adverse reactions when compared with older children and adults. Whenever a patient is transfused, he/she should be closely monitored for signs of a reaction. Often, a potential reaction is noted by a change in vital signs, respiratory status, or skin manifestations (e.g., rash, hives). Typically, these changes present early in the transfusion, but they may occur at any point. The Joint Commission recommends monitoring vital signs pre-transfusion, within 15 minutes of initiation, and within 1 hour of transfusion end [171]. Hospital policies are based on these guidelines but may differ with respect to each other.

Febrile Nonhemolytic Transfusion Reactions

Febrile nonhemolytic transfusion reactions (FNHTRs) are characterized by fever, chills, and diaphoresis. These reactions are believed to result from the release of pyrogenic cytokines by leukocytes within the plasma during storage. The incidence of FNHTRs has decreased dramatically since the implementation of prestorage leukoreduction of RBCs and platelet products in 1999. Whereas FNHTRs occurred in approximately 10% of transfusions in the past, the incidence for all products since the introduction of leukoreduction is now 0.1% to 3% (approximately 0.2% for prestorage leukoreduction) [22, 23]. When FNHTR is suspected, the transfusion should be stopped. While FNHTR is typically self-limited, it is important to investigate the possibility of more serious reactions. A sample of blood from the patient may be sent for DAT, plasma hemoglobin quantification, serum lactate dehydrogenase, bilirubin level and/or urine blood to ensure that the patient is not experiencing a hemolytic transfusion reaction. The transfusion service may repeat the crossmatch between the RBC unit and a post-transfusion patient sample to ensure there is no new unexpected incompatibility. Bacterial contamination should be assessed via cultures of the transfused product and the patient's blood; empiric antibiotic therapy may be warranted. Most FNHTRs respond to antipyretics, and meperidine may be used for rigors [172, 173].

Allergic Transfusion Reactions

Allergic transfusion reactions (ATRs) are marked by urticaria and itching, but can include flushing, bronchospasm, and anaphylaxis in severe cases. For mild or localized cutaneous cases, the transfusion can be continued once symptoms have subsided; this is the only scenario in which transfusion can be reinitiated with the same unit after a reaction. Severe allergic reactions (anaphylactoid or anaphylactic reactions) may require treatment with corticosteroids and/or epinephrine. The same blood unit should never be restarted in severe cases, even after symptoms have abated. Leukoreduction does not decrease the incidence of ATRs as it has for FNHTRs [23]. Premedication with antihistamines with or without steroids is recommended for ATRs. Because these reactions are caused by an antibody response in a sensitized recipient to soluble plasma proteins within the blood product, washed RBCs and platelets may be used for severe or recurrent ATRs nonresponsive to medication. Severe ATRs leading to anaphylaxis can be caused by the development of anti-IgA antibodies in recipients who are IgA-deficient. In these instances, IgA-deficient–plasma products may be obtained, but require the use of rare donor registries [174]. In patients of Asian descent, haptoglobin deficiency may also be associated with severe ATRs [175].

The use of platelets in additive solution (PAS) resulted in decreased incidence of ATRs and FNHTRs in one adult study, presumably due to decrease in donor plasma content in the blood products [176]. However, neonates represented only 1.8% of the study population. Other retrospective reports describing PAS use have included children and neonates, but overall the effect of PAS platelets in neonates requires further study [177].

Hemolytic Reactions

Acute hemolytic transfusion reactions are rare in neonates, partly due to the absence of naturally occurring isoagglutinins before 4 months of age, but also due to the practice in some NICUs of transfusing neonates with group O blood. Although there are case reports of anti-RhE and anti-Kell formation in infants as young as 18 days of life, the majority of reports support the infrequency of RBC alloimmunization and delayed hemolytic transfusion reactions (DHTRs) in infants less than 4 months of age due to their immunologic immaturity [178, 179]. A cohort study of 1641 neonates and children up to the age of 3 years found no alloimmunization cases within the first 6 months of life. The authors concluded that after initial testing, repeat antibody screening, and cross-matching during the first 4 months of life could be safely omitted [180]. This approach also reduces iatrogenic blood loss due to repeated laboratory sample draws.

A phenomenon known as "T-activation" can cause immune-mediated hemolysis in neonates, which can range from minor to severe and fatal, if not recognized. Removal of *N*-acetyl neuraminic (sialic) acid residues from the O-linked oligosaccharides on glycophorins (A, B, and C) on RBC membranes by neuraminidases produced by bacteria, particularly *Clostridium bacteroides* and *Streptococcus pneumoniae*, results in activation of the normally masked Thompsen–Friedenreich (T) cryptantigen on the red-cell surface of the neonate. Transfusion of adult blood containing naturally occurring anti-T antibodies into neonates with T-activation can present with evidence of intravascular hemolysis following transfusion of blood products, or unexplained failure to achieve the expected post-transfusion hemoglobin increment. T-activation has been reported mainly in neonates with necrotizing enterocolitis, especially in those with severe disease requiring surgical intervention, but also in septic infants with other surgical problems [181]. Routine cross-matching techniques will not detect the polyagglutination due to T-activation when monoclonal ABO antiserum is used. Minor cross-matching of neonatal T-activated red cells with donor anti-T-containing serum may show agglutination, but this is not performed routinely. Infants with discrepancies in forward and reverse blood typing and evidence of hemolysis on smear should be suspected of T-antigen activation. The diagnosis is confirmed by specific agglutination tests using peanut lectin *Arachis hypogea* and *Glycine soja*, but such reagents may not be readily available. Further hemolysis may be prevented by using washed RBC and platelets, and low-titer anti-T plasma if available [181, 182]. Exchange transfusion with plasma-reduced components may be necessary for infants with severe ongoing hemolysis. The clinical significance of hemolysis

mediated by anti-T and the need to avoid plasma transfusion in these patients remains a topic of discussion [183].

Numerous nonimmunologic causes of hemolysis can occur in neonates, such as exposure of RBCs to thermal and mechanical stresses (see RBC section), co-administering incompatible fluids and/or drugs, and the transfusion of abnormal donor RBCs (i.e., G6PD deficiency) [184, 185].

Donor Leukocyte Effects

The presence of donor leukocytes in blood products can contribute to HLA alloimmunization, which can complicate future medical interventions by increasing transplant graft failure rate or contribute to platelet refractoriness. Another described phenomenon is transfusion-related immunomodulation (TRIM), a process in which leukocytes, cytokines, stored RBCs, or other biological response mediators alter the recipient's immune system. Both effects are improved, although not eliminated, by pre-storage leukoreduction of blood products [186, 187]. The effectiveness of other interventions to address TRIM (e.g., washing) has not been established [188]. The characteristics and impact of TRIM in critically ill pediatric patients are under investigation [189].

Transfusion-Related Acute Lung Injury

The passive transfusion of blood containing leukoagglutinins (HLA or neutrophil antibodies) directed against the recipient's leukocytes initiates complement activation with microvascular lung injury. This condition termed transfusion-related acute lung injury (TRALI) typically manifests with non-cardiogenic pulmonary edema, severe hypoxemia, hypotension, fever, and transient leukopenia within 6 hours of transfusion. TRALI has been well documented in the pediatric population, but is reported only rarely in neonates partly because of the difficulty in distinguishing the acute respiratory distress that accompanies the syndrome from other causes of respiratory deterioration [188]. High-volume plasma products (FFP, apheresis platelets, GCs) account for the majority of severe TRALI cases, and multiparous women are the most commonly implicated donors [190]. Use of high-volume plasma products from men, women who have never been pregnant, or previously pregnant women who have tested negative for HLA antibodies has dramatically decreased the incidence of TRALI [191]. A case has been reported of a 4-month-old girl who experienced TRALI within 2 hours of completion of a RBC transfusion from her mother. HLA antibodies were identified in the mother's serum demonstrating the possible role of HLA antibodies in the pathogenesis of TRALI in the setting of a designated blood transfusion between mother and infant [192]. TRALI has been documented as complicating granulocyte transfusions in neonates [159, 160].

Transfusion-Associated Circulatory Overload

Transfusion-associated circulatory overload (TACO) is defined as acute respiratory distress associated with signs of fluid overload, including tachycardia, hypertension, pulmonary edema, positive fluid balance, or elevated levels of brain natriuretic peptides. It contributes to deaths attributable to transfusion. Neonates are at risk because their small blood volume may not accommodate rapid or large volume transfusions. Other risk factors include pre-existing cardiac or renal dysfunction, and hospitalization in the intensive care unit [193]. The presentations of TACO and TRALI are similar, and both may be difficult to differentiate from the patient's underlying disease. Diuretics may be helpful in supporting patients affected by TACO. Preventative options include anticipating blood needs in order to transfuse smaller aliquots at a lower rate, selecting lower-volume alternatives (e.g., volume reduced units or factor concentrates), and closely monitoring the fluid balance [194].

Transfusion-Associated Graft-versus-Host Disease

Transfusion-associated graft-versus-host disease (TAGVHD) occurs due to the proliferation and engraftment of viable donor lymphocytes in an immunosuppressed or immunodeficient transfusion recipient who does not recognize the cells as being foreign and is unable to reject them. Similarities in HLA antigens facilitate engraftment and, therefore, this phenomenon is much more likely to occur when family members serve as blood donors or when the population is relatively homogeneous. Infants at high risk of TAGVHD include those receiving transfusions

from blood relatives, those receiving IUTs, those receiving postnatal transfusions who had received IUTs, those receiving large volumes transfusions (i.e., exchange transfusion), and those with primary cell-mediated immunodeficiency disease [195–198]. Although there exists no "standard of care" regarding irradiation of blood products for infants without TAGVHD risk factors, some institutions adopt universal irradiation policies, whereby all infants less than 4 months of age receive irradiated cellular blood products so as to avoid TAGVHD in patients with an undiagnosed immunodeficiency. Other transfusion centers irradiate all cellular blood products given to preterm infants with birth weights ≤1.0 to 1.2 kg [199]. The known and presumed indications for irradiation of blood components for neonates are listed in Table 20.3.

The clinical signs and symptoms of TAGVHD typically present 3 to 30 days following transfusion of a leukocyte replete cellular component, and include fever; generalized, erythematous rash with/without progression to desquamation; diarrhea; hepatitis (mild to fulminant liver failure); respiratory distress; and severe pancytopenia resulting from graft T lymphocyte-induced hematopoietic progenitor cell death. The mortality rate is approximately 90% in the pediatric population, mostly as a result of bone marrow hypoplasia. Treatment supportive, as there exists no effective curative therapy [178].

TAGVHD can be abrogated by pretransfusion gamma irradiation of all cellular blood components at 2,500 cGy. The shelf life of irradiated red cells is 28 days; however, no data currently exists on the safety in the neonatal population of gamma irradiated RBCs that are stored for this amount of time [200]. Because potassium and free hemoglobin increase after irradiation and storage of RBCs, it is preferable to irradiate cellular blood products close to administration time for neonates, who may not be able to tolerate high potassium loads; this is often referred to as irradiation on issue.

Transfusions and Necrotizing Enterocolitis

Another concern linked to RBC transfusions is the development of neonatal NEC; several retrospective studies have demonstrated a temporal association between the two. They report that 25%–38% of NEC cases occur within 48 hours of RBC transfusion and that the risk of transfusion-associated NEC increases with decreasing gestational age of the infant [201–204]. Blau et al. found a convergence of transfusion-associated NEC at 31 weeks' gestation, the age of presentation of O_2 toxicity and other neovascularization syndromes [202]. In another retrospective report, Singh et al. displayed a strong association of transfusion within 24 hours and NEC (OR = 7.60, p = 0.001), a significant albeit decreased association for transfusion within 48 hours (OR = 5.55, p = 0.001), and a statistically insignificant (absent) association for transfusion within 96 hours (OR = 2.13, p = 0.07) in their multivariate analysis [205]. Although attempts were made to minimize the confounding effects of multiple variables, the effect of infants' nadir hematocrit level on the risk of developing NEC remained statistically significant, making it impossible to separate the influence of hematocrit and RBC transfusion.

However, other studies suggest that RBC transfusions may be an epiphenomenon with respect to NEC rather than a contributor to the pathogenesis of disease. Bednarek et al. reported that there was no significant difference in the incidence of NEC between high versus low hematocrit threshold transfusion practices among six NICUs [8], and the PINT trial did not show a difference in the incidence of NEC between the low versus high hematocrit transfusion threshold groups [14]. In a meta-analysis of the published literature on transfusions and NEC, increased RBC transfusions were associated with lower rates of NEC. Thus, the direction of effect of RBC transfusions on NEC in randomized trials was opposite to that seen in observational studies [206]. Keir and colleagues performed a separate systematic review and did not find an association between transfusions and NEC [18]. A meta-analysis of 17 observational studies reported similar results, with the caveat that these studies were predominantly of low-to-moderate quality [207]. One recent prospective study of 598 very low birth weight infants found that severe anemia (hemoglobin <8 g/dL), but not RBC transfusion, was associated with an increased risk of NEC. Thus, prevention of severe anemia may be more important than avoidance of RBC transfusion alone [208]. The temporal relationship observed between RBC transfusion and neonatal NEC may represent reverse causation, whereby clinical instability from evolving NEC leads to RBC transfusion prior to the formal diagnosis of

NEC. A prospective, multicenter observational cohort study of infants with birth weight less than or equal to 1250 g is underway to investigate the associations between RBC transfusion, product irradiation, anemia, and intestinal oxygenation and injury that lead to NEC [209].

Metabolic Adverse Reactions

Neonates, especially extremely premature infants, are vulnerable to metabolic irregularities resulting from blood transfusion due to immaturity of many of their organ systems, which are responsible for metabolizing and excreting compounds within blood components. Glucose imbalances, hyperkalemia, and hypocalcemia are the most common metabolic derangements related to transfusion.

Continuous glucose infusion rates (GIR) of >3–4 (mg/kg)/min are often required in preterm infants to maintain glucose balance. Hypoglycemia may occur during transfusion of small volumes of CPDA-1 or AS-1 RBCs if dextrose-containing intravenous infusion is interrupted, as GIRs supplied solely from the RBC product are approximately 0.2 (mg/kg)/min for CPDA-1 RBCs and 0.5 (mg/kg)/min for Adsol preserved AS-1 RBCs. It has been reported that approximately 15% of preterm infants receiving AS-1 preserved RBCs, and 64% of infants receiving CPDA-1 preserved RBCs require supplemental dextrose infusions as a result of hypoglycemia [37, 210]. Conversely, the glucose load for an exchange transfusion can be quite high, which can cause asymptomatic hyperglycemia (see Table 20.4). Rebound hypoglycemia can occur after exchange transfusions in infants resulting from an increased intra-procedural insulin surge. The incidence of hypoglycemia, either during or after exchange transfusions, has been reported to range from 1.4% to 3.6% in neonates regardless of whether group-O WB or reconstituted WB is used [211, 212]. Preventive measures for hypoglycemia entail frequent monitoring of blood glucose by bedside blood glucose meters during transfusions in infants at risk for glucose imbalances, and transfusing RBCs through a second line while continuing the maintenance fluids infusion at a lower rate.

Inhibition of the red-cell membrane-bound ATP pump during extended storage causes leakage of intracellular potassium, resulting in K^+ levels of 0.03–0.05 mEq/mL in the supernatant plasma at 42 days of storage. Conversely, after

Table 20.4 Dose of anticoagulant-preservative additives in transfused small-volume transfusion and exchange transfusion

Additive	CPDA-1 RBCs[*]		AS-1 RBCs[**]		Exchange transfusion (w/ reconstituted WB)[***]		Toxic dose (potential)
	(mg/kg)	((mg/kg)/hr)	(mg/kg)	((mg/kg)hr)	(mg/mL)	(mg/kg)	(mg/kg)
Dextrose	39	13	86	29	5.6	358	240/hour
Sodium	2.5	0.8	28	9.3	1.0	64	137/day
Citrate	9.1	3.0	6.5	2.2	2.7	173	180/hour
Phosphate	1.9	0.6	1.3	0.4	0.16	10	>60/day
Adenine	0.3	0.1	0.7	0.2	0.04	26	15/day
Mannitol	0	0	22	7.3	0.22	14	360/day

Notes: Small-volume transfusion assumes 10 mL/kg transfusion over 3 hours.

[*]CPDA-1 RBC Hct: 80%.

[**]AS-1 RBC Hct: 60%.

[***]One-volume exchange transfusion assumes TBV ~80 mL/kg, and reconstituted WB final Hct 50%–60%. Modified from refs [21, 210].

35 days of storage of CPDA-1 preserved RBCs, K^+ levels in the plasma approximates to 0.07–0.08 mEq/mL. Small-volume transfusions (15 mL/kg) of the CPDA-1 stored (Hct: 70%) and AP stored (Hct: 60%) RBCs supply a potassium dose of 0.3–0.4 mEq/kg and 0.3 mEq/kg, respectively [198]. Given the daily potassium requirement of approximately 2–3 mEq/kg, simple RBC transfusions given over 2–4 hours should not cause hyperkalemia. Multiple reports have confirmed the safety of transfusing dedicated RBC units at 10–15 mL/kg volumes over 2–4 hours to their expiration date (35 or 42 days), even in VLBW infants [19, 35, 36].

Life-threatening hyperkalemia has been reported in circumstances when RBC transfusions (fresh and old) have been administered rapidly (10–20 mL/kg over 10–15 minutes) to neonates with concurrent low cardiac output states, when given through a central line directly into the inferior vena cava, and when irradiated >24 hours prior to infusion [213]. Reconstituted fresh WB (<7 days old) is often recommended for large-volume transfusions and rapid small-volume transfusions because large amounts of rapidly administered (old) RBCs, can cause toxic K^+ concentrations [21]. When reconstituted fresh WB is unavailable for large-volume transfusions, the RBC units can be either washed or volume reduced (Hct: 80%) prior to reconstitution. In addition, rapidly transfusing RBCs through hand-held syringes using ≥23-gauge needles has been

shown to cause hemolysis, and is therefore discouraged [185]. Coordination with the transfusion service is critical when transfusions are being arranged for neonates at high risk of hyperkalemia, so that proper selection and preparation of the RBC units can be ensured.

Premature infants are vulnerable to hypocalcemia resulting from transfusion of citrate enriched blood, due to immaturity of their liver and kidney function, and the low amount of skeletal muscle mass. Furthermore, sick neonates often have comorbid conditions, such as acidosis and hypothermia, which may predispose to hypocalcemia by decreasing citrate clearance through the kidney and liver [210]. The amount of citrate infused into a neonate during a small-volume transfusion is very unlikely to cause hypocalcemia; however, the citrate load during an exchange transfusion (or massive transfusion) can reach high enough levels to lead to symptomatic hypocalcemia (Table 20.4). Symptomatic hypocalcemia is one of the most common serious side effects encountered among infants undergoing exchange transfusions with reported incidences in the range 5%–8% depending on the health status of the infant and exchange transfusion indication [212]. Preventive measures for hypocalcemia include: monitoring ionized calcium levels and/or QT intervals throughout exchange transfusion procedures, and aggressively correcting other metabolic abnormalities which may potentiate symptoms of hypocalcemia [210].

Effect of Plasticizers

The toxicity associated with the use of the plasticizer 2-(diethylhexyl)phthalate (DEHP) in blood storage bags has been debated in the transfusion medicine community for over 50 years. DEHP is added to polyvinylchloride plastic storage blood bags to increase bag flexibility, RBC survival, and oxygen permeability for platelet storage. DEHP also stabilizes RBC membranes, which prevents hemolysis and alteration during refrigerated storage. Due to its desirable structural properties, it is also widely used in medical plastics as well as in food storage and household products [214]. Critically ill neonates exposed to endotracheal tubes, orogastric tubes, intravenous tubing, and blood products can have DEHP exposures that exceed safe levels by 3–5 orders of magnitude [215].

Although no short- or long-term complications have been determined in infants, animal studies raise concerns about possible effects on hepatocellular, pulmonary, and reproductive function and potential carcinogenicity in the developing infant. There is evidence that DEHP exerts detrimental effects on the endocrine system by acting as an androgen antagonist and an estrogen agonist. While DEHP is broken down in the gastrointestinal tract to some extent, transfusions bypass this protection. At particular risk for toxicity are neonates receiving high volume transfusions, such as neonatal RBC exchange, during extracorporeal membrane oxygenation (ECMO), and during massive transfusion [216, 217].

Manufacturers have attempted to find suitable alternatives to DEHP. For example, butyrul-n-trihexyl-citrate leaches from the plastic at a slower rate, exhibits lower toxicity, and provides similar antihemolytic effects [218]. Other DEHP-free storage containers are at various stages of development throughout the world. However, a recent survey identified barriers to widespread implementation including decreased quality of blood products stored in non-DEHP plastics, higher price, shorter shelf-life, and ongoing debate about the evidence of DEHP toxicity [219].

Transfusion-Transmitted Infections

The potential risk of transfusion transmitted infections in the USA has been dramatically reduced by extensive donor screening and laboratory testing. The addition of HIV and HCV nucleic-acid testing (NAT) in 1999 to serological testing has further decreased the risk of transfusion transmission by shortening the window periods from time of acute infection to the detection of laboratory markers of infection [220]. Furthermore, since the first case of transfusion acquired-WNV (TA-WNV) recognized in 2002, implementation of WNV NAT in 2003 has prevented widespread WNV transmission via the blood supply. In the past decade, nationwide testing for *Trypanosoma cruzi* and Zika virus has been implemented. Nonetheless, infectious risks are not negligible, and therefore should be discussed with the parents of the infant as part of the consent process prior to any blood transfusion. The current estimated post-transfusion infectious risks are noted in Table 20.5. Efforts are ongoing to continue improving the safety of the blood supply [221].

Current transfusion-transmitted disease testing for allogeneic blood donation includes hepatitis B virus surface antigen (HBsAg), hepatitis B core antibody (anti-HBc), anti-hepatitis C antibody (anti-HCV), antibody to HIV-1 and HIV-2 (anti-HIV-1/2), antibody to human T-lymphotropic virus (HTLV-I and HTLV-II), serology for syphilis and *T. cruzi* (Chagas disease), and nucleic acid testing (NAT) for HIV-1, HIV-2, HCV, HBV, West Nile virus (WNV), and Zika virus (ZIKV) [222, 223]. In addition, some regions also screen for babesia while all platelets undergo bacterial culture because their storage at room temperature increases the risk of contamination.

HIV/AIDS

Nearly all cases of HIV infection acquired from blood transfusions in the USA occurred before 1985, when the implementation of routine serological screening for HIV in blood donors, and effective viral inactivation methods for plasma derived clotting factor concentrates became available. Asymptomatic HIV infection has been identified as late as 5–9.5 years post-transfusion in cohorts of neonates transfused before routine donor screening for HIV antibody were tested [224].

Nowadays, the risk of HIV transmission from blood transfusion is less than 1 in 2.1 million because of improved donor history screening and the advent of NAT testing in the late 1990s, which decreased the estimated window period to about 9 days [225].

Table 20.5 Risks of transfusion-transmitted infections

Infectious agent	Infectious risk
Bacterial contamination risk *(Yersinia enterocolitica, Escherichia coli, Brucella)*	
Platelets	1 in 2,500
RBCs	1 in 38,500
Septic transfusion reaction risk	
Platelets	1 in 100,000–200,000
RBCs	1 in 250,000
HIV	1 in 2.3 million
Hepatitis A	1 in 10 million
Hepatitis B	1 in 2 million
Hepatitis C	1 in 2 million
HTLV-I/II	1 in 3 million
West Nile virus	<1 in 3 million
Syphilis	Virtually nonexistent; theoretical risk from platelets stored at room temperature
Chagas disease (*T. cruzi*)	Extremely low*
Malaria	<1 in 3 million
CMV	<1 in 3 million
Babesiosis (*Babesia microti*)	Extremely low**
Creutzfeldt–Jakob disease	No cases reported in US; theoretical risk
Zika virus	<1 in 3 million***

Notes: *Although approximately 1 in 25,000–50,000 US donors are seropositive, only 7 cases of transfusion transmitted *T. cruzi* in USA/Canada.

* But may be as high as 1 in 1,800 in highly endemic areas (Upper Midwest and NE USA). A recent guidance from the Food and Drug Administration recommends implementation of NAT testing in endemic regions by May 2020 [268].

*** Based on sample of 466,834 donations tested between September 19 and November 30, 2016.

Bold: Serologic and/or NAT testing done on all allogeneic blood donations.

References [220, 223, 238, 269, 270].

Hepatitis B

Transfusion-acquired hepatitis B in neonates bears a 70% risk of chronic carrier state, which is similar to that of perinatally acquired infection. This contrasts the 5%–10% chronic carrier rate in adults with HBV infection, likely a result of the neonate's immature immune system. Additionally, whereas acute HBV infection is symptomatic in about 50% of adults, HBV infection acquired in infancy and early childhood is more often asymptomatic [226].

Hepatitis C

Acute hepatitis C virus (HCV) infection is often asymptomatic, but chronic viremia exceeds 60% with approximately 20% of those with untreated chronic hepatitis developing cirrhosis within two decades [227]. Cirrhosis carries a 1%–5% risk of hepatocellular carcinoma within 20 years of diagnosis [178]. Long-term outcome of HCV infection is dependent upon the route of transmission, age when infected, sex, and coexisting morbidities. A 35 year long-term follow up study of 31 adults with transfusion-acquired HCV at birth suggest a milder disease with slower progression to hepatic fibrosis in transfusion-acquired HCV at birth, than those who acquire HCV in early adulthood [228]. A recently reported look-back study of previously transfused infants and children found an 88% persistent HCV viremia rate at 10 years post transfusion in individuals with silent infection (positive anti-HCV serology). This contrasts previously reported pediatric HCV clearance rates of 45% and 42% at 19.5 and 35 years post-transfusion respectively, which implied that, unlike adults, pediatric patients may clear HCV over time [229]. Although the degree of inflammation and fibrosis in liver biopsies of treatment naive children has been shown to be milder than in adults with chronic active hepatitis, some have reported 12% of patients with significant liver fibrosis at 13 years post-infection [230]. Therefore, it is important for pediatricians to identify HCV-silently infected individuals to prevent the long-term effects of HCV infection. Effective therapies using direct-acting antiviral agents are available for HCV-infected children [231].

Cytomegalovirus

Among tested pathogens, CMV is unique in that donor positivity does not lead to deferral. In fact, CMV is widespread in blood donors, with seropositivity rates in the range 30%–70%. Older donors have higher rates. Viral genome has been detected in the white blood cells of CMV-seropositive individuals, and even CMV-seronegative donors may harbor latent CMV infection in their mononuclear cells. Post-transfusion CMV infection in LBW infants born to seronegative mothers causes a serious clinical syndrome of fever, respiratory distress, hepatosplenomegaly, and cytopenias and may result in death [183]. Disseminated CMV infection has been described in a full-term infant following ECMO [184]. Risk factors for neonatal transfusion-acquired CMV (TA-CMV) include birth weight <1,200 grams, exposure to at least 50 mL of blood, and maternal CMV seronegativity. CMV-seronegative blood or leukocyte-reduced blood is recommended for transfusions in all low birth weight infants born to seronegative mothers or those with unknown serostatus and for intrauterine transfusions [185].

Current third-generation leukocyte reduction filters provide WBC reduction to less than 5×10^6 total WBCs per unit, in accordance to AABB standards [1]. A key study showed that equivalent rates of TA-CMV infection were found for CMV-seronegative units and leuko-reduced units transfused to allogeneic hematopoietic stem cell transplant patients (1.4% vs. 2.4% respectively) [232]. A prospective multicenter birth cohort study revealed that transfusion of leuko-reduced, CMV-seronegative blood products effectively prevented transmission of CMV to very low birth weight infants. In fact, acquisition of CMV in the patient population was primarily

through maternal breast milk [233]. Together with other reports, the findings support the notion that leuko-reduced blood products are "CMV safe." Some experts have argued that leukocyte-reduction alone is sufficient [234] and others have published that TA-CMV is vanishingly rare [235]. However, no formal consensus on the debate of equivalency has been developed [236], leading some to advise against the elimination of "dual inventories" of blood products for CMV-seronegative and seropositive units. Nonetheless, variable strategies for preventing TT-CMV currently exist depending on the number of high-risk patients treated at a given center, the regional donor demographics and seropositivity rate, and product availability.

West Nile Virus

West Nile virus (WNV), a mosquito-borne virus, was first detected in the United States in 1999, with the first cases of TA-WNV occurring in 2002. Neuroinvasive disease occurs in 20% of infected individuals with worse sequelae in the immunocompromised and elderly. Following implementation of WNV NAT on donation multipools in 2003, there were approximately nine WNV transfusion transmissions in the subsequent 2 years, representing window period donations [237]. With implementation of the more sensitive individual NAT during periods of higher WNV activity, the risk of transfusion transmission has markedly decreased [238]. Although perinatal transmission and infection through breastmilk have been reported and implicated in neonatal cases WNV infection respectively, there currently exist no clear cases of TA-WNV in the neonatal population [239].

Zika Virus

Zika virus (ZIKV) is a flavivirus first discovered in the Zika Forest in Uganda in 1947. For many years, the virus caused sporadic outbreaks in Africa before gradually moving east. Several Pacific islands were affected in 2013–2014. In 2016, the virus appeared in South America and rapidly spread. The virus is transmitted by the *Aedes* mosquito and therefore shows more activity during the summer months. Transfusion-transmitted infection has been documented [240].

Unlike other flaviviruses, ZIKV has been associated with microcephaly and other fetal abnormalities when placental transmission occurs in an acutely infected pregnant woman and is currently under intense study [241]. Of concern for blood supply safety, about 80% of infected patients are asymptomatic. Thus, there was a great risk of a viremic blood donation and transmission to a susceptible donor without suitable laboratory detection. Blood collections were temporarily halted in areas with local virus transmission (e.g., Puerto Rico). In the fall of 2016, NAT screening of all donations in the United States was implemented under an investigation new drug protocol. During a period of about 2 months, 5 of 466,834 donations tested for ZIKV RNA were found to be positive [223]. The FDA cleared the first approved ZIKV detection test based on viral RNA in the plasma of blood donors in October 2017. The estimated risk per transfusion unit stands at less than 1 in 3 million [238].

Emerging Pathogens

The transfusion community maintains continuous attention to emerging infections such as babesiosis, variant Creutzfeldt–Jakob Disease (vCJD), chikungunya, dengue fever, and malaria. Despite extensive donor screening and laboratory testing, new infectious agents can still be transmitted through blood transfusions [238].

Transmission of babesiosis and malaria has been reported in neonates within endemic areas such as the northeast United States and Africa, respectively [242, 243]. Healthy patients transfused with blood contaminated with *Babesia microti* often do not get sick; however, transfusion-transmitted *Babesia* can be a significant cause of transfusion-related morbidity and mortality, especially for premature infants. Neonatologists in endemic areas should have a high index of suspicion for babesiosis in premature infants exposed to blood transfusions because infection is minimized but not eliminated through current blood bank practices [242]. At this time, blood products collected in United States regions with high prevalence of the disease (e.g., Minnesota, Wisconsin, Massachusetts, and Connecticut) are tested for *Babesia* by a nucleic acid detection test [244]. However, implementation of nationwide testing has thus far not been mandated due to cost-effectiveness considerations [245, 246].

Pathogen reduction/inactivation offers the advantage of eliminating the risk of infection with any nucleic acid-containing agent, which includes viruses, bacteria, protozoa, and fungi (prions excluded). However, current pathogen reduction/ techniques using nucleic acid-inactivating agents are still under investigation because no single technique has proved to be effective for all blood components [247].

Pathogen Reduction/Pathogen Inactivation

Current screening approaches are reactive in nature and depend on pathogen identification, characterization of infectious markers, and development of detection assays. While this iterative approach has provided very high blood supply safety, it does require some time to implement for each emerging pathogen.

Pathogen reduction/inactivation (PR/PI) is an all-encompassing term for a variety of methods (e.g., photochemical activation or solvent detergent treatment) that may be applied to blood following collection in order to confer broad protection against multiple infectious agents by countering proliferation and contamination [247]. Many of these technologies target DNA or cell membranes and are effective across different classes of pathogens (e.g., viruses, bacteria, and parasites, but not prions), offering the ability to interdict agents that are known to be transfusion-transmissible as well as emerging pathogens that pose uncertain risks to the blood supply.

The appeal of pathogen reduction is that it is a proactive approach to blood safety that inactivates pathogens instead of only screening for their presence. Although developed to complement current testing, PR could ultimately prove to be an alternative to testing. If widely effective, PR could reduce the number of donor deferrals due to disease risk factors. Since PR/PI inactivates white blood cells, it may provide additional benefits such as TA-GVHD prevention and alloimmunization reduction [248, 249]. However, concerns remain that PR/PI's detrimental effect on platelet and plasma function may lead to increased bleeding risk in susceptible patients such as trauma victims [250].

Two different methodologies of photochemical activation which have been more extensively studied will be briefly described but others are at various stages of development. Thus far, these technologies have been applied only to platelets and plasma. Platelets are of primary concern since their storage at 22–26 °C heightens their risk of contamination. No photochemical activation process is currently in clinical use for RBCs; these present an obstacle due to hemoglobin's absorption.

INTERCEPT® and Mirasol® Systems

The only photochemical activation platform approved by the FDA at the time of writing is the INTERCEPT® system (Cerus, Concord, CA, USA). This technique uses amotosalen, which can intercalate between DNA bases. In the presence of activation by UVA light, this molecule irreversibly cross-links with the DNA, thus preventing DNA transcription and cellular reproduction [251]. After INTERCEPT® treatment, an adsorption step removes excess amotosalen; only a tiny quantity remains [252].

INTERCEPT® is widely used for platelets and plasma and is approved in the United States and European Union for this purpose [253, 254]. The technology is effective against viruses, bacteria, and protozoans. However, breakthrough transmission has been reported with hepatitis A virus (HAV), hepatitis E virus (HEV), parvovirus B19, poliovirus, and certain spore-forming and/or fast-growing bacteria [255, 256].

However, of the published studies with INTERCEPT® platelets, few children have been included. A large European prospective hemovigilance study of INTERCEPT®-treated platelets following 19,175 transfusions in 2,441 patients demonstrated a low incidence of acute transfusion reactions and a safety profile in line with conventional platelet components. Only 46 of the patients were neonates (<28 days of age) who received a range of 1 to 9 platelet transfusions while 242 were children (<18 years of age) who received a range of 1 to 66 transfusions, which was similar in number to the adults. No adverse events occurred in the neonatal patients. Pediatric patients experienced similar rates of acute transfusion reactions (3.7%, $p = 0.179$) and severe adverse events (0.4%, $p = 0.550$) compared to adults. None of the severe adverse events were judged to be related to INTERCEPT®-treated platelets [257].

The Mirasol® (TerumoBCT, Lakewood, CO, USA) system uses riboflavin as a photosensitizer compound with UVB light. Riboflavin readily traverses lipid membranes and then intercalates nonspecifically with nucleic acids. Upon exposure to UVB light, intercalated riboflavin modified guanine

residues promote the generation of oxygen radicals [258, 259]. Since riboflavin and its byproducts are naturally occurring, no additional steps for removal following treatment are believed to be necessary [260]. Mirasol® has shown efficacy against a wide variety of pathogens that pose a risk of transfusion transmission [247, 261, 262].

A Cochrane review that evaluated 10 randomized control trials (9 with INTERCEPT®, 1 with Mirasol®) showed no difference in clinically significant bleeding or severe bleeding between recipients of pathogen reduced platelets compared to control platelets. When evaluated, all-cause mortality, product utilization, and adverse events were also not increased [263, 264]. Clinical trials performed with INTERCEPT®-treated plasma have shown no difference in clinical efficacy when compared to standard FFP [265]. A European prospective hemovigilance study of INTERCEPT®-treated platelets following 19,175 transfusions in 2,441 patients demonstrated a low incidence of acute transfusion reactions and a safety profile in line with conventional platelet components. Forty-six of the patients were neonates (<28 days of age) who received a range of 1 to 9 platelet transfusions while 242 were children (<18 years of age) who received a range of 1 to 66 transfusions [257].

Ongoing Monitoring of PR

The use of PR/PI blood products is slowly increasing throughout the world. Many countries in Europe have broadly implemented PR/PI technology. At the same time, its long-term effects are not fully characterized. This is particularly important for neonates, who have the longest life expectancy of treated patients. If it is determined that certain patient groups, such as neonatal patients, should not receive large amounts of blood products with psoralens or other photoactivators, then hospital-based transfusion services have the challenge of operationalizing two inventories. The PIPPP study (Pathogen Inactivated Platelets use in Pediatric Patients: The International Experience) will query regional pediatric centers using PR/PI platelets about transfusion numbers, patient ages, adverse events, and transfusion reactions. The hope is that this study will bring to light a more expansive representation of PR/PI blood product usage in children and infants that is not represented in the available literature [266].

Future Directions

Neonatal transfusion practices remain highly variable across institutions due to a paucity of evidence-based guidelines. Cure and colleagues recently identified several key areas requiring additional research, including ideal parameters for assessing the need for transfusion beyond cell counts as well as markers for assessing transfusion efficacy and long-term outcomes, methods of gathering and compiling epidemiologic data on neonatal transfusions, and blood management strategies for neonates, especially with regard to safety of pathogen-inactivated products [267]. The authors propose that additional translational studies and clinical randomized controlled trials are needed to address these questions along with large, centralized repositories for collection and analysis of data. The NIH has recently launched REDS-IV-P (available online at https://bit.ly/34C 2WvU) to respond to many of the unanswered issues on neonatal and pediatric transfusion practice.

Summary of Key Points

- Leukoreduction, donor selection criteria, and improved infectious disease screening have contributed to a very safe blood supply. Pathogen reduction/inactivation may help address the threat of emerging diseases.
- Nevertheless, transfusions still carry infectious and non-infectious risks, and should therefore be administered carefully and judiciously. Rapid, large volume transfusions, in particular, can lead to metabolic derangements. Product modifications such as irradiation or volume reduction can help reduce the risks of certain complications.
- During all transfusions, patients must be closely monitored for signs and symptoms of transfusion reactions.
- Current neonatal transfusion practices are guided by the gestational age and clinical status of the patient, but remain highly variable across institutions due to lack of evidence-based studies for many blood components.
- Recent clinical trials have contributed toward understanding of neonatal transfusion triggers and clinical outcomes, but ongoing and future trials are needed for further clarification of

these parameters as well as identification of viable alternatives to blood products.

- Increasing availability of both plasma-derived and recombinant factor concentrates has led to replacement of plasma products in the treatment of certain clinical conditions and additional applications in the management of neonates on extracorporeal life support.

References

1. Ooley PW, ed. *Standards for Blood Banks and Transfusion Services*, 31st ed. (Bethesda, MD: AABB Press, 2018), p. 122.

2. Wong EC, Punzalan RC. Neonatal and pediatric transfusion practice. In Fung MK, ed. *Technical Manual of the American Association of Blood Banks* 19th ed. (Bethesda, MD: AABB Press, 2017) pp. 613–40.

3. Stockman JA, 3rd. Anemia of prematurity. Current concepts in the issue of when to transfuse. *Pediatr Clin North Am* 1986;**33**(1):111–28.

4. Wong EC, Roseff SD, King KE. *Pediatric Transfusion: A Physician's Handbook*, 4th ed. (Bethesda, MD: AABB Press, 2015).

5. Jakacka N, Snarski E, Mekuria. S. Prevention of iatrogenic anemia in critical and neonatal care. *Adv Clin Exp Med*, 2016;**25**(1):191–7.

6. Widness JA. Treatment and prevention of neonatal anemia. *NeoReviews* 2008;**9**(11):e526–33.

7. Del Vecchio A, Franco C, Petrillo F, D'Amato G. Neonatal transfusion practice: When do neonates need red blood cells or platelets? *Am J Perinatol* 2016;**33**(11):1079–84.

8. Bednarek FJ, Weisberger S, Richardson DK, et al. Variations in blood transfusions among newborn intensive care units. SNAP II Study Group. *J Pediatr* 1998;**133**(5):601–7.

9. Alverson DC. The physiologic impact of anemia in the neonate. *Clin Perinatol* 1995; **22**(3):609–25.

10. Ramasethu J, Luban NLC. Red cell transfusions in the newborn. *Semin Neonatol* 1999;**4**:5–16.

11. Pichler G, Wolf M, Roll C, et al. Recommendations to increase the validity and comparability of peripheral measurements by near infrared spectroscopy in neonates. 'Round table', section of haematology, oxygen transport and microcirculation, 48th annual meeting of ESPR, Prague 2007. *Neonatology* 2008;**94**(4):320–2.

12. Greisen G. Is near-infrared spectroscopy living up to its promises? *Semin Fetal Neonatal Med* 2006;**11** (6):498–502.

13. Strauss RG. How I transfuse red blood cells and platelets to infants with the anemia and

thrombocytopenia of prematurity. *Transfusion* 2008;48(2):209–17.

14. Kirpalani H, Whyte RK, Andersen C, et al. The Premature Infants in Need of Transfusion (PINT) study: A randomized, controlled trial of a restrictive (low) versus liberal (high) transfusion threshold for extremely low birth weight infants. *J Pediatr* 2006;**149**(3):301–7.

15. Bell EF, Strauss RG, Widness JA, et al. Randomized trial of liberal versus restrictive guidelines for red blood cell transfusion in preterm infants. *Pediatrics* 2005;**115**(6):1685–91.

16. Nopoulos PC, Conrad AL, Bell EF, et al. Long-term outcome of brain structure in premature infants: Effects of liberal vs restricted red blood cell transfusions. *Arch Pediatr Adolesc Med* 2011;**165**(5):443–50.

17. Whyte RK, Kirpalani H, Asztalos EV, et al. Neurodevelopmental outcome of extremely low birth weight infants randomly assigned to restrictive or liberal hemoglobin thresholds for blood transfusion. *Pediatrics* 2009;**123**(1):207–13.

18. Keir A, Pal S, Trivella M, et al. Adverse effects of red blood cell transfusions in neonates: A systematic review and meta-analysis. *Transfusion* 2016;**56**(11):2773–80.

19. Jain R, Jarosz C. Safety and efficacy of AS-1 red blood cell use in neonates. *Transfus Apher Sci* 2001;**24**(2):111–15.

20. Strauss RG, Burmeister LF, Johnson K, et al. Feasibility and safety of AS-3 red blood cells for neonatal transfusions. *J Pediatr* 2000;**136**(2):215–19.

21. Luban NL, Strauss RG, Hume HA. Commentary on the safety of red cells preserved in extended-storage media for neonatal transfusions. *Transfusion* 1991;**31**(3):229–35.

22. King KE, Shirey RS, Thomas SK, et al. Universal leukoreduction decreases the incidence of febrile nonhemolytic transfusion reactions to RBCs. *Transfusion* 2004;**44**(1):25–9.

23. Paglino JC, Pomper GJ, Fisch GS, et al. Reduction of febrile but not allergic reactions to RBCs and platelets after conversion to universal prestorage leukoreduction. *Transfusion* 2004;**44**(1):16–24.

24. Leukocyte reduction and ultraviolet B irradiation of platelets to prevent alloimmunization and refractoriness to platelet transfusions. The Trial to Reduce Alloimmunization to Platelets Study Group. *N Engl J Med* 1997;**337**(26):1861–9.

25. Paul DA, Leef KH, Locke RG, et al. Transfusion volume in infants with very low birth weight: A randomized trial of 10 versus 20 ml/kg. *J Pediatr Hematol Oncol* 2002;**24**(1):43–6.

26. Luban NL, Mikesell G, Sacher RA. Techniques for warming red blood cells packaged in different containers for neonatal use. *Clin Pediatr (Phila)* 1985;**24**(11):642–4.

27. Bandarenko N, King K, eds. Blood components. In *Blood Transfusion Therapy: A Physician's Handbook* (Bethesda, MD: AABB, 2017).

28. Luban NL. Massive transfusion in the neonate. *Transfus Med Rev* 1995;**9**(3):200–14.

29. Manno CS, Hedberg KW, Kim HC, et al. Comparison of the hemostatic effects of fresh whole blood, stored whole blood, and components after open heart surgery in children. *Blood* 1991;**77**(5):930–6.

30. Friesen RH, Perryman KM, Weigers KR, et al. A trial of fresh autologous whole blood to treat dilutional coagulopathy following cardiopulmonary bypass in infants. *Paediatr Anaesth* 2006;**16**(4):429–35.

31. Mou SS, Giroir BP, Moliter-Kirsch EA, et al. Fresh whole blood versus reconstituted blood for pump priming in heart surgery in infants. *N Engl J Med* 2004;**351**(16):1635–44.

32. Gruenwald CE, McCrindle BW, Crawford-Lean L, et al. Reconstituted fresh whole blood improves clinical outcomes compared with stored component blood therapy for neonates undergoing cardiopulmonary bypass for cardiac surgery: A randomized controlled trial. *J Thorac Cardiovasc Surg* 2008;**136**(6):1442–9.

33. Widness JA, Seward VJ, Kromer IJ, et al. Changing patterns of red blood cell transfusion in very low birth weight infants. *J Pediatr* 1996;**129**(5):680–7.

34. Strauss RG. Transfusion therapy in neonates. *Am J Dis Child* 1991;**145**(8):904–11.

35. Lee DA, Slagle TA, Jackson TM, et al. Reducing blood donor exposures in low birth weight infants by the use of older, unwashed packed red blood cells. *J Pediatr* 1995;**126**(2):280–6.

36. Strauss RG, Burmeister LF, Johnson K, et al. AS-1 red cells for neonatal transfusions: A randomized trial assessing donor exposure and safety. *Transfusion* 1996;**36**(10):873–8.

37. Goodstein MH, Locke RG, Wlodarcyzk D, et al. Comparison of two preservation solutions for erythrocyte transfusions in newborn infants. *J Pediatr* 1993;**123**(5):783–8.

38. Strauss RG, Villhauer PJ, Cordle DG. A method to collect, store and issue multiple aliquots of packed red blood cells for neonatal transfusions. *Vox Sang* 1995;**68**(2):77–81.

39. Chambers LA. Evaluation of a filter-syringe set for preparation of packed cell aliquots for neonatal transfusion. *Am J Clin Pathol* 1995;**104**(3):253–7.

40. Mangel J, Goldman M, Garcia C, et al. Reduction of donor exposures in premature infants by the use of designated adenine-saline preserved split red blood cell packs. *J Perinatol* 2001;**21**(6):363–7.

41. Liu EA, Mannino FL, Lane TA. Prospective, randomized trial of the safety and efficacy of a limited donor exposure transfusion program for premature neonates. *J Pediatr* 1994;**125**(1):92–6.

42. Baud O, Lacaze M, Masmonteil-Lion A, et al. Single blood donor exposure programme for preterm infants: A large open study and an analysis of the risk factors to multiple donor exposure. *Eur J Pediatr* 1998;**157**(7):579–82.

43. Wang-Rodriguez J, Mannino FL, Liu E, et al. A novel strategy to limit blood donor exposure and blood waste in multiply transfused premature infants. *Transfusion* 1996;**36**(1):64–70.

44. Fergusson DA, Hébert P, Hogan DL, et al. Effect of fresh red blood cell transfusions on clinical outcomes in premature, very low-birth-weight infants: The ARIPI randomized trial. *JAMA* 2012;**308**(14):1443–51.

45. Nickel RS, Josephson CD. Neonatal transfusion medicine: Five major unanswered research questions for the twenty-first century. *Clin Perinatol* 2015;**42**(3):499–513.

46. Lacroix J, Hébert P, Fergusson DA, et al. Age of transfused blood in critically ill adults. *N Engl J Med* 2015;**372**(15):1410–18.

47. Steiner ME, Ness PM, Assmann SF, et al. Effects of red-cell storage duration on patients undergoing cardiac surgery. *N Engl J Med* 2015;**372**(15):1419–29.

48. Dhabangi A, Ainomugisha B, Cserti-Gazdewich C, et al. Effect of transfusion of red blood cells with longer vs shorter storage duration on elevated blood lactate levels in children with Severe anemia: The TOTAL randomized clinical trial. *JAMA* 2015;**314**(23):2514–23.

49. Heddle NM, Cook RJ, Arnold DM, et al. Effect of short-term vs. long-term blood storage on mortality after transfusion. *N Engl J Med* 2016;**375**(20):1937–45.

50. Carson, JL, Guyatt G, Heddle NM, et al. Clinical practice guidelines from the AABB: Red blood cell transfusion thresholds and storage. *JAMA* 2016;**316**(19):2025–35.

51. Tobian AA, Heddle NM, Wiegmann TL, Carson JL. Red blood cell transfusion: 2016 clinical practice guidelines from AABB. *Transfusion* 2016;**56**(10):2627–30.

52. Strauss, RG, et al. Randomized trial assessing the feasibility and safety of biologic parents as RBC donors for their preterm infants. *Transfusion*, 2000;**40**(4):450–6.

53. Strauss RG, Barnes A Jr., Blanchette VS, et al. Directed and limited-exposure blood donations for infants and children. *Transfusion* 1990;**30**(1):68–72.

54. Jacquot C, Seo A, Miller PM, et al. Parental versus non-parental-directed donation: An 11-year experience of infectious disease testing at a pediatric tertiary care blood donor center. *Transfusion* 2017;**57**(11):2799–803.

55. Elbert C, Strauss RG, Barrett F, et al. Biological mothers may be dangerous blood donors for their neonates. *Acta Haematol* 1991;**85**(4):189–91.

56. Fasano R, Luban NL. Blood component therapy. *Pediatr Clin North Am* 2008;**55**(2):421–45, ix.

57. Mainie P. Is there a role for erythropoietin in neonatal medicine? *Early Hum Dev* 2008;**84**(8):525–32.

58. Shannon KM, Keith JF 3rd, Mentzer WC, et al. Recombinant human erythropoietin stimulates erythropoiesis and reduces erythrocyte transfusions in very low birth weight preterm infants. *Pediatrics* 1995;**95**(1):1–8.

59. Maier RF, Obladen M, Seigalla P, et al. The effect of epoetin beta (recombinant human erythropoietin) on the need for transfusion in very-low-birth-weight infants. European Multicentre Erythropoietin Study Group. *N Engl J Med* 1994;**330**(17):1173–8.

60. Meyer MP, et al. Recombinant human erythropoietin in the treatment of the anemia of prematurity: Results of a double-blind, placebo-controlled study. *Pediatrics* 1994;**93**(6 Pt 1):918–23.

61. Meyer MP, Sharma E, and Carsons M. Recombinant erythropoietin and blood transfusion in selected preterm infants. *Arch Dis Child Fetal Neonatal Ed* 2003;**88**(1):F41–5.

62. Ohls RK, Ehrenkranz RA, Wright LL, et al. Effects of early erythropoietin therapy on the transfusion requirements of preterm infants below 1250 grams birth weight: A multicenter, randomized, controlled trial. *Pediatrics* 2001;**108**(4):934–42.

63. Von Kohorn I, Ehrenkranz RA. Anemia in the preterm infant: Erythropoietin versus erythrocyte transfusion–it's not that simple. *Clin Perinatol* 2009;**36**(1):111–23.

64. Aher S, Ohlsson A. Late erythropoietin for preventing red blood cell transfusion in preterm and/or low birth weight infants. *Cochrane Database Syst Rev* 2006;**3**:CD004868.

65. Aher S, Ohlsson A. Early versus late erythropoietin for preventing red blood cell transfusion in preterm and/or low birth weight infants. *Cochrane Database Syst Rev* 2006;**3**:CD004865.

66. Ohlsson A, Aher SM. Early erythropoietin for preventing red blood cell transfusion in preterm and/or low birth weight infants. *Cochrane Database Syst Rev* 2006;**3**:CD004863.

67. Fischer HS, Reibel NJ, Bührer C, Dame C. Prophylactic early erythropoietin for neuroprotection in preterm infants: A meta-analysis. *Pediatrics* 2017;**139**(5):e20164317.

68. Luban NL. Management of anemia in the newborn. *Early Hum Dev* 2008;**84**(8):493–8.

69. Eichler H, Schaible T, Richter E, et al. Cord blood as a source of autologous RBCs for transfusion to preterm infants. *Transfusion* 2000;**40**(9):1111–17.

70. Imura K, Kawahara H, Kitayama Y, et al. Usefulness of cord-blood harvesting for autologous transfusion in surgical newborns with antenatal diagnosis of congenital anomalies. *J Pediatr Surg* 2001;**36**(6):851–4.

71. Brune T, Garritsen H, Hentschel R, et al. Efficacy, recovery, and safety of RBCs from autologous placental blood: Clinical experience in 52 newborns. *Transfusion* 2003;**43**(9):1210–16.

72. Garritsen HS, Brune T, Louwen F, et al. Autologous red cells derived from cord blood: Collection, preparation, storage and quality controls with optimal additive storage medium (Sag-mannitol). *Transfus Med* 2003;**13**(5):303–10.

73. Bifano EM, Dracker RA, Lorah K, et al. Collection and 28-day storage of human placental blood. *Pediatr Res* 1994;**36**(1 Pt 1):90–4.

74. Aladangady N, McHugh S, Aitchison TC, et al. Infants' blood volume in a controlled trial of placental transfusion at preterm delivery. *Pediatrics* 2006;**117**(1):93–8.

75. Rabe H, Reynolds G, Diaz-Rossello J. Early versus delayed umbilical cord clamping in preterm infants. *Cochrane Database Syst Rev* 2004;**4**: CD003248.

76. Rabe H, Reynolds G, Diaz-Rossello J. A systematic review and meta-analysis of a brief delay in clamping the umbilical cord of preterm infants. *Neonatology* 2008;**93**(2):138–44.

77. Hosono S, Mugishima H, Fujita H, et al. Umbilical cord milking reduces the need for red cell transfusions and improves neonatal adaptation in infants born at less than 29 weeks' gestation: A randomised controlled trial. *Arch Dis Child Fetal Neonatal Ed* 2008;**93**(1):F14–19.

78. Rabe H, Jewison A, Alvarez RF, et al. Milking compared with delayed cord clamping to increase placental transfusion in preterm neonates: A randomized controlled trial. *Obstet Gynecol* 2011;**117**(2 Pt 1):205–11.

79. Rabe H, Gyte GM, Díaz-Rossello JL, Duley L. Effect of timing of umbilical cord clamping and other strategies to influence placental transfusion at preterm birth on maternal and infant outcomes. *Cochrane Database Syst Rev* 2012;**8**: CD003248.

80. Christensen RD, Carroll PD, Josephson CD. Evidence-based advances in transfusion practice in neonatal intensive care units. *Neonatology* 2014;**106**(3):245–53.

81. Kc A, Rana N, Målqvist M, et al. Effects of delayed umbilical cord clamping vs early clamping on anemia in infants at 8 and 12 months: A randomized clinical trial. *JAMA Pediatr* 2017;**171**(3):264–70.

82. ACOG Committee on Obstetric Practice. Committee Opinion No. 684: Delayed umbilical cord clamping after birth. *Obstet Gynecol* 2017;**129** (1):e5–e10.

83. Osborn HH, Henry G, Wax P, et al. Theophylline toxicity in a premature neonate: Elimination kinetics of exchange transfusion. *J Toxicol Clin Toxicol* 1993;**31**(4):639–44.

84. Sancak R, Kucukoduk S, Tasdemir HA, et al. Exchange transfusion treatment in a newborn with phenobarbital intoxication. *Pediatr Emerg Care* 1999;**15**(4):268–70.

85. Lawe JE. Successful exchange transfusion of an infant for AIHA developing late in mother's pregnancy. *Transfusion* 1982;**22**(1):66–8.

86. Motta M, Cavazza A, Migliori C, Chirico G. Autoimmune haemolytic anaemia in a newborn infant. *Arch Dis Child Fetal Neonatal Ed* 2003;**88** (4):F341–2.

87. Lorch V, Jones FS, Hoersten IR. Treatment of hyperkalemia with exchange transfusion. *Transfusion* 1985;**25**(4):390–1.

88. Vemgal P, Ohlsson A. Interventions for non-oliguric hyperkalaemia in preterm neonates. *Cochrane Database Syst Rev* 2007;**1**:CD005257.

89. Mathur NB, Subramanian BK, Sharma VK, et al. Exchange transfusion in neutropenic septicemic neonates: Effect on granulocyte functions. *Acta Paediatr* 1993;**82**(11):939–43.

90. Alpay F, Sarici SU, Okutan V, et al. High-dose intravenous immunoglobulin therapy in neonatal immune haemolytic jaundice. *Acta Paediatr* 1999;**88**(2):216–19.

91. Mukhopadhyay K, Murki S, Narang A, et al. Intravenous immunoglobulins in rhesus hemolytic disease. *Indian J Pediatr* 2003;**70** (9):697–9.

92. Walsh SA, Yoa N, Khuffash A, et al. Efficacy of intravenous immunoglobulin in the management of haemolytic disease of the newborn. *Ir Med J* 2008;**101**(2):46–8.

93. Zwiers C, Scheffer-Rath ME, Lopriore E, de Haas M, Liley HG. Immunoglobulin for alloimmune hemolytic disease in neonates. *Cochrane Database Syst Rev* 2018;**3** CD003313.

94. Ip S, Chung M, Kulig J, et al. An evidence-based review of important issues concerning neonatal hyperbilirubinemia. *Pediatrics* 2004;**114**(1): e130–53.

95. Dash N, Kumar P, Sundaram V, Attri SV. Pre exchange albumin administration in neonates with hyperbilirubinemia: A randomized controlled trial. *Indian Pediatr* 2015. **52**(9):763–7.

96. Ramasethu J. Exchange transfusions. In MacDonald MG, Ramasethu R, eds. *Atlas of Procedures in Neonatology* (Philadelphia, PA: JB Lippincott, 2002).

97. van de Bor M, Benders MJ, Dorrepaal A, et al. Cerebral blood volume changes during exchange transfusions in infants born at or near term. *J Pediatr* 1994;**125**(4):617–21.

98. Patra K, Storfer-Isser A, Siner B, et al. Adverse events associated with neonatal exchange transfusion in the 1990s. *J Pediatr* 2004;**144** (5):626–31.

99. Chima RS, Johnson LH, Bhutani BK. Evaluation of adverse events due to exchange transfusions in term and near-term newborns (abstract). *Pediatric Research* 2001;**49**:324.

100. Steiner LA, Bizzarro MJ, Ehrenkranz RA, Gallagher PG. A decline in the frequency of neonatal exchange transfusions and its effect on exchange-related morbidity and mortality. *Pediatrics* 2007;**120**(1):27–32.

101. Chitty HE, Ziegler N, Savoia H, Doyle LW, Fox LM. Neonatal exchange transfusions in the 21st century: A single hospital study. *J Paediatr Child Health* 2013;**49**(10):825–32.

102. Werner EJ. Neonatal polycythemia and hyperviscosity. *Clin Perinatol* 1995;**22** (3):693–710.

103. Black VD, Lubchenco LO, Koops BL, et al. Neonatal hyperviscosity: Randomized study of effect of partial plasma exchange transfusion on long-term outcome. *Pediatrics* 1985;**75** (6):1048–53.

104. Delaney-Black V, Camp BW, Lubchenco LO, et al. Neonatal hyperviscosity association with lower achievement and IQ scores at school age. *Pediatrics* 1989;**83**(5):662–7.

105. Wong W, Fok TF, Lee CH, et al. Randomised controlled trial: Comparison of colloid or crystalloid for partial exchange transfusion for treatment of neonatal polycythaemia. *Arch Dis Child Fetal Neonatal Ed* 1997;**77**(2):F115–18.

106. Schimmel MS, Bromiker R, Soll RF. Neonatal polycythemia: Is partial exchange transfusion justified? *Clin Perinatol* 2004;**31**(3):545–53, ix-x.

107. Patil S, Saini SS, Kumar P, Shah R. Comparison of intra-procedural pain between a novel continuous arteriovenous exchange and conventional pull-push techniques of partial exchange transfusion in neonates: A randomized controlled trial. *J Perinatol* 2014;**34**(9):693–7.

108. Moise KJ Jr. Management of rhesus alloimmunization in pregnancy. *Obstet Gynecol* 2008;**112**(1):164–76.

109. Moise KJ Jr., Argoti PS. Management and prevention of red cell alloimmunization in pregnancy: A systematic review. *Obstet Gynecol* 2012;**120**(5):1132–9.

110. Zwiers, C, van der Bom JG, van Kamp IL, et al. Postponing early intrauterine transfusion with intravenous immunoglobulin treatment: The PETIT study on severe hemolytic disease of the fetus and newborn. *Am J Obstet Gynecol* 2018;**219** (3):291.e1–291.e9.

111. Zwiers C, van Kamp I, Oepkes D, Lopriore E. Intrauterine transfusion and non-invasive treatment options for hemolytic disease of the fetus and newborn: A review on current management and outcome. *Expert Rev Hematol* 2017;**10**(4):337–44.

112. Moise KJ. Red blood cell alloimmunization in pregnancy. *Semin Hematol* 2005;**42**(3):169–78.

113. Van Kamp IL, Klumper FJ, Oepkes D, et al. Complications of intrauterine intravascular transfusion for fetal anemia due to maternal red-cell alloimmunization. *Am J Obstet Gynecol* 2005;**192**(1):171–7.

114. Hallak M, Moise KJ Jr., Hesketh DE, et al. Intravascular transfusion of fetuses with rhesus incompatibility: Prediction of fetal outcome by changes in umbilical venous pressure. *Obstet Gynecol* 1992;**80**(2):286–90.

115. Lindenburg IT, van Kamp IL, Oepkes D. Intrauterine blood transfusion: Current indications and associated risks. *Fetal Diagn Ther* 2014;**36**(4):263–71.

116. Janssens HM, de Haan MJ, van Kamp IL, et al. Outcome for children treated with fetal intravascular transfusions because of severe blood group antagonism. *J Pediatr* 1997;**131** (3):373–80.

117. De Boer IP, Zeestraten EC, Lopriore E, et al. Pediatric outcome in Rhesus hemolytic disease treated with and without intrauterine transfusion. *Am J Obstet Gynecol* 2008;**198**(1):54 e1–4.

118. Oepkes D, Adama van Scheltema P. Intrauterine fetal transfusions in the management of fetal anemia and fetal thrombocytopenia. *Semin Fetal Neonatal Med* 2007;**12**(6):432–8.

119. Pacheco LD, Berkowitz RL, Moise KJ Jr., et al. Fetal and neonatal alloimmune thrombocytopenia: A management algorithm based on risk stratification. *Obstet Gynecol* 2011;**118**(5):1157–63.

120. Sola-Visner M, Sallmon H, Brown R. New insights into the mechanisms of nonimmune thrombocytopenia in neonates. *Semin Perinatol* 2009;**33**(1):43–51.

121. Andrew M, Vegh P, Caco C, et al. A randomized, controlled trial of platelet transfusions in thrombocytopenic premature infants. *J Pediatr* 1993;**123**(2):285–91.

122. Stanworth SJ, Clarke P, Watts T, et al. Prospective, observational study of outcomes in neonates with severe thrombocytopenia. *Pediatrics* 2009;**124**(5):e826–34.

123. Muthukumar P, Venkatesh V, Curley A, et al. Severe thrombocytopenia and patterns of bleeding in neonates: Results from a prospective observational study and implications for use of platelet transfusions. *Transfus Med* 2012;**22** (5):338–43.

124. von Lindern JS, Khodabux CM, Hack KE, et al. Long-term outcome in relationship to neonatal transfusion volume in extremely premature infants: A comparative cohort study. *BMC Pediatr* 2011;**11**:48.

125. Borges JP, dos Santos AM, da Cunha DH, et al. Restrictive guideline reduces platelet count thresholds for transfusions in very low birth weight preterm infants. *Vox Sang* 2013;**104** (3):207–13.

126. von Lindern JS, Hulzebos CV, Bos AF, et al. Thrombocytopaenia and intraventricular haemorrhage in very premature infants: A tale of two cities. *Arch Dis Child Fetal Neonatal Ed* 2012;**97**(5):F348–52.

127. Curley A, Stanworth SJ, Willoughby K, et al. Randomized trial of platelet-transfusion thresholds in neonates. *N Engl J Med* 2019;**380** (3):242–51.

128. Sparger KA, Assmann SF, Granger S, et al. Platelet transfusion practices among very-low-birth-weight infants. *JAMA Pediatr* 2016;**170** (7):687–94.

129. Kelton JG. Idiopathic thrombocytopenic purpura complicating pregnancy. *Blood Rev* 2002;**16** (1):43–6.

130. Payne SD, Resnik R, Moore TR, Hedriana HL, Kelly TF. Maternal characteristics and risk of severe neonatal thrombocytopenia and intracranial hemorrhage in pregnancies complicated by autoimmune thrombocytopenia. *Am J Obstet Gynecol* 1997;**177**(1):149–55.

131. van der Lugt NM, van Kampen A, Walther FJ, Brand A, Lopriore E. Outcome and management in neonatal thrombocytopenia due to maternal idiopathic thrombocytopenic purpura. *Vox Sang* 2013;**105**(3):236–43.

132. Roberts I, Stanworth S, Murray NA. Thrombocytopenia in the neonate. *Blood Rev* 2008;**22**(4):173–86.

133. Lieberman L, Greinacher A, Murphy MF, et al. Fetal and neonatal alloimmune thrombocytopenia: Recommendations for evidence-based practice, an international approach. *Br J Haematol* 2019;**185**(3):549–62.

134. Ghevaert C, Campbell K, Walton J, et al. Management and outcome of 200 cases of fetomaternal alloimmune thrombocytopenia. *Transfusion* 2007;**47**(5):901–10.

135. Roseff SD, Luban NL, Manno CS. Guidelines for assessing appropriateness of pediatric transfusion. *Transfusion* 2002;**42**(11):1398–413.

136. Angiolillo A, Luban NL. Hemolysis following an out-of-group platelet transfusion in an 8-month-old with Langerhans cell histiocytosis. *J Pediatr Hematol Oncol* 2004;**26**(4):267–9.

137. Cid J, Lozano M. Risk of Rh(D) alloimmunization after transfusion of platelets from D+ donors to D- recipients. *Transfusion* 2005;**45**(3):453; author reply 453–4.

138. Cid J, Lozano M, Ziman A, et al. Low frequency of anti-D alloimmunization following D+ platelet transfusion: The Anti-D Alloimmunization after D-incompatible Platelet Transfusions (ADAPT) study. *Br J Haematol* 2015;**168**(4):598–603.

139. Delaney M, Svensson AM, Lieberman L. Perinatal issues in transfusion practice. In Fung MK, ed. *Technical Manual of the American Association of Blood Banks*, 19th ed. (Bethesda, MD: AABB Press, 2017), pp. 599–612.

140. Kiefel V, Bassler D, Kroll H, et al. Antigen-positive platelet transfusion in neonatal alloimmune thrombocytopenia (NAIT). *Blood* 2006;**107**(9):3761–3.

141. Baker JM, Shehata N, Bussel J, et al. Postnatal intervention for the treatment of FNAIT:

A systematic review. *J Perinatol* 2019;**39** (10):1329–39.

142. Sidhu RS, Le T, Brimhall B, Thompson H. Study of coagulation factor activities in apheresed thawed fresh frozen plasma at 1–6 degrees C for five days. *J Clin Apher*, 2006;**21**(4):224–6.

143. Robitaille N, Hume HA. Blood components and fractionated plasma products: Preparations, indications, and administration. In Arceci RJ, Hann IM, Smith OP, eds. *Pediatric Hematology* (Malden, MA: Blackwell, 2006), pp. 693–706.

144. Hellstern P. Solvent/detergent-treated plasma: Composition, efficacy, and safety. *Curr Opin Hematol* 2004;**11**(5):346–50.

145. Riedler GF, Haycox AR, Duggan AK, Dakin HA. Cost-effectiveness of solvent/detergent-treated fresh-frozen plasma. *Vox Sang* 2003;**85**(2):88–95.

146. Keir AK, Stanworth SJ. Neonatal plasma transfusion: An evidence-based review. *Transfus Med Rev* 2016;**30**(4):174–82.

147. Acunas BA, Peakman M, Liossis G, et al. Effect of fresh frozen plasma and gammaglobulin on humoral immunity in neonatal sepsis. *Arch Dis Child Fetal Neonatal Ed* 1994;**70**(3):F182–7.

148. Desborough M, Sandu R, Brunskill SJ, et al. Fresh frozen plasma for cardiovascular surgery. *Cochrane Database Syst Rev* 2015;7:CD007614.

149. Fasano R, Luban NL. Blood component therapy. *Pediatr Clin North Am* 2008; 421–45, ix.

150. Carr R. Neutrophil production and function in newborn infants. *Br J Haematol* 2000;**110** (1):18–28.

151. Sandberg K, Fasth A, Berger A, et al. Preterm infants with low immunoglobulin G levels have increased risk of neonatal sepsis but do not benefit from prophylactic immunoglobulin G. *J Pediatr* 2000;**137**(5):623–8.

152. Price TH, Boeckh M, Harrison RW, et al. Efficacy of transfusion with granulocytes from G-CSF/dexamethasone-treated donors in neutropenic patients with infection. *Blood* 2015;**126** (18):2153–61.

153. Marfin AA, Price TH. Granulocyte transfusion therapy. *J Intensive Care Med* 2015;**30**(2):79–88.

154. Pammi M, Brocklehurst P. Granulocyte transfusions for neonates with confirmed or suspected sepsis and neutropenia. *Cochrane Database Syst Rev* 2011;10:CD003956.

155. Carr R, Modi N, Dore C. G-CSF and GM-CSF for treating or preventing neonatal infections. *Cochrane Database Syst Rev* 2003;3:CD003066.

156. Ohlsson A, Lacy JB. Intravenous immunoglobulin for suspected or proven infection in neonates. *Cochrane Database Syst Rev* 2015;3:CD001239.

157. Cairo MS, Worcester CC, Rucker RW, et al. Randomized trial of granulocyte transfusions versus intravenous immune globulin therapy for neonatal neutropenia and sepsis. *J Pediatr* 1992;**120**(2 Pt 1):281–5.

158. Mohan P, Brocklehurst P. Granulocyte transfusions for neonates with confirmed or suspected sepsis and neutropaenia. *Cochrane Database Syst Rev* 2003;4:CD003956.

159. O'Connor JC, Strauss RG, Goeken NE, Knox LB. A near-fatal reaction during granulocyte transfusion of a neonate. *Transfusion* 1988;**28** (2):173–6.

160. Zylberberg R, Schott RJ, Fort J, Roberts J, Friedman R. Sudden death following white cell transfusion in a premature infant. *J Perinatol*, 1987;**7**(2):90–2.

161. Dutcher JP, Kendall J, Norris D, et al. Granulocyte transfusion therapy and amphotericin B: Adverse reactions? *Am J Hematol* 1989;**31**(2):102–8.

162. Freidman DF, Montenegro LM. Extracorporeal membrane oxygenation and cardiopulmonary bypass. In Hillyer CD, Strauss RG, Luban NL, eds. *Handbook of Pediatric Transfusion Medicine* (London: Elsevier Academic Press, 2004), pp. 181–9.

163. Dalton HJ, Reeder R, Garcia-Filion P, et al. Factors associated with bleeding and thrombosis in children receiving extracorporeal membrane oxygenation. *Am J Respir Crit Care Med* 2017;**196** (6):762–71.

164. Thomas J, Kostousov V, Teruya J. Bleeding and thrombotic complications in the use of extracorporeal membrane oxygenation. *Semin Thromb Hemost* 2018;**44**(1):20–9.

165. Mok YH, Lee JH, Cheifetz IM. Neonatal extracorporeal membrane oxygenation: Update on management strategies and long-term outcomes. *Adv Neonatal Care* 2016;**16**(1):26–36.

166. Sawyer AA, Wise L, Ghosh S, Bhatia J, Stansfield BK. Comparison of transfusion thresholds during neonatal extracorporeal membrane oxygenation. *Transfusion* 2017;**57** (9):2115–20.

167. Bjerke HS, Kelly RE Jr., Foglia RP, Barcliff L, Petz L. Decreasing transfusion exposure risk during extracorporeal membrane oxygenation (ECMO). *Transfus Med* 1992;**2**(1):43–9.

168. Wong TE, Delaney M, Gernsheimer T, et al. Antithrombin concentrates use in children on extracorporeal membrane oxygenation:

A retrospective cohort study. *Pediatr Crit Care Med* 2015;**16**(3):264–9.

169. Todd Tzanetos DR, Myers J, Wells T, et al. The use of recombinant antithrombin III in pediatric and neonatal ECMO patients. *ASAIO J* 2017;**63**(1):93–8.

170. Punzalan RC, Gottschall JL. Use and future investigations of recombinant and plasma-derived coagulation and anticoagulant products in the neonate. *Transfus Med Rev* 2016;**30**(4):189–96.

171. DeYoung Sullivan K, Vu T, Richardson G, Castillo E, Martinez F. Evaluating the frequency of vital sign monitoring during blood transfusion: An evidence-based practice initiative. *Clin J Oncol Nurs* 2015;**19**(5):516–20.

172. Kennedy LD, Case LD, Hurd DD, Cruz JM, Pomper GJ. A prospective, randomized, double-blind controlled trial of acetaminophen and diphenhydramine pretransfusion medication versus placebo for the prevention of transfusion reactions. *Transfusion* 2008;**48**(11):2285–91.

173. Sanders RP, Maddirala SD, Geiger TL, et al. Premedication with acetaminophen or diphenhydramine for transfusion with leucoreduced blood products in children. *Br J Haematol* 2005;**130**(5):781–7.

174. Vamvakas EC. Allergic and anaphylactic reactions. In Popovsky MA, ed. *Transfusion Reactions* 3rd ed. (Bethesda, MD: AABB Press, 2007), pp. 105–56.

175. Shimada E, Tadokoro K, Watanabe Y, et al. Anaphylactic transfusion reactions in haptoglobin-deficient patients with IgE and IgG haptoglobin antibodies. *Transfusion* 2002;**42**(6):766–73.

176. Cohn CS, Stubbs J, Schwartz J, et al. A comparison of adverse reaction rates for PAS C versus plasma platelet units. *Transfusion* 2014;**54**(8):1927–34.

177. Kojima S, Yanagisawa R, Tanaka M, Nakazawa Y, Shimodaira S. Comparison of administration of platelet concentrates suspended in M-sol or BRS-A for pediatric patients. *Transfusion* 2018;**58**(12):2952–8.

178. Wong EC, Luban NL, *Hazards of transfusion*. In Hann IM, Arceci RJ, Smith OP, eds. *Pediatric Hematology* (Malden, MA: Blackwell Publishing, 2006), pp. 724–44.

179. Strauss RG, Cordle DG, Quijana J, Goeken NE. Comparing alloimmunization in preterm infants after transfusion of fresh unmodified versus stored leukocyte-reduced red blood cells. *J Pediatr Hematol Oncol* 1999;**21**(3):224–30.

180. Turkmen T, Qiu D, Cooper N, et al. Red blood cell alloimmunization in neonates and children up to 3 years of age. *Transfusion* 2017;**57**(11):2720–6.

181. Ramasethu J, Luban N. T activation. *Br J Haematol* 2001;**112**(2):259–63.

182. Fasano RM, Paul WM, Pisciotto PT. Complications of neonatal transfusion. In Popovsky MA, ed. *Transfusion Reactions* 4th ed. (Bethesda, MD: AABB Press, 2012) pp. 471–518.

183. Roseff SD. Cryptantigens: Time to uncover the real significance of T-activation. *Transfusion* 2017;**57**(11):2553–7.

184. Holman P, Blajchman MA, Heddle N. Noninfectious adverse effects of blood transfusion in the neonate. *Transfus Med Rev* 1995;**9**(3):277–87.

185. Miller MA, Schlueter AJ. Transfusions via hand-held syringes and small-gauge needles as risk factors for hyperkalemia. *Transfusion* 2004;**44**(3):373–81.

186. Jackman RP, Deng X, Bolgiano D, et al. Leukoreduction and ultraviolet treatment reduce both the magnitude and the duration of the HLA antibody response. *Transfusion* 2014;**54**(3):672–80.

187. Fergusson D, Hébert PC, Lee SK, et al. Clinical outcomes following institution of universal leukoreduction of blood transfusions for premature infants. *JAMA* 2003;**289**(15):1950–6.

188. Crawford TM, Andersen CC, Hodyl NA, Robertson SA, Stark MJ. The contribution of red blood cell transfusion to neonatal morbidity and mortality. *J Paediatr Child Health* 2019;**55**(4):387–92.

189. Muszynski JA, Spinella PC, Cholette JM, et al. Transfusion-related immunomodulation: Review of the literature and implications for pediatric critical illness. *Transfusion* 2017;**57**(1):195–206.

190. Sanchez R, Toy P. Transfusion related acute lung injury: A pediatric perspective. *Pediatr Blood Cancer* 2005;**45**(3):248–55.

191. Kopko PM and Popovsky MA. Transfusion related acute lung injury. In Popovsky MA, ed. *Transfusion Reactions*, (Bethesda, MD: AABB Press, 2007), pp. 207–28.

192. Yang X, Ahmed S, Chandrasekaran V. Transfusion-related acute lung injury resulting from designated blood transfusion between mother and child: A report of two cases. *Am J Clin Pathol* 2004;**121**(4):590–2.

193. De Cloedt, L, Savy N, Gauvin F, et al. Transfusion-associated circulatory overload in

ICUs: A scoping review of incidence, risk factors, and outcomes. *Crit Care Med* 2019;**47**(6):849–56.

194. Pendergrast J, Armali C, Cserti-Gazdewich C, et al. Can furosemide prevent transfusion-associated circulatory overload? Results of a pilot, double-blind, randomized controlled trial. *Transfusion* 2019;**59**(6):1997–2006.

195. Flidel O, Barak Y, Lifschitz-Mercer B, Frumkin A, Mogilner BM. Graft versus host disease in extremely low birth weight neonate. *Pediatrics* 1992;**89**(4 Pt 1):689–90.

196. Funkhouser AW, Vogelsang G, Zehnbauer B, et al. Graft versus host disease after blood transfusions in a premature infant. *Pediatrics*, 1991;**87**(2):247–50.

197. Sanders MR, Graeber JE. Posttransfusion graft-versus-host disease in infancy. *J Pediatr* 1990;**117**(1 Pt 1):159–63.

198. Strauss RG. Data-driven blood banking practices for neonatal RBC transfusions. *Transfusion* 2000;**40**(12):1528–40.

199. Delaney M. How I reduce the risk of missed irradiation transfusion events in children. *Transfusion* 2018;**58**(11):2517–21.

200. Davey RJ, McCoy NC, Yu M, et al. The effect of prestorage irradiation on posttransfusion red cell survival. *Transfusion* 1992;**32**(6):525–8.

201. Josephson CD, Wesolowski A, Bao G, et al. Do red cell transfusions increase the risk of necrotizing enterocolitis in premature infants? *J Pediatr* 2010;**157**(6): 972–8, e1–3.

202. Blau J, Calo JM, Dozor D, et al. Transfusion-related acute gut injury: Necrotizing enterocolitis in very low birth weight neonates after packed red blood cell transfusion. *J Pediatr* 2011;**158**(3):403–9.

203. Paul DA, Mackley A, Novitsky A, et al. Increased odds of necrotizing enterocolitis after transfusion of red blood cells in premature infants. *Pediatrics* 2011;**127**(4):635–41.

204. Baxi AC, Josephson CD, Iannucci GJ, Mahle WT. Necrotizing enterocolitis in infants with congenital heart disease: The role of red blood cell transfusions. *Pediatr Cardiol* 2014;**35**(6):1024–9.

205. Singh R, Visintainer PF, Frantz ID 3rd, et al. Association of necrotizing enterocolitis with anemia and packed red blood cell transfusions in preterm infants. *J Perinatol* 2011;**31**(3):176–82.

206. Kirpalani H, Zupancic JA. Do transfusions cause necrotizing enterocolitis? The complementary role of randomized trials and observational studies. *Semin Perinatol* 2012;**36**(4):269–76.

207. Garg P, Pinotti R, Lal CV, Salas AA. Transfusion-associated necrotizing enterocolitis in preterm infants: An updated meta-analysis of observational data. *J Perinat Med* 2018;**46**(6):677–85.

208. Patel RM, Knezevic A, Shenvi N, et al. Association of red blood cell transfusion, anemia, and necrotizing enterocolitis in very low-birth-weight infants. *JAMA* 2016;**315**(9):889–97.

209. Marin T, Patel RM, Roback JD, et al. Does red blood cell irradiation and/or anemia trigger intestinal injury in premature infants with birth weight</= 1250 g? An observational birth cohort study. *BMC Pediatr* 2018;**18**(1):270.

210. Pisciotto PT, Luban NLC. Complications of neonatal transfusion. In Popovsky MA, ed. *Transfusion Reactions*, (Bethesda, MD: AABB Press, 2007), pp. 459–500.

211. Yigit S, Gursoy T, Kanra T, et al. Whole blood versus red cells and plasma for exchange transfusion in ABO haemolytic disease. *Transfus Med* 2005;**15**(4):313–18.

212. Jackson JC. Adverse events associated with exchange transfusion in healthy and ill newborns. *Pediatrics* 1997;**99**(5):E7.

213. Lee AC, Reduque LL, Luban NL, et al. Transfusion-associated hyperkalemic cardiac arrest in pediatric patients receiving massive transfusion. *Transfusion* 2014;**54**(1):244–54.

214. Shaz BH, Grima K, Hillyer CD 2-(Diethylhexyl) phthalate in blood bags: Is this a public health issue? *Transfusion* 2011;**51**(11):2510–17.

215. Mallow EB, Fox MA. Phthalates and critically ill neonates: Device-related exposures and non-endocrine toxic risks. *J Perinatol* 2014;**34**(12):892–7.

216. Sampson J, de Korte D. DEHP-plasticised PVC: Relevance to blood services. *Transfus Med*, 2011;**21**(2):73–83.

217. Jaimes R 3rd, Swiercz A, Sherman M, Muselimyan N, Marvar PJ, Posnack NG. Plastics and cardiovascular health: phthalates may disrupt heart rate variability and cardiovascular reactivity. Am J Physiol Heart Circ Physiol. 2017 Nov 1;**313**(5):H1044-H1053.

218. Snyder EL, Hedberg SL, Napychank PA, et al. Stability of red cell antigens and plasma coagulation factors stored in a non-diethylhexyl phthalate-plasticized container. *Transfusion* 1993;**33**(6):515–19.

219. van der Meer PF, Devine DV, Biomedical Excellence for Safer Transfusion (BEST) Collaborative. Alternatives in blood operations when choosing non-DEHP bags. *Vox Sang* 2017;**112**(2):183–4.

220. Katz L, Dodd R. Transfusion-transmitted diseases. In Shaz BH, Hillyer CD, Roshal M, Abrams CS, eds. *Transfusion Medicine and Hemostasis: Clinical and Laboratory Aspects*, 2nd ed. (London: Elsevier, 2013).

221. Jacquot C, Delaney M. Efforts toward elimination of infectious agents in blood products. *J Intensive Care Med* 2018;33(10):543–50.

222. Stramer SL, Galel SA. Infectious disease screening. In Fung MK ed. *Technical Manual of the American Association of Blood Banks* 18th ed. (Bethesda, MD: AABB Press, 2017), pp. 161–205.

223. Williamson PC, Linnen JM, Kessler DA, et al. First cases of Zika virus-infected US blood donors outside states with areas of active transmission. *Transfusion* 2017;57(3pt2):770–8.

224. Lieb LE, Mundy TM, Goldfinger D, et al. Unrecognized human immunodeficiency virus type 1 infection in a cohort of transfused neonates: A retrospective investigation. *Pediatrics*, 1995;95(5):717–21.

225. Zou S, Dorsey KA, Notari EP, et al. Prevalence, incidence, and residual risk of human immunodeficiency virus and hepatitis C virus infections among United States blood donors since the introduction of nucleic acid testing. *Transfusion* 2010;50(7):1495–504.

226. Schillie S, Walker T, Veselsky S, et al. Outcomes of infants born to women infected with hepatitis B. *Pediatrics* 2015;135(5):e1141–7.

227. Seeff LB, Hollinger FB, Alter HJ, et al. Long-term mortality and morbidity of transfusion-associated non-A, non-B, and type C hepatitis: A National Heart, Lung, and Blood Institute collaborative study. *Hepatology* 2001;33(2):455–63.

228. Casiraghi MA, De Paschale M, Romanò L, et al. Long-term outcome (35 years) of hepatitis C after acquisition of infection through mini transfusions of blood given at birth. *Hepatology* 2004;39(1):90–6.

229. Luban NL, Colvin CA, Mohan P, Alter HJ. The epidemiology of transfusion-associated hepatitis C in a children's hospital. *Transfusion* 2007;47(4):615–20.

230. Goodman ZD, Makhlouf HR, Liu L, et al. Pathology of chronic hepatitis C in children: Liver biopsy findings in the Peds-C Trial. *Hepatology* 2008;47(3):836–43.

231. Karnsakul W, Schwarz KB. Management of hepatitis C infection in children in the era of direct-acting antiviral agents. *J Viral Hepat* 2019;26(9):1034–9.

232. Bowden RA, Slichter SJ, Sayers M, et al. A comparison of filtered leukocyte-reduced and cytomegalovirus (CMV) seronegative blood products for the prevention of transfusion-associated CMV infection after marrow transplant. *Blood* 1995;86(9):3598–603.

233. Josephson CD, Caliendo AM, Easley KA, et al. Blood transfusion and breast milk transmission of cytomegalovirus in very-low-birth-weight infants: A prospective cohort study. *JAMA Pediatr* 2014;168(11):1054–62.

234. Strauss RG. Optimal prevention of transfusion-transmitted cytomegalovirus (TTCMV) infection by modern leukocyte reduction alone: CMV sero/antibody-negative donors needed only for leukocyte products. *Transfusion* 2016;56(8):1921–4.

235. Goldfinger D, Burner JD. You can't get CMV from a blood transfusion: 2017 Emily Cooley award lecture. *Transfusion* 2018;58(12):3038–43.

236. AABB, Clinical Transfusion Medicine Committee, Heddle NM, Boeckh M, et al. AABB Committee Report: Reducing transfusion-transmitted cytomegalovirus infections. *Transfusion* 2016;56(6 Pt 2):1581–7.

237. Stramer SL, Fang CT, Foster GA, et al. West Nile virus among blood donors in the United States, 2003 and 2004. *N Engl J Med* 2005;353(5):451–9.

238. Busch MP, Bloch EM, Kleinman S. Prevention of transfusion-transmitted infections. *Blood* 2019;133(17):1854–64.

239. O'Leary DR, Kuhn S, Kniss KL, et al. Birth outcomes following West Nile virus infection of pregnant women in the United States: 2003–2004. *Pediatrics* 2006;117(3):e537–45.

240. Plourde AR, Bloch EM. A literature review of zika virus. *Emerg Infect Dis* 2016;22(7):1185–92.

241. Shirley DT, Nataro JP. Zika virus infection. *Pediatr Clin North Am* 2017;64(4):937–51.

242. Simonsen KA, Harwell JI, Lainwala S. Clinical presentation and treatment of transfusion-associated babesiosis in premature infants. *Pediatrics* 2011;128(4):e1019–24.

243. Glanternik JR, Baine IL, Rychalsky MR, et al. A cluster of cases of Babesia microti among neonates traced to a single unit of donor blood. *Pediatr Infect Dis J* 2018;37(3):269–71.

244. Moritz ED, Winton CS, Tonnetti L, et al. Screening for Babesia microti in the US blood supply. *N Engl J Med* 2016;375(23):2236–45.

245. Goodell AJ, Bloch EM, Krause PJ, Custer B. Costs, consequences, and cost-effectiveness of strategies for Babesia microti donor screening of the US blood supply. *Transfusion* 2014;54(9):2245–57.

246. Ward SJ, Stramer SL, Szczepiorkowski ZM. Assessing the risk of Babesia to the United States blood supply using a risk-based decision-making

approach: Report of AABB's Ad Hoc Babesia Policy Working Group (original report). *Transfusion* 2018;**58**(8):1916–23.

247. Prowse CV. Component pathogen inactivation: A critical review. *Vox Sang* 2013;**104**(3):183–99.

248. Kleinman S, Stassinopoulos A. Risks associated with red blood cell transfusions: Potential benefits from application of pathogen inactivation. *Transfusion* 2015;**55**(12):2983–3000.

249. Cid J. Prevention of transfusion-associated graft-versus-host disease with pathogen-reduced platelets with amotosalen and ultraviolet A light: A review. *Vox Sang* 2017;**112**(7):607–13.

250. Hess JR, Pagano MB, Barbeau JD, Johannson PI. Will pathogen reduction of blood components harm more people than it helps in developed countries? *Transfusion* 2016;**56**(5):1236–41.

251. Kaiser-Guignard J, Canellini G, Lion N, et al. The clinical and biological impact of new pathogen inactivation technologies on platelet concentrates. *Blood Rev* 2014;**28**(6):235–41.

252. Ciaravino V, McCullough T, Cimino G. The role of toxicology assessment in transfusion medicine. *Transfusion* 2003;**43**(10):1481–92.

253. Musso D, Richard V, Broult J, Cao-Lormeau VM. Inactivation of dengue virus in plasma with amotosalen and ultraviolet A illumination. *Transfusion* 2014;**54**(11):2924–30.

254. Irsch J, Seghatchian J. Update on pathogen inactivation treatment of plasma, with the INTERCEPT Blood System: Current position on methodological, clinical and regulatory aspects. *Transfus Apher Sci* 2015;**52**(2):240–4.

255. Hauser L, Roque-Afonso AM, Beylouné A, et al. Hepatitis E transmission by transfusion of Intercept blood system-treated plasma. *Blood* 2014;**123**(5):796–7.

256. Schmidt M, Hourfar MK, Sireis W, et al. Evaluation of the effectiveness of a pathogen inactivation technology against clinically relevant transfusion-transmitted bacterial strains. *Transfusion* 2015;**55**(9):2104–12.

257. Knutson F, Osselaer J, Pierelli L, et al. A prospective, active haemovigilance study with combined cohort analysis of 19,175 transfusions of platelet components prepared with amotosalen-UVA photochemical treatment. *Vox Sang* 2015;**109**(4):343–52.

258. Cardo LJ, Salata J, Mendez J, Reddy H, Goodrich R. Pathogen inactivation of Trypanosoma cruzi in plasma and platelet concentrates using riboflavin and ultraviolet light. *Transfus Apher Sci* 2007;**37**(2):131–7.

259. Goodrich RP, Edrich RA, Li J, Seghatchian J. The Mirasol PRT system for pathogen reduction of platelets and plasma: An overview of current status and future trends. *Transfus Apher Sci* 2006;**35**(1):5–17.

260. Perez-Pujol S, Tonda R, Lozano M, et al. Effects of a new pathogen-reduction technology (Mirasol PRT) on functional aspects of platelet concentrates. *Transfusion* 2005;**45**(6):911–19.

261. Tonnetti L, Proctor MC, Reddy HL, Goodrich RP, Leiby DA. Evaluation of the Mirasol pathogen [corrected] reduction technology system against Babesia microti in apheresis platelets and plasma. *Transfusion* 2010;**50**(5):1019–27.

262. Aubry M, Richard V, Green J, Broult J, Musso D Inactivation of Zika virus in plasma with amotosalen and ultraviolet A illumination. *Transfusion* 2016;**56**(1):33–40.

263. Butler C, Doree C, Estcourt LJ, et al. Pathogen-reduced platelets for the prevention of bleeding. *Cochrane Database Syst Rev* 2013;(3):CD009072.

264. Amato M, Schennach H, Astl M, et al. Impact of platelet pathogen inactivation on blood component utilization and patient safety in a large Austrian Regional Medical Centre. *Vox Sang* 2017;**112**(1):47–55.

265. Hubbard T, Backholer L, Wiltshire M, Cardigan R, Ariëns RA. Effects of riboflavin and amotosalen photoactivation systems for pathogen inactivation of fresh-frozen plasma on fibrin clot structure. *Transfusion* 2016;**56**(1):41–8.

266. Jacquot C, Delaney M. Pathogen-inactivated blood products for pediatric patients: Blood safety, patient safety, or both? *Transfusion* 2018;**58**(9):2095–101.

267. Cure P, Bembea M, Chou S, et al. 2016 proceedings of the National Heart, Lung, and Blood Institute's scientific priorities in pediatric transfusion medicine. *Transfusion* 2017;**57**(6):1568–81.

268. US FDA. Recommendations for reducing the risk of transfusion-transmitted babesiosis: guidance for industry. US Department of Health and Human Services Food and Drug Administration Center for Biologics Evaluation and Research. 2019. Available online at www.fda.gov/media/114847/download.

269. Hong H, Xiao W, Lazarus HM, et al. Detection of septic transfusion reactions to platelet transfusions by active and passive surveillance. *Blood* 2016;**127**(4):496–502.

270. Stramer SL, Notari EP, Krysztof DE, Dodd RY. Hepatitis B virus testing by minipool nucleic acid testing: Does it improve blood safety? *Transfusion* 2013;**53**(10 Pt 2):2449–58.

Chapter 21

Neonatal Leukemia

Erin M. Guest, Catherine Garnett, Irene Roberts, and Alan S. Gamis

Introduction

Leukemia in the neonatal period is very rare and can present as early as the day of birth [1, 2]. Acute leukemia arises from clonal changes in hematopoietic precursor cells. In neonatal leukemia, defined as leukemia presenting in the first month after birth, these clonal abnormalities initiate during fetal development [3]. A backtracking molecular study of infants and young children who developed leukemia beyond the neonatal period demonstrated that the same clonal mutations found in the leukemia were also present in neonatal blood spots [4]. Though some epidemiologic studies have suggested that maternal intake of certain foods may contribute, the genetic and environmental risk factors for infant leukemia are not well understood [5–7]. One exception is the observation that an identical twin of an infant with acute lymphoblastic leukemia has a nearly 100% chance of developing the same type of leukemia [8, 9]. In contrast, the genetic risk factors associated with myeloproliferative neoplasms among neonates are better defined [10]. Neonates with Down syndrome are at risk of transient myeloproliferative disorder (TMD) [11] and neonates with Noonan syndrome or related Ras pathway disorders may present with juvenile myelomonocytic leukemia (JMML) [10]. Both TMD and JMML have the potential to be serious and life-threatening. Recognition of the presenting features of neonatal leukemia is important, as early initiation of therapy may prevent rapid progression of disease.

Acute Lymphoblastic Leukemia

The incidence of acute lymphoblastic leukemia (ALL) in infants under 1 year of age is 2.1 cases per 100,000 age-adjusted US population, or about 100 cases per year in the US [12]. ALL is slightly more common among female infants with a female to male ratio of 1.6:1 [12]. Age less than 3 months at diagnosis, rearrangement of the *KMT2A* gene (*KMT2A*-r) on chromosome 11q23, hyperleukocytosis at presentation, and poor response to prednisone therapy are adverse prognostic factors [13–16]. Congenital ALL diagnosed in the first month of life accounts for a minority of cases and is associated with a poor prognosis, with less than 20% overall survival [17].

A hallmark feature of infant ALL is extreme hyperleukocytosis. The white blood cell (WBC) count is typically above 100,000/μL and may be greater than 1,000,000/μL, with lymphoblasts representing the majority of nucleated cells. Alternatively, the leukemia may be of ambiguous lineage, with features of both lymphoblasts and myeloblasts, and therefore is thought to be derived from a very early multipotent hematopoietic precursor cell. Anemia and thrombocytopenia result from poor bone marrow production of other cell lineages. Hepatomegaly and splenomegaly, secondary to infiltration by lymphoblasts, may be associated with liver dysfunction, massive abdominal enlargement, and respiratory insufficiency. Infants with ALL may be lethargic and hemodynamically unstable at presentation, secondary to poor cerebral vascular flow, electrolyte abnormalities, hypoglycemia, or other metabolic derangements. Tumor lysis syndrome, acute renal failure, and disseminated intravascular coagulation (DIC) are oncologic emergencies associated with new onset neonatal ALL. Central nervous system involvement with leukemia, in the form of bulging fontanelle, papilledema, seizures,

Neonatal Hematology, Pathogenesis, Diagnosis, and Management of Hematologic Problems, 3rd edition, ed. Pedro A. de Alarcón, Eric J. Werner, Robert D. Christensen, and Martha C. Sola-Visner. Published by Cambridge University Press. © Cambridge University Press 2021.

cranial nerve palsies, or lymphoblasts detected in the cerebrospinal fluid, is common in infants with ALL. Skin infiltration, known as leukemia cutis, is also common and appears as blue to purple, nontender nodules scattered over the scalp, face, trunk, and extremities. It may be mistaken for excessive bruising and sometimes is the chief complaint that prompts initial evaluation.

The evaluation of a neonate with suspected ALL should include assessment for acute problems requiring immediate intervention (Table 21.1). The diagnosis of ALL is generally apparent by clinical presentation and peripheral blood analysis, but a bone marrow aspirate is helpful to obtain adequate material for cytogenetic studies. If the patient is too unstable to undergo a bone marrow procedure, then peripheral blood may be substituted for all of the necessary diagnostic studies. A lumbar puncture for cerebrospinal fluid testing and administration of intrathecal

Table 21.1 Evaluation of neonates with suspected leukemia

Evaluation
History and physical with particular attention to neurological status, cranial nerve deficits, and leukemia cutis
Check for dysmorphism suggestive of Down syndrome or Noonan syndrome
Complete blood count, differential, morphology by peripheral blood smear
Peripheral blood cytogenetics or FISH for trisomy 21 if Down syndrome suspected
Basic metabolic profile, serum phosphorus
Hepatic function panel
Lactate dehydrogenase
Uric acid level
Prothrombin time, partial thromboplastin time, fibrinogen
Blood group/type and alloantibody screen
Blood culture if fever or other signs of sepsis
Bone marrow aspirate for morphologic, flow cytometric, cytogenetic, and molecular testing*
Cerebrospinal fluid assessment for leukemic blasts**
Consider CXR, abdominal USS and/or echocardiogram to assess for effusions/ascites
Genetic testing: GATA1 mutation analysis if TMD suspected; RAS pathway gene mutation analysis if Noonan syndrome, NF1 and/or JMML suspected

*May substitute peripheral blood if patient is too unstable to undergo a bone marrow procedure

**Instill intrathecal chemotherapy during diagnostic lumbar puncture

chemotherapy should be completed prior to the initiation of systemic chemotherapy. Leukemic infiltrates may be seen on a biopsy of a skin nodule, but skin biopsy is not necessary if the diagnosis is established by other means and the rash is typical of leukemia cutis.

Initial stabilization measures may include intravenous hydration, respiratory support with supplemental oxygen or mechanical ventilation, and pressor support. If the neonate is hemodynamically or neurologically unstable and has hyperleukocytosis with WBC count >100,000/μL then corticosteroid therapy should be initiated promptly and a cytoreductive procedure such as manual whole blood exchange or leukapheresis should be considered on a case-by-case basis [18, 19]. The goal of early intervention is to reduce the hyperviscosity associated with hyperleukocytosis and minimize end organ damage. Corticosteroid therapy is the mainstay of anti-leukemia induction therapy. Methylprednisolone or prednisone is given as single agent therapy for up to 7 days prior to cytotoxic chemotherapy [20]. Blood product transfusions should be given to support the hemodynamic status and correct DIC. Caution should be used because cellular blood products may further increase blood viscosity and risk cerebrovascular events. Platelet transfusions may accelerate DIC. Allopurinol should be started to prevent excess uric acid formation. If the uric acid is elevated and/or if the patient has acute renal dysfunction then administration of rasburicase, a recombinant urate-oxidase enzyme, is necessary to prevent irreversible renal damage. Even in the absence of elevated uric acid or serum creatinine, rasburicase should be considered to prevent tumor lysis syndrome with the initiation of corticosteroid therapy. It is important to note that rasburicase is contraindicated in patients with known glucose-6-phosphate dehydrogenase (G6PD) deficiency as it can precipitate severe acute hemolysis. Once the patient is stable, large bore central lines such as pheresis catheters should be removed as soon as possible to avoid catheter-associated thrombosis.

Treatment of neonatal ALL involves corticosteroid therapy and multi-agent cytotoxic chemotherapy. The total duration of therapy is typically 2 years for both boys and girls. Induction therapy lasts for 5 weeks and is a high risk time period for complications, including toxic mortality [21–23]. Invasive infections are particularly problematic among infants undergoing myelosuppressive therapy. Unfortunately, clinical trials have consistently demonstrated that adding more chemotherapy leads to increased toxicities without improving survival outcomes [24, 25]. The majority of infants enter into a temporary remission, followed by early relapse within 1–2 years. Relapsed infant ALL is quite chemoresistant and carries a very poor prognosis [26]. Hematopoietic stem cell transplant (HSCT) can be curative in first remission or following relapse, but is associated with a high mortality rate and many infants still experience relapse post HSCT [27–30].

Rearrangement of *KMT2A*, formerly known as *MLL*, is the primary clonal abnormality present in nearly all cases of congenital ALL and is the driver of leukemogenesis [31]. It is associated with lack of CD10 expression on the surface of the lymphoblasts. The *KMT2A* gene encodes for MLL protein, a histone methyltransferase involved with regulation of gene expression. The most common translocation partner of *KMT2A* in neonatal ALL is *AFF1* (*AF4*), denoted as t(4;11)(q21;q23), though many other partners of *KMT2A* have been described [32]. As yet, no clinical drug is available to specifically target *KMT2A*-r. Overexpression of *FLT3*, which encodes for a receptor tyrosine kinase, is characteristic of ALL with *KMT2A*-r and was the target of a novel therapeutic in the Children's Oncology Group trial, AALL0631 (NCT00557193) [33]. The Children's Oncology Group trial, AALL15P1 (NCT02828358), is investigating the safety and efficacy of azacitidine, a DNA demethylating agent, in conjunction with chemotherapy for infants with ALL. Immunotherapy approaches are also being trialed and may prove to be of benefit to infants if results show increased cure rates and/or decreased need for chemotherapy.

The rate of event-free survival (EFS) of neonatal ALL with *KMT2A*-r is less than 20% [17]. Among all infants less than age 1 year with *KMT2A*-r ALL, the EFS is approximately 40% [20, 34, 35]. In contrast, infant ALL that lacks *KMT2A*-r is associated with an EFS of >70% [20, 35–37]. As noted previously, relapsed infant ALL is characterized by a very poor second remission rate and the majority of patients succumb to progressive leukemia [38]. Neonates with ALL tend to have lower first remission rates than older infants. Refractory disease, as evidenced by poor response to the first week of prednisone or persistent positive residual disease in the bone marrow during treatment, is indicative of a high risk of leukemia progression [15, 39]. In contrast, neonates who enter into a quick remission and have no detectable residual disease at the end of induction have the best chance of long-term cure.

Neonates with ALL who survive to the age of 3 years without relapse may be presumed to be cured of the ALL. Late relapses are uncommon. Survivors, particularly those treated with cranial radiation therapy and/or HSCT, are at risk of complications of therapy, including growth delay, diminished cognitive ability, cardiomyopathy, secondary acute myeloid leukemia, infertility, and other long-term health problems [40, 41]. Despite these risks, survivors may experience normal growth and development with relatively minimal late effects and normal fertility. As treatments improve with time, more children and adults will survive neonatal ALL and the late effects will become better defined for this cohort.

Acute Myeloid Leukemia

Acute myeloid leukemia (AML) has been reported to be slightly more common than ALL in the infant age range, although it is also extremely rare [42, 43]. The male to female ratio is nearly equal, at 1.1:1 [12]. Excluding AML related to Down syndrome, there are no consistent predisposing genetic or environmental risk factors for neonatal presentation of AML [43]. Similar to ALL in infants, AML in infants frequently involves *KMT2A*-r as the driving molecular abnormality. The most common translocation in infant AML is t(9;11)(p21;q23) involving the partner gene *MLLT3* (*AF9*) [44]. The prognosis of infant AML with *KMT2A*-r may be related to the partner gene as well as the breakpoint of *KMT2A* [45]. Acute megakaryoblastic leukemia with t(1;22)(p13;q13) which leads to fusion of RBM15-MKL1, is also seen with increased frequency in congenital AML and is associated with an intermediate prognosis [46].

Neonates with AML may present with extensive extramedullary involvement [47]. Leukemia cutis is seen in at least 25%–30% of cases of neonatal AML and its appearance is similar to leukemia cutis of neonatal ALL [48]. Hyperleukocytosis, anemia, thrombocytopenia, hepato(spleno)megaly, and central nervous system involvement are also common features between neonatal AML and ALL

[1]. In the case of AML, the circulating clonal population consists of aberrant myeloblasts, typically with monoblastic or megakaryoblastic morphologic features [2, 42, 49]. Neonates with AML are at risk of rapid progression to respiratory failure, neurologic deterioration, hemodynamic instability, DIC, and multisystem organ failure. Tumor lysis syndrome is also a risk, but somewhat less prominent in AML than ALL. A rare phenomenon of spontaneous regression of AML has been described in very young infants, particularly those with t(8;16)(p11.2;p13.3), which results in *KAT6A-CREBBP* fusion [50, 51]. As a result, some clinical trials require infants to be at least 1 month of age or to have evidence of symptomatic or progressive AML for enrolment and initiation of therapy.

The initial workup of a neonate with suspected AML is the same as that of ALL (see Table 21.1). A bone marrow aspirate should be performed unless the baby is too unstable to undergo the procedure. Early interventions include intravenous hydration, cardiopulmonary support, and transfusion of blood products as necessary to promote hemodynamic stability, prevent bleeding and correct DIC. Rapid initiation of broad-spectrum antibiotics should be a priority if fever or other signs of sepsis are present. Leukapheresis should be strongly considered for infants with hyperleukocytosis, defined as WBC count above 100,000/μL, and/or signs of life-threatening organ dysfunction due to involvement of AML [52]. Cerebrovascular events and bleeding complications of DIC are oncologic emergencies associated with hyperleukocytosis in patients with newly diagnosed AML.

Infants with AML are typically treated on the same chemotherapy protocols as older children [53]. The protocols consist of blocks of highly intensive, myelosuppressive chemotherapy. The current treatment in the US is based upon the outcomes of infants treated on the Children's Oncology Group trial AAML0531 (NCT00372593), and includes five courses of cytarabine-based chemotherapy and gemtuzumab ozogamicin in the first course [54]. The total duration of treatment is approximately 6 months. Among infants in AAML03P1 (NCT00070174) and AAML0531, treatment with gemtuzumab ozogamicin, an anti-CD33 directed antibody-drug conjugate, was safe and associated with favorable disease outcomes [55]. HSCT is incorporated into the treatment of infants and children with AML and certain high-risk features

of cytogenetics or response, such as detection of residual disease following the first course of therapy.

The event-free survival of neonates with symptomatic or progressive AML requiring treatment has been reported in the range of 40%–50% [42, 53]. Infants are at high risk of death due to toxicities such as pulmonary or sepsis complications during the induction phases of chemotherapy [23]. Therefore, it is important to keep infants with AML hospitalized until evidence of count recovery following each cycle of chemotherapy. Among survivors of neonatal AML, there is potential for significant late effects of therapy, including secondary malignancies, although the risks are not well defined due to the rarity of neonatal leukemia [40, 53].

Juvenile Myelomonocytic Leukemia

Juvenile myelomonocytic leukemia (JMML) is a rare clonal myeloproliferative disorder, driven by Ras pathway overactivation, with the potential to be rapidly progressive and fatal in young children [56]. When JMML presents in the neonatal period, it is often associated with Noonan syndrome, and is sometimes referred to as JMML-like myeloproliferative disorder of Noonan syndrome (NS/MPD) [10]. The diagnosis of JMML is based on specific clinical and genetic criteria [57, 58].

JMML can be difficult to recognize initially because the clinical findings may overlap with other conditions, such as sepsis [59]. Splenomegaly is a key diagnostic feature. Hepatomegaly, lymphadenopathy, rash, fever, and bleeding may also result from organ infiltration, anemia, and thrombocytopenia. In cases with very early presentation of severe anemia, hydrops may be present. In the peripheral blood, the total absolute monocyte count must be greater than 1000/μL and it may be much higher, and the total WBC count is typically also elevated while the blast percentage is less than 20%. A peripheral blood smear demonstrates increased myeloid precursor cells, including blast cells and abnormal monocytes. A bone marrow aspirate should be obtained, if possible, to rule out acute leukemia. Cytogenetic testing must be performed to show absence of the *BCR/ABL* rearrangement in the clonal population. Monosomy 7 or other chromosomal abnormalities may be present. In older infants and children, the hemoglobin F percentage may be increased for age but this test may be less informative in neonates with physiologic high hemoglobin F.

With recent advances in genomic understanding of JMML, the diagnostic criteria now incorporate genetic findings. Somatic mutation in *PTPN11*, *KRAS*, or *NRAS*, clinical diagnosis of neurofibromatosis type 1 (NF1) or germ line *NF1* mutation, or germ line *CBL* mutation or loss of heterozygosity of *CBL* are each diagnostic oncogenetic findings [10]. Individuals with Noonan syndrome and *PTPN11*, *KRAS*, or *NRAS* mutation and patients with *CBL* mutation harbor a germ line mutation in the Ras pathway [60, 61]. Interestingly, the JMML-like polyclonal myeloproliferation of NS/MPD or of germ line *CBL* mutation is similar to transient myeloproliferative disorder of Down syndrome, in that it usually resolves spontaneously [62, 63]. In contrast infants and children with NF1-associated JMML always require hematopoietic stem cell transplant (HSCT) and the disease is associated with high relapse rates as well as high disease-related mortality [64]. For this reason, it is critical to determine if a neonate with JMML or a JMML-like picture has a germ line oncogenetic driver mutation. Of note, even some germ line mutations of Noonan syndrome or of *CBL* may lead to a more rapidly progressive disease in the neonate [65, 66]. As part of the diagnostic workup, molecular testing mutations in the aforementioned Ras pathway genes must be completed on both somatic (peripheral blood or bone marrow) and germ line (e.g., buccal swab) samples. Genetic counseling and molecular testing should be offered for parents and siblings of patients with germ line mutations.

The prognosis for infants and children with JMML is dependent upon age at diagnosis, with older children at higher risk, and cytogenetic factors [64, 67]. The majority of neonates with NS/MPD survive, with spontaneous resolution of the disorder. Among all infants less than 1 year of age with JMML, the rate of disease free survival is approximately 50% and the primary reason for treatment failure is relapse following HSCT [64]. Chemotherapy alone is not curative of JMML but it may be used for control of symptoms related to organ infiltration while awaiting definitive therapy with HSCT [58]. A "watch and wait" strategy is recommended for patients with certain oncogenetic variants [58]. The risk of myeloid malignancies does not appear to be increased for patients with Noonan syndrome who recover from NS/MPD [56, 66].

Down Syndrome Associated Leukemia and Transient Myeloproliferative Disorder

Background

Neonates with Down syndrome (trisomy 21) are especially susceptible to a leukemic disorder variously named transient myeloproliferative disorder (TMD), transient abnormal myelopoiesis (TAM), and transient leukemia of Down syndrome (TL-DS) [68–71]. These terms all refer to the same disorder and for simplicity, the term TMD is used throughout this chapter. TMD is often referred to as a preleukemic condition since retrospective and prospective studies show that the majority of cases spontaneously resolve without chemotherapy and without progressing to full blown leukemia [71, 72]. TMD always has a myeloid phenotype. Indeed, acute lymphoblastic leukemia has never been reported in a child with Down syndrome under the age of 12 months [73]. Importantly, despite the label "transient," some affected neonates with TMD will develop fulminant, progressive leukemic blast cell infiltration of major organs, which is sometimes fatal. Up to 20% of survivors will ultimately develop a full blown acute myeloid leukemia of Down syndrome (ML-DS) [71, 72, 74]. It is therefore extremely important to be able to recognize TMD in neonates with Down syndrome, to diagnose it accurately and promptly and to monitor it effectively. Fortunately, recent advances in our understanding of the pathogenesis and natural history have allowed the development of consensus guidelines to help achieve these goals [11].

Pathogenesis and Epidemiology

Key to our understanding of TMD has been the discovery of the link to mutations in a single gene (*GATA1*). We now know that the blood cells in all neonates with TMD carry mutations in the *GATA1* gene [69, 71, 75–78]. From a scientific point of view, the association between *GATA1* mutations and trisomy 21 provides a unique model in which to study the development of leukemia in children with Down syndrome. From a clinical perspective, the discovery of *GATA1* mutations has provided a molecular test to confirm the diagnosis of TMD (see later) and it helps us understand the natural history of TMD and its evolution to ML-DS. The mutations in the GATA1 gene cause the production of a GATA1 protein that is shorter (Gata1s) than the normal GATA1 protein. GATA1s is responsible for TMD although we still do not fully understand the mechanism [69, 75, 77, 79].

Clinical, pathologic and genetic studies show that GATA1 mutations are not inherited; instead they are acquired at some time during fetal life [69, 76]. They can be detected in cord blood, neonatal peripheral blood or on neonatal blood spots [69]. GATA1 mutations only cause TMD in neonates with trisomy 21, i.e., those who have typical features of Down syndrome or in neonates with mosaic Down syndrome [72, 77]. Furthermore, if very sensitive detection methods are used, 25%–30% of all neonates with DS have GATA1 mutations at birth, although only ~1 in 3 with GATA1 mutation (i.e., 10% overall) will have clinical features of TMD [71]. GATA1 mutations are never acquired after birth and they disappear in the first 3–12 months of life except in children with Down syndrome who go on to develop ML-DS [69, 76]. Therefore, GATA1 mutations contribute to the pathogenesis of both TMD and ML-DS. The reason(s) for the high frequency of GATA1 mutations in Down syndrome and how the combination with trisomy 21 causes neonatal TMD and ML-DS is unknown but remains an area of very active research.

Retrospective studies of the prevalence of TMD, carried out before GATA1 mutational analysis was available, are based on a clinical or hematologic diagnosis of TMD. These studies found that TMD affects ~10% of neonates with Down syndrome [68, 70, 72]. The only available prospective study published to date, the Oxford Down Syndrome Cohort Study, included a cohort of babies with Down syndrome who had a blood count, blood smear, and GATA1 mutation analysis in the first week of life whether or not they had any clinical signs of TMD [71]. Taking this unbiased approach, the study found a similar prevalence of TMD based on clinical and hematologic features (9%), but identified a much higher frequency of GATA1 mutations overall (28%). Thus, the majority of neonates with GATA1 mutations did not have clear clinical or hematologic evidence of TMD and were termed "silent

TAM (TMD)." The clinical significance of silent TMD is discussed below (see Table 21.2). Even though the GATA1 gene is on the X chromosome, there is no gender difference in the rate or severity of TMD. TMD has been reported in all ethnic groups with no apparent differences between groups [71, 80].

Clinical Features of TMD

The clinical features of transient myeloproliferative disorder are presented in Table 21.2. The classical clinical features of TMD are hepatomegaly, with or without splenomegaly; pleural and/or pericardial effusion and/or ascites; skin rash; and jaundice. In practice, only a minority of neonates will have all of these features. Overall, clinically severe TMD (liver failure/fibrosis, ascites, pleural/pericardial effusion, renal failure and/or coagulopathy) affects 10%–30% of babies with TMD [71, 72, 74, 80]. The skin rash in TMD is typically papular or vesiculopustular, although skin nodules have occasionally been reported [81].

It is important not to rely on clinical signs alone to make a diagnosis of TMD. In particular, the presence of jaundice is a very poor diagnostic indicator of TMD because ~50% of neonates with DS but without any evidence of TMD will have jaundice [71]. In addition, neonates with TMD who have a very florid, typical hematologic picture of TMD with high numbers of circulating blasts, may have none of the typical clinical features of the disease. This heterogeneity of clinical presentations means that a blood count and blood smear are essential to make a diagnosis of TMD and also to plan management (see below). Most of the clinical features of TMD are caused by tissue or organ infiltration by leukemic blasts. However, splenomegaly, which is found in 30% of cases, is often due to portal venous obstruction [82]. Splenic infiltration is rarely reported [83, 84].

TMD typically presents at birth or during the first few days after birth. Later presentations are usually because the diagnosis was not considered (and a blood count and blood smear not performed) in the first few days of life rather than because the clinical features appear late. However, in a small proportion of cases signs of liver fibrosis and associated liver failure, including conjugated hyperbilirubinemia and/or coagulopathy, may progress from mild, clinically insignificant features at birth to severe disease 2–3 weeks later. Around 4% of

Table 21.2 Clinical and hematologic features of TMD

Clinical features of TMD	% of TMD cases in which features seen	Additional comments
Jaundice	70%	Very common, but also seen in around 50% of DS neonates without TMD
Hepatomegaly	40%	
Splenomegaly	30%	Often due to portal venous obstruction and more commonly in association with hepatomegaly than in isolation. Splenic infiltration rare.
Pleural and/or pericardial effusion and/or ascites	25%	
Skin rash	11%	Typically, papular and/or vesiculopapular. May be non-specific. Rashes also seen in DS without TMD.
Bleeding	10%	Secondary to multiple causes including thrombocytopenia, liver failure, coagulopathy (disseminated intravascular coagulation).
Hepatic fibrosis +/− failure	~5%	
Hydrops fetalis	<5%	Need to exclude TMD but other causes should be considered in a neonate with DS.
Hematological features of TMD		
Leukocytosis	50%	Common but not diagnostic. Also seen in many DS neonates without TMD and normal in at least a third of TMD cases.
Circulating blast cells	>20%	Peripheral blood blasts are common in DS neonates both with and without TMD. Importance of GATA1 mutational analysis to confirm diagnosis of TMD, particularly if blast % is <20%.
Thrombocytopenia	50%	Common but not diagnostic to TMD. Occurs at a similar frequency in DS neonates without a GATA1 mutation and neonates with TMD may have a normal platelet count or, in some cases, thrombocytosis.
Neutrophilia	10%–15%	Neutrophilia is also seen in ~25% of DS neonates without a GATA1 mutation. Increased basophil and myelocyte counts also reported.
Eosinophilia	10%–16%	
Anemia	5%–10%	Since uncommon as a TMD-related feature, consider other causes of anemia

Note: Based on data from Klusmann et al. [72] and Roberts et al. [71]; and unpublished data.

neonates with TMD present with hydrops fetalis, although this is not a specific sign of TMD as there are other causes of hydrops in neonates with Down syndrome, including cardiac disease and infection [83]. TMD may also occasionally present in fetal life when it usually leads to intrauterine or neonatal death [72, 74, 85].

Hematologic Features of TMD

Table 21.2 shows the most common (and the most reliable) hematologic findings in TMD are a raised leukocyte count and the presence of increased blast cells on a peripheral blood smear. Typically, neutrophils, basophils and myelocytes are also increased

[71] and a small proportion of neonates with TMD have eosinophilia [86]. There is no difference in platelet count between neonates with and without TMD. This is because trisomy 21 itself causes thrombocytopenia. Indeed, the frequency of thrombocytopenia is ~50% in neonates with Down syndrome whether or not they have TMD. Furthermore, a proportion of neonates with TMD have a raised platelet count (>400 × 10⁹/L). Therefore, it is important to recognize that the absence of thrombocytopenia does not exclude TMD and, equally, that the presence of thrombocytopenia does not identify babies at increased likelihood of having TMD. Giant platelets and megakaryocyte

cytoplasmic fragments are commonly seen on the blood smear in neonates with TMD presumably because the acquired *GATA1* mutation interferes with normal platelet and megakaryocyte development. The hematocrit and hemoglobin are normal in the majority of neonates with TMD; very few affected neonates are anemic [71, 74].

Blast cells in TMD are extremely pleomorphic. They range from typical myeloblasts with few distinguishing features to characteristic megakaryoblasts with "blebby" cytoplasm to very large cells with a high nuclear to cytoplasmic ratio, which are sometimes binucleate. The percentage of blast cells in TMD is best determined by manual examination of a peripheral smear. In addition, as blast cells often disappear quickly, smears from a sample collected on day 7 of life may look relatively normal. It is therefore important to arrange for blood smear evaluation as soon as possible after birth.

Diagnosis and Definition of TMD and Silent TMD

The WHO Classification of tumors of hematopoietic and lymphoid tissues defines TMD as "increased peripheral blood blast cells in a neonate with Down syndrome" without recommending a threshold value for the percentage of blast cells [87]. Since the Oxford Down Syndrome Cohort Study found that ~98% of all neonates with Down syndrome had peripheral blood blasts, whether or not they had a *GATA1* mutation, the "presence of blasts" alone is insufficient to make a diagnosis of TMD. A more practical approach is to integrate information from the blood count, blood smear and mutational analysis of the *GATA1* gene in order to make a reliable diagnosis of TMD [71]. Thus, the most useful diagnostic tests for TMD are a complete blood count to look for leukocytosis, a peripheral blood smear to estimate the percentage of blasts, and *GATA1* mutation analysis for all cases where the diagnosis is uncertain. There is no evidence that carrying out a bone marrow aspiration conveys any useful additional information [72, 74, 80]. In exceptional cases, e.g., in neonates who present late with clinical features which could be consistent with TMD (e.g., liver failure), bone marrow aspiration for morphology and *GATA1* mutation analysis

may be useful if no peripheral blood blasts can be seen at that stage.

The identification of a high frequency of acquired *GATA1* mutations in Down syndrome neonates without clinical or hematologic features of TMD (blasts ≤10%) has led to the designation silent TMD. One reason neonates present with silent TMD is delayed assessment for peripheral blasts after the first week of life, as the blast percentage often falls rapidly after birth. Since both TMD and silent TMD may evolve to ML-DS before the age of 4 years, the only way to identify all those at risk of ML-DS, is to screen all neonates with Down syndrome for *GATA1* mutations using sensitive techniques, such as next generation sequencing [71]. Given the resource implications of this approach and the low risk of ML-DS in silent TMD (~1%), recent guidelines suggest discussing this with parents and screening only where there is diagnostic difficulty [11].

Differential Diagnosis of TMD

The most useful clinical indicator of TMD in neonates with typical features of Down syndrome is hepatomegaly with or without splenomegaly. As mentioned above, these signs are not specific to TMD and other causes of hepato(spleno)megaly should always be considered, including congenital infection, metabolic disorders, hemangiomas and neonatal hepatitis. For neonates with Down syndrome who have hepato(spleno)megaly, the most useful discriminating investigation is a blood smear since none of these differential diagnoses will give rise to large numbers (>20%) circulating blast cells. Where the blast cells are less prominently increased (10%–20%), *GATA1* mutation analysis will be needed to establish the diagnosis accurately.

The most useful hematologic indicators of TMD are leukocytosis and increased blast cells, although only a blast percentage of >20% is specific for TMD. The most important differential diagnosis of leukocytosis and increased blast cells in a neonate with Down syndrome is a leukemoid reaction. The usual cause of this is neonatal sepsis or prematurity. It is important to note that maternal chorioamnionitis is a frequent trigger of preterm labor and may lead to marked leukocytosis and increased blast cells even in the absence of bacterial infection in the neonate; this appearance tends to be even more prominent in neonates with Down syndrome. In our experience the percentage of blast cells in a leukemoid reaction never exceeds 20% in a neonate with Down syndrome or 8% in a neonate without Down syndrome. Other causes of leukocytosis and increased blast cells in a neonate are rare and include congenital acute lymphoblastic leukemia or acute myeloid leukemia, metastatic neuroblastoma, and NS/MPD. Typically, the most difficult differential diagnosis is the presence of typical clinical and hematologic features of TMD in a neonate with no clinical features of Down syndrome. In such cases, mosaic Down syndrome should always be considered and peripheral blood cytogenetic analysis performed.

Natural History of TMD and Evolution to MI-DS

The early outcome of TMD is strongly linked to the presence or absence of clinical evidence of severe disease. The majority of cases of TMD resolve spontaneously within a few weeks or months of birth [71, 72, 74]. The Children's Oncology Group (COG) study reported spontaneous resolution at a median of 36 days (range 2–126) in almost all (99%) of neonates without severe disease (which they defined as life-threatening symptoms; discussed below under Treatment) [74]. Similar results have been noted in the Oxford Down Syndrome Cohort Study [71]. Clinical and hematologic evidence of spontaneous resolution of TMD may still be followed by subsequent ML-DS, as discussed below, and follow up of all cases of TMD, whether they appear to resolve or not, is therefore essential.

For mildly affected neonates with TMD, there are no reports of TMD-related death. The early mortality rate (within 6 months) is much higher in those that are severely affected. In the study by Klusmann et al., e.g., all seven neonates with liver fibrosis and all six neonates with renal failure died [72]. Although not all of the deaths can be directly attributed to TMD (e.g., co-existing severe congenital anomalies), TMD is an important cause of perinatal death in Down syndrome and prompt diagnosis is essential. The usual cause of TMD-related death is progressive hepatopathy with conjugated hyperbilirubinemia, often accompanied by disseminated intravascular coagulation and multi-organ failure. Liver biopsies in such cases typically show severe cholestasis, diffuse hepatic fibrosis, and infiltration with leukemic blast cells [88]. Other causes of TMD-related death include hydrops fetalis and cardiorespiratory failure due to pleural or pericardial effusion and/or infection [72, 74, 80, 89].

The median age at diagnosis of ML-DS is 12–18 months [72, 74, 80]. It is uncommon to proceed straight from TMD-phase disease to ML-DS. More often, the clinical and hematologic signs of TMD resolve completely so that the blood count is completely restored to normal [71, 72, 80]. Often the first sign of impending transformation is a fall in the platelet count which may be accompanied by a progressive anemia and/or neutropenia. Although the majority of cases of ML-DS present this way, occasional cases evolve straight from the proliferative TMD phase of the disease into a typical leukemia with large numbers of blasts cells but few, if any, of the typical features of TMD – immature myeloid cells (myelocytes, band cells), giant platelets and megakaryocyte fragments. In rare cases, ML-DS may present in the fetus or neonate with extreme hyperleukocytosis and almost 100% blast cells. Such cases have *GATA1* mutations and have presumably acquired additional mutations in utero although this has not yet been specifically documented.

The estimated risk of a neonate with TMD subsequently developing ML-DS varies in different studies and lies somewhere between 11% and 23% depending on the type of study. If inclusion is based on a clinical diagnosis of TMD, and hence more severe cases, the risk of ML-DS is 20%–22% [72, 74, 80, 89]; if all babies with TMD are included, as in the Oxford Down Syndrome Cohort Study, the risk is lower (11%) [71]. The factors that determine whether a neonate with TMD will progress to ML-DS are not fully understood. Data from the Oxford Down Syndrome Cohort Study, which has followed >70 babies with silent TMD, shows that the risk of developing ML-DS in this group was very low (1%–2%) compared to a risk of ~10% in neonates with TMD [71].

Fetal presentation of TMD is uncommon, with fewer than 5% of neonatal cases already diagnosed before birth. In such cases, TMD is generally identified through abnormalities on fetal ultrasound scanning, usually in the third trimester. The most common abnormalities are hepatomegaly and/or splenomegaly (80%), fetal hydrops (31%), and pericardial effusion(23%); ascites, pleural effusion, and peripheral edema have also been reported [90]. Fetal blood sampling shows leukocytosis with increased blast cells; thrombocytopenia and abnormal liver function are also reported [90]. A recent review of 39 published cases found a fairly high rate of intrauterine or early neonatal death (41%) although 14/39 children (39%) were still alive at follow up despite the high frequency of severe disease [90]. Importantly, spontaneous resolution of TMD may begin before birth and so the need for premature delivery of an affected fetus has to be considered on a case by case basis, based on clinical signs and evidence of deterioration.

Management of TMD

Most neonates with TMD do not require specific treatment as, in nearly all, spontaneous regression will ensue (Fig. 21.1). However, all cases of TMD require careful monitoring to identify those most at risk of early death as a result high disease burdens and associated organ damage. Recent consensus guidelines from UK pediatric hematologists and neonatologists adapted the COG study approach of defining a list of life-threatening symptoms as

a way to identify neonates most at risk of early death and therefore most likely to benefit from treatment, including hyperleukocytosis (WBC >100 × 10⁹/l), severe liver disease, pleural/pericardial effusions and coagulopathies (Table 21.3) [11]. In line with this, they recommended the following investigations to assess and monitor disease severity: peripheral blood count and blood smear, renal and liver function tests (including conjugated bilirubin), coagulation screen, chest X-ray, echocardiogram and abdominal ultrasound.

The only chemotherapeutic agent with evidence of clinical value in TMD is cytarabine. As TMD blasts are extremely sensitive to cytarabine [91, 92], very low doses are usually effective in reducing the peripheral blood blasts and leukemic involvement of affected tissues. In the most recent trial (TMD Prevention 2007; TMD07), Flasinski and colleagues showed that low-dose, subcutaneous or intravenous cytarabine (1.5 mg/kg per day for 7 days) reduced mortality in TMD compared to historic controls [93]. At this dose, toxicity was acceptable but it is important to note that higher doses (e.g., 3.3 mg/kg as used in a previous study [74]) carry high rates of

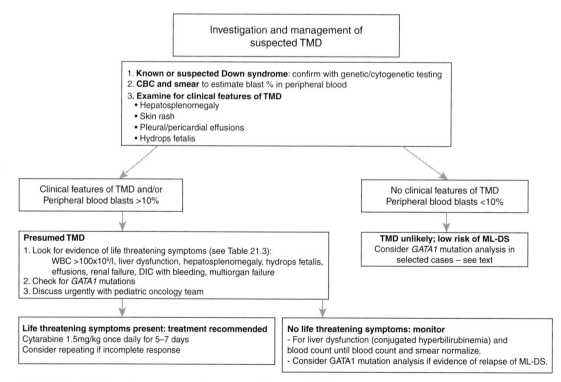

Fig. 21.1 Investigation and management of a neonate with suspected TMD.

Table 21.3 Life threatening symptoms of TMD: indications for treatment

Symptom
White cell count >100 × 10^9/l, signs of hyperviscosity
Liver dysfunction: conjugated bilirubin >83 µmol/l, ascites, massive hepatomegaly
Hepatosplenomegaly (beyond umbilicus or causing respiratory or feeding compromise)
Hydrops fetalis
Pleural or pericardial effusions
Renal failure
Coagulopathy with bleeding/evidence of disseminated intravascular coagulation
Multi-organ failure

Note: Adapted from Gamis et al. [74] and Tunstall et al. [11].

hematologic toxicity. Exchange transfusion has been used to manage hyperleukocytosis in ML-DS. Although exchange transfusion may be a rapid way to reduce the WBC count in neonates with leukostasis, there is no evidence of any advantage over cytarabine and there are insufficient data to determine the value of this approach.

All cytarabine-treated babies should be closely monitored for cytarabine-associated neutropenia and sepsis, as well as disease response. In some cases, a single course of cytarabine is not sufficient to control TMD entirely. In a small proportion of cases, repeat courses of cytarabine should be considered to achieve control where severe liver dysfunction persists [94]. There is no evidence that neonates with mosaic Down syndrome respond any differently to cytarabine than neonates with clinical Down syndrome and therefore the same indications and dose should be used. It is important to note that hepatomegaly may take several months to resolve even in the absence of residual disease. There is currently no evidence that treatment of TMD with cytarabine prevents subsequent ML-DS and there is therefore no indication to treat asymptomatic TMD [74, 93].

It is advisable to follow all neonates with TMD whether or not they are treated with cytarabine. Apart from clinical assessment, the most useful tests for monitoring are complete blood count and peripheral smear; the smear may identify small numbers of blast cells when the blood count is normal or only mildly abnormal. Attention should be paid to the platelet count, as a drop in platelets is often the first sign of impending ML-DS. Serial monitoring of *GATA1* mutations to look for minimal residual disease (MRD) has not been shown to be useful, but no systematic studies using sensitive methodology have yet been reported. Since the majority of cases of ML-DS present before the age of 2 years, it would be reasonable to monitor the blood count and smear more frequently (every 2–3 months) for the first 2 years of life and reduce to 6 monthly until the age of 4 years if the blood count is normal. Significant blood count abnormalities, particularly thrombocytopenia, should prompt consideration of *GATA1* mutation analysis and a bone marrow aspirate with a trephine biopsy if fibrosis makes bone marrow aspiration technically difficult. Presentation of ML-DS after the age of 4 years is exceptionally rare [68, 95, 96]. Neonates with mosaic Down syndrome are at the same risk of subsequent progression to ML-DS as those with clinical Down syndrome and they should therefore be monitored in the same way.

Given the small number of case reports, no clear guidance is available regarding the best way to manage TMD in utero [90]. Management has been based on supportive care, such as intrauterine transfusion of red cells and/or platelets. There are no reports of intrauterine therapy with cytarabine.

References

1. van der Linden MH, Creemers S, Pieters R. Diagnosis and management of neonatal leukaemia. *Semin Fetal Neonatal Med* 2012;**17**(4):192–5.

2. Roberts I, Fordham NJ, Rao A, Bain BJ. Neonatal leukaemia. *Br J Haematol* 2018;**182**(2):170–84.

3. Ford AM, Ridge SA, Cabrera ME, et al. In utero rearrangements in the trithorax-related oncogene in infant leukaemias. *Nature* 1993;**363** (6427):358–60.

4. Gale KB, Ford AM, Repp R, et al. Backtracking leukemia to birth: Identification of clonotypic gene fusion sequences in neonatal blood spots. *Proc Natl Acad Sci USA* 1997;**94**(25):13950–4.

5. Valentine MC, Linabery AM, Chasnoff S, et al. Excess congenital non-synonymous variation in leukemia-associated genes in MLL-infant leukemia: A Children's Oncology Group report. *Leukemia* 2014;**28**(6):1235–41.

6. Bueno C, Montes R, Catalina P, Rodriguez R, Menendez P. Insights into the cellular origin and

etiology of the infant pro-B acute lymphoblastic leukemia with MLL-AF4 rearrangement. *Leukemia* 2011;**25**(3):400 –10.

7. Spector LG, Xie Y, Robison LL, et al. Maternal diet and infant leukemia: The DNA topoisomerase II inhibitor hypothesis: A report from the children's oncology group. *Cancer Epidemiol Biomarkers Prev* 2005;**14**(3):651–5.

8. Greaves MF, Maia AT, Wiemels JL, Ford AM. Leukemia in twins: Lessons in natural history. *Blood* 2003;**102**(7):2321–33.

9. Chuk MK, McIntyre E, Small D, Brown P. Discordance of MLL-rearranged (MLL-R) infant acute lymphoblastic leukemia in monozygotic twins with spontaneous clearance of preleukemic clone in unaffected twin. *Blood* 2009;**113**(26):6691–4.

10. Hasle H. Myelodysplastic and myeloproliferative disorders of childhood. *Hematology Am Soc Hematol Educ Program* 2016;**2016**(1):598–604.

11. Tunstall O, Bhatnagar N, James B, et al. Guidelines for the investigation and management of transient leukaemia of Down Syndrome. *Br J Haematol* 2018;**182**(2):200–11.

12. Noone AM, Howlader N, Krapcho M, et al. SEER Cancer Statistics Review, 1975–2015, based on November 2017 SEER data submission (Bethesda, MD: National Cancer Institute, 2018). Available online at https://seer.cancer.gov/csr/1975_2015.

13. Guest EM, Stam RW. Updates in the biology and therapy for infant acute lymphoblastic leukemia. *Curr Opin Pediatr* 2017;**29**(1):20–6.

14. Hilden JM, Dinndorf PA, Meerbaum SO, et al. Analysis of prognostic factors of acute lymphoblastic leukemia in infants: Report on CCG 1953 from the Children's Oncology Group. *Blood* 2006;**108**(2):441–51.

15. Dordelmann M, Reiter A, Borkhardt A, et al. Prednisone response is the strongest predictor of treatment outcome in infant acute lymphoblastic leukemia. *Blood* 1999;**94**(4):1209–17.

16. Pui CH, Ribeiro RC, Campana D, et al. Prognostic factors in the acute lymphoid and myeloid leukemias of infants. *Leukemia* 1996;**10**(6):952–6.

17. van der Linden MH, Valsecchi MG, De Lorenzo P, et al. Outcome of congenital acute lymphoblastic leukemia treated on the Interfant-99 protocol. *Blood* 2009;**114**(18):3764–8.

18. Nguyen R, Jeha S, Zhou Y, et al. The role of leukapheresis in the current management of hyperleukocytosis in newly diagnosed childhood acute lymphoblastic leukemia. *Pediatr Blood Cancer* 2016;**63**(9):1546–51.

19. Runco DV, Josephson CD, Raikar SS, et al. Hyperleukocytosis in infant acute leukemia: A role

for manual exchange transfusion for leukoreduction. *Transfusion* 2018;**58**(5):1149–56.

20. Pieters R, Schrappe M, De Lorenzo P, et al. A treatment protocol for infants younger than 1 year with acute lymphoblastic leukaemia (Interfant-99): An observational study and a multicentre randomised trial. *Lancet* 2007;**370** (9583):240–50.

21. Salzer WL, Jones TL, Devidas M, et al. Decreased induction morbidity and mortality following modification to induction therapy in infants with acute lymphoblastic leukemia enrolled on AALL0631: A report from the Children's Oncology Group. *Pediatr Blood Cancer* 2015;**62** (3):414–18.

22. Salzer WL, Jones TL, Devidas M, et al. Modifications to induction therapy decrease risk of early death in infants with acute lymphoblastic leukemia treated on Children's Oncology Group P9407. *Pediatr Blood Cancer* 2012;**59**(5):834–9.

23. Tomizawa D, Tawa A, Watanabe T, et al. Appropriate dose reduction in induction therapy is essential for the treatment of infants with acute myeloid leukemia: A report from the Japanese Pediatric Leukemia/Lymphoma Study Group. *Int J Hematol* 2013;**98**(5):578–88.

24. Tomizawa D. Recent progress in the treatment of infant acute lymphoblastic leukemia. *Pediatr Int* 2015;**57**(5):811–19.

25. Kotecha RS, Gottardo NG, Kees UR, Cole CH. The evolution of clinical trials for infant acute lymphoblastic leukemia. *Blood Cancer J* 2014;**4**: e200.

26. Driessen EM, de Lorenzo P, Campbell M, et al. Outcome of relapsed infant acute lymphoblastic leukemia treated on the interfant-99 protocol. *Leukemia* 2016;**30**(5):1184–7.

27. Biondi A, Rizzari C, Valsecchi MG, et al. Role of treatment intensification in infants with acute lymphoblastic leukemia: Results of two consecutive AIEOP studies. *Haematologica* 2006;**91**(4):534–7.

28. Dreyer ZE, Dinndorf PA, Camitta B, et al. Analysis of the role of hematopoietic stem-cell transplantation in infants with acute lymphoblastic leukemia in first remission and MLL gene rearrangements: A report from the Children's Oncology Group. *J Clin Oncol* 2011;**29** (2):214–22.

29. Koh K, Tomizawa D, Moriya Saito A, et al. Early use of allogeneic hematopoietic stem cell transplantation for infants with MLL gene-rearrangement-positive acute lymphoblastic leukemia. *Leukemia* 2015;**29**(2):290–6.

30. Mann G, Attarbaschi A, Schrappe M, et al. Improved outcome with hematopoietic stem cell

transplantation in a poor prognostic subgroup of infants with mixed-lineage-leukemia (MLL)-rearranged acute lymphoblastic leukemia: Results from the Interfant-99 Study. *Blood* 2010;**116**(15):2644–50.

31. Sanjuan-Pla A, Bueno C, Prieto C, et al. Revisiting the biology of infant t(4;11)/MLL-AF4+ B-cell acute lymphoblastic leukemia. *Blood* 2015;**126** (25):2676–85.

32. Meyer C, Burmeister T, Groger D, et al. The MLL recombinome of acute leukemias in 2017. *Leukemia* 2018;**32**(2):273–84.

33. Brown P, Levis M, Shurtleff S, et al. FLT3 inhibition selectively kills childhood acute lymphoblastic leukemia cells with high levels of FLT3 expression. *Blood* 2005;**105**(2):812–20.

34. Dreyer ZE, Hilden JM, Jones TL, et al. Intensified chemotherapy without SCT in infant ALL: Results from COG P9407 (Cohort 3). *Pediatr Blood Cancer* 2015;**62**(3):419–26.

35. Tomizawa D, Koh K, Sato T, et al. Outcome of risk-based therapy for infant acute lymphoblastic leukemia with or without an MLL gene rearrangement, with emphasis on late effects: A final report of two consecutive studies, MLL96 and MLL98, of the Japan Infant Leukemia Study Group. *Leukemia* 2007;**21** (11):2258–63.

36. Nagayama J, Tomizawa D, Koh K, et al. Infants with acute lymphoblastic leukemia and a germline MLL gene are highly curable with use of chemotherapy alone: Results from the Japan Infant Leukemia Study Group. *Blood* 2006;**107** (12):4663–5.

37. De Lorenzo P, Moorman AV, Pieters R, et al. Cytogenetics and outcome of infants with acute lymphoblastic leukemia and absence of MLL rearrangements. *Leukemia* 2014;**28**(2):428–30.

38. Tomizawa D, Koh K, Hirayama M, et al. Outcome of recurrent or refractory acute lymphoblastic leukemia in infants with MLL gene rearrangements: A report from the Japan Infant Leukemia Study Group. *Pediatr Blood Cancer* 2009;**52**(7):808–13.

39. Van der Velden VH, Corral L, Valsecchi MG, et al. Prognostic significance of minimal residual disease in infants with acute lymphoblastic leukemia treated within the Interfant-99 protocol. *Leukemia* 2009;**23**(6):1073–9.

40. Leung W, Hudson M, Zhu Y, et al. Late effects in survivors of infant leukemia. *Leukemia* 2000;**14** (7):1185–90.

41. Kaleita TA, Reaman GH, MacLean WE, Sather HN, Whitt JK. Neurodevelopmental outcome of infants with acute lymphoblastic leukemia: A Children's Cancer Group report. *Cancer* 1999;**85**(8):1859–65.

42. Bresters D, Reus AC, Veerman AJ, van Wering ER, van der Does-van den Berg A, Kaspers GJ. Congenital leukaemia: The Dutch experience and review of the literature. *Br J Haematol* 2002;**117** (3):513–24.

43. Isaacs H, Jr. Fetal and neonatal leukemia. *J Pediatr Hematol Oncol* 2003;**25**(5):348–61.

44. Balgobind BV, Raimondi SC, Harbott J, et al. Novel prognostic subgroups in childhood 11q23/MLL-rearranged acute myeloid leukemia: Results of an international retrospective study. *Blood* 2009;**114**(12):2489–96.

45. Emerenciano M, Meyer C, Mansur MB, Marschalek R, Pombo-de-Oliveira MS. The distribution of MLL breakpoints correlates with outcome in infant acute leukaemia. *Br J Haematol* 2013;**161**(2):224–36.

46. Dastugue N, Lafage-Pochitaloff M, Pages MP, et al. Cytogenetic profile of childhood and adult megakaryoblastic leukemia (M7): A study of the Groupe Francais de Cytogenetique Hematologique (GFCH). *Blood* 2002;**100** (2):618–26.

47. Bayoumy M, Wynn T, Jamil A, et al. Prenatal presentation supports the in utero development of congenital leukemia: A case report. *J Pediatr Hematol Oncol* 2003;**25**(2):148–52.

48. Resnik KS, Brod BB. Leukemia cutis in congenital leukemia. Analysis and review of the world literature with report of an additional case. *Arch Dermatol* 1993;**129**(10):1301–6.

49. Ishii E, Oda M, Kinugawa N, et al. Features and outcome of neonatal leukemia in Japan: Experience of the Japan infant leukemia study group. *Pediatr Blood Cancer* 2006;**47**(3):268–72.

50. Barrett R, Morash B, Roback D, et al. FISH identifies a KAT6A/CREBBP fusion caused by a cryptic insertional t(8;16) in a case of spontaneously remitting congenital acute myeloid leukemia with a normal karyotype. *Pediatr Blood Cancer* 2017;**64**(8):26450.

51. Coenen EA, Zwaan CM, Reinhardt D, et al. Pediatric acute myeloid leukemia with t(8;16)(p11; p13), a distinct clinical and biological entity: A collaborative study by the International-Berlin-Frankfurt-Munster AML-study group. *Blood* 2013;**122**(15):2704–13.

52. Creutzig U, van den Heuvel-Eibrink MM, Gibson B, et al. Diagnosis and management of acute myeloid leukemia in children and adolescents: Recommendations from an international expert panel. *Blood* 2012;**120** (16):3187–205.

53. Creutzig U, Zimmermann M, Bourquin JP, et al. Favorable outcome in infants with AML after intensive first- and second-line treatment: An AML-BFM study group report. *Leukemia* 2012;**26**(4):654–61.

54. Gamis AS, Alonzo TA, Meshinchi S, et al. Gemtuzumab ozogamicin in children and adolescents with de novo acute myeloid leukemia improves event-free survival by reducing relapse risk: Results from the randomized phase III Children's Oncology Group trial AAML0531. *J Clin Oncol* 2014;**32**(27):3021–32.

55. Guest EM, Aplenc R, Sung L, et al. Gemtuzumab ozogamicin in infants with AML: Results from the Children's Oncology Group trials AAML03P1 and AAML0531. *Blood* 2017;**130**(7):943–5.

56. Chang TY, Dvorak CC, Loh ML. Bedside to bench in juvenile myelomonocytic leukemia: Insights into leukemogenesis from a rare pediatric leukemia. *Blood* 2014;**124**(16):2487–97.

57. Arber DA, Orazi A, Hasserjian R, et al. The 2016 revision to the World Health Organization classification of myeloid neoplasms and acute leukemia. *Blood* 2016;**127**(20):2391–405.

58. Locatelli F, Niemeyer CM. How I treat juvenile myelomonocytic leukemia. *Blood* 2015;**125**(7):1083–90.

59. Lee ML, Yen HJ, Chen SJ, et al. Juvenile myelomonocytic leukemia in a premature neonate mimicking neonatal sepsis. *Pediatr Neonatol* 2016;**57**(2):149–52.

60. Niemeyer CM, Kang MW, Shin DH, et al. Germline CBL mutations cause developmental abnormalities and predispose to juvenile myelomonocytic leukemia. *Nat Genet* 2010;**42**(9):794–800.

61. Perez B, Mechinaud F, Galambrun C, et al. Germline mutations of the CBL gene define a new genetic syndrome with predisposition to juvenile myelomonocytic leukaemia. *J Med Genet* 2010;**47**(10):686–91.

62. Matsuda K, Shimada A, Yoshida N, et al. Spontaneous improvement of hematologic abnormalities in patients having juvenile myelomonocytic leukemia with specific RAS mutations. *Blood* 2007;**109**(12):5477–80.

63. Matsuda K, Taira C, Sakashita K, et al. Long-term survival after nonintensive chemotherapy in some juvenile myelomonocytic leukemia patients with CBL mutations, and the possible presence of healthy persons with the mutations. *Blood* 2010;**115**(26):5429–31.

64. Locatelli F, Nollke P, Zecca M, et al. Hematopoietic stem cell transplantation (HSCT) in children with juvenile myelomonocytic leukemia (JMML): Results of the EWOG-MDS/EBMT trial. *Blood* 2005;**105**(1):410–19.

65. Mason-Suares H, Toledo D, Gekas J, et al. Juvenile myelomonocytic leukemia-associated variants are associated with neo-natal lethal Noonan syndrome. *Eur J Hum Genet* 2017;**25**(4):509–11.

66. Strullu M, Caye A, Lachenaud J, et al. Juvenile myelomonocytic leukaemia and Noonan syndrome. *J Med Genet* 2014;**51**(10):689–97.

67. Flotho C, Kratz CP, Bergstrasser E, et al. Genotype-phenotype correlation in cases of juvenile myelomonocytic leukemia with clonal RAS mutations. *Blood* 2008;**111**(2):966–7; author reply 7–8.

68. Zipursky A. Transient leukaemia–a benign form of leukaemia in newborn infants with trisomy 21. *Br J Haematol* 2003;**120**(6):930–8.

69. Ahmed M, Sternberg A, Hall G, et al. Natural history of GATA1 mutations in Down syndrome. *Blood* 2004;**103**(7):2480–9.

70. Pine SR, Guo Q, Yin C, et al. Incidence and clinical implications of GATA1 mutations in newborns with Down syndrome. *Blood* 2007;**110**(6):2128–31.

71. Roberts I, Alford K, Hall G, et al. GATA1-mutant clones are frequent and often unsuspected in babies with Down syndrome: identification of a population at risk of leukemia. *Blood* 2013;**122**(24):3908–17.

72. Klusmann JH, Creutzig U, Zimmermann M, et al. Treatment and prognostic impact of transient leukemia in neonates with Down syndrome. *Blood* 2008;**111**(6):2991–8.

73. Buitenkamp TD, Izraeli S, Zimmermann M, et al. Acute lymphoblastic leukemia in children with Down syndrome: A retrospective analysis from the Ponte di Legno study group. *Blood* 2014;**123**(1):70–7.

74. Gamis AS, Alonzo TA, Gerbing RB, et al. Natural history of transient myeloproliferative disorder clinically diagnosed in Down syndrome neonates: A report from the Children's Oncology Group Study A2971. *Blood* 2011;**118**(26):6752–9; quiz 996.

75. Hitzler JK, Cheung J, Li Y, Scherer SW, Zipursky A. GATA1 mutations in transient leukemia and acute megakaryoblastic leukemia of Down syndrome. *Blood* 2003;**101**(11):4301–4.

76. Yoshida K, Toki T, Okuno Y, et al. The landscape of somatic mutations in Down syndrome-related myeloid disorders. *Nat Genet* 2013;**45**(11):1293–9.

77. Alford KA, Reinhardt K, Garnett C, et al. Analysis of GATA1 mutations in Down syndrome transient

myeloproliferative disorder and myeloid leukemia. *Blood* 2011;**118**(8):2222–38.

78. Malinge S, Chlon T, Dore LC, et al. Development of acute megakaryoblastic leukemia in Down syndrome is associated with sequential epigenetic changes. *Blood* 2013;**122**(14):e33–43.

79. Wechsler J, Greene M, McDevitt MA, et al. Acquired mutations in GATA1 in the megakaryoblastic leukemia of Down syndrome. *Nat Genet* 2002;**32**(1):148–52.

80. Massey GV, Zipursky A, Chang MN, et al. A prospective study of the natural history of transient leukemia (TL) in neonates with Down syndrome (DS): Children's Oncology Group (COG) study POG-9481. *Blood* 2006;**107** (12):4606–13.

81. Winckworth LC, Chonat S, Uthaya S. Cutaneous lesions in transient abnormal myelopoiesis. *J Paediatr Child Health* 2012;**48**(2):184–5.

82. Gamis AS, Smith FO. Transient myeloproliferative disorder in children with Down syndrome: clarity to this enigmatic disorder. *Br J Haematol* 2012;**159** (3):277–87.

83. Smrcek JM, Baschat AA, Germer U, Gloeckner-Hofmann K, Gembruch U. Fetal hydrops and hepatosplenomegaly in the second half of pregnancy: A sign of myeloproliferative disorder in fetuses with trisomy 21. *Ultrasound Obstet Gynecol* 2001;**17**(5):403–9.

84. Yagihashi N, Watanabe K, Yagihashi S. Transient abnormal myelopoiesis accompanied by hepatic fibrosis in two infants with Down syndrome. *J Clin Pathol* 1995;**48**(10):973–5.

85. Heald B, Hilden JM, Zbuk K, et al. Severe TMD/ AMKL with GATA1 mutation in a stillborn fetus with Down syndrome. *Nat Clin Pract Oncol* 2007;**4** (7):433–8.

86. Maroz A, Stachorski L, Emmrich S, et al. GATA1s induces hyperproliferation of eosinophil precursors in Down syndrome transient leukemia. *Leukemia.* 2014;**28**(6):1259–70.

87. Swerdlow SN, Campo E, Pileri SA, et al., eds. *WHO Classification of Tumours of Haematopoietic and Lymphoid Tissues*, revised 4th ed. (Lyon: IARC, 2017).

88. Miyauchi J, Ito Y, Kawano T, Tsunematsu Y, Shimizu K. Unusual diffuse liver fibrosis accompanying transient myeloproliferative disorder in Down's syndrome: A report of four autopsy cases and proposal of a hypothesis. *Blood* 1992;**80**(6):1521–7.

89. Muramatsu H, Kato K, Watanabe N, et al. Risk factors for early death in neonates with Down syndrome and transient leukaemia. *Br J Haematol* 2008;**142**(4):610–15.

90. Tamblyn JA, Norton A, Spurgeon L, et al. Prenatal therapy in transient abnormal myelopoiesis: A systematic review. *Arch Dis Child Fetal Neonatal Ed* 2016;**101**(1):F67–71.

91. Taub JW, Huang X, Matherly LH, et al. Expression of chromosome 21-localized genes in acute myeloid leukemia: Differences between Down syndrome and non-Down syndrome blast cells and relationship to in vitro sensitivity to cytosine arabinoside and daunorubicin. *Blood* 1999;**94** (4):1393–400.

92. Zwaan CM, Kaspers GJ, Pieters R, et al. Different drug sensitivity profiles of acute myeloid and lymphoblastic leukemia and normal peripheral blood mononuclear cells in children with and without Down syndrome. *Blood* 2002;**99** (1):245–51.

93. Flasinski M, Scheibke K, Zimmermann M, et al. Low-dose cytarabine to prevent myeloid leukemia in children with Down syndrome: TMD Prevention 2007 study. *Blood Adv* 2018;**2** (13):1532–40.

94. Park MJ, Sotomatsu M, Ohki K, et al. Liver disease is frequently observed in Down syndrome patients with transient abnormal myelopoiesis. *Int J Hematol* 2014;**99**(2):154–61.

95. Hasle H, Abrahamsson J, Arola M, et al. Myeloid leukemia in children 4 years or older with Down syndrome often lacks GATA1 mutation and cytogenetics and risk of relapse are more akin to sporadic AML. *Leukemia* 2008;**22**(7):1428–30.

96. Uffmann M, Rasche M, Zimmermann M, et al. Therapy reduction in patients with Down syndrome and myeloid leukemia: The international ML-DS 2006 trial. *Blood* 2017;**129** (25):3314–21.

Chapter 22

Neonatal and Perinatal Solid Tumors

Kevin F. Ginn, Jaszianne A. Tolbert, Glenson Samuel, J. Allyson Hays, and Alan S. Gamis

Introduction

Solid tumors in neonates can arise anywhere in the body and present unique challenges to clinicians. Benign tumors are most common [1], and are typically less amenable to chemotherapy or radiation and more in need of surgical approaches. Radiation's role in childhood cancer is diminishing as better chemotherapeutic approaches are developed and its use in neonates is rare due to its devastating long-term toxicity. Finally, differences in neonatal physiology imparts a variable upon chemotherapy pharmacokinetics that is difficult to fully control and frequently results in greater toxicity. These factors, combined with the biology of the tumors uniquely seen in the neonate, worsen the survival for neonates with cancer. This chapter acquaints the clinician with the array of tumors most commonly found in the infant <28 days of age (Table 22.1).

Epidemiology

Fortunately, tumors in newborns are rare. Among infants less than 1 year of age, 13% of malignancies are diagnosed in the first month of life with an incidence of 30–36 cases per million neonates [2, 3], which is significantly less than the overall 233 cases per million children <1 year of age [2]. The distribution of tumors seen in neonates is quite different than seen in older children (Table 22.2). Solid tumors outside the central nervous system (CNS) make up the majority of neonatal tumors [4, 5], and quite the opposite distribution is seen in older children [6]. Other entities found in infants typically not

included in the tumor registries include vascular tumors and histiocytic disorders and these are briefly discussed in this chapter. Overall survival (OS) is worse in neonates either due to inability to give optimal therapies, differences in tumor biology or potentially due to decisions to forgo therapy when chance of cure or good quality of life is perceived as low by family and/or providers. Recent SEER analyses found a 5 year OS of 60.3% (95% CI, 56.2%–64.4%) with the highest survival seen in those with solid tumors (71.2%) versus leukemias (39.1%), and CNS tumors (15%)[4], and all significantly worse than in children ages 1–14 years whose 5 year OS is 80.6% [7]. Some exceptions exist, e.g., infants with neuroblastoma whose tumors are significantly less likely to contain the adverse MYCN oncogene and which frequently have the unique characteristic of spontaneous regression not seen in older children.

When encountering a neonatal solid tumor one must consider the possibility of a genetic predisposition and certainly the family will want information regarding this potential association. In a large pediatric series 8.5% of pediatric cancer cases were associated with a germline mutation in a cancer predisposition gene [8]. As techniques and genetic data improve, we may find a higher association. The most important first step is obtaining a detailed family history followed by full assessment of any additional clinical features pointing toward an associated syndrome. Screening tools are available to help determine the need for further work-up and referral to genetics [9].

Neonatal Hematology, Pathogenesis, Diagnosis, and Management of Hematologic Problems, 3rd edition, ed. Pedro A. de Alarcón, Eric J. Werner, Robert D. Christensen, and Martha C. Sola-Visner. Published by Cambridge University Press. © Cambridge University Press 2021.

Table 22.1 Neonatal tumors by location (not all discussed in this chapter)

Brain tumors	Cardiac tumors	Pulmonary/thoracic tumors
Teratoma	Rhabdomyoma	Pleuropulmonary blastoma
Astrocytoma (glioma)	Teratoma	Congenital cystic adenomatoid malformation
Medulloblastoma	Fibroma	Bronchopulmonary malformation
Choroid plexus papilloma	Vascular tumor	Pulmonary arteriovenous malformation
Choroid plexus carcinoma	Purkinje cell tumor	Pulmonary myofibroblastic tumor
Ependymoma	Myxoma	Chest wall hamartoma
Atypical teratoid/rhabdoid tumor	**Adrenal tumors**	Bronchogenic cyst
Supratentorial embryonal tumors	Adrenal hemorrhage	Pulmonary sequestration, intrapulmonary and
Juvenile xanthogranuloma	Subdiaphragmatic extralobar	extrapulmonary
	pulmonary sequestration	Neuroblastoma
	Neuroblastoma	
Head and neck tumors	**Liver tumors**	**Gastric tumors**
Thyroglossal duct	Hemangioma	Teratoma
Branchial cleft cyst	Hemangioendothelioma	Hamartoma
Lymphangioma	Mesenchymal hamartoma	**Ovarian tumors**
Hemangioma	Hepatoblastoma	Ovarian cysts
Vascular malformations	Metastatic neuroblastoma	Granulocytic sarcoma
Lingual thyroid	Histiocytic disorders	Teratoma
Congenital epulis	**Renal tumors**	Germ cell tumor
Ranula and other cystic lesions	Hydronephrosis	**Testicular tumors**
Teratoma (epignathus)	Polycystic kidney disease	Scrotal hematoma
Dermoid cyst	Congenital mesoblastic	Hematocele
Fibromatosis coli	nephroma	Hydrocele
Fibromatoses	Wilms tumor	Hernia
Rhabdomyosarcoma	Rhabdoid tumor of the	Testicular torsion
Retinoblastoma	kidney	Yolk sac tumor
Neuroblastoma	Clear cell sarcoma of the	Gonadoblastoma
	kidney	Teratoma
		Hamartoma

Peripheral Nerve Tumors and Adrenal Masses

Neuroblastoma, the most common extracranial malignant tumor in infants, has an incidence in the neonatal period of 17–19.7 per million live births [10–12]. The true incidence may be vastly underestimated as a number of infants are never symptomatic and tumors spontaneously regress as shown in past newborn screening studies [13, 14]. Neuroblastomas and their more benign histologic variants, ganglioneuroblastoma and ganglioneuroma, originate from neural crest cells and most commonly arise in the adrenal glands but may present anywhere along the sympathetic chain. Infants frequently present with abdominal distention due to a mass but clinical presentation varies depending upon tumor location. Some may present with Horner syndrome or paralysis due to compression of neurovascular structures, with hepatomegaly due to metastatic disease or with respiratory distress related to a posterior mediastinal tumor. Metastatic lesions, such as a blueberry muffin rash, periorbital and other bone lesions, or

bone marrow involvement with cytopenias may be the initial presentation rather than the primary tumor. Other manifestations may include refractory hypertension and diarrhea due to tumor secretion of hormones such as norepinephrine and vasoactive intestinal peptide [15].

Diagnosis and staging includes CT (abdominal lesions) or MRI (paraspinous lesions) and biopsy if feasible. Neuroblastomas concentrate meta-iodo-benzyl-guanidine (MIBG), thus an MIBG scan should be performed if available [16]. Urinary catecholamines, homovanillic acid (HVA), and vanillylmandelic acid (VMA), should be obtained and are elevated in more than 90% of patients. Bone marrow examination completes the staging evaluation [17].

Neuroblastoma treatment is based on risk including age, stage of disease, and tumor features such as histology, DNA ploidy, 11q aberration, and MYCN amplification [18]. The International Neuroblastoma Risk Group (INRG) stages disease based on metastatic disease (stage M), image defined features suggestive of resectability in those without metastatic disease (L1 or L2) or

383

Table 22.2 Distribution of solid tumors found in neonatal studies with comparison to older children

				Source			
	Alfaar et al. [4] SEER (1973–2007)	Parkes et al. [5] Midlands, UK (1960–1989)	Desandes et al. [3] France (2000–2009)	Rao et al. [1] Glasgow (1955–1999)	Total (solid tumors)	Ries et al. [6] SEER (1975–1995)**
Age group	<1 month	<1 month	<28 days	<28 days	<1 month	<15 yrs
Total (N)	**615**	**99**	**285**	**83**	**879**	**19,845**
Solid tumors – N (% of all tumors)	**454 (74%)**	**86 (86%)**	**256**	**83**	**879**	**(51.7%)**
% of non-CNS solid tumors						
Peripheral nerve tumors (including neuroblastoma)	38%	17%	52%	17%	38%	21%
Germ cell (including teratomas)	37%	53%*	32%	40%	37%	10%**
Soft tissue	11%	9%	9%	16%	11%	27%***
Renal tumors	4%	8%	2%	16%	5%	17%
Retinal tumors	6%	2%	3%	–	4%	8%
Hepatic tumors	2%	7%	1%	5%	2%	4%
Other	2%	2%	–	7%	2%	10%
CNS tumors – N (% of all tumors)	**68 (11%)**	**5 (5% total)**	**29**	**-**	**-**	**(20.2%)******
Leukemias/lymphomas – N (% of all tumors)	**93 (15%)**	**8 (8%)**	**N/A**	**-**	**-**	**(42.2%)**
Lymphoid	(3.6%)					(24.7%)
Myeloid	(7.3%)					(6.8%)
Unspecified or lymphoreticular	(4.2%)					(10.7%)

Notes: * These were all reported as teratomas

** Does not include borderline malignancies such as teratomas

*** Includes both soft tissue (7%) and bone (4.5%) sarcomas

**** Does not include benign/low grade brain tumors

patients <18 months of age with metastatic disease but no bone involvement (MS) [17, 19]. MYCN amplification confers high risk regardless of other factors and requires intensive chemotherapy, radiation when able and immunotherapy [18, 20]. When MYCN amplification is not present (90% of infants), subsequent treatment ranges from surgery alone to the intensive therapy just described depending upon other risk features [18]. Spontaneous regression is a unique possibility in infants with neuroblastoma [21]. When a small adrenal mass is the sole manifestation, expectant observation has been successful with 100% survival and sparing 81% eventual surgery [22]. Infants with stage MS may also experience spontaneous regression of their tumors. In one Children's Oncology Group study, 55% required only supportive care; however, some may develop respiratory compromise due to extensive liver involvement and require chemotherapy and/or radiation therapy as symptomatic infants under 2 months of age are at the highest risk of mortality [23, 24].

While prognosis is similar in neonates and older infants with neuroblastoma of similar biologic features, the overall prognosis in infants is superior to older children as most lesions in this age group are lower stage, respond well to therapy and, in some cases, spontaneously regress [25–27]. The 5 year OS approaches 80% for children less than 1 year at diagnosis and >95% for infants with neuroblastoma without MYCN amplification [25, 28].

Benign adrenal masses are common occurrences in the prenatal and newborn period and are commonly adrenal hemorrhage or subdiaphragmatic extralobar pulmonary sequestration (SEPS) [29]. Though the majority of these lesions spontaneously regress, it is important to distinguish them from adrenal malignancies such as neuroblastoma [29]. **Adrenal hemorrhage** is the most common neonatal adrenal mass and may present unilaterally or bilaterally [29]. Most adrenal hemorrhages spontaneously resolve, thus careful observation is sufficient.

Subdiaphragmatic extralobar pulmonary sequestration (SEPS) is a rare congenital anomaly composed of nonfunctioning pulmonary tissue. These sequestrations may be found within the lung or below the diaphragm and have similar ultrasound appearance to neuroblastoma. Prenatally detected neuroblastoma is 2.5 times more common than SEPS [30]. SEPS are identified in the second trimester and are usually left-sided echogenic masses; neuroblastomas are identified in the third trimester and are usually right-sided cystic masses [30]. In fact, approximately 25% of neuroblastomas diagnosed in the perinatal or neonatal age are cystic [27].

Non-CNS Germ Cell Tumors

Germ cell tumors (GCT) are a heterogeneous group of benign and malignant neoplasms derived from primordial germ cells. In neonates, they are the most common neoplasm accounting for 35%–40% of all tumors in the first month of life [31]. In order of prevalence, the most common histologic subtypes of germ cell tumors in the neonate include teratoma (mature or immature), yolk sac tumor and choriocarcinoma [32]. Though most are benign in the neonatal period, there remains a high morbidity rate due to hydrops, premature delivery, and peri-operative and post-surgical anatomical defects.

Teratoma is the most common GCT in neonates. Teratomas are equally divided between mature and immature histologic types, the latter having a higher incidence of yolk sac components [32]. Most teratomas are extra-gonadal and frequently occur in the sacrococcygeal region but may arise in any midline location. Sacrococcygeal teratomas (SCT) present as an extrapelvic mass protruding between the coccyx and rectum. Hereditary SCT, which are less common, are almost always presacral and may be an isolated finding or part of the Currarino triad (presacral tumor, anorectal malformations, and sacral anomaly) [33]. Hereditary SCT are less likely to contain malignant elements [32]. Treatment generally consists of complete, early surgical resection often with coccygectomy taking extreme care to avoid tumor rupture and spillage which may lead to serious life threatening bleeding complications [24]. Congenital head and neck teratomas, though infrequent (4%), may present unique challenges including potential need for ex-utero intrapartum treatment (EXIT) to establish a patent airway [34]. In addition to surgery, platinum-based chemotherapy protocols have been successful in SCT with malignant features [24]. After treatment, monitoring for recurrence with physical exams and serum tumor markers (if elevated at diagnosis) is paramount as most recurrences occur within 3 years.

Yolk sac tumor (YST) is the most common malignant GCT in infancy [32]. Other synonymous terms for YST include endodermal sinus tumor, orchioblastoma, Teilum's tumor, and clear cell adenocarcinoma [35]. On macroscopic exam, these tumors often appear cystic and yellow with areas of hemorrhage, necrosis and liquefaction [35]. Alpha fetoprotein (AFP) is typically elevated at diagnosis and should raise the suspicion for malignant yolk sac components even in those with teratomas. It is important to remember that AFP at birth is significantly higher than normal adult ranges and thus an infant's AFP levels must be compared to infant norms until greater than 1 year of age [36]. Successful treatment outcomes involve surgical resection and in rare cases platinum-based chemotherapy.

Choriocarcinoma is a rare tumor in neonates that is highly fatal if left untreated. In neonates, choriocarcinoma is thought to arise as metastatic disease from a focus of choriocarcinoma in the placenta. Patients often present with anemia, failure to thrive, hepatomegaly, respiratory distress, and seizures. Evaluation should include measurement of human chorionic gonadotrophin (β-hCG) which is often markedly elevated [37]. Unlike most GCT, surgical resection alone is not curative and is not recommended upfront due to friability of the tumor and potential for bleeding. Whereas a high mortality was historically seen in affected neonates, more modern approaches with platinum-containing multi-agent chemotherapy has improved survival [35].

Soft Tissue Tumors

Sarcomas are of mesenchymal origin and are the fifth most prevalent malignancy in infants with an incidence of 1.6/100,000 in children less than 1 year of age [38]. In neonates they comprise 11% of non-CNS solid tumors. Age correlates strongly with the epidemiological pattern and clinical behavior of various soft tissue sarcomas (STS) within the pediatric population [39]. Neonates experience a uniquely different distribution of soft tissue tumors as compared to older patients with only one-third of neonatal STS comprising rhabdomyosarcoma followed by infantile fibrosarcoma [4, 40].

Rhabdomyosarcoma (RMS) in newborns comprise only 1%–2% of all RMS patients and are rarely diagnosed prenatally. Clinical symptoms vary and are dependent upon mass effect on surrounding organs by these rapidly proliferating tumors. Based on the Intergroup Rhabdomyosarcoma Studies (IRS), approximately 40% of RMS occur in the head and neck region, followed by the genitourinary tract (slightly less than 25%), and then extremities (approximately 20%) [41]. Within the neonatal period, tumors in the face or neck region may be misdiagnosed as vascular tumors or oropharyngeal teratomas. Twenty percent of patients at diagnosis have regional lymph node involvement and distant metastases commonly involving the lungs, bone marrow, and bones. The presence of metastatic skin lesions and early metastatic brain lesions are more common in neonatal RMS [42].

Sufficient tumor tissue is required for complete characterization. Histologically RMS is grouped into two main subgroups: embryonal (ERMS) and alveolar (ARMS). ERMS has a better prognosis than ARMS which is characterized by the t(2;13) or t(1;13) chromosomal translocations [43]. Diagnostic workup includes MRI or CT scan of the primary lesion, chest CT, bone scan, and bone marrow evaluation. These tumors are rarely resectable at diagnosis. Therapeutic management is divided into systemic (chemotherapy) and localized therapy (surgery and/or radiation therapy). Chemotherapy varies based on the site and stage of tumor, but in order to minimize toxicity dose-modifications are made in the management of neonatal RMS. Overall, the IRS Group reported a 3 year OS of 49% in newborns [44], and in the SEER database a 5 year OS of 38% [39].

Fibroblastic-myofibroblastic tumors are relatively frequent soft tissue tumors in children less than 1 year of age. Morphology frequently mimics sarcomas and their histology may be inconsistent with clinical findings making the diagnosis difficult. These tumors frequently present as large unresectable tumors posing a therapeutic challenge to surgeons and oncologists. Current therapeutic strategies involve a multidisciplinary approach with the use of systemic therapies to reduce sequelae of radical surgery.

Fibromatosis is a major subgroup of fibroblastic-myofibroblastic tumors and can occur in three forms: solitary, multicentric, or generalized. Solitary fibromatosis can occur at a multitude of sites; surgery is the mainstay of treatment and local recurrence is likely with incomplete resection. Unresectable tumors may be monitored closely for regression. Systemic therapy is often necessary for lesions in precarious locations or those that are progressive and/or symptomatic. Low-dose chemotherapy may play a role in the management of aggressive fibromatosis; however, the role for adjuvant chemotherapy remains unclear. Therapy may also be initiated with non-cytotoxic agents such as anti-inflammatory agents or hormonal therapy [45]. If possible, deferment of chemotherapy or radiation therapy is most advantageous until these children are older. Desmoid type fibromatosis can be sporadic or can arise within the setting of familial adenomatosis polyposis (FAP) including the Gardner's variant. Potential drivers of tumorigenesis involve mutations of beta-catenin, CTNNB1, and the APC gene on chromosome 5q21 [46]. Typically, these tumors are deep-seated masses without a pseudocapsule and are located within musculo-aponeurotic structures (neck, chest, extremities, abdominal wall) rendering them difficult to resect. Even with wide resection, recurrence rate is high.

Hemangiopericytomas (HPC), now termed as myofibroma, are rapidly growing, highly vascularized soft tissue neoplasms of pericytic origin. These usually arise in the lower extremities or pelvis. Congenital hemangiopericytoma represent about one-third of pediatric HPCs, and are considered a distinct entity from the adult form of the disease. Most infantile hemangiopericytomas are benign. These tumors may regress but often require multimodal therapeutic approaches including surgery, chemotherapy, and radiotherapy if they possess aggressive features [47–49].

Infantile fibrosarcoma (IFS) is classified as a soft tissue tumor with an intermediate prognosis. They represent approximately 5%–10% of sarcomas in children younger than 12 months [50, 51]. Sixty percent of cases are diagnosed before 3 months of age, with 30%–50% of these noted at birth or diagnosed in utero [40, 52]. The translocation t(12;15) with the transcript ETV6-NTRK3 is characteristic for IFS [53]. IFS generally present as an enlarging non-inflammatory mass and are often highly vascular with ulceration. Typical locations for IFS are within the soft tissue of the extremities (66% of cases), followed by the trunk (25%), and then head and neck (7%) [51]. Distant metastases are rare and prognosis is favorable with greater than 80% survival [50, 54]. Tumors not primarily resectable may be monitored for spontaneous regression. Chemotherapy may be considered in an effort to render tumors more easily resectable. Vincristine and actinomycin (VA) are the chemotherapeutic agents of choice however more intensive therapy may be needed [54].

Leiomyosarcoma behaves benignly in the neonatal period. These tumors frequently arise in the intestines and may present with aseptic chemical peritonitis due to gut perforation with meconium peritonitis or intestinal obstruction. Management is surgical [55].

Central Nervous System Tumors

Central nervous system (CNS) tumors are the most common solid tumor in pediatrics, most commonly are low grade gliomas and most commonly arise in the posterior fossa [56]. In contrast, neonatal CNS tumors are extremely rare making up 0.5%–1.9% of all pediatric brain tumors [57], are more frequently supratentorial, and are most commonly teratomas [58]. Prenatal ultrasound may identify CNS tumors prior to birth due to enlarged head circumference, abnormal brain or skull development or visualization of the tumor itself. Prenatal MRI may be utilized to better image the mass and allow for safer delivery planning [59]. Survival for neonatal CNS tumors is very poor. A California center reviewed 250 cases and showed a 28% survival with 21% of deaths being stillbirths. For the most commonly encountered tumor, teratomas, only 12% survived [60]. Tumors that are identified prior to 30 weeks' gestation have nearly 100% mortality [59].

Teratomas, more frequent outside of the CNS, are the most common intracranial neoplasm representing up to 50% of cases. Teratomas most commonly arise in the midline (i.e., pineal or suprasellar region) but may occur in the cerebral hemispheres or cerebellum. A solid and cystic mass with mineralization (calcifications) may be identified on imaging with more invasive, larger masses with more significant solid components pointing towards a more immature, malignant form [59]. Serum and/or cerebrospinal fluid (CSF) tumors markers such as AFP and β-hCG may aid in the diagnosis and if elevated point to a malignant component [61]. These tumors may grow very large leading to poor cerebral development, macrocephaly, and commonly result in fetal demise [62]. Rarely, surgically removed mature teratomas may result in long-term survival [63].

Gliomas arise from multiple cells of origin anywhere in the brain or spine and include astrocytic tumors, oligodendroglial tumors, oligoastrocytic tumors, and ependymal tumors. Histologic grading ranges from WHO Grade I (most commonly pilocytic astrocytoma) to WHO Grade IV (most commonly glioblastoma) [64]. Molecular profiling is increasingly incorporated into the comprehensive diagnosis and helps classify these entities into various prognostic groups with many new therapeutic targets [65]. Low grade gliomas are the most common CNS tumor in pediatrics and they most commonly arise in the posterior fossa [56]. In contrast, gliomas are the second most common CNS tumor in neonates, more commonly arise in the cerebral hemispheres, are 1.5 times more likely to be higher grade, and often present with macrocephaly, hydrocephalus and hemorrhage [66]. In a large series overall survival for astrocytic tumors was 30%; however, if separating low grade and high grade tumors, the survival ranges from 90% to 20%, respectively [58, 60, 66]. Complete surgical resection of low-grade gliomas is considered curative. For unresectable tumors, options increasingly include use of targeted agents after molecular profiling [67]; however, traditional chemotherapy approaches remain first line. In neonates, radiation is not a viable option.

Subependymal giant cell astrocytoma (SEGA) may present in the neonatal period with hydrocephalus or a large mass in up to 2% of patients with tuberous sclerosis complex (TSC) and these patients more commonly have TSC2/PKD1 mutations [68]. Surgical resection remains the preferred treatment for SEGA, however, treatment with mTOR inhibitors (Everolimus) can be attempted where results in older pediatric patients have shown around 80% of patients had a 50% or more reduction in tumor volume [69]. Tumor size reduction may lead to safer surgical options.

Embryonal tumors include medulloblastoma, atypical teratoid rhabdoid tumor (ATRT) and the group formally classified as primitive neuroectodermal tumor (PNET) [65]. In neonates, the most common embryonal tumors are medulloblastoma and ATRT and both are aggressive tumors with high frequency of CNS metastasis. Up to 66% of patients with congenital rhabdoid tumors have been reported to have rhabdoid tumor predisposition syndrome due to germline SMARCB1 or rarely SMARCA4 mutations and must be screened

for synchronous malignant rhabdoid tumors of the kidney and soft tissues [70, 71]. Unless a gross total resection can be achieved in a patient without metastatic disease palliative care may be warranted without therapy given the poor prognosis [71]. Even with aggressive treatment the survival rate is approximately 40% [72]. Medulloblastomas by definition arise from the cerebellum and have been divided into multiple molecular subgroups with infant tumors most commonly falling into the sonic hedgehog (SHH) subtype [73]. For infants with medulloblastoma, Gorlin syndrome (nevoid basal cell carcinoma syndrome) due to mutations in PTCH1 in the SHH pathway must be considered as a predisposing factor [74]. Molecular profiling and classic clinical staging such as metastatic disease state and extent of resection both play a role in prognostication. Although radiation is effective, it is avoided in the youngest patients and treatment instead includes only aggressive chemotherapy approaches often including high dose chemotherapy with autologous stem cell rescue. The outcome with this approach has been reported to result in 5 year OS as high as 76% [75]. Although radiation in infants is avoided these patients are still left with significant neurocognitive dysfunction [76, 77].

Choroid plexus tumors arise in the ventricles and are divided into three WHO Grades: WHO Grade I choroid plexus papilloma, WHO Grade II atypical choroid plexus papilloma, and WHO Grade III choroid plexus carcinoma [64]. Choroid plexus tumors may be identified by ultrasound imaging showing the intraventricular mass or present with massive hydrocephalus due to overproduction of CSF [78, 79]. Choroid plexus papillomas may be treated with surgical resection alone; however, choroid plexus carcinomas require aggressive chemotherapy even after complete resection and survival is poor [80]. Patients with choroid plexus carcinoma have a high risk of a germline mutation in TP53 (Li–Fraumeni syndrome) and should undergo genetic screening [81].

Renal Tumors

Renal neoplasms comprise 7% of all neonatal tumors [82]. Congenital mesoblastic nephroma is most prevalent followed in incidence by the malignant tumors Wilms tumor, rhabdoid tumor, and clear cell sarcoma.

Congenital mesoblastic nephroma is the most common renal mass in neonates accounting for approximately 60% of cases [82–84]. It is a tumor predominantly of infants (median age 1–2 months) presenting typically as a unilateral large mass often associated with polyuria, hypertension, hypercalcemia, and occasionally congestive heart failure [85]. Prenatal diagnosis of CMN is seen in 15% of cases [84]. Metastatic disease is rare primarily occurring with relapse [86]. Histologically three subtypes are recognized: classical (most common), cellular, and mixed (least common) [83, 84]. The cellular subtype is often (58%) characterized by the translocation t(12;15) (p13p15), a fusion of *ETV6* and *NTRK3* genes that is also seen in infantile fibrosarcoma [87]. Treatment is complete surgical resection (achieved in >80%) via radical nephrectomy which is curative in more than 90% of cases [83, 84, 86]. Chemotherapy is reserved for large unresectable tumors or after relapse (most common among cellular subtypes) [88, 89]. Surgical complications are frequent (23%) and half of deaths due to CMN are associated with surgical complications occurring primarily in the youngest patients, emphasizing the need for care in experienced centers [84, 90]. Infants younger than 2 months with stage III tumors (incomplete resection or tumor spillage) may be observed as later recurrence is typically retrievable with surgery and/or chemotherapy [84].

Wilms' tumor is the most common pediatric renal tumor but represents only 20% of neonatal renal tumors [83, 86]. Occurrence is often sporadic though a small percentage of diagnoses are associated with congenital syndromes (Beckwith–Wiedemann, WAGR, and Denys–Drash) [82, 91]. Tumors may be unilateral or bilateral (rare) and typically present as a palpable abdominal mass with or without associated abdominal pain, distention, and hypertension. Almost all bilateral Wilms' tumors contain nephrogenic rests but in unilateral Wilms' tumor these abnormal foci increase the risk of developing bilateral Wilms' tumor and must be carefully monitored [92]. Histologic subtypes include favorable and anaplastic histology though the latter is rarely seen in neonates. Treatment often involves radical nephrectomy, adjuvant chemotherapy and in cases of tumor spillage, radiation to the primary tumor site. Cure rates are >90% with poorer outcomes seen in patients with metastatic disease, anaplastic histology and other unfavorable

prognostic factors [86]. For those with stage I (completely resected with no capsular invasion) favorable histology tumors weighing <550 g, chemotherapy may be deferred to use only in those who recur [93].

Rhabdoid tumor of the kidney (RTK) is a rare but lethal disease seen in 11% of neonates with renal tumors [83, 94]. Universal to RTK is the loss of function of the *SMARCB1/INI1* gene located on chromosome 22q11.2 resulting in *INI1* negative immunostaining. This mutation is germline in 25% of patients [95]. Patients usually present with an abdominal mass and associated fever and hematuria. Often advanced stage disease is present at diagnosis due to the high potential for brain, bone, liver, abdominal, and lung metastasis [83, 86]. The high prevalence of brain metastases (26%) mandates early imaging [83]. Treatment generally follows high risk renal tumor protocols with surgical resection, chemotherapy, and radiation. Despite treatment, outcome is poor with survival in neonates <10%–20% [83, 86, 94].

Clear cell sarcoma of the kidney (CCSK) is a rare (<2%–3%) diagnosis in the neonate. Present in nearly all cases is the *BCOR* mutation [96]. Patients typically present with palpable abdominal mass with associated hypertension, hematuria, and abdominal pain. This aggressive tumor often metastasizes to bone but may also involve brain, lungs, and liver [89]. Treatment involves complete surgical resection, chemotherapy, and radiation [83]. Outcomes for neonates with CCSK are superior to that of older children as most neonates who are treated survive [83], though prognostic information is limited in this group.

Retinoblastoma

Retinoblastoma is the most common tumor of the eye in children and accounts for 1%–3% of all childhood malignancies [97]. In neonates, retinoblastoma almost exclusively occurs in offspring of parents with retinoblastoma 1 (RB1) gene mutation of chromosome 13q14.2. Older infants and children may be noted to have leukocoria, strabismus, and lack of red reflex. Differential diagnoses of leukocoria includes congenital cataracts, toxocariasis, retinopathy of prematurity, persistent fetal vasculature, retinal detachment, and vitreous hemorrhage [98]. The American Association of

Ophthalmic Oncologists and Pathologists recommends children without a family history undergo red reflex testing at routine visits until 5 years of age, at which time the retina is mature.

Recommendations for children with RB1 mutation or positive family history include more frequent examinations [99]. RB1 testing may be performed upon delivery or prenatally via amniocentesis between 16 and 33 weeks' gestation [100]. Children with RB1 mutation may have unilateral tumors but the other eye may become affected. Bilateral retinoblastoma tends to occur in children with germline mutation and is typically seen in younger patients (14–16 months) than unilateral retinoblastoma (29–30 months) [101–103]. Children with suspected retinoblastoma need an MRI to determine extent of disease including evaluation for possible trilateral retinoblastoma with pineal involvement.

Treatment, based upon the degree of retrievable vision and extent of disease, includes enucleation of the eye, intravenous chemotherapy, and intravitreal chemotherapy. Infants greater than 3 months of age may receive intra-arterial chemotherapy via the ophthalmic artery. Bridge therapy with intravenous carboplatin until 3 months of age and 6 kilograms in weight has successfully been utilized for neonates [104]. Overall survival exceeds 90% [4, 105].

Children with RB1 mutation are predisposed to secondary malignancies including STS and breast cancers. The American Association of Cancer Research has published recommendations for surveillance [106].

Hepatic Tumors

Hepatic tumors are uncommon in the perinatal period accounting for only 2%–7% of solid tumors [107–109]. Benign tumors such as infantile hemangioma and mesenchymal hamartoma are more predominant than malignant tumors during this period.

Infantile hemangiomas are the most common benign tumors of the liver in the fetus and neonate and often present as multiple liver lesions [110, 111]. These highly vascular tumors are characterized by rapid proliferation in the neonatal period followed by a slower period of involution during childhood. Though benign, they may lead to serious complications including consumptive coagulopathy, severe anemia, and high output cardiac

failure. Treatment and outcomes are detailed in the section on Vascular Tumors.

Mesenchymal hamartoma is the second most common benign tumor of the liver in fetuses and neonates and presents as a multicystic liver mass [112]. These fluid-filled masses are characterized by rapid growth and expansion often leading to abdominal distention, respiratory distress, and compression of surrounding vessels and organs [113]. Severe, life-threatening complications such as fetal hydrops, congestive heart failure, and still birth may also occur [113]. Treatment consists of surgical resection when feasible. If surgery is not an option then close ultrasound monitoring until surgery can take place is warranted [114, 115]. One study showed 76% survival with surgery compared to 64% survival for all patients with mesenchymal hamartoma [112].

Hepatoblastomas are the most common primary hepatic malignancy [116]. though most hepatic malignancies in the fetus and neonate are actually metastatic lesions from other tumor sites. Neuroblastoma, GCT, renal tumors, RMS, and leukemias are some of the malignancies that can metastasize to the liver [117].

Hepatoblastoma incidence has increased possibly owing to increased survival of preterm and low birth weight infants and their associated increased risk of hepatoblastoma [118, 119]. These tumors often present as a firm, palpable mass with associated abdominal distention and pain. Hepatoblastoma may be associated with genetic syndromes such as Beckwith–Wiedemann, Li–Fraumeni, FAP, and trisomy 18, thus a comprehensive family history and genetic testing is indicated [120]. AFP levels are elevated in approximately 70% of cases, while lower AFP levels are associated with more aggressive features and poorer outcomes [121]. Thrombocytosis may also be present as part of a paraneoplastic effect. Treatment consists of surgical resection alone for well-differentiated fetal histology hepatoblastoma, but pre-operative platinum-based chemotherapy may be utilized to reduce tumor volume. Patients with other histologic subtypes of hepatoblastoma all receive chemotherapy regardless of extent of resection. Liver transplantation is reserved for patients with unresectable disease after neoadjuvant chemotherapy [122, 123]. Past studies suggested worse outcomes in neonates with hepatoblastoma but more recent cooperative group trials have significantly improved outcomes which are now comparable to or better than older children with current 5 year OS in excess of 85%–90% [112, 124, 125].

Vascular Tumors

Vascular tumors are the most common soft tissue and subcutaneous neoplasm in infants. Differentiating amongst the various types of vascular tumors and more importantly between vascular tumors and sarcomas may be difficult [126]. In neonates, the primary vascular tumors are benign congenital hemangiomas that arise prenatally and are present at birth, benign infantile hemangiomas that arise late in the first month from pre-existing telangectasias or areas of skin discoloration, and borderline, locally aggressive kaposiform hemangioendotheliomas and their variant tufted angiomas.

Hemangiomas are a benign neoplasm with a predilection to arise in the head and neck region. Cutaneous infantile hemangiomas (IH) are the most common benign vascular tumor of infancy occurring in 4%–5% of infants, are more prevalent in premature infants and commonly manifest at the age of 3–6 weeks [127, 128]. An initial phase of rapid proliferation lasting an average of 5 months followed by a slow involutional phase occurring over years is typical [129, 130]. IH is not associated with coagulopathies. Diagnosis is typically clinical with biopsies rarely needed; however, histopathology should include GLUT1 as endothelial cells in IH express GLUT1, whereas congenital hemangiomas do not. Underlying malformations should be ruled out, e.g., PHACE syndrome [131]. Visceral hemangiomas, most frequently involving the liver, should be sought in infants with more than five cutaneous hemangiomas [130]. Most hemangiomas require no intervention, but in functional impairment or dramatic aesthetic concerns, may require treatment [132, 133]. Beta blockers, such as propranolol [134], are most commonly utilized in the setting of diffuse or multifocal hepatic hemangiomas displaying symptoms such as high cardiac output failure or profound hypothyroidism. Other medical treatment options include steroids, laser therapy, excision, and in diffuse visceral lesions, even cyclophosphamide or vincristine have been used [135, 136]. If medical management is unsuccessful liver transplant may be indicated [137]. Vascular cutaneous lesions present at birth are most frequently congenital hemangiomas (CH) [130, 138]. These tumors present at birth, typically regress and do not grow further unless internal hemorrhage occurs. Coagulopathy has been associated with these types of hemangioma. Therapy for CH typically is supportive but may require embolization or surgery.

Kaposiform hemangioendothelioma (KHE) (and the variant **tufted angioma**) is an extremely rare aggressive vascular neoplasm, with 60% of cases occurring within the neonatal period. KHE are commonly located in the retroperitoneum and deep soft tissues of the extremities (83% of the cases) [139]. Superficial soft tissues, scalp, neck, chest wall, and mediastinum involvement have also been reported. KHE is most often solitary. Infants with KHE frequently (70%) experience the consumptive coagulopathic Kasabach–Merritt phenomenon (thrombocytopenia, hypofibrinogenemia, elevated d-dimers). Patients with larger visceral tumors have a 40%–50% mortality rate [40]. MRI is preferred as the imaging modality and if feasible histologic confirmation is advised. Treatment varies based upon severity of the case. Due to size, site, and involvement of several tissue planes, there is often an inability to safely resect these tumors. Initial medical treatment is most commonly corticosteroids [140], followed by vincristine [141]. Other therapeutic options include antiplatelet therapy [142], interferon-alpha [143], anti-fibrinolytic therapy, chemotherapy, propranolol [144], embolization [145], and sirolimus as a monotherapy or in combination with steroids [146]. Even with therapy, KHE often do not fully regress and may recur [147].

Histiocytic Disorders

Histiocytic diseases are defined by clonal proliferation of histiocytes, which are normal cells in the skin and bone marrow, leading to tissue destruction, cytokine release, and variable clinical appearance. This family of disorders includes Langerhans cell histiocytosis, hemophagocytic lymphohistiocytosis, juvenile xanthogranulomatous disease, and sinus histiocytosis with massive lymphadenopathy/Rosai–Dorfman. These are rare in the general population, but especially so in the neonatal period. Of the histiocytic disorders, the most common in infants include Langerhans cell histiocytosis and hemophagocytic lymphohistiocytosis.

Langerhans cell histiocytosis (LCH) most commonly presents with skin rash (50%) and bone lesions (10%) [148]. In neonates skin involvement is more prevalent, present in 86%–92% [149]. The neonate may present with "blueberry muffin rash" or other skin findings that may self-resolve. This has been referred to in the past by a variety of names including congenital self-healing reticulohistiocytosis, histiocytosis X, and Hashimoto-Pritzker syndrome. The differential diagnosis includes seborrheic dermatitis, diaper dermatitis, and chronic otitis media. The rash of LCH is a diagnostic challenge as it has varying appearance of vesiculo-pustules, molluscum, or petechial rash and can be nonspecific. Subcutaneous nodules of LCH present similarly to neuroblastoma, congenital leukemia, mastocytosis, and vascular lesions. When presenting as vesicles or bullae, LCH of the skin appears similar to erythema toxicum, herpes simplex or varicella infection, miliaria cystallina or rubra, neonatal pustular melanosis or incontinentia pigmenti [148]. Children have the potential to develop disseminated disease. Most concerning is involvement of risk organs which include liver, spleen, and bone marrow but disease may also commonly involve lungs, lymph nodes, and other tissues. Current nomenclature is to define the organ systems involved, either single system or multisystem and include risk organ involvement status. Incidence in the neonatal period is estimated at one to two cases per million [150]. Of neonates enrolled on LCH trials, 59% had multisystem involvement [149]. Biopsy of an LCH lesion may demonstrate CD1a positivity, S100 positivity and Langerin/CD207 positivity by immunohistochemistry. In young children, there is a more severe form of the disease that includes skin, risk organs, and the central nervous system which was previously called Letterer–Siwe disease. In neonates with multisystem involvement the 5 year OS was 57%, lower than in those with single system involvement (94% 5 year OS) and worse than older children with multisystem involvement [149, 151]. Treatment of LCH may include topical agents for isolated skin disease or systemic chemotherapy for multisystem disease. Surveillance for disease reactivation is imperative for up to five years following diagnosis [152].

Hemophagocytic lymphohistiocytosis (HLH) classically presents as fevers, failure to thrive, hepatomegaly, splenomegaly, liver failure, thrombo-cytopenia, and hydrops in the neonatal period [151]. Fever and hypertriglyceridemia may be less common in neonatal HLH as compared to older children, thus one must have a high index of suspicion [153]. Primary (familial) and secondary (acquired) HLH have similar presentations and are often difficult to distinguish. Positive family history may be of assistance and often other children were born with rapid decline and typically death occurs without specific therapy. Most common genetic mutations are in the *Perforin*, *Syntaxin* and *Munc* genes though a good portion of children with suspected primary HLH do not have an identified mutation to date [154]. Clinical diagnosis may be made by either genetic confirmation of pathogenic mutation or five of the eight clinical criteria: fever, lymphadenopathy, hepatomegaly or splenomegaly, elevated ferritin >500 ng/mL, serum triglyceride level >265 mg/dL or fibrinogen <150 mg/dL, hemophagocytosis on pathologic specimen, elevated serum interleukin 2 level >2,400 units/mL, and impaired natural killer (NK) cell activity. With HLH-directed therapy, survival in all ages is approximately 61% [155, 156]. In neonates the few reports have noted less optimistic outcomes between 26%–40% [151, 153]. Given the nonspecific clinical appearance of children with HLH, other diagnoses including sepsis and immune deficiencies must be considered.

Juvenile xanthogranuloma (JXG) typically presents as a cutaneous yellow nodule or papule that is most commonly located on the head, upper trunk, or neck. JXG makes up 20% of histiocytic diagnoses at birth in one review, however, the median age of diagnosis is 2 years [151, 157]. Natural history of the disease is slow resolution over a period of 3 to 6 years [158]. Cutaneous disease is most common with deep seated lesions less so (27% of neonates). Lesions can be seen in the liver, lung, soft tissue, spleen, eye, and brain. JXG lesions may present similarly to hematoma, LCH, myofibroma, sarcoma, and IH [158]. Ocular disease is more common in children less than 2 years of age and presentations may include unilateral hyphema, glaucoma, or exophthalmos [157]. Treatment is usually supportive, however, intervention may be required for those with systemic disease [151]. Screening ophthalmologic exams to monitor for ocular involvement is recommended until the age of 2 years [157].

Treatment of Neonates with Cancer

The pharmacokinetic (PK) characteristics of chemotherapy is important in understanding therapeutic and toxic effects in patients. Commonly used anticancer drugs have been shown to exhibit large amounts of pharmacokinetic variability among individuals. This is particularly true in the pediatric population [159–161]. Pharmacokinetic properties such as absorption, distribution, metabolism, and elimination are rapidly changing in the neonate and may alter the distribution of a drug [162]. Larger extracellular and total-body water spaces in neonates may result in lower plasma levels of drugs when the drugs are administered in a weight-based fashion [162]. As such, the challenge in treating the youngest patients lies in balancing the need to achieve therapeutic drug exposures while avoiding serious and sometimes life-threatening toxicities. Standard dosing guidelines for infants are available for a limited number of drugs, thus it is critical that careful monitoring for side effects and accorded dose adjustments be performed for each individual patient [163].

Radiation therapy is avoided in the neonate due to its potential to disrupt the growth and development of normal tissues. Neonates in particular are susceptible to the adverse effects of radiation due to the overall immaturity of their organs and tissues [164, 168]. Standard treatment protocols most often avoid or delay radiation in this population, however, if radiation cannot be avoided, restricted field, with low-dose opposed radiation should be used [164, 165].

Conclusion

Although most tumors in neonates are benign, malignancies do occur. The treatment of benign tumors ranges from observation to aggressive resection. The treatment of neonates with cancer can be difficult and complicated. Neonates, due to their immaturity and physiology, are at increased risk of side effects from chemotherapy and radiation. Because of the rarity of malignant tumors in the neonate and the complexities of administering chemotherapy and radiation therapy to the newborn, neonates with these disorders should be referred to specialized centers experienced in the care of neonates with cancer.

References

1. Rao S, Azmy A, Carachi R. Neonatal tumours: A single-centre experience. *Pediatr Surg Int* 2002;**18** (5–6):306–9.

2. Gurney J, Smith M, Ross J. Cancer among infants. InRies L, Smith MA, Gurney JG, et al. eds. *Cancer Incidence and Survival among Children and Adolescents: United States SEER Program 1975–1995*, Vol. NIH Pub. No. 99–4649. (Bethesda, MD: National Cancer Institute, SEER Program, 1999).

3. Desandes E, Guissou S, Ducassou S, Lacour B. Neonatal solid tumors: Incidence and survival in France. *Pediatr Blood Cancer* 2016;**63**(8):1375–80.

4. Alfaar AS, Hassan WM, Bakry MS, Qaddoumi I. Neonates with cancer and causes of death; lessons from 615 cases in the SEER databases. *Cancer Med* 2017;**6**(7):1817–26.

5. Parkes SE, Muir KR, Southern L, et al. Neonatal tumours: A thirty-year population-based study. *Med Pediatr Oncol* 1994;**22**(5):309–17.

6. Ries L, Percy C, Bunin G. Introduction. InRies L, Smith MA, Gurney JG, et al. eds. *Cancer Incidence and Survival among Children and Adolescents: United States SEER Program 1975–1995*, Vol. NIH Pub. No. 99–4649. (Bethesda, MD: National Cancer Institute, SEER Program,1999).

7. Smith MA, Seibel NL, Altekruse SF, et al. Outcomes for children and adolescents with cancer: Challenges for the twenty-first century. *J Clin Oncol* 2010;**28**(15):2625–34.

8. Zhang J, Walsh MF, Wu G, et al. Germline mutations in predisposition genes in pediatric cancer. *N Engl J Med* 2015;**373** (24):2336–46.

9. Jongmans, MC, Loeffen JL, Waanders E, et al. Recognition of genetic predisposition in pediatric cancer patients: an easy-to-use selection tool. *Eur J Med Genet* 2016;**59**(3):116–25.

10. Chandrasekaran A. Neonatal solid tumors. *Pediatr Neonatol*, 2018;**59**(1):65–70.

11. Bader JL, Miller RW. US cancer incidence and mortality in the first year of life. *Am J Dis Child* 1979;**133**(2):157–9.

12. Parkes S, Muir KR, Southern L, et al. Neonatal tumours: A thirty-year population-based study. *Med Pediatr Oncol* 1994;**22**(5):309–17.

13. Yamamoto K, Ohta S, Ito E, et al. Marginal decrease in mortality and marked increase in incidence as a result of neuroblastoma screening at 6 months of age: Cohort study in seven prefectures in Japan. *J Clin Oncol* 2002;**20** (5):1209–14.

14. Barrette S, Bernstein ML, Robison LL, et al. Incidence of neuroblastoma after a screening program. *J Clin Oncol* 2007;**25**(31):4929–32.

15. Puyo A, Levin G, Armando I, Barontini M. Total plasma dopamine/norepinephrine ratio in catecholamine-secreting tumors. Its relation to hypertension. *Hypertension* 1988;**11**(2 Pt 2):I202–6.

16. Maris JM, Hogarty MD, Bagatell R, Cohn SL. Neuroblastoma. *Lancet* 2007;**369**(9579):2106–20.

17. Monclair T, Brodeur GM, Ambros PF, et al. The International Neuroblastoma Risk Group (INRG) Staging System: An INRG Task Force Report. *J Clin Oncol* 2009;**27**(2):298–303.

18. Cohn, SL, Pearson AD, London WB, et al. The International Neuroblastoma Risk Group (INRG) Classification System: An INRG Task Force Report. *J Clin Oncol* 2009;**27**(2):289–97.

19. Ora I, Eggert A. Progress in treatment and risk stratification of neuroblastoma: impact on future clinical and basic research. *Semin Cancer Biol* 2011;**21**(4):217–28.

20. Canete, A, Gerrard M, Rubie H, et al. Poor survival for infants with MYCN-amplified metastatic neuroblastoma despite intensified treatment: The International Society of Paediatric Oncology European Neuroblastoma Experience. *J Clin Oncol* 2009;**27**(7):1014–19.

21. Hero, B, Simon T, Spitz R, et al. Localized infant neuroblastomas often show spontaneous regression: Results of the prospective trials NB95-S and NB97. *J Clin Oncol*, 2008;**26**(9):1504–10.

22. Nuchtern, JG, London WB, Barnewolt CE, et al. A prospective study of expectant observation as primary therapy for neuroblastoma in young infants: A Children's Oncology Group Study. *Ann Surg* 2012;**256**(4):573–80.

23. Nickerson, HJ, Matthay KK, Seeger RC, et al. Favorable biology and outcome of stage IV-S neuroblastoma with supportive care or minimal therapy: A Children's Cancer Group study. *J Clin Oncol*, 2000;**18**(3):477–86.

24. Rescorla, FJ, Sawin RS, Coran AG, Dillon PW, Azizkhan RG. Long-term outcome for infants and children with sacrococcygeal teratoma: A report from the Childrens Cancer Group. *J Pediatr Surg* 1998;**33**(2):171–6.

25. Fernandez, K, Solid tumors in the neonatal period. *NeoReviews* 2014;**15**(2):e56-e68.

26. Moppett J, Haddadin I, Foot AB. Neonatal neuroblastoma. *Arch Dis Child Fetal Neonatal Ed* 1999;**81**(2):F134–7.

27. Isaacs H, Jr. Fetal and neonatal neuroblastoma: Retrospective review of 271 cases. *Fetal Pediatr Pathol* 2007;**26**(4):177–84.

28. De Bernardi B, Gerrard M, Boni L, et al. Excellent outcome with reduced treatment for infants with disseminated neuroblastoma without MYCN gene amplification. *J Clin Oncol* 2009;**27**(7):1034–40.

29. Nadler EP, Barksdale EM. Adrenal masses in the newborn. *Semin Pediatr Surg* 2000;**9**(3):156–64.

30. Curtis MR, Mooney DP, Vaccaro TJ, et al. Prenatal ultrasound characterization of the suprarenal mass: Distinction between neuroblastoma and subdiaphragmatic extralobar pulmonary sequestration. *J Ultrasound Med* 1997;**16**(2):75–83.

31. Isaacs H, Jr. Congenital and neonatal malignant tumors. A 28-year experience at Children's Hospital of Los Angeles. *Am J Pediatr Hematol Oncol* 1987;**9**(2):121–9.

32. Isaacs H, Jr. Perinatal (fetal and neonatal) germ cell tumors. *J Pediatr Surg* 2004;**39**(7):1003–13.

33. Gopal M, Turnpenny PD, Spicer R. Hereditary sacrococcygeal teratoma–not the same as its sporadic counterpart! *Eur J Pediatr Surg* 2007;**17**(3):214–6.

34. Dharmarajan H, Rouillard-Bazinet N, Chandy BM. Mature and immature pediatric head and neck teratomas: A 15-year review at a large tertiary center. *Int J Pediatr Otorhinolaryngol* 2018;**105**:43–7.

35. Frazier AL, Weldon C, Amatruda J. Fetal and neonatal germ cell tumors. *Semin Fetal Neonatal Med* 2012;**17**(4):222–30.

36. Wu JT, Book L, Sudar K. Serum alpha fetoprotein (AFP) levels in normal infants. *Pediatr Res*, 1981;**15**:50–2.

37. Blohm ME, Gobel U. Unexplained anaemia and failure to thrive as initial symptoms of infantile choriocarcinoma: A review. *Eur J Pediatr* 2004;**163**(1):1–6.

38. Ferrari A, Sultan I, Huang TT, et al. Soft tissue sarcoma across the age spectrum: A population-based study from the Surveillance Epidemiology and End Results database. *Pediatr Blood Cancer* 2011;**57**(6):943–9.

39. Sultan I, Casanova M, Al-Jumaily U, et al. Soft tissue sarcomas in the first year of life. *Eur J Cancer* 2010;**46**(13):2449–56.

40. Ferrari A, Orbach D, Sultan I, Casanova M, Bisogno G. Neonatal soft tissue sarcomas. *Semin Fetal Neonatal Med* 2012;**17**(4):231–8.

41. Güra A, Tezcan G, Karagüzel G, Cevikol C, Oygür N. An unusual localization of embryonal rhabdomyosarcoma in a neonate. *Turk J Pediatr* 2007;**49**(1):82–4.

42. Rodriguez-Galindo C, Hill DA, Onyekwere O, et al. Neonatal alveolar rhabdomyosarcoma with

skin and brain metastases. *Cancer* 2001;**92**
(6):1613–20.

43. De Giovanni C, Landuzzi L, Nicoletti G, Lollini PL,
Nanni P. Molecular and cellular biology of
rhabdomyosarcoma. *Future Oncol* 2009;**5**
(9):1449–75.

44. Lobe TE, Wiener ES, Hays DM, et al. Neonatal
rhabdomyosarcoma: The IRS experience. *J Pediatr
Surg* 1994;**29**(8):1167–70.

45. Lackner H, Urban C, Kerbl R, Schwinger W,
Beham A. Noncytotoxic drug therapy in children
with unresectable desmoid tumors. *Cancer*
1997;**80**(2):334–40.

46. Domont J, Salas S, Lacroix L, et al. High frequency
of beta-catenin heterozygous mutations in
extra-abdominal fibromatosis: A potential
molecular tool for disease management. *Br
J Cancer* 2010;**102**(6):1032–6.

47. Ferrari A, Casanova M, Bisogno G, et al.
Hemangiopericytoma in pediatric ages: A report
from the Italian and German Soft Tissue Sarcoma
Cooperative Group. *Cancer* 2001;**92**(10):2692–8.

48. Staples JJ, Robinson RA, Wen BC, Hussey DH.
Hemangiopericytoma: The role of radiotherapy.
Int J Radiat Oncol Biol Phys 1990;**19**(2):445–51.

49. Rodriguez-Galindo C, Ramsey K, Jenkins JJ, et al.
Hemangiopericytoma in children and infants.
Cancer 2000;**88**(1):198–204.

50. Cecchetto, G, Carli M, Alaggio R, et al.
Fibrosarcoma in pediatric patients: Results of the
Italian Cooperative Group studies (1979–1995).
J Surg Oncol 2001;**78**(4):225–31.

51. Orbach, D, Rey A, Oberlin O, et al. Soft tissue
sarcoma or malignant mesenchymal tumors in the
first year of life: experience of the International
Society of Pediatric Oncology (SIOP) Malignant
Mesenchymal Tumor Committee. *J Clin Oncol*
2005;**23**(19):4363–71.

52. Coffin, CM, Jaszcz W, O'Shea PA, Dehner LP. So-
called congenital-infantile fibrosarcoma: does it
exist and what is it? *Pediatr Pathol* 1994;**14**
(1):133–50.

53. Bourgeois JM, Knezevich SR, Mathers JA,
Sorensen PH. Molecular detection of the
ETV6-NTRK3 gene fusion differentiates congenital
fibrosarcoma from other childhood spindle cell
tumors. *Am J Surg Pathol* 2000;**24**(7):937–46.

54. Orbach D, Rey A, Cecchetto G, et al. Infantile
fibrosarcoma: management based on the
European experience. *J Clin Oncol* 2010;**28**
(2):318–23.

55. Hwang ES, Gerald W, Wollner N, Meyers P, La
Quaglia MP. Leiomyosarcoma in childhood and
adolescence. *Ann Surg Oncol* 1997;**4**(3):223–7.

56. Ostrom QT, Gittleman H, Farah P, et al. CBTRUS
statistical report: Primary brain and central
nervous system tumors diagnosed in the United
States in 2008–2012. *Neuro Oncol* 2015;**17**(Suppl
4):iv1–iv62.

57. Buetow PC, Smirniotopoulos JG, Done S.
Congenital brain tumors: A review of 45 cases.
AJNR Am J Neuroradiol 1990. **11**(4):793–9.

58. Isaacs H, Jr. I. Perinatal brain tumors: A review of
250 cases. *Pediatr Neurol*, 2002;**27**(4):249–61.

59. Severino M, Schwartz ES, Thurnher MM, et al.
Congenital tumors of the central nervous system.
Neuroradiol J 2010;**52**(6):531–48.

60. Isaacs H, Jr. II. Perinatal brain tumors: A review of
250 cases. *Pediatr Neurol* 2002;**27**(5):333–42.

61. Huang X, Zhang R, Zhou LF. Diagnosis and
treatment of intracranial immature teratoma.
Pediatr Neurosurg 2009;**45**(5):354–60.

62. Arslan E, Usul H, Baykal S, et al. Massive
congenital intracranial immature teratoma of the
lateral ventricle with retro-orbital extension:
A case report and review of the literature. *Pediatr
Neurosurg* 2007;**43**(4):338–42.

63. Im, SH, Wang KC, Kim SK, et al. Congenital
intracranial teratoma: Prenatal diagnosis and
postnatal successful resection. *Med Pediatr Oncol*
2003;**40**(1):57–61.

64. Louis DN, Ohgaki H, Wiestler OD, et al. The 2007
WHO classification of tumours of the central
nervous system. *Acta Neuropathol* 2007;**114**
(2):97–109.

65. Louis, DN, Perry A, Reifenberger G, et al. The 2016
World Health Organization Classification of
Tumors of the Central Nervous System: A
summary. *Acta Neuropathol* 2016;**131**(6):803–20.

66. Isaacs H, Jr. Perinatal (fetal and neonatal)
astrocytoma: A review. *Childs Nerv Syst* 2016;**32**
(11):2085–2096.

67. Nageswara Rao AA, Packer RJ. Advances in the
management of low-grade gliomas. *Curr Oncol
Rep* 2014;**16**(8):398.

68. Kotulska K, Borkowska J, Mandera M, et al.
Congenital subependymal giant cell astrocytomas
in patients with tuberous sclerosis complex. *Childs
Nerv Syst* 2014;**30**(12):2037–42.

69. Franz DN, Agricola K, Mays M, et al.
Everolimus for subependymal giant cell
astrocytoma: 5-year final analysis. *Ann Neurol*
2015;**78**(6):929–38.

70. Nemes K, Bens S, Bourdeaut F, et al. Rhabdoid
tumor predisposition syndrome. In Adam MP,
Ardinger HH, Pagon RA, et al., eds. *GeneReviews®*
(Seattle, WA: University of Washington, 1993).

71. Nemes K, Clément N, Kachanov D, et al. The extraordinary challenge of treating patients with congenital rhabdoid tumors: A collaborative European effort. *Pediatr Blood Cancer* 2018;**65**(6): e26999.

72. Schrey D, Carceller Lechón F, Malietzis G, et al. Multimodal therapy in children and adolescents with newly diagnosed atypical teratoid rhabdoid tumor: Individual pooled data analysis and review of the literature. *J Neurooncol* 2016;**126**(1):81–90.

73. Cavalli, FMG, Remke M, Rampasek L, et al. Intertumoral heterogeneity within medulloblastoma subgroups. *Cancer Cell*, 2017;**31**(6):737–54 e6.

74. Thalakoti S, Geller T. Basal cell nevus syndrome or Gorlin syndrome. *Handb Clin Neurol* 2015;**132**:119–28.

75. Lafay-Cousin L, Smith A, Chi SN, et al. Clinical, pathological, and molecular characterization of infant medulloblastomas treated with sequential high-dose chemotherapy. *Pediatr Blood Cancer* 2016;**63**(9):1527–34.

76. Lafay-Cousin L, Fay-McClymont T, Johnston D, et al. Neurocognitive evaluation of long term survivors of atypical teratoid rhabdoid tumors (ATRT): The Canadian registry experience. *Pediatr Blood Cancer* 2015;**62**(7):1265–9.

77. Lafay-Cousin L, Bouffet E, Hawkins C, et al. Impact of radiation avoidance on survival and neurocognitive outcome in infant medulloblastoma. *Curr Oncol* 2009;**16**(6):21–8.

78. Nimjee SM, Powers CJ, McLendon RE, Grant GA, Fuchs HE. Single-stage bilateral choroid plexectomy for choroid plexus papilloma in a patient presenting with high cerebrospinal fluid output. *J Neurosurg Pediatr* 2010;**5**(4):342–5.

79. Fujimura M, Onuma T, Kameyama M, et al. Hydrocephalus due to cerebrospinal fluid overproduction by bilateral choroid plexus papillomas. *Childs Nerv Syst* 2004;**20**(7):485–8.

80. Gopal P, Parker JR, Debski R, Parker JC Jr. Choroid plexus carcinoma. *Arch Pathol Lab Med* 2008;**132**(8):1350–4.

81. Gozali, AE, Britt B, Shane L, et al. Choroid plexus tumors; management, outcome, and association with the Li–Fraumeni syndrome: The Children's Hospital Los Angeles (CHLA) experience, 1991–2010. *Pediatr Blood Cancer* 2012;**58**(6):905–9.

82. Powis M. Neonatal renal tumours. *Early Hum Dev* 2010;**86**(10):607–12.

83. Isaacs H Jr. Fetal and neonatal renal tumors. *J Pediatr Surg* 2008;**43**(9):1587–95.

84. England RJ, Haider N, Vujanic GM, et al. Mesoblastic nephroma: A report of the United Kingdom Children's Cancer and Leukaemia Group (CCLG). *Pediatr Blood Cancer* 2011;**56**(5):744–748.

85. Lee EY. CT imaging of mass-like renal lesions in children. *Pediatr Radiol* 2007;**37**(9):896–907.

86. van den Heuvel-Eibrink MM, Grundy P, Graf N, et al. Characteristics and survival of 750 children diagnosed with a renal tumor in the first seven months of life: A collaborative study by the SIOP/GPOH/SFOP, NWTSG, and UKCCSG Wilms tumor study groups. *Pediatr Blood Cancer* 2008;**50**(6):1130–34.

87. Vokuhl C, Nourkami-Tutdibi N, Furtwängler R, et al. ETV6–NTRK3 in congenital mesoblastic nephroma: A report of the SIOP/GPOH nephroblastoma study. *Pediatr Blood Cancer* 2018;**65**(4):e26925.

88. Patel Y, Mitchell CD, Hitchcock RJ. Use of sarcoma-based chemotherapy in a case of congenital mesoblastic nephroma with liver metastases. *Urology* 2003;**61**(6):1260.

89. Glick RD, Hicks MJ, Nuchtern JG, et al. Renal tumors in infants less than 6 months of age. *J Pediatr Surg* 2004;**39**(4):522–5.

90. Gooskens S, Houwing ME, Vujanic GM, et al. Congenital mesoblastic nephroma 50 years after its recognition: A narrative review. *Pediatr Blood Cancer* 2017;**64**(7):e26437.

91. Royer-Pokora B. Genetics of pediatric renal tumors. *Pediatr Nephrol* 2013;**28**(1):13–23.

92. Beckwith JB, Nephrogenic rests and the pathogenesis of Wilms tumor: Developmental and clinical considerations. *Am J Med Genet* 1998;**79**(4):268–73.

93. Fernandez CV, Perlman EJ, Mullen EA, et al. Clinical outcome and biological predictors of relapse after nephrectomy only for very low-risk Wilms tumor: A report from Children's Oncology Group AREN0532. *Ann Surg* 2017;**265**(4):835–40.

94. Tomlinson GE, Breslow NE, Dome J, et al. Rhabdoid tumor of the kidney in the National Wilms' Tumor Study: Age at diagnosis as a prognostic factor. *J Clin Oncol* 2005;**23**(30):7641–5.

95. Eaton, KW, Tooke LS, Wainwright LM, et al. Spectrum of SMARCB1/INI1 mutations in familial and sporadic rhabdoid tumors. *Pediatr Blood Cancer*, 2011;**56**(1):7–15.

96. Ueno-Yokohata H, Okita H, Nakasato K, et al. Consistent in-frame internal tandem duplications of BCOR characterize clear cell sarcoma of the kidney. *Nat Genet* 2015;**47**(8):861.

97. Cronin KA, Ries LA, Edwards BK. The Surveillance, Epidemiology, and End Results (SEER) Program of the National Cancer Institute. *Cancer* 2014;**120**(Suppl 23):3755–7.

98. Wan MJ, VanderVeen DK. Eye disorders in newborn infants (excluding retinopathy of prematurity). *Arch Dis Child Fetal Neonatal Ed* 2015;**100**(3):F264-9.

99. Skalet AH, Gombos DS, Gallie BL, et al. Screening children at risk for retinoblastoma: Consensus Report from the American Association of Ophthalmic Oncologists and Pathologists. *Ophthalmology* 2018;**125**(3):45358.

100. Soliman SE, Dimaras H, Khetan V, et al. Prenatal versus postnatal screening for familial retinoblastoma. *Ophthalmology* 2016;**123**(12):2610–17.

101. Hurwitz, R, et al. Retinoblastoma. In Pizzo P, Poplack D, eds. *Principles and Practice of Pediatric Oncology*, (Philadelphia, PA: Lippincott Williams & Wilkins, 2011), pp. 809–37.

102. Draper GJ Sanders BM, Brownbill PA, Hawkins MM. Patterns of risk of hereditary retinoblastoma and applications to genetic counselling. *Br J Cancer* 1992;**66**(1):211–9.

103. Abramson, DH, Frank CM, Susman M, et al. Presenting signs of retinoblastoma. *J Pediatr* 1998;**132**(3 Pt 1):505–8.

104. Gobin YP, Dunkel IJ, Marr BP, et al. Combined, sequential intravenous and intra-arterial chemotherapy (bridge chemotherapy) for young infants with retinoblastoma. *PLoS One*, 2012;**7**(9):e44322.

105. Desandes E, Guissou S, Ducassou S, Lacour B. Neonatal solid tumors: Incidence and survival in France. *Pediatr Blood Cancer* 2016;**63**(8):1375–80.

106. Kamihara J, Bourdeaut F, Foulkes WD, et al. Retinoblastoma and neuroblastoma predisposition and surveillance. *Clin Cancer Res* 2017;**23**(13):e98–e106.

107. Isaacs H. *Tumors of the Fetus and Infant: An Atlas*, 2nd ed. (New York: Springer,2013).

108. Weinberg AG, Finegold MJ. Primary hepatic tumors in childhood. In Finegold MJ, ed. *Pathology of Neoplasia in Children and Adolescents* (Philadelphia, PA: WB Saunders, 1986), pp. 333–65.

109. von Schweinitz D. Neonatal liver tumours. *Semin Neonatol* 2003;**8**(5):403–10.

110. Boon LM, Burrows PE, Paltiel HJ, et al. Hepatic vascular anomalies in infancy: A twenty-seven-year experience. *J Pediatr* 1996;**129**(3):346–54.

111. Cohen RC, Myers NA. Diagnosis and management of massive hepatic hemangiomas in childhood. *J Pediatr Surg* 1986;**21**(1):6–9.

112. Isaacs H, Jr. Fetal and neonatal hepatic tumors. *J Pediatr Surg* 2007;**42**(11):1797–803.

113. DeMaioribus CA, Lally KP, Sim K, Isaacs H, Mahour GH. Mesenchymal hamartoma of the liver. A 35-year review. *Arch Surg* 1990;**125**(5):598–600.

114. Stringer MD, Alizai NK. Mesenchymal hamartoma of the liver: A systematic review. *J Pediatr Surg* 2005;**40**(11):1681–90.

115. Anil G, Fortier M, Low Y. Cystic hepatic mesenchymal hamartoma: The role of radiology in diagnosis and perioperative management. *Br J Radiol* 2011;**84**(1001):e91–4.

116. Hiyama E. Pediatric hepatoblastoma: Diagnosis and treatment. *Transl Pediatr* 2014;**3**(4):293–9.

117. Fernandez-Pineda I, Cabello-Laureano R. Differential diagnosis and management of liver tumors in infants. *World J Hepatol* 2014;**6**(7):486–95.

118. Oue T, Kubota A, Okuyama H, et al. Hepatoblastoma in children of extremely low birth weight: a report from a single perinatal center. *J Pediatr Surg* 2003;**38**(1):134–7; discussion 134–7.

119. Kapfer SA, Petruzzi MJ, Caty MG. Hepatoblastoma in low birth weight infants: An institutional review. *Pediatr Surg Int* 2004;**20**(10):753–6.

120. Pizzo P, Poplack D. *Principles and Practice of Pediatric Oncology*, 6th ed. (Philadelphia, PA: Lippincott Williams & Wilkins,2011).

121. De Ioris M, Brugieres L, Zimmermann A, et al. Hepatoblastoma with a low serum alpha-fetoprotein level at diagnosis: The SIOPEL group experience. *Eur J Cancer* 2008;**44**(4):545–50.

122. Davidoff, AM, Fernandez-Pineda I, Santana VM, Shochat SJ. The role of neoadjuvant chemotherapy in children with malignant solid tumors. *Semin Pediatr Surg* 2012;**21**(1):88–99.

123. Perilongo G, Shafford E, Maibach R, et al. Risk-adapted treatment for childhood hepatoblastoma. final report of the second study of the International Society of Paediatric Oncology–SIOPEL 2. *Eur J Cancer* 2004;**40**(3):411–21.

124. Trobaugh-Lotrario AD, Chaiyachati BH, Meyers RL, et al. Outcomes for patients with congenital hepatoblastoma. *Pediatr Blood Cancer* 2013;**60**(11):1817–25.

125. Dall'Igna P, Brugieres L, Christin AS, et al. Hepatoblastoma in children aged less than six months at diagnosis: A report from the SIOPEL group. *Pediatr Blood Cancer* 2018;**65**(1):e26791.

126. Wassef M, Blei F, Adams D, et al. Vascular anomalies classification: Recommendations from the International Society for the Study of Vascular Anomalies. *Pediatrics* 2015;**136**(1): e203-e214.

127. Darrow DH, Greene AK, Mancini AJ, Nopper AJ. Diagnosis and management of infantile hemangioma: Executive summary. *Pediatrics* 2015;**136**(4):786–91.

128. Munden A, Butschek R, Tom WL, et al. Prospective study of infantile haemangiomas: Incidence, clinical characteristics and association with placental anomalies. *Br J Dermatol* 2014;**170**(4):907–13.

129. Bruckner AL, Frieden IJ. Hemangiomas of infancy. *J Am Acad Dermatol* 2003;**48**(4):477–93; quiz 494–6.

130. Darrow, DH, Greene AK, Mancini AJ, et al. Diagnosis and management of infantile hemangioma. *Pediatrics* 2015; **136**(4):e1060–e1104.

131. Metry D, Heyer G, Hess C, et al. Consensus statement on diagnostic criteria for PHACE syndrome. *Pediatrics* 2009;**124**(5):1447–56.

132. Buckmiller L, Dyamenahalli U, Richter GT. Propranolol for airway hemangiomas: case report of novel treatment. *Laryngoscope* 2009;**119**(10):2051–4.

133. Keller RG, Patel KG. Evidence-based medicine in the treatment of infantile hemangiomas. *Facial Plast Surg Clin North Am* 2015;**23**(3):373–92.

134. Mazereeuw-Hautier J, Hoeger PH, Benlahrech S, et al. Efficacy of propranolol in hepatic infantile hemangiomas with diffuse neonatal hemangiomatosis. *J Pediatr* 2010;**157**(2):340–2.

135. Wasserman JD, Mahant S, Carcao M, Perlman K, Pope E. Vincristine for successful treatment of steroid-dependent infantile hemangiomas. *Pediatrics* 2015;**135**(6):e1501–5.

136. Vlahovic A, Simic R, Djokic D, Ceran C. Diffuse neonatal hemangiomatosis treatment with cyclophosphamide: A case report. *J Pediatr Hematol Oncol* 2009;**31**(11):858–60.

137. Sundar Alagusundaramoorthy S, Vilchez V, Zanni A, et al. Role of transplantation in the treatment of benign solid tumors of the liver: a review of the United Network of Organ Sharing data set. *JAMA Surg* 2015;**150**(4):337–42.

138. North, PE, Waner M, James CA, et al. Congenital nonprogressive hemangioma: A distinct clinicopathologic entity unlike infantile hemangioma. *Arch Dermatol* 2001;**137**(12):1607–20.

139. Subash A, Senthil GK, Ramamoorthy R, Appasamy A, Selvarajan N. Kaposiform hemangioendothelioma with Kasabach–Merritt phenomenon in a neonate of life- and limb-threatening nature: A case report. *J Indian Assoc Pediatr Surg* 2015;**20**(4):194–6.

140. Arunachalam P, Kumar VR, Swathi D. Kasabach–Merritt syndrome with large cutaneous vascular tumors. *J Indian Assoc Pediatr Surg* 2012;**17**(1):33–6.

141. Fahrtash F, McCahon E, Arbuckle S. Successful treatment of kaposiform hemangioendothelioma and tufted angioma with vincristine. *J Pediatr Hematol Oncol* 2010;**32**(6):506–10.

142. Fernandez-Pineda I, Lopez-Gutierrez JC, Chocarro G, Bernabeu-Wittel J, Ramirez-Villar GL. Long-term outcome of vincristine-aspirin-ticlopidine (VAT) therapy for vascular tumors associated with Kasabach–Merritt phenomenon. *Pediatr Blood Cancer* 2013;**60**(9):1478–81.

143. Acharya S, Pillai K, Francis A, Criton S, Parvathi VK. Kasabach–Merritt syndrome: Management with interferon. *Indian J Dermatol*, 2010;**55**(3):281–3.

144. Filippi L, Tamburini A, Berti E, et al. Successful propranolol treatment of a kaposiform hemangioendothelioma apparently resistant to propranolol. *Pediatr Blood Cancer* 2016;**63**(7):1290–2.

145. Chiu YE, Drolet BA, Blei F, et al. Variable response to propranolol treatment of kaposiform hemangioendothelioma, tufted angioma, and Kasabach–Merritt phenomenon. *Pediatr Blood Cancer* 2012;**59**(5):934–8.

146. Hammill AM, Wentzel M, Gupta A, et al. Sirolimus for the treatment of complicated vascular anomalies in children. *Pediatr Blood Cancer* 2011;**57**(6):1018–24.

147. Schaefer BA, Wang D, Merrow AC, Dickie BH, Adams DM. Long-term outcome for kaposiform hemangioendothelioma: A report of two cases. *Pediatr Blood Cancer* 2017;**64**(2):284–6.

148. Krafchik B, Pope E, Walsch SRA. *Histiocytosis of the skin in children and adults*. In Weitzman S, Egeler MR, eds. *Histiocytic Disorders of Children and Adults* (Cambridge, UK: Cambridge University Press, 2005), pp. 130–53.

149. Minkov M, Prosch H, Steiner M, et al. Langerhans cell histiocytosis in neonates. *Pediatr Blood Cancer* 2005;**45**(6):802–7.

150. Stein SL, Paller AS, Haut PR, Mancini AJ. Langerhans cell histiocytosis presenting in the neonatal period: A retrospective case series. *Arch Pediatr Adolesc Med* 2001;**155**(7):778–83.

151. Isaacs H, Jr. Fetal and neonatal histiocytoses. *Pediatr Blood Cancer* 2006;**47**(2):123–9.

152. Ladisch S, Jaffe E. The histiocytoses. In Pizzo P, Poplack D, eds. *Principles and Practice of Pediatric Oncology* (Philadelphia, PA: Lippincott, 2006).

153. Suzuki N, Morimoto A, Ohga S, et al. Characteristics of hemophagocytic lymphohistiocytosis in neonates: a nationwide survey in Japan. *J Pediatr* 2009;**155**(2):235–8, e1.

154. Janka GE. Familial and acquired hemophagocytic lymphohistiocytosis. *Annu Rev Med* 2012;**63**:233–46.

155. Henter JI, Horne A, Aricó M, et al. HLH-2004: Diagnostic and therapeutic guidelines for hemophagocytic lymphohistiocytosis. *Pediatr Blood Cancer* 2007;**48**(2):124–31.

156. Bergsten, E, Horne A, Aricó M, et al. Confirmed efficacy of etoposide and dexamethasone in HLH treatment: Long-term results of the cooperative HLH-2004 study. *Blood* 2017;**130**(25):2728–38.

157. Weitzman S, Whitlock J. Uncommon histiocytic disorder: The non-Langerhans cell histiocytosis. In Weitzman S, Egeler MR, eds. *Histiocytic Disorders of Children and Adults* (Cambridge, UK: Cambridge University Press, 2005), pp. 293–320.

158. Oza VS, Stringer T, Campbell C, et al. Congenital-type juvenile xanthogranuloma: A case series and literature review. *Pediatr Dermatol* 2018;**35**(5):582–7.

159. Yule SM, Boddy AV, Cole M, et al. Cyclophosphamide pharmacokinetics in children. *Br J Clin Pharmacol* 1996;**41**(1):13–19.

160. Periclou AP, Avramis VI. NONMEM population pharmacokinetic studies of cytosine arabinoside after high-dose and after loading bolus followed by continuous infusion of the drug in pediatric patients with leukemias. *Cancer Chemother Pharmacol* 1996;**39**(1–2):42–50.

161. McLeod HL, Relling MV, Crom WR, et al. Disposition of antineoplastic agents in the very young child. *Br J Cancer Suppl* 1992;**18**:S23–9.

162. Kearns, GL, Abdel-Rahman SM, Alander SW, et al. Developmental pharmacology: Drug disposition, action, and therapy in infants and children. *N Engl J Med* 2003;**349**(12):1157–67.

163. Hutson JR, Weitzman S, Schechter T, et al. Pharmacokinetic and pharmacogenetic determinants and considerations in chemotherapy selection and dosing in infants. *Expert Opin Drug Metab Toxicol* 2012;**8**(6):709–722.

164. Weitzman S, Grant R. Neonatal oncology: diagnostic and therapeutic dilemmas. *Semin Perinatol* 1997;**21**(1):102–11.

165. Littman P, D'Angio GJ. Radiation therapy in the neonate. *Am J Pediatr Hematol Oncol* 1981;**3**(3):279–85.

Chapter

23 Disorders of the Fetomaternal Unit

Eric J. Werner, Nancy C. Chescheir, and Randall G. Fisher

Introduction

The fetal–placental–maternal unit can produce significant abnormalities in the neonate's hematologic health at birth. A newborn can have disorders of white blood cells, red blood cells, or platelets, or any combination thereof. Neonatal cytopenias can result from dilution, peripheral destruction, or a defect in cellular production [1]. Maternal illness can be the cause of such abnormalities (Table 23.1). Close communication between the obstetrical provider and the pediatrician is important. This can allow for anticipation of a problem in order to mitigate the consequences, or to discover the cause if an unexpected cytopenia is detected.

Thrombocytopenia

While only 1%–5% of all neonates will have a platelet count below 150,000/µl, as many as 35% of infants admitted to the neonatal intensive care unit will have this finding [2]. The most common cause of early onset thrombocytopenia is chronic fetal hypoxemia such as occurs with intrauterine

preeclampsia and its variants, and uncontrolled diabetes. While the pediatrician should be open to other diagnostic possibilities, this type of thrombocytopenia is usually self-limited and mild and results from a bone marrow effect with a resulting decrease in megakaryocytes.

Additional causes related to the maternal–fetal unit include immune-mediated disorders such as neonatal alloimmune thrombocytopenia caused by isoimmunization of the mother against specific platelet antigens. Mothers with autoantibodies against platelet antigens can pass those antibodies transplacentally to the infant resulting in neonatal thrombocytopenia. Other causes include intrauterine infections, and neonatal sepsis.

Anemia

Neonatal anemia, defined as a hemoglobin or hematocrit more than two standard deviations below the mean for gestational age can occur due to blood loss, diminished production or increased destruction of red blood cells.

Blood loss can occur prior to delivery in the setting of twin-to-twin transfusion syndrome

Table 23.1 Causes of cytopenia in the newborn related to the fetomaternal unit

	Thrombocytopenia	Anemia	Neutropenia
Maternal sepsis	XX	XX	XX
Preeclampsia/eclampsia	XX		XX
Immune disorders	XX	XX	XX
Congenital infection	XX	XX	XX
Diabetes mellitus	X	XX	XX
Fetal growth restriction Neonatal lupus erythematosis	XX X		XX X

Neonatal Hematology, Pathogenesis, Diagnosis, and Management of Hematologic Problems, 3rd edition, ed. Pedro A. de Alarcón, Eric J. Werner, Robert D. Christensen, and Martha C. Sola-Visner. Published by Cambridge University Press. © Cambridge University Press 2021.

(TTTS), placental abruption or fetal-to-maternal hemorrhage (FMH). During delivery, blood loss can occur due to transplacental-incision during Cesarean delivery or with internal neonatal bleeding. Infants who suffer rapid, large volume losses typically present with acute distress and shock while those with chronic blood loss anemia may be without symptoms other than pallor. Decreased red blood cell (RBC) production due to abnormalities in the fetal–placental–maternal unit is most commonly related to maternal infections, such as with parvovirus B19 which suppresses the RBC progenitor cells, or Kell isoimmunization which behaves similarly.

Of the three mechanisms for neonatal anemia, increased RBC destruction is the most common. Immune-mediated hemolysis can result from RBC antigens such as D, Duffy, and other irregular antibodies, autoimmune disorders such as neonatal lupus, and maternal infection [3]. Intrinsic red cell disorders such as enzymopathies, membrane defects, hemoglobin disorders, mechanical destruction as seen in vascular disorders or DIC should also be considered in the infant with hemolysis.

Neutropenia

The most common variety of congenital neutropenia is decreased white blood cell (WBC) production related to maternal gestational hypertension. In this case, there is neither a left shift nor any morphologic abnormalities. Gestational hypertension-associated neutropenia is usually self-limited by day 5. An additional perinatal cause of congenital neutropenia is bacterial infection, resulting in accelerated neutrophil use, accompanied by a left shift and morphologic changes such as toxic granulation, vacuolization and Döhle bodies. In this case, the neutropenia resolves as the infection resolves. Finally, neonatal neutropenia can be caused by antineutrophil antibodies from the mother, as occurs with maternal systemic lupus erythematosus or in alloimmune neonatal neutropenia, a disorder similar to red blood cell isoimmunization except that the antibodies are directed against neutrophils, which leads to their destruction [4].

Placental Causes of Anemia

Placental abnormalities may lead to fetal blood loss (Table 23.2).

Table 23.2 Causes of fetal blood loss

Placental
Abruptio placenta
Placenta previa (if fetal vessels are torn)
Placental laceration at operative delivery
Umbilical-vessel injury during amniocentesis
Umbilical-cord rupture

Transfusion syndromes
Fetomaternal transfusion
Fetofetal transfusion (twin–twin transfusion)

Abruptio Placenta and Placenta Previa

While the majority of blood loss with placenta previa or abruptio placenta is maternal, fetal blood loss can also occur [5, 6]. The frequency of neonatal anemia requiring transfusion increases with the severity of maternal bleeding [7]. Vaginal blood can be tested for fetal hemoglobin using the Apt test [8]. Vaso previa is a relatively rare phenomenon where fetal vessels within membranes, either due to a velamentous insertion of the vessels or bridging vessels from the main body of the placenta to a succenturiate lobe overlie the cervical os. The risk of severe fetal hemorrhage with delivery is very high with vasa previa and can be improved with antenatal diagnosis [9].

Placental or umbilical cord damage can cause neonatal anemia. For instance, umbilical cord blood rupture may occur [10], especially with traumatic delivery or vasa previa. Surgical laceration of the placenta, as may occur with cesarean section, may cause significant fetal blood loss. Vascular anomalies of the umbilical cord can lead to neonatal anemia [8]. Although uncommon, a traumatic amniocentesis or cordocentesis can result in significant fetal hemorrhage [11].

Infants who have experienced acute hemorrhage during fetal life present with clinical features of acute anemia: pallor, hypovolemia, and hypotension. Unlike patients with hemolytic disorders, these infants do not typically develop hyperbilirubinemia. A hemoglobin measurement immediately following birth often does not accurately reflect the severity of the bleeding. Furthermore, because capillary blood counts are generally higher than central measurements, especially in the acidotic infant, they may underestimate anemia [12]. The management of such infants initially consists of volume replacement, usually with volume expanders such as Ringer's lactate or normal saline. Red blood cell transfusion may be indicated for large fetal blood loss.

Fetomaternal Bleeds

Small quantities of fetal erythrocytes pass into the maternal circulation in the majority of pregnancies [13]. In approximately 98% of pregnancies, less than 2 ml of fetal cells are found in the maternal blood. However, in about 0.1%–0.3% of pregnancies, this volume exceeds 20–30 ml [14, 15]. In a retrospective analysis of a large database of deliveries, Christensen et al. found an incidence of FMH of 1:9160 live births [16].

The estimated acute fetal blood loss can be calculated based on the number of fetal erythrocytes in the mother's blood (see below) and may be underestimated with chronic bleeding or blood group incompatibility. The presence of pregnancy complications, preeclampsia, cesarean section, maternal trauma, placement of an intrauterine pressure catheter, or complicated delivery have been reported to cause significant fetomaternal bleeding [13, 17]. Massive fetomaternal hemorrhage can cause symptomatic anemia or even fetal demise [18, 19]. Chronic fetomaternal bleeding can cause nonimmune hydrops [20]. The presence of symptomatic anemia is dependent upon both the amount of and the time course of the hemorrhage, i.e., a large acute bleed presents with hypovolemic shock, whereas chronic bleeding may present with pallor or congestive heart failure.

Diagnosis

The usual approach is to examine maternal blood for fetal erythrocytes using the Kleihauer–Betke stain or flow-cytometric techniques [21, 22]. These two techniques correlate well [23, 24], but there are data to show that anti Hb F flow cytometry has greater precision [25] and some laboratories may only offer one of these tests. Anti-D flow cytometry is only useful in the setting of a mother who is D antigen negative and a fetus who is D antigen positive. The formula used to determine the amount of fetal blood in the maternal circulation is [26]:

% fetal RBCs × maternal blood volume = volume of fetal blood in maternal circulation.

Variations of this formula have been reported and a normal fetal Hct should be assumed rather than

the actual fetal Hct as a massive FMH may cause severe fetal anemia [27].

Because fetal cells may be cleared quickly from the maternal circulation, delay in assessment may prevent the identification, or underestimate the volume, of fetal blood lost into the maternal circulation, especially if there is a blood-group incompatibility between the infant and mother. False-positive results of Kleihauer–Betke testing can occur if the mother has an increased percentage of hemoglobin F in her own cells, as may occur with the hereditary persistence of fetal hemoglobin, aplastic anemia, or use of cancer chemotherapy [28]. Combined antibody flow cytometry may occasionally useful in this setting [27]. Fetal ultrasound abnormalities and/or non-stress test may not be reliably sensitive to the identification of fetal anemia but Doppler studies of fetal middle cerebral artery (MCA) flow velocity are a useful technique to identify fetal anemia [29–31]. Fetal tachycardia and/or a sinusoidal wave pattern on fetal heart rate may be suggestive of fetal anemia [31, 32].

Management

As with acute hemorrhage, the initial management of the neonate with acute severe fetomaternal bleeding is volume expansion using isotonic crystalloid solutions and possibly red blood cell transfusion. Chronic bleeding, not resulting in severe or symptomatic anemia, can be managed with iron supplementation.

Outcomes

Rubod found that massive fetomaternal hemorrhage accounted for 1.6% of all fetal deaths identified over a 7 year review in two university hospitals for an overall rate of 1.3 deaths from this disorder per 10,000 live births [33]. Risk factors for adverse neonatal outcomes include an initial neonatal hemoglobin <4 g/dL, or an estimated fetal blood loss of >20 ml/kg [15, 33, 34]. Similarly, there was a 71% rate of adverse outcomes in Christensen's series with risk factors including an initial Hb < 5 g/dL or birth at less than 35 weeks gestational age [16]. When the calculated fetal blood loss is corrected for the estimated fetoplacental blood volume, there is good correlation with the fetal/neonatal hemoglobin concentration [15].

Twin–Twin Transfusion Syndrome

Essentially all monochorionic placentas have intraplacental anastomatic vessels joining the circulation of one twin to the other. In the normal monochorionic, diamniotic twin placenta there is a mean of eight such anastomoses [35]. These anastomoses are the basis for many of the complications unique to this type of twinning. While this physical characteristic is fundamental to these disorders, the pathophysiological basis is as yet poorly understood. The nomenclature for these disorders is changing, with the umbrella term considered by many to be twin–twin transfusion syndrome (TTTS). Within this is what many still call twin-to-twin transfusion syndrome (the term used in this chapter) while others use twin oligohydramnios polyhydramnios syndrome (TOPS), twins anemia polycythemia syndrome (TAPS), and acute twin–twin transfusion syndrome.

Within monochorionic diamniotic placentas there can be arterio-arteriolar (AA), veno-venous (VV), and aterio-venous (AV) anastomosis. The AA and VV anastomosis allow for bidirectional flow, while the AV anastomosis allow for only unidirectional flow. It is the arterio-venous anastomoses that are the cause of these pathologic conditions. In fact, the presence of many arterio-arterio anastomoses is relatively protective against TTTS [36].

Twin–twin transfusion syndrome occurs in 5.5%–17.5% of monochorionic, diamniotic monozygotic twins [36]. It results from imbalanced blood traversing from the donor twin to the recipient twin through arterio-venous anastomoses. The donor twin develops anemia, hypovolemia, oliguria, and oligohydramnios while the recipient twin develops polycythemia, hypervolemia, polyuria, polyhydramios and in severe forms, hydrops fetalis. The hormonal response includes activation of the renin-angiotensin system in the donor, with increase tubular reabsorption, increased angiotensin 2 production, worsening oligohydramnios and vasoconstriction [37].

The increased blood volume of the recipient twin increases atrial pressure, resulting in cardiac atrial natriuretic peptide synthesis. The hormonal response ultimately suppresses antidiuretic hormone production due to increased glomerular filtration rate and a decrease in tubular reabsorption, resulting in an increase in urine production and resulting polyhydramnios. Because the donor's angiotensin 2 crosses through the anastomosis to the recipient, there can be hypertensive microangiopathy in both twins [37].

Historically, neonatal TTTS was diagnosed when there was a >5 g/dl difference in hemoglobin concentration and a >20% difference in birth weight between the twins. These criteria are no longer used as they may be present in both monochorionic twins without TTTS and in dichorionic twins [36]. TTTS can develop rapidly or indolently, and at various times in pregnancy and as such, after 16 weeks, ultrasound examination of monochorionic diamniotic twins is recommended every other week [38]. The goal is to identify those twins at high risk of extreme prematurity, fetal or neonatal death, or neurologic injury so that in utero intervention, or delivery if appropriate, can be offered.

Sonographic findings include discordant fetal growth with abnormal amniotic fluid volumes, inability to visualize the bladder or stomach of the smaller twin, a large and possibly hydropic twin with polyhydramnios and a persistently full bladder. Fetal Doppler is useful as well to help predict outcomes. Severely abnormal umbilical artery Doppler findings, such as absent or reversal of the end diastolic flow of the cord of the donor predicts a high risk of perinatal death. Measurement of the peak systolic velocity in the middle cerebral artery (MCA) is useful is used to determine the presence and degree of fetal anemia. Staging systems using these findings, and in some centers fetal echocardiogram findings, are used to predict outcomes and to determine interventions [39].

In 2004, Senat and colleagues reported a randomized trial of selective fetal laser ablation of fetoscopically identified placental surface anastomosis versus amnioreduction of the polyhydramniotic sac [40]. There was a significant improvement in the survival of at least one twin on day 28 of life (76% vs. 56%) and a lower risk of neurologic injury among survivors (6% vs. 15%) in those who underwent laser intervention. Since this trial, modifications in the instrumentation and technique have further improved outcomes. The current most commonly used method is the so-called Solomon technique which was developed to decrease the risk of incomplete closure of significant anastomoses which could lead to recurrent TTTS or twin anemia polycythemia syndrome (TAPS). In the Solomon technique, after selective laser ablation of identified anastomoses, the placental equator is lasered to attempt to completely separate the two circulations. The Solomon technique reduces the persistence of anastomoses after selective laser ablation from 34% to 19%, recurrent TTTS from 7% to 1% and TAPS from 16% to 3%, without increased complications [41]. This technique is the preferred approach. For patients without access to laser therapy or who present after 26–28 weeks, serial amnioreduction may be used.

Twin Anemia Polycythemia Syndrome

Twin anemia polycythemia syndrome (TAPS) occurs most commonly after laser therapy for TTTS but can occur spontaneously. Very small, <1 mm diameter, AV anastomoses are required for TAPS to occur. Through these very small connections, chronic low volume transfusion occurs. Flow has been measured using Doppler technology to be 5–15 ml/24 hours [35]. There are a variety of definitions for TAPS but in general, there are large intertwin differences in hemoglobin levels without polyhydramnios and oligohydramnios. Prenatally, the diagnosis is made when the peak systolic velocity of the MCA in the anemic fetus is >1.5 multiples of the median (MoM; corrected for gestational age) and < 1.0 MoM in the polycythemic one. Postnatally, the diagnosis is made when there is an intertwin hemoglobin difference of ≥8 g/dL and at least one of the following: small residual anastomoses identified on the placental surface using a vessel-injection technique OR a reticulocyte count ratio of >1.7:

(reticulocyte count ratio = reticulocyte (donor)/ reticulocyte (recipient)).

Robyr reports that in 12/13 such cases, the original recipient twin became the donor [42]. Persistent hemoglobin differences after laser therapy is considered a failure of the ablation and have been significantly reduced in frequency with the Solomon technique, but still can occur. Close observation with twice weekly MCA Doppler studies is recommended after laser therapy to detect either recurrent TTTS or TAPS. Treatment depends on gestational age and whether a repeat laser treatment is possible. Without the polyhydramnios to improve visibility fetoscopically, a repeat procedure can be quite difficult. Other therapies which have been suggested include either of both intrauterine transfusion for the anemic fetus with partial exchange transfusion for the polycythemic fetus to decrease the hypercoagulation problems [43].

Acute Intertwin Transfusion

Another relatively rare form of TTTS occurs when there is an acute transfusion of a significant volume of blood from one twin to the other at the time of delivery. While the diagnosis may be suggested by a difference in hemoglobin concentration, it should be recognized that in acute blood loss, hypovolemia may precede anemia. The donor infants may require early intervention with volume expanders and/or blood transfusion [36].

When one of a monochorionic twin pair dies in utero, that fetal–placental unit becomes a low pressure sink for the surviving twin. Via the anastomosis, there can be an immediate exsanguination from the surviving twin, resulting in acute anemia and hypovolemia with resulting death, or possible intracerebral and renal ischemic injury. The neonatal hematologic status will depend at least in part on how remote from the event that delivery occurs.

Clinical Manifestations

Most infants with TTTS are born early and suffer complications of prematurity. Following laser therapy, prematurity is still a problem, occurring in 17% prior to 28 weeks, 30% before 32 weeks and 50% before 34 weeks [37]. The neonatal findings will then not only reflect the placental anastomosis-mediated diseases, but also the consequences of prematurity.

In a study of patients treated in their center, Verbeek et al. looked at the hematologic outcomes of the donor and recipient twins as to whether they had been treated conservatively (expectant management or serial amnioreduction), treated with complete laser coagulation [44]. In addition, they assessed those treated with complete laser coagulation but who had persistent TTTS or TAPS. The results, shown in Table 23.3 show the incidence of anemia in the donor twin and polycythemia in the recipient twin by whether the twins were treated conservatively, had a complete laser, had persistent TTTS after laser (incomplete

Table 23.3 Requirement for transfusion (donor twin) or partial exchange transfusion (recipient twin) on day 1 in TTTS

	Transfusion day 1 donor	Partial exchange transfusion day 1 recipient
TTTS Conservative treatment	33% (14 of 43)	24% (10 of 42)
TTTS with laser treatment	5% (13 of 251)	1% (2 of 252)
TTTS + TAPS	55% (26 of 47)	35% (16 of 46)

Notes: TTTS, twin-to-twin transfusion syndrome
TAPS, twin anemia–polycythemia syndrome
Adapted from [44].

Table 23.4 Neonatal hematologic outcome in TTTS, TAPS, and acute TTTS

	Anemia	Polycythemia	Either twin pair
TTTS conservative	32	24	42
TTTS incomplete laser (TAPS)	55	35	78
TTTS Complete laser	5	1	7
Spontaneous TAPS	82	53	82
Acute peripartum TTTS	28	28	55

Note: Adapted from [44].

laser), spontaneous TAPS, or acute peripartum TTTS. Table 23.4 shows the need for blood transfusions in donor twins and plasma exchange transfusion in recipient twins if treated conservatively or having persistent TTTS or TAPS, but much lower rates for twin pairs treated successfully.

In addition to plethora, a number of other systems may be involved in the recipient. Cardiac findings include biventricular hypertrophy and tricuspid regurgitation [45]. Hyperviscosity secondary to polycythemia perhaps with the addition of vasoconstriction due to activation of the renal angiostensin system can result in vascular occlusion which may manifest with limb necrosis [46, 47]. Broadbent identified 16 cases of postnatal limb ischemia in one of a twin pair [48]. In nine cases, TTTS was identified and in all the limb ischemia occurred in the recipient twin. In the remaining cases, sepsis was the cause in one and TTTS was neither reported nor excluded in the others [48]. Hypoxic/ischemic events have also been noted [39].

The donor twin may exhibit cutaneous erythropoiesis (manifested as blueberry-muffin rash [49, 50], neutropenia [51], and/or renal failure [52, 53]. Thrombocytopenia, usually self-limited, occurs more commonly in neonates affected by TAPS than in uncomplicated monochorionic twins [44].

Neonatal Management

The type of antenatal therapy, if any, and results of post procedure can inform the neonatologist and hematologist of the most likely concerns for the neonate. The maternal fetal medicine and obstetrical teams should discuss this with in detail prior to delivery with the neonatologist. Depending on the acuity process preceding delivery, one or both of the neonates may be very non-euvolemic.

Postnatally, the donor twin may require volume expansion. If the twin is severely hypovolemic and/or anemic, then red blood cell transfusion may be indicated. Glucose infusions may be necessary for hypoglycemia in the donor twin. Long-term iron supplementation should be administered to the donor twin. The recipient twin should be evaluated for complications of the polycythemia/hyperviscosity syndrome, such as respiratory distress, jitteriness, seizures, hypocalcemia, hypoglycemia, and hyperbilirubinemia.

The affected twin may require partial exchange transfusion. The complications and management of the polycythemia/hyperviscosity syndrome are discussed in Chapter 11.

Placental Tumors

In neonatal anemia with no obvious explanation, pathologic examination of the placenta may provide an explanation and should be requested promptly prior to disposal of the placenta. Disorders that alter the fetal vascular integrity of the placenta can cause significant fetal blood loss, either as FMH or potentially into the amniotic fluid, depending on the site of the abnormality. Chorioangiomas are the most common placental tumour and are typically small, single and of no significant consequence [54]. Giant placental chorioangioma, typically defined as greater than 4 cm in size, however, can cause microangiopathic hemolytic anemia, thrombocytopenia, and non-immune hydrops fetalis [55, 56]. Multiple chorioangiomas (also known as chorioangiomatosis) are extremely rare and have been associated with severe anemia, thrombocytopenia and fetal growth restriction [57]. Despite their similar morphology, in a case-controlled survey study, infantile hemagiomas were not seen in increased frequency in infants of pregnancies complicated by placental chorioangiomas [58].

Choriocarcinoma within the placenta is extremely rare, and can cause fetal to maternal hemorrhage, as well as metastatic fetal and maternal disease. Intraplacental choriocarcinoma is accompanied by FMH quite frequently and can results in fetal anemia and death [59, 60]. These rare tumors may present with cutaneous nodules that can be mistaken for hemagiomas [61].

Fetal Growth Restriction

A variety of maternal or placental conditions can cause fetal growth restriction (FGR). In general, maternal vasculopathies (systemic or local) can result in poor placental development, which ultimately results in FGR. Examples of maternal systemic vasculopathic disorders include: hypertension, long-standing diabetes, and lupus and lupus-like disorders. The neonatal hematologic effects of these disorders on the fetus may by compounded if the maternal disease results in fetal growth restriction. Local vasculopathies, such as Müllerian abnormalities in the uterus or uterine fibroids may result in placentation in an area of abnormal maternal vasculature.

In the face of abnormal gas and nutrient exchange with placental insufficiency, there are many adaptive mechanisms. Blood flow to vital structures, such as the fetal brain, adrenal gland, heart, and placenta are preserved at the expense of normal perfusion of the bone marrow, lungs, gut, and musculature. This redistribution of blood flow results in cerebral vasodilation, peripheral vasoconstriction, and increased end-diastolic pressure in the ventricles. The hematologic effects, including polycythemia, thrombocytopenia and neutropenia, in the growth restricted fetus can vary and seem to be related to the severity of the fetal hypoxemia [62]. Elevated nucleated RBCs (adjusted for gestational age) are a marker for intrauterine hypoxia [63, 64].

Fetal Doppler measurements have been correlated with abnormal hematologic profiles in the FGR neonate. Critically abnormal umbilical artery Doppler studies (such as absent end diastolic flow or reversed diastolic flow) are evidence of very high resistance of flow through the placenta. Increases in the degree of pulsatility in the middle cerebral artery suggest cerebral vasodilation. In a study of 100 small for gestational age fetuses, Martinelli et al. showed that abnormal umbilical artery Doppler results correlated positively with elevations in neonatal nucleated RBC levels and negatively with platelet and white blood cell counts [65]. Similarly, Baschat and colleagues have shown that crucially abnormal umbilical artery Doppler measurements in the FGR fetus are associated with increasing nucleated RBC levels [66]. This group hypothesize that progressive fetal hypoxemia triggers the release of erythropoietin and RBC production and release at both intramedullary and extramedullary sites [67]. Furthering this point, they later showed that rate of progression of fetal Doppler abnormalities correlated with increased NRBCs and decreased Hb and platelets in the newborn after delivery [68].

There is also an effect on platelets. Stimulation of some antiplatelet factor by fetal acidosis, hypoxemia, or hypotension has been invoked by Baschat et al. as the mechanism to explain the 10 fold higher rate of neonatal thrombocytopenia in the growth-restricted fetus with absent or reversed umbilical artery Doppler measurement [66].

Diabetes

Maternal diabetes can have profound effects on fetal development. Maternal diabetes may predate the pregnancy or can develop during pregnancy (gestational diabetes). It is estimated that 0.2%–0.3% of pregnancies are affected by pre-existing diabetes mellitus and 1%–5% are affected by gestational diabetes [69]. Reported problems in infants of diabetic mothers (IDM) include decreased survival and increased rates of prematurity and frequency of both small for gestational age (SGA) and large for gestational age (LGA), although the LGA group predominates. Insulin does not cross the placenta, and hence maternal hyperglycemia causes fetal hyperglycemia and resultant fetal hyperinsulinemia. Polycythemia and thrombosis are the most significant hematologic complications in the IDM.

Polycythemia in Infants of Diabetic Mothers

Infants of diabetic mothers have an increased incidence of polycythemia [70, 71]. Mimouni and colleagues found that the incidence of polycythemia (venous hematocrit (Hct) ≥65% at 2 hours of age) in IDMs was 29% versus 6% for infants matched for gestational age, mode of delivery, and Apgar scores [72]. The hematocrit of the infant did not correlate with maternal glycosylated hemoglobin levels but did correlate with neonatal hypoglycemia. In contrast, Cordero et al. identified polycythemia in only 5% of IDMs in their cohort, although Hb were not done specifically at 2 hours and only done in roughly half of their cohort [73]. Green and colleagues found that the hematocrit of IDMs correlated with maternal glycosylated hemoglobin levels at term (average gestation 38 weeks) but not at 36 weeks' gestational age [74]. This may suggest that the maternal glucose control in late gestation has the greatest influence on the incidence of polycythemia.

Several factors may contribute to polycythemia in the IDM. Fetal hyperglycemia causes fetal hyperinsulinemia and insulin itself may promote erythropoiesis [75, 76]. Widness and colleagues found that the umbilical-vein erythropoietin concentrations were elevated in IDMs and correlated with maternal HbA1c levels taken the month before delivery [77]. Fetal erythropoietin concentrations correlate with fetal insulin levels [78].

Nucleated RBC levels, which may be a marker of fetal hypoxia, are also elevated in the IDM [79, 80]. There is a delayed switch from gamma- to beta-chain production in the IDM [81, 82]. Cetin et al. found a correlation between maternal β-hydroxybutyrate levels at 34–36 weeks and polycythemia in their newborns [83].

The complications of the polycythemia/hyperviscosity syndrome such as hypocalcemia, hypoglycemia, and hyperbilirubinemia should be expected and managed (see Chapter 11).

Thrombosis in Infants of Diabetic Mothers

The incidence of thrombosis, especially renal-vein thrombosis, is increased in IDMs [71]. Clinical manifestations of renal vein thrombosis may include shock, vomiting, hematuria, and a palpable kidney. Both venous and arterial thrombosis can occur in the IDM. While reported cases of peripartum gangrene of the limb are rare, 22% of one series were reported to be in IDMs [84]. One study found an association of perinatal arterial ischemic stroke with gestational diabetes [85].

It is likely that the increased incidence of thrombosis in the IDM is multifactorial. Polycythemia causes increased blood viscosity. Birth trauma, in part caused by macrosomia, may lead to vessel damage. Both platelet and plasma factors place the IDM at increased risk for thrombosis. Hathaway and colleagues suggested that there is increased platelet consumption [86]. Stuart and colleagues documented increased platelet reactivity and platelet endoperoxide formation in diabetic mothers and transiently in their infants [87]. Umbilical arteries from IDMs born to mothers with elevated HbA1c values produce significantly less prostacyclin, a potent inhibitor of platelet aggregation, than those obtained from control infants or IDMs of mothers with normal values for HbA1c [88]. Sarkar et al. found that protein C levels were lower in IDMs-either gestational diet controlled or insulin dependent, but there was no difference in the frequency of factor V Leiden, prothrombin gene mutation P20210A, methylenetetrahydrofolate reductase C677 T, or other common genetic risk factors [89]. Easa and Coen failed to find a difference in the prothrombin time, activated partial thromboplastin time, fibrinogen, factors V, X, or XII, or von Willebrand antigen [90]. Ironically, they found slightly lower levels for factor VIII and increased levels of antithrombin. Antiplasmin concentrations are increased in mothers with diabetes and their infants [91]. Elevated levels of homocysteine, a known risk factor for thrombosis have also been reported in IDM [92].

Thrombocytopenia in Infants of Diabetic Mothers

Mild thrombocytopenia is seen in IDM [86, 90]. The mean platelet count in IDMs was shown to be lower than in matched controls and did not correlate with maternal glycemic control [80]. Usually, no specific therapy is indicated.

Immunologic Changes in Infants of Diabetic Mothers

A few reports of immunologic abnormalities in IDMs have been reported, but their significance is not yet clear. Mehta and Petrova reported decreased neutrophil chemotaxis, random motility and chemiluminescence in IDM when compared to neonatal controls [93]. Infants of IDDM and gestational diabetes have reduced natural killer cells compared to healthy controls [94]. Roll et al. reported decreased numbers of both T and B lymphocytes in infants of insulin-dependent mothers [95].

Hypertensive Disorders of Pregnancy

Maternal hypertensive disorders (MH) is a well-recognized and potentially serious complication. Hypertension in pregnancy is divided into four categories: (1) preeclampsia/eclampsia, (2) chronic hypertension, (3) chronic hypertension with superimposed preeclampsia, and (4) gestational hypertension. Gestational hypertension is defined in women who develop elevated blood pressure without proteinuria after 20 weeks of gestation without symptoms of preeclampsia or eclampsia [96]. Risk factors for preeclampsia are noted in Table 23.5.

Eclampsia is diagnosed when a woman with preeclampsia develops new onset of seizures or altered mental status. HELLP (hemolysis, elevated liver enzymes, and low platelets) syndrome is considered by most to be a variant of severe preeclampsia and is diagnosed in the presence of maternal hemolysis, elevated liver enzymes and

Table 23.5 Risk factors for preeclampsia

Nulliparity
Extremes of maternal age
Multiple gestation
Chronic hypertension
Pre-existing diabetes mellitus
Collagen-vascular disease
African American
Antiphospholipid syndrome
Obesity
Prior pregnancy with preeclampsia
Nephropathy

low maternal platelets, usually with hypertension and proteinuria.

Neutropenia in Infants of Hypertensive Mothers

Although the association of neonatal neutropenia with maternal hypertensive disorders (particularly preeclampsia and its variants) is well established, there are conflicting data regarding the epidemiology of the association, risks of neonatal sepsis, and possible mechanisms.

In their classic paper defining the normal neonatal neutrophil count, Manroe and colleagues demonstrated a high incidence of neutropenia in the infants of the mothers with maternal hypertension (IMH) [97]. Since that time, other studies have demonstrated a 40%–50% incidence of neutropenia in infants of mothers with gestaional hypertension (IGH), using Manroe's data for the normal range [98–100]. Doron and colleagues found an incidence of 48% using normative data developed for premature infants [101]. Of 95 extremely low birth weight (ELBW) infants found to have an ANC <1,000 per microliter in the first 3 days of life (from a total cohort of 388 infants) 68% were either SGA or IGH [102]. Smaller (<1,500 g), more premature (<30 weeks' gestational age), and/or cesarean-section-delivered IGH are more likely to have neutropenia. The incidence of neutropenia increases with the severity of maternal hypertension [99, 101]. In contrast, some have failed to find an increased incidence of neutropenia in premature IGH compared with matched controls also using normative data developed for premature infants [103].

In a small series, Bolat et al. found neutropenia in 18 of 31 (58%) IMH vs. 6% in a control group. The neutropenia was mild in eight, moderate in six, and severe in four of the infants. Lymphopenia was noted in 36% of these infants and 19% of the control group [104].

It is yet unclear if it is the maternal hypertension or the SGA status of the infant that is the primary contributor to neonatal neutropenia and thrombocytopenia. Christensen et al. did a retrospective review of all infants born SGA with an absolute neutrophil count <1,000/mcL born within a large health system [105]. They excluded from analysis infants with other known causes of neutropenia including early-onset sepsis. Six percent of tested SGA infants had early-onset neutropenia vs. 1% of gestational-age matched controls. The I/T ratio of these infants was within the reference range and their neutrophil counts increased to the reference range by day 7. Sixty-four percent of these infants also had thrombocytopenia. The neutropenia was not independently associated with maternal hypertension beyond their SGA status [105]. In contrast, Bizerea found that neutropenia occurred in 33% of SGA infants of hypertensive mothers and 23% of AGA infants of hypertensive mothers as opposed to only 2.6% of SGA controls [106].

Koenig and Christensen identified decreased neutrophil production, perhaps due to an inhibitor of myelopoiesis, as the cause of neutropenia in the IMH [100]. Other possible causes of decreased white cell production in fetuses of hypertensive women include: a neutrophil production inhibitor in the placenta or in fetal blood; the erythrocyte steal phenomena with intrauterine hypoxemia in which there is a shift towards red cell production; down regulation of white cell production due to placental dysfunction; and FAS-FAS ligand interaction abnormalities [107]. Some studies have shown this neutropenia to last for less than 72 hours [98, 100], while another study reported more prolonged neutropenia [108]. Compared with infants with sepsis-induced neutropenia, the neutropenia in IMH occurs earlier in life and does not have an increased ratio of immature to total neutrophils [99]. Yet, Saini et al. reported that the expression of surface adhesion markers, indicating neutrophil activation, was increased in infants of preeclamptic mothers [109].

There have been conflicting studies as to whether the neutropenia in IMH is associated with an increased risk of infection. Doron and colleagues reported an increased rate of bacterial infection in the first 48 hours of life in neutropenic compared with non-neutropenic IMH [101]. Other studies have shown an increased incidence of late-onset infection, usually after the neutropenia had resolved [99, 100]. Stoll reported from a review of the National Institute of Child Health and Human Development Neonatal Research Network that the presence of maternal hypertension/preeclampsia actually decreased the risk of neonatal infection [110]. Sharma et al. did a retrospective study of IMH [107]. The vast majority of neutropenic children were born prematurely, 86.4% of those from multiple gestations and 80% of the singletons. In this series, only the neutropenic multiple-gestation infants were at increased risk of sepsis compared to non-neutropenic multiples; this was not true of singletons [107].

Neutropenia in IMH may respond to granulocyte colony stimulating factor injections [111]. However, the need for routine use of this medication in the uninfected preterm infant with neutropenia has not been demonstrated to be necessary [103, 112]. Sixteen percent of the infants in Christensen's series were treated with IVIg or G-CSF without an effect on outcome [105].

Thrombocytopenia in Infants of Mothers with Hypertensive Disorders of Pregnancy

Thrombocytopenia in neonates that presents in the first 72 hours of life is often found in the setting of placental insufficiency and maternal hypertension is a common cause. According to Chakravorty et al., this form of thrombocytopenia is usually benign and is rarely severe, uncommonly results in a rapid drop in platelet count and usually does not require treatment [113]. Early onset thrombocytopenia that differs from this pattern warrants further work up regarding etiology [114].

While thrombocytopenia is seen in 15%–36% of IMH [98–100, 104, 115), it is often but not always mild. In a prospective study from India, platelet counts were assessed in 97 IMH [116]. Of these, 36.1% had thrombocytopenia and in 20% the platelet count was <30,000/µL. Thrombocytopenia was significantly more likely in male children (OR 2.54, CI 1.08–5.95), with a trend towards increased risk associated with prematurity and low birth weight [116]. In a study of thrombocytopenia in hospitalized neonates, McPherson and Juul, using combined data for SGA and IMH, found the percentage of uninfected neonates with thrombocytopenia was higher in SGA/IMH vs. AGA infants for gestational ages <27 weeks (80% vs. 30%); 27<30 weeks (50% vs. 13%) and 30<34 weeks (30% vs. 8%) [117]. Most of their cases of thrombocytopenia attributed to SGA/IMH resolved within 2 weeks. In an analysis of ELBW infants, Christensen found that SGA or IMH was the most common diagnosed cause of thrombocytopenia, accounting for 37% of all cases [118]. There are similar rates of thrombocytopenia for infants born to mothers with HELLP as compared with maternal eclampsia/preeclampsia [119–121]. Disseminated intravascular coagulation (DIC) has been reported in IMH whose mothers' platelet counts were <50,000/μl [115]. In studies to determine the etiology of thrombocytopenia in IMH, Tsao et al. showed that soluble fms-like tyrosine kinase 1 levels were higher in IMH and inversely correlated with infant platelet counts [122]. Infants with high levels of soluble fms-like tyrosine kinase 1 were more likely to have lower platelet counts, maternal preeclampsia and to be SGA [122]. Thrombopoietin levels did not differ between infants of mothers with and without MH [123]. Megakaryocytopoeitic defects have been postulated [124].

Polycythemia in Infants of Hypertensive Mothers

An increased incidence of polycythemia in IMH has been reported [125]. Brazy and colleagues found the mean hemoglobin level to be 5% higher in IMH [115]. The recommendations regarding the management of polycythemia are outlined in Chapter 11.

Autoimmune Syndromes

Neonatal Lupus Erythematosus

The neonatal lupus erythematosus (NLE) syndrome is believed to be due to the transplacental passage of autoantibodies, usually anti-Ro (SS-A) or anti-La (SS-B). Irreversible congenital heart block arising in the second trimester is the most devastating complication of the NLE syndrome. Cutaneous manifestations of NLE often begin after birth. Other complications include hepatitis and occasionally neurologic manifestations, including seizures.

Transient thrombocytopenia has been noted in roughly 10% of infants with NLE [126, 127]. Zuppa et al. followed 50 infants identified with anti-SS/Ro antibodies at birth; 90% of the antibodies resolved by 9 months of age [128]. Anemia was found in 2% at birth, 24% at 3 months, and 12% at 6 months. Neutropenia was found in 4% at birth, 24% at 3 months, 12% at 6 months, and 2% at 9 months. Thrombocytopenia was found in 2% at birth and none thereafter. None of the hematologic findings in Zuppa's series caused complications or required treatment [128]. Hariharan and colleagues reported a case of NLE-associated microangiopathic anemia with severe thrombocytopenia that responded to intravenous gammaglobulin and corticosteroid treatment [129]. Recently, a newborn with a perinatal stroke was described who along with his mother had anti-SS/Ro antibodies [130]. There are multiple new agents available for management of individuals with autoimmune disease. Pediatricians should be aware of recommendations regarding the use of such agents in pregnancy and lactation as they develop [131].

Antiphospholipid Antibody Syndrome

An association between the presence of anticardiolipin antibodies and recurrent fetal loss has been well described. The presence of these antibodies in the mother may increase the risk for fetal growth restriction [132]. The presence of anticardiolipin antibody and/or the lupus anticoagulant is associated with an increased risk of maternal venous and arterial thrombosis, although the majority are venous. The cause of the increased thrombosis is not certain, but it appears to be related to platelet activation in the maternal circulation. The IgG isotype of the anticardiolipin antibody can cross the placenta [133].

There have been numerous case reports of fetal and neonatal thrombosis with the maternal antiphospholipid syndrome including the CNS vessels, renal vasculature, vena cava, and aorta [134]. Boffa and Lachassinne described 16 episodes of neonatal thrombosis in infants of mothers with APL: 13 (of 16) were arterial and 8 (of 16) were strokes [135].

The presence of the anticardiolipin antibodies in the newborn is usually transient but may persist for months due to the half-life of transplacentally acquired maternal IgG [136]. Persistent antiphospholipid antibodies have been reported in a cohort of infants with perinatal stroke [137].

Neonatal thrombosis associated with this syndrome should be managed as described in Chapter 19.

Maternal Malignancy

Cancer complicates approximately 1 in 1,000 pregnancies [138–140]. The potential effect of cancer treatment on the fetus, raises serious questions for the management of the mother with cancer [141]. Such cases should be referred whenever possible to a center with the full range of resources and knowledge available to provide the best possible outcomes for the mother and infant.

The most common cancers requiring systemic treatment during pregnancy include breast, ovarian and cervical cancer, lymphoma, leukemia, and sarcoma [138–140]. Chemotherapeutic agents and radiation therapy have been used to treat cancer during pregnancy and several reviews of this topic and specific malignancies are available [138, 142–144].

Antineoplastic agents used to treat cancer can cross the placenta, albeit that maternal pharmacodynamics and placental factors may affect and likely decrease fetal drug exposure [143]. There are differences in both the fetal and maternal physiology that might affect the toxicity of these agents [145, 146]. There is an increase in fetal malformations if chemotherapy in the first trimester [138, 142–144], but the relative risk of chemotherapy-induced malformation appears to decrease significantly when it is administered after the first trimester [139]. Infants exposed to chemotherapy during the second and third trimesters may be at increased risk for preterm birth [147, 148] and/or fetal growth restriction [149]. Maternal chemotherapy may cause fetal functional toxicity. Idarubicin-induced fetal cardiotoxicity has been reported [150], but a longer-term follow up study did not find cardiac issues in 26 infants exposed to anthracycline in utero [147]. Myelosuppressive chemotherapy may cause neonatal pancytopenia which may be present at birth or develop in the first few days of life [151], and hence some authors have recommended trying to avoid myelosuppressive chemotherapy after the 35th week of gestation [143].

Much still needs to be learned about the effects of newer chemotherapeutic agents on the fetus. For example, while infrequently studied in infants of mothers treated with rituximab, neonatal B cell depletion has been reported [152]. Pediatricians will need to follow the evolving literature regarding specific agents to determine what if any modifications to care will need to occur for infants exposed in utero.

There is limited, but growing, long-term follow up of children whose mothers were treated with chemotherapy [143, 147, 153]. In a follow-up study of 157 products of intrauterine chemotherapy exposure after the first trimester for maternal cancer (first exposure at 20.1±5.7 weeks) there was no increase in congenital anomalies, preterm delivery, or growth restriction when compared with general population norms [153]. The rate of congenital malformations and long term complications was not increased in survivors of maternal breast cancer reported in a long term registry [154]. Amant et al. failed to find neurocognitive long-term effects [147]. While such studies will need to continue, in particular as new anti-cancer therapies are used, the available data allows the pediatrician to share optimism with the family when a mother has been treated with chemotherapy while pregnant.

The topic of radiation administered during pregnancy has been reviewed [155, 156]. Fetal growth restriction, microcephaly, eye, and central nervous system (CNS) abnormalities are the predominant complications of intrauterine exposure to ionizing radiation in humans [157]. Hematopoietic, hepatic, renal, and cutaneous effects of radiation therapy have been reported when the fetus is exposed to radiation late in gestation. Factors that affect fetal dose include size of the radiation field, the target dose, the distance from the field edge to the fetus, shielding measures, radiation machine used, and leakage [155, 158, 159]. The pediatrician should be cognizant of potential fetal radiation exposure and include this on their problem list for long-term monitoring as the literature on such exposed infants evolves.

Placental Metastases

While primary placental malignancies arise from gestational trophoblastic neoplasia including partial and complete hydatiform moles and choriocarcinoma, maternal malignancy rarely spreads to the fetus or the placenta [160]. In 2002, Walker et al. reviewed 68 cases of maternal malignancy metastatic to the fetus (21%) and placenta (79%) [161]. Malignant melanoma is the most common malignancy to metastasize to products of conception, followed by breast cancer, leukemia/lymphoma, and lung cancer [161]. Hurley et al. describe a case where the mother died shortly of non-Hodgkins lymphoma shortly after delivery while the infant was diagnosed with a histologically identical tumor at 2 months of age [162]. Hence, the placenta should be carefully examined in cases of known maternal malignancy.

Maternal Medications

There is a vast array of medications, including prescription drugs, non-prescription medications, herbal supplements, native and traditional remedies, and others, that a mother may take during pregnancy. A few examples of medications that may affect the newborn's hematologic status are noted below. Whenever a neonate presents with early-onset hematologic abnormalities, a careful history of maternal medication use should be obtained with an understanding of placental transfer and potential hematologic consequences.

Effects on Hemostasis

Vitamin K deficiency is seen in 10%–66% of newborns whose mothers have been treated with anticonvulsants, including phenobarbital, phenytoin, and carbamazepam [163–165]. Hemorrhagic disease of the newborn with intraventricular hemorrhage has been reported. The coagulopathy can be reversed with vitamin K administration. While there have been recommendations for pregnant women taking enzyme-inducing anti-epileptic drugs to receive prenatal vitamin K prior to delivery [166], an assessment of the evidence could not confirm or refute the efficacy of this practice [167]. Vitamin K deficiency can also be caused by maternal warfarin ingestion, rifampicin, and isoniazid [168].

As described above, cancer chemotherapeutic agents can cause neonatal thrombocytopenia. Heparin-induced thrombocytopenia (HIT) occurs in a small percentage of individuals treated with heparin. It is manifested by mild thrombocytopenia and, paradoxically, an increased risk for thrombosis. HIT is caused by an antibody directed against the heparin–platelet factor 4 complex. HIT occurs in pregnant women; since the HIT antibody is an IgG antibody that is transported transplacentally, it has been found in cord blood [169].

The risk of venous thromboembolism increases four to five fold during pregnancy and even more in the 3 months following delivery [170]. Low molecular weight heparin and occasionally unfractionated heparin have been the mainstays of management and do not cross the placenta. Other than the potential for HIT as above, they should not affect neonatal hemostasis [170]. Both warfarin and direct thrombin inhibitors cross the placenta and warfarin has been associated with a fetal embryopathy. At this point, direct thrombin inhibitors are not recommended for use in pregnancy [170]. Women with very high thrombotic risk such as those with mechanical heart valves or HIT should be managed by a multidisciplinary team and the pediatrician should be aware of such treatment. Pediatricians should be aware that warfarin may be used in women with mechanical heart valves and be prepared to manage infants exposed in utero [170, 171].

Effects on Red Blood Cells

Glucose-6-phosphate dehydrogenase (G-6-PD) deficiency is by far the most prevalent genetically transmitted erythrocyte enzymopathy, with millions of individuals affected. Fetal hemolysis in G-6-PD deficient fetuses can be triggered by maternal ingestion of compounds known to induce hemolysis in deficient RBCs, including naphthalene, fava beans (broad beans), and several medications such as aspirin, some antimalarials, several sulfonamids, and others. The neonatal manifestations of G-6-PD deficiency are described in Chapter 10.

Anemia and thrombocytopenia was seen in 10/13 infants whose mothers received natalizumab for multiple sclerosis during pregnancy [172]. As more biologic and biosimilar agents are used for a variety of conditions, the pediatrician will need to stay current on potential hematologic toxicities in the newborn.

Effects on Leukocytes

Barak and colleagues reported that infants whose mothers received antenatal administration of betamethasone within 36 hours of delivery had higher leukocyte and neutrophil counts than control infants, and that this effect lasted for up to 7 days [173]. However, the role of antenatal betamethasone exposure in causing leukemoid reactions and their potential sequelae in small infants is less clear. Leukemoid reactions have been noted in infants whose mothers received antenatal dexamethasone [174]. Juul and colleagues found neutrophilia in 28% but also neutropenia in 26% of infants <32 weeks gestational age with antenatal betamethasone exposure [175]. Of 6 infants <34 weeks gestational age with leukemoid reaction in the first 4 days of life, four had antenatal betamethasone exposure within 48 hours of birth [176].

Maternal Nutritional Deficiencies

Anemia in pregnancy is defined as a Hb <11.0 g/dL or a Hct <33% during the first or third trimester or a Hb <10.5 g/dL or a Hct <32% in the second trimester [177, 178]. Nutritional anemias in pregnancy may have important clinical ramifications for both the mother and the developing fetus [178, 179].

Maternal Iron Deficiency Anemia

In 2011, the global prevalence of iron deficiency anemia was estimated to be 38% and in high income countries about 25% [180]. During pregnancy, the mother and the fetus both require iron. The mother's blood volume increases, both the red cell volume and the plasma volume. The fetus requires iron for use in many cellular processes as well as for red cell production. The average daily requirement for absorbed iron during pregnancy is 4.4 mg/day and increases from 0.8 mg/day in the first 10 weeks to 7.5 mg/day in the last 10 weeks [181]. Iron is required to support the additional red cell volume in the mother, the fetal red cell volume, placental requirements, average daily losses and average perinatal blood loss with delivery [179]. The fetal iron endowment is 75 mg/kg [182]. Iron deficiency may be caused by inadequate nutritional intake, excessive blood losses, including those of preceding pregnancies, or a combination of these problems. In addition to maternal iron deficiency and perinatal blood loss, factors that increase erythropoiesis in the fetus such as maternal diabetes, maternal smoking and fetal growth restriction may be associated with fetal iron deficiency through increased iron demands by the erythron leaving less iron for other tissues [183, 184]. After birth, the supply of iron in breast milk for exclusively breast-fed infants is critical.

It would seem, therefore, that there would be clarity about the benefits of identifying pregnant women with iron deficiency anemia and treating them. The American College of Obstetricians and Gynecologists has recommended (and this was reaffirmed in 2017) that all pregnant women should be screened for anemia during pregnancy and that those with IDA should be supplemented [185]. Contrary to this, the United States Preventive Service Taskforce report in 2015 concluded that the "current evidence is insufficient to assess the balance of benefits and harms of routine iron supplementation for pregnant women or for screening for iron deficiency anemia" [186]. They cited an absence of any study that evaluated the direct effects of routine screening in asymptomatic women on either maternal health or birth outcomes, even though there is evidence that a pregnant woman's blood counts and indices are improved with these measures.

Many studies of pregnancy outcomes, both maternal and neonatal, have been done in developing countries and may not be generalizable to high income countries. Data regarding the direct effect on neonatal anemia is not robust. There is conflicting data about the association of maternal iron deficiency anemia even indirectly with factors that influence neonatal health. The majority of iron transfer to the fetus occurs late in the 3rd trimester [187]. As such, any association of maternal iron deficiency anemia with preterm birth could influence total body iron for the infant.

In a meta-analysis done to evaluate the population attributable fraction of maternal anemia to poor birth outcomes, Rahman et al. found significant associations with low birth weight (RR 1.31, 95% CI 1.13–1.51), preterm birth (RR 1.63, 95% CI 1.33–2.01), perinatal mortality (RR 1.51, 95% CI 1.30–1.76), and neonatal mortality (RR 2.72, 95% Ci 1.19–6.25) [180]. They calculated that the population attributable fraction in low and middle income countries of maternal anemia to be 12% for low birth weight, 19% for preterm birth and 18% for perinatal mortality.

Counter to that, the Cochrane Collaboration in 2015 analyzed 61 randomized, or quasi-randomized trials to assess the association of maternal preventive iron supplementation on maternal and neonatal outcomes [188]. They found much of the work to be of low quality. Supplementation did significantly reduce maternal anemia at term by 70% (RR 0.30, 95% CI 0.19–0.46), iron deficiency anemia by 67% (RR 0.33, 95% CI 0.16–0.69) and iron deficiency at term (RR 0.43, 95% CI 0.27–0.66). They did report that low quality data showed a reduction in low birth weight babies (8.4% in supplemented patients, 10.3% in unsupplemented patients), they did not find a significant difference in preterm births. Similarly, in a retrospective cohort from a birth registry in the Aberdeen region of Scotland, investigators found no increased rate of premature births [189].

Diagnosis of Iron Deficiency

The diagnosis of iron deficiency can be difficult, because many standard diagnostic measures can be affected by pregnancy. Low ferritin values typically do indicate iron deficiency, however, ferritin is an acute-phase reactant whose levels may increase with many disorders, so a normal ferritin value does not exclude iron deficiency. While levels <12–15 ng/mL are typically used to indicate iron deficiency, higher values may have greater sensitivity [178]. The ratio of serum iron to iron-binding capacity (iron-saturation ratio) can be affected by inflammation, diurnal variation, and acute iron ingestion and is subject to significant variability. The soluble transferrin receptor increases with iron deficiency and is not affected by inflammation [178], and has been used by some to estimate incidence of iron deficiency with pregnancy [190], but is not specific for iron deficiency as levels also increase with ineffective erythropoiesis and may not be routinely evaluable. One small study found that low reticulocyte hemoglobin content correlated well with other measures of iron deficiency in pregnant women [191]. This test may also not be routinely available. Measurements of iron sufficiency and nutrition in the neonate are discussed in greater detail in Chapter 8.

Maternal Iron Status and Infant Iron Status

The effect of maternal iron deficiency on maternal and fetal health has been reviewed [192]. The fetus is quite effective at extracting iron from its mother, even when her iron stores are depleted. There is no correlation between the maternal and neonatal hemoglobin concentrations at birth [192]. Recent studies show that in fact infants born to mothers with iron deficiency likely have decreased iron stores, absorb greater amounts of supplemental iron and are more likely to develop iron deficiency later in infancy [193].

In view of the demonstration that neonatal iron deficiency may have significant impacts beyond anemia, such as neurodevelopment, understanding the impact of maternal iron deficiency on neonatal iron stores is relevant to their care. The neonatal ferritin levels are higher than the mothers in the absence of fetal blood loss, indicating that the placenta is capable of transporting iron across a gradient. The 5th percentile for ferritin for a term infant has been defined as <40 ng/ml and increases during gestation [194].

While the newborn's hemoglobin concentration may not be affected unless the mother is very anemic, maternal iron supplementation during pregnancy may improve the infant's hemoglobin levels later in life [193, 195]. Delayed cord clamping to >180 seconds after delivery has been shown to decrease iron deficiency at 3–6 months of age [196, 197].

Folate

Folate is a required cofactor in many one-carbon-transfer reactions. Such reactions are components of the purine and thymidine synthetic pathways and, hence, affect DNA synthesis. Because this step is critical for hematopoiesis, folate deficiency can be a cause of anemia, thrombocytopenia, and neutropenia. Folates are also important in the degradation of histidine and homocysteine. Folate is found in many foods, especially leafy vegetables, fruits, and yeast. It is also found in human and cow's milk, but it is very low in goat's milk [198].

In addition to diet, several other factors can affect maternal folate levels. Excessive cooking inactivates folate. Methotrexate, pyrimethamine, and trimethoprim inhibit dihydrofolate reductase and interfere with the production of 5,6,7,8-tetrahydrofolic acid, the active form of folate in one-carbon transfers [199]. Women with hemolytic anemias, tropical or nontropical sprue, other malabsorptive states, as well as those taking anticonvulsive medications and high-dose oral contraceptives have increased folate requirements [199]. Folate deficiency is also seen in women who have undergone bariatric surgery [178].

Folate deficiency in unsupplemented pregnant women is common but may be masked by concomitant iron deficiency. Maternal folate deficiency is associated with an increased risk for fetal neural-tube defects, and fetal growth restriction [200]. Current recommended daily intake for women of childbearing age for folate is 400 µg/day [201]. Folate is transported against a gradient in the placenta and cord levels of plasma folate are higher than maternal levels [199]. In many areas of the world, including North America, folate is added to foods to decrease the incidence of preconceptual maternal folate deficiency and subsequent neural tube defects, however, this is not done universally [202].

Because of the preferential transport of folate to the fetus, deficiency in the immediate newborn period is unlikely. Neonates of mothers with even severe megaloblastic anemia have normal hemoglobin concentrations [203]. Postnatal events such as hemolysis, infection, malnutrition, diarrhea, and liver disease increase the likelihood of folate deficiency in the neonate [199]. The diagnosis should be suspected in the malnourished infant with persistent anemia, especially when associated with thrombocytopenia and/or neutropenia. Bone-marrow examination may reveal megaloblastic hematopoiesis, and hypersegmented neutrophils may be seen on the peripheral blood smear. The diagnosis is confirmed by reduced serum or erythrocyte folate concentrations. Erythrocyte folate levels would be expected to decline more slowly than serum folate levels [199]. Total plasma homocysteine levels may be elevated in folate deficiency.

Cobalamin deficiency should be sought is patients diagnosed with folate deficiency as cobalamin deficiency causes reduced erythrocyte folate concentrations [199], and folate treatment may improve the hematologic parameters but neurologic damage may progress [204]. Inherited disorders of folate metabolism, in particular hereditary folate malabsorption, may affect folate levels or mimic folate deficiency [205].

Treatment

Infants with folate deficiency will respond to folate supplementation. Often doses as low as 200–500 µg may be sufficient, but higher doses may be necessary in cases of intestinal malabsorption syndromes. Doses of 50–200 µg/kg have been recommended for infants [205]. Folate may also be added to hyperalimentation solutions.

Cobalamin

Cobalamin, or vitamin B12, is a cofactor in the conversion of homocysteine to methionine and methylmalonyl coenzyme A to succinyl coenzyme A. The former reaction is critical for creation of intracellular polyglutamated tetrahydrofolate, the functional metabolite of folic acid. Hence, cobalamin deficiency impairs DNA synthesis. In addition to megaloblastic anemia, a peripheral neuropathy with degeneration of the lateral and posterior columns of the spinal cord can occur.

Cobalamin is present primarily in foods of animal origin [206]. A complex series of reactions leads to the absorption and distribution of cobalamin in humans. Intrinsic factor, produced in saliva and gastric juice, combines in the gastrointestinal tract with cobalamin and facilitates binding to a specific receptor in the ileum. The complex is then absorbed, metabolized, and transported through the blood by transcobalamin II [199].

The RDA for cobalamin for pregnant women is 2.6 µg/day and for lactating women 2.8 µg/day [207]. There is preferential transport of cobalamin from the mother to the fetus [207]. While this causes a decline in maternal serum cobalamin levels during pregnancy, the fetal cobalamin content of 50 µg is but a small fraction of the usual maternal stores. Neonatal serum cobalamin levels are higher than maternal levels [208], but fall over the first 6 weeks of age [209]. Maternal cobalamin levels correlate with neonatal levels in infants of mothers with omnivorous diets [209].

Cobalamin deficiency in pregnant women is very common in many underdeveloped areas of the world including the Latin America, sub-Saharan Africa and South Asia [210]. Unlike folate, vitamin B12 is not routinely added to foods. Pernicious anemia is the most common cause of severe vitamin B12 deficiency [206]. Maternal dietary deficiency, due to vegetarian/vegan diets without supplementation may lead to eventual infantile B12 deficiency [211, 212], especially if the infants are exclusively breast fed [206]. In addition to nutritional deficits, other potential causes of maternal B12 deficiency include pernicious anemia, gastrectomy or gastric bypass surgery, ileal resection, inflammatory bowel disease, tropical sprue, gastritis, fish tapeworm infestation, sprue, intestinal bacterial overgrowth, or medications that block vitamin B12 absorption such as metformin or gastric acid inhibitors [199, 206, 210, 213].

Maternal B-12 deficiency is associated with an increased risk for adverse perinatal outcomes including early miscarriage, spontaneous abortion and neural tube defects [210]. It is important to obtain a nutritional, surgical, and medication history from the mother of an infant suspected of having B12 deficiency, however, mothers may be deficient in this vitamin without a history of veganism and without diagnostic abnormalities on their blood counts [214].

Hematologic manifestations of vitamin B12 deficiency include anemia, which is often macrocytic, thrombocytopenia, leucocytopenia and hypersegmented neutrophils [199, 204]. However, cobalamin deficiency was not seen in a series of infants and children with red cell macrocytosis [215]. Bone marrow megaloblastic changes may be seen [204]. Serum cobalamin levels are usually low, but can lack sensitivity and specificity. Additionally, folate deficiency can cause reduced serum cobalamin levels [204]. Therefore, especially in the absence of megaloblastic changes, the diagnosis is confirmed with metabolic markers of functional cobalamin deficiency including elevated homocysteine and methylmalonic acid levels [199]. Nonspecific findings of cobalamin deficiency include elevation of the serum lactate dehydrogenase (LDH), hyperbilirubinemia, and an elevated ferritin [204].

In addition to hematologic findings, symptoms of vitamin B12 deficiency in the infant can include neurologic manifestation that can be severe including hypotonia, neurodevelopmental delay, tremors, hyperirritability, and cerebral atrophy. These may not be fully reversible [199, 206, 214]. Hypogammaglobulinemia has been seen as well [216].

Other causes of B12 deficiency in an infant include malabsorption from resection of the terminal ileum as may occur with necrotizing enterocolitis or congenital disorders that affect cobalamin absorption such as intrinsic factor deficiency, Imerslund–Gräsbeck syndrome or transcobalamin II deficiency [199]. Congenital disorders of cobalamin metabolism may present with similar findings but normal cobalamin levels [199].

Treatment

The treatment of the infant with cobalamin deficiency depends in part on the degree of anemia. Severe anemia should be treated with slow transfusion, as rapid response to cobalamin is unlikely. Rapid transfusion in the severely anemic child may precipitate or aggravate congestive heart failure. Low initial doses, e.g., 0.2 µg/kg, of cyanocobalamin may be given subcutaneously [199]. Serum potassium levels should be monitored carefully, and potassium treatment initiated if indicated, as hypokalemia may develop, especially if large doses of cobalamin are administered. Unless there is documentation of a nutritional etiology for the cobalamin deficiency, the infant should be studied for a defect in cobalamin absorption, transport, or metabolism [199].

Intrauterine Infection

On occasion, the fetus can acquire bacterial, viral, or protozoal infections transplacentally from the mother (Table 23.6). This section will focus on the diagnosis and hematologic manifestations of perinatal infections. Anemia, thrombocytopenia, leukocyte abnormalities, and coagulation abnormalities are common in the fetus with intrauterine infection. As it is not yet possible to rapidly differentiate viral from bacterial infection in the newborn, the initial therapy for most of these patients will usually include empirical antibiotics. Unless specifically stated, the management of the hematologic problems found in these infants is outlined in other chapters. The reader is referred to other references, such as the Red Book®: *2018–2021 Report of the Committee on*

Table 23.6 Intrauterine infections

Protozoal	
	Toxoplasmosis
Bacterial	
	Syphilis
Viral	
	Cytomegalovirus
	Rubella
	Enterovirus
	Herpes simplex
	Parvovirus B19
	Human immunodeficiency virus

Infectious Diseases (31st edition) from the American Academy of Pediatrics [217], for specific recommendations regarding the treatment of infants with congenital infections.

Congenital Protozoal Infection

Toxoplasmosis

Toxoplasma gondii is a protozoal feline parasite that can infect humans and other animals. In almost all cases of fetal infection, the susceptible mother has experienced a primary infection that goes unnoticed. Immunocompromised mothers can transmit reactivated disease to the fetus. Maternal primary infection late in pregnancy increases the likelihood of fetal infection, but the consequences of late-gestation fetal infection are fewer [218]. Antibiotic treatment of the mother decreases the likelihood of fetal infection [218]. Toxoplasma infection in the newborn has been reviewed [218, 219].

In recent years, the prevalence of toxoplasmosis is decreasing both in the United States and in Europe [218, 220]. In France it has been estimated to be 2.9 cases per 10,000 live births while in the US it is about 0.5 cases per 10,000 live births. [220].

Clinical manifestations in symptomatic patients include seizures, hydrocephalus, chorioretinitis, fever, hepatomegaly, splenomegaly, and jaundice. Neonatal disease can be generalized or limited to the CNS. Generalized disease appears to be limited to those infants infected in the first two trimesters. The majority of infants with congenital toxoplasmosis have asymptomatic or subclinical disease [218].

Diagnosis

The diagnosis of congenital toxoplasmosis can be based on demonstration of the organism, serologic studies, or antigen testing. Histologic demonstration and/or tissue culture of the organism can be accomplished on several tissues or fluids, including the placenta and amniotic fluid [218]. Serologic tests include the Sabin–Feldman dye test, indirect hemagglutination, the indirect fluorescent antibody test, enzyme-linked immunosorbent assay (ELISA) tests, and others. The sensitivity and availability of these assays vary significantly between laboratories. There are several issues to consider when using humoral

responses to diagnose congenital toxoplasmosis. Specific IgG in neonatal serum can be acquired transplacentally from the mother; hence, in the first few months of life, a single positive test for IgG does not confirm neonatal infection. Persistent or rising IgG titers in the infant are considered diagnostic but require serial testing over the first several months of life.

Testing for toxoplasma-specific IgM can be done by several different methods. The IFA test is significantly less sensitive than either the ELISA or the ISAGA; in congenitally infected neonates, the IFA is positive in only 25% versus 75% if ELISA is used. The IFA test can also be rendered falsely negative by high-titer maternal IgG, and is often falsely positive in the presence of rheumatoid factor or antinuclear antibody. The double-sandwich ELISA avoids these pitfalls. Measurement of IgA and IgE is at least comparable to IgM for diagnosing neonatal infection; occasionally, an infant born to a mother with IgA or IgM antibodies to toxoplasmosis will have a transiently false-positive IgA antibody test [221]. While a positive immunoglobulin M (IgM) or IgA serologic test for *Toxoplasma* in the newborn should be considered diagnostic for congenital toxoplasmosis, the fetus does not begin to make specific antibody until after the 15th to 20th week of gestation. The clinician should also know that most readily available commercial antibody tests for toxoplasmosis are not consistently reliable. In general, it is best to involve infectious diseases trained physicians early in the process and to send serology to a known reliable laboratory for testing.

Polymerase chain reaction (PCR) has been shown to have very high sensitivity and specificity for *Toxoplasma* [222]. PCR testing of amniotic fluid was shown to have a sensitivity of 64% and a specificity of 100% for the prenatal diagnosis of congenital toxoplasmosis [223]. Peripheral blood leukocytes and cerebrospinal fluid (CSF) amongst others can also be tested by PCR for *Toxoplasma* [217]. Often, a combination of tests is necessary to confirm infection.

Hematologic Manifestations of Congenital Toxoplasmosis

Anemia has been reported in 4%–64% of infants with congenital toxoplasmosis and is present in most symptomatic infants [224–226]. The incidence of anemia reflects the presence of other manifestations. For instance, 77% of a referral population with symptomatic generalized disease had anemia, as opposed to only 10% of infants identified through serologic screening [218, 225]. The presence of increased nucleated RBCs and reticulocytosis indicate that the anemia is due to hemolysis [224]. Congenital toxoplasmosis can cause nonimmune hydrops [227].

Thrombocytopenia can be seen in symptomatic infection. Alford and colleagues found thrombocytopenia in 10% of prospectively identified infants [225]. Hohlfeld and colleagues found thrombocytopenia in 26% of fetuses with congenital toxoplasmosis studied by fetal-blood sampling [228].

Leukocyte abnormalities have been described in congenital toxoplasmosis. Eighteen percent of infants with generalized disease had eosinophilia [218]. Hohlfeld and colleagues found leukocytosis and eosinophilia in 7% and 9%, respectively, of infected fetuses [222]. Infected infants had lower levels of CD4 lymphocytes and a lower ratio of CD4 to CD8 lymphocytes than uninfected infants of mothers with gestational toxoplasmosis [229].

Congenital Bacterial Infection

Syphilis

Congenital syphilis caused by the spirochete *Treponema pallidum* was one of the first recognized perinatal infections. In the USA, risk factors for congenital syphilis include young maternal age, low socioeconomic status, parental drug use, sexual promiscuity, and inadequate prenatal care [230]. Unfortunately, syphilis is once again on the rise in America [217]. In the UK, low maternal infection rates were noted in the mid 1990s. Risk factors identified in the UK included being born abroad, non-white ethnicity, and living near London [231]. High rates of gestational syphilis have also been reported from Bolivia (4.3%), and aboriginal Australia (28%). Rates declined slightly in only 54 of 132 countries from 2012 to 2016; declines were substantive in only five of these countries [232] .

Clinical Manifestations

In endemic areas, the incidence of maternal syphilis infection in mothers of stillbirths is significantly greater than in mothers of live births. The probability of congenital syphilis and stillbirth is highest with secondary syphilis and early latent disease; the risk of disease is much lower in maternal late latent disease [233, 234]. Syphilis is a cause of stillbirth, nonimmune hydrops [233], and intrauterine growth retardation [234]. Many organs can be involved with congenital syphilis, and several clinical patterns of disease have been noted, including asymptomatic infection, maculopapular skin rash, mucoid and occasionally bloody rhinitis ("snuffles"), jaundice with hepatomegaly, monocytosis or lymphocytosis, hemolytic anemia, lytic bone lesions, nephritic syndrome, and neurosyphilis (which in newborns is often manifested only by a positive CSF VDRL) [234]. Congenital syphilis has been reviewed [230, 235].

Diagnosis

The diagnosis of congenital syphilis may require a high index of suspicion in the absence of obvious clinical stigmata of the disease. Maternal infection is often asymptomatic. Even if the characteristic chancres appear, they may be non-painful and hidden from sight. In one study of 155 women with syphilis during pregnancy, infection was asymptomatic in 121 (78%) [236]. Maternal screening serologies performed early in pregnancy will miss infection later in gestation. This is the basis for the recommendation that all pregnant women be screened for syphilis in the first trimester and again at the start of the third trimester. Women at high risk or who reside in high-prevalence areas should also be screened again at delivery [235]. High-risk women should also be screened at 28–32 weeks [233]. Placental abnormalities, such as the presence of plasma cells, may suggest the diagnosis of maternal infection. *The Red Book®: 2018–2021 Report of the Committee on Infectious Diseases* from the American Academy of Pediatrics notes that no newborn should be discharged from the hospital without determination of the mother's serologic status for syphilis [217].

Diagnostic tests for the infant include X-ray examinations, tests for the organism, serologic tests, and, recently, PCR assays. Non-treponemal tests have long been used as screening tests for syphilis. The venereal disease research lab (VDRL) and rapid plasma reagin (RPR) identify antibody against cardiolipin. The RPR may be the more sensitive test for serum, but only the VDRL is recommended for detection in the CSF [227]. If the infant's serum antibody titer is higher than the mother's, a presumptive diagnosis of congenital infection is made, but it is important to use the same assay performed in the same laboratory. Problems with non-treponemal assays include a relatively high false-negative rate in early, latent, and tertiary syphilis, a potential for a false-negative reaction with very high titers of antibody (the "prozone phenomenon"), and false-positive results caused by acute processes such as hepatitis, lymphoma, viral infection, malaria, endocarditis, or connective tissue disease [233]. Chronic biologic false-positive reactions can be caused by drug abuse or systemic diseases such as chronic hepatitis or collagen vascular disease, especially systemic lupus erythematosus. Women with false-positive RPRs will almost always have negative specific treponemal tests (see below). Wharton jelly contamination can cause a false-positive non-treponemal antibody test from cord blood [217]. Testing cord-blood sera may be less sensitive than testing neonatal serum at 2 to 3 days of age [237]. Non-treponemal antibody titers decrease over time with successful treatment [217].

Specific treponemal antibody tests are also used; these include the fluorescent treponemal antibody absorption test (FTA-ABS) and the microhemagglutination *T. pallidum* (MHA-TP) test. These tests have a sensitivity of 75%–85% in early syphilis and 100% for later diagnosis [234]. Because these tests usually remain positive, even in treated patients, the presence of a positive test does not prove active disease and thus cannot be used to monitor response to therapy. Unless the disease is early, a negative test excludes the diagnosis. Because false-positive tests can be caused by infection with non-pallidum treponemes, treponemal antibody tests should be combined with a non-treponemal test [233]. Some institutions reverse the traditional order of testing, starting with treponemal testing such as the MHA-TP and then do RPRs only on those who screen positive. This "reverse testing algorithm" offers no obvious benefit to the clinician and sometimes results in confusion. Potentially exposed babies are still screened with RPR of serum, and VDRL of CSF.

Hematologic Features of Congenital Syphilis

Whitaker and Sartain described nine infants with congenital syphilis [238]. Eight had anemia. They observed that infants with the largest spleens had the most severe anemia, but splenectomy failed to resolve the anemia in one of these infants. Infants presenting in the first week of life have typical features of hemolysis; i.e., hyperbilirubinemia, increased reticulocyte counts, and peripheral blood-smear findings of polychromasia and increased numbers of nucleated RBCs. Hemolysis appeared to be most rapid in the first week of life. Hemoglobin levels generally became normal after 3 months of age. While hyperbilirubinemia is common, most infants have elevation of both the direct and indirect fractions of bilirubin.

Thrombocytopenia was found in 28% of South African infants with congenital syphilis [239]. Whitaker and Sartain documented thrombocytopenia in five of seven infants in whom platelet counts were performed [238]. Platelet counts as low as 17,000–20,000/μL were seen in both series. Thrombocytopenia is secondary to decreased survival, not to inadequate production of platelets. It is important to note that in some cases thrombocytopenia may be the only manifestation of congenital syphilis [230]. Neutrophilia with a left shift in the differential count was seen in 33% of Whitaker's series. One infant had both vacuolization of the granulocytes and 5% peripheral blast forms that resolved in the first week of life [238]. Lymphocytosis or monocytosis and even leukemoid reaction may occur [240]. Rarely, a baby with congenital syphilis may develop paroxysmal cold hemoglobinuria [241]. Hemophagocytosis has also been described [242].

Congenital Viral Infections

Cytomegalovirus

Approximately 1% (range 0.2%–2.2%) of newborns are infected by cytomegalovirus (CMV) [243–245]. Maternal seropositivity rates vary with location and socioeconomic status. Females in developing countries or of lower socioeconomic status are more likely to become infected with CMV early in life and to be seropositive before pregnancy [245]. While most symptomatic intrauterine infections occur with primary infection in the mother [248], they may also occur in infants of seropositive mothers; in some studies, this rate was as high as 1%–2% [249].

Infants can also be infected during delivery from exposure to maternal secretions, and postnatally from breast milk of infected mothers, via blood transfusion, or from exposure to infected individuals [246]. Perinatally and postnatally acquired CMV infections are generally asymptomatic, but symptoms resembling congenital CMV may develop in premature neonates, particularly in those with a birth weight of less than 1,500 grams [247].

At birth, the majority of infants infected with CMV as fetuses are asymptomatic. In a study of 197 infants with congenital CMV, only 18% of infants showed signs of the disorder, and all of these were born to mothers with primary infection [248]. Severe generalized congenital CMV disease occurs in about half of symptomatic babies. CMV infection in the mother is more likely to have CNS sequelae when infection occurs in the first trimester [249]. Babies infected in utero with CMV may be born prematurely or have fetal growth restriction. Signs of symptomatic congenital CMV include petechiae, hepatomegaly, splenomegaly, and jaundice [250]. Neurologic problems are often prominent and include microcephaly, lethargy, poor suck, and seizures [250]. Intracerebral calcifications, generally periventricular, are a sequela of congenital infection [250]. Chorioretinitis is the most common ophthalmologic finding, but optic neuritis, cataracts (more common in rubella infection), and colobomas may be seen [250, 251]. Multiple other organs can be affected and infants may present with the classic "blueberry-muffin rash" due to dermal hematopoiesis [48]. Survival and/or long-term outcome of symptomatic infants is very poor.

Most infants with congenital CMV infection are asymptomatic at birth, but sequelae may appear in later life. Approximately 10%–15% of infants with congenital CMV infection who are asymptomatic at birth develop significant mental retardation or hearing deficit within the first 5 years of life [250].

Diagnosis

The demonstration of symptomatic CMV in infants of seropositive mothers indicates that maternal IgG cannot be used to exclude perinatal CMV infection [252, 253]. Diagnosis in the fetus can be challenging. While ultrasound abnormalities consistent with CMV combined with positive maternal serologies strongly support the diagnosis of intrauterine infection, a normal ultrasound does not exclude either congenital infection or sequelae [254]. IgG avidity assays are available; these are helpful in establishing the diagnosis of primary CMV infection in the mother because avidity is low for approximately 18–20 weeks after primary infection [254]. Early in gestation, infants are incapable of producing IgM [255]. Furthermore, even if the infected fetus does produce specific CMV IgM it may disappear before delivery [256]. The most sensitive techniques for prenatal diagnosis are viral culture from amniotic fluid and detection of CMV DNA via PCR, although this may be less sensitive in fetuses under 21 weeks' gestation or less than 6 weeks from maternal infection [257]. Symptomatic congenital CMV may develop even though amniotic fluid PCR failed to demonstrate the presence of the virus, and the severity of congenital CMV disease in babies is not predictable by amniotic fluid viral load [258].

Postnatally, the diagnosis is now being established most commonly by salivary PCR, which is a rapid, sensitive, and non-invasive test. More traditional testing by cell culture of urine or other body fluids or tissues is time consuming, expensive, and requires expertise, and thus is being supplanted by PCR methodology [259, 260].

Hematologic Manifestations of Congenital CMV

Thrombocytopenia and petechiae are common in symptomatic infants [250]. Hohlfeld and colleagues found that 36% of infants with congenital CMV had thrombocytopenia, and that 38% of these had a platelet count below 50,000/μL [228]. In another study, 62/81 (77%) of babies with generalized CMV disease had a platelet count below 100,000/μL, and 42/81 (53%) had a platelet count less than 50,000/μL [252]. Several observations suggest there is accelerated platelet destruction with congenital CMV. Consumptive coagulopathy and thrombosis have been noted in infants with congenital CMV [261, 262]. Apparent immune thrombocytopenia following congenital CMV infection has been reported [263]. Hypersplenism may also contribute to the shortened platelet lifespan. However, human CMV infection can also impair megakaryocyte viability [264]. Hence, decreased platelet production may contribute to the thrombocytopenia. Thrombocytopenia, with or without petechiae, may persist for weeks to months in some affected babies. On rare occasions, petechiae may be the only sign of congenital CMV infection.

Hemolytic anemia is a common finding in infants with symptomatic CMV [250]. Erythroblastosis, polychromasia and abnormal RBC morphology may be seen in the peripheral blood of infants with congenital CMV [244, 262]. Contributing factors include RBC membrane damage and hypersplenism [265]. Autoimmune hemolytic anemia is a complication of infantile CMV [266]. CMV has been shown to infect hematopoietic precursors, and hence decreased erythrocyte production may play a role [267]. CMV may cause hydrops fetalis [268].

Leukocyte abnormalities are common. Atypical lymphocytosis can be seen [269]. Neutropenia following congenital CMV infection has been reported [270].

Rubella

Rubella is a member of the togavirus family. It has a worldwide distribution, but vaccination has dramatically decreased the prevalence of viral infection in the developed world. Maternal infection is usually confirmed serologically. However, epidemics still occur even in developed countries and an estimated 100,000 cases of congenital rubella syndrome occur annually [271]. Positive rubella-specific IgM is a good indication of a recent maternal infection, but false-positive and false-negative tests may be seen [272]. Maternal reinfection may occur, and while risk of fetal infection is small, estimated at <5%, and the risk of congenital defects is even smaller, it is not absent [273, 274]. The development of fetal embryopathic changes is highest with first trimester infection and decreases over the first two trimesters [272, 275].

Not all congenitally infected newborns are symptomatic, and defects, especially deafness, can develop over time. In most cases, however, infection in the newborn is suspected on clinical grounds. The common manifestations of congenital rubella syndrome include fetal growth restriction, hepatosplenomegaly, congenital heart disease (most commonly patent ductus arteriosus or pulmonary valvular stenosis), meningoencephalitis, mental retardation, bony lucencies on X-ray, sensorineural hearing loss, interstitial pneumonitis, and ophthalmologic findings, including cataracts, retinopathy, and/or congenital glaucoma [276]. These infants may also present with the blueberry-muffin rash of dermal erythropoiesis. Of these findings, the major defects (and the defects that most characterize congenital rubella syndrome) are heart defects, eye defects (cataracts, glaucoma, or microphthalmia), and deafness.

Diagnosis

Viral culture and PCR should be attempted; the virus is most readily detected in specimens from the pharynx or nasal swab specimens but it can also be found in conjunctival scrapings, cerebrospinal fluid, blood, or urine specimens [272, 276]. Congenital rubella is a chronic infection; viral shedding usually persists for months [272]. Virus may be cultured from the CNS of infants with encephalitis [276]. Rubella-specific IgM from the infant is a strong indicator of congenital rubella, but false-positive tests can occur with rheumatoid factor, parvovirus IgM, or heterophile antibodies [272]. Rubella-specific IgM persists for a longer time in the infant with congenital rubella syndrome [277]. Passive rubella IgG from the mother should decrease by about one dilution per month and be absent by 6–10 months; stable or increasing rubella-specific IgG in the baby over the course of several months usually indicates congenital infection [272]. PCR of amniotic fluid has been used to diagnose rubella in the fetus of infected mothers [276, 278].

Hematologic Manifestations of Congenital Rubella

Decreased platelet counts are seen in the congenital rubella syndrome (CRS) [276]. Petechiae and purpura are noted in 29%–100% of such infants [279, 280]. Cooper and colleagues reported that 17% of infants with congenital rubella had platelet counts below 20,000/μL [281]. Bone marrow studies from thrombocytopenic infants with congenital rubella showed decreased megakaryopoiesis with a shift to more juvenile megakaryocytes [280, 282]. Splenic sequestration may be a contributing factor. DIC has been reported [262]. Thrombocytopenia may be a marker of severe of congenital rubella syndrome [283].

Anemia is noted in less than 20% of babies with congenital rubella; it may be present at birth or develop over the first month [280, 281]. There are several features that suggest hemolysis. Peripheral blood smears show abnormal red-cell morphology and increased numbers of normoblasts. The reticulocyte count is increased. The bone marrow usually shows accelerated erythropoiesis with an increased erythroid:myeloid ratio [282]. Decreased RBC survival has been documented [280]. One report, however, described a transient bone marrow (BM) hypoplasia in an infant with congenital rubella [284]. Leukopenia and leukocytosis have been noted in patients with congenital rubella [280]. Lymphadenopathy has been noted in approximately 20% of patients. Hepatomegaly and/or splenomegaly are common in symptomatic infants [281].

Herpes Simplex

Herpes simplex virus (HSV), like all members of the herpesvirus family, establishes latency after acute infection and then may reactivate periodically, sometimes with symptoms and sometimes without. There are two distinct antigenic types of HSV. Although an old paradigm holds that HSV-1 usually infects the oral region while HSV-2 typically involves the genital region, there is much overlap in both the epidemiologic and clinical manifestations of the two viruses. Acquisition generally occurs through intimate contact. Seropositivity to HSV-2 parallels the onset of sexual activity [285]. Older serologic tests did not distinguish reliably between HSV-1 and HSV-2, but more recently approved assays are able to do so [286]. Unless the exposure was recent, a negative serologic test should exclude prior infection in the mother [287]. Recommendations for the diagnosis of neonatal HSV infection include surface swab specimen (mouth, nasopharynx, conjunctivae, and anus) HSV PCR, vesicular PCR, and CSF and blood PCR [288]. Cell culture may still be available in some places, but most institutions have replaced cell cultures with PCR testing. Most infants with congenital HSV are born to asymptomatic mothers [285]. Factors that increase the risk of neonatal infection include primary maternal infection during gestation, infection late in gestation (preventing the transmission of maternal HSV-specific antibody to the fetus), the use of fetal scalp electrodes, and prolonged rupture of membranes [285].

The incidence of perinatal HSV in the USA is approximately 11–33 per 100,000 live births [285]. Infection of the neonate can occur in utero, during delivery, or postnatally. Intrauterine transmission is uncommon but may cause signs and symptoms similar to those of other congenital infections, such as toxoplasmosis and CMV, or it may cause unusual skin manifestations that are not readily recognized as herpetic [289]. More commonly, the newborn is exposed to virus from maternal genital fluids during delivery [285]. Perinatal HSV usually presents in the first month of life, with two-thirds of cases presenting in the first week [290]. Infection may also occur with exposure to infected caregivers, including mothers, fathers, and other providers [285, 291]. Perinatal infections are classified as localized disease to the skin, eyes, and mucous membranes (often called "SEM" disease); encephalitis with or without SEM involvement; and disseminated disease [285]. Disseminated disease is often fatal and may involve the liver, lungs, heart, CNS, skin, and other organs.

Diagnosis

In the absence of skin vesicles, the diagnosis of disseminated neonatal HSV can be challenging. After 24 hours of age, swab specimens of conjunctivae, nasopharynx, and rectum should not be positive for HSV by either PCR or culture unless the neonate is infected. When skin lesions are present, the diagnosis can be confirmed by rupturing vesicles, scraping the base of the vesicles, and submitting the specimens to the laboratory for PCR testing (or viral culture, where available). Treatment should be instituted at the first suspicion of HSV disease. Cerebrospinal fluid cultures are often falsely negative, even in the presence of significant encephalitis, and therefore PCR is the gold standard for diagnosing CNS disease [288, 292]. Studies show a broad range of sensitivity for CSF PCR in HSV encephalitis [285]; acyclovir should be continued if there are other features strongly suggestive of HSV CNS disease, such as focal seizures, abnormalities localized to the temporal lobes on imaging studies, or paroxysmal lateralizing epileptiform discharges ("PLEDS") on electroencephalography. Elevation of liver enzymes may be an early clue to the diagnosis of disseminated disease in febrile neonates [293].

Hematologic Manifestations of Congenital Herpes Simplex

DIC has been reported repeatedly in congenital HSV infection [262, 294, 295]. In 1970, Miller and colleagues reviewed the available literature on fatal neonatal HSV [296]. Abnormal bleeding was noted in 22 of 54 cases and abnormal coagulation studies were reported in 7 of 10 studied cases [296]. Hepatic disease can contribute to the coagulopathy. The presence of DIC increases the infant's risk of dying from neonatal HSV [290].

Enterovirus

The *Enterovirus* genus, including Coxsackie viruses, echoviruses, polioviruses, and enteroviruses, consists of non-enveloped, single-stranded negative-sense RNA viruses [297]. They are common causes of illness in humans. In the immunocompetent host, infections are generally self-limited and benign. However, serious sequelae, such as paralytic polio, may occur. Enterovirus disease is most prevalent in the summer and the fall.

While transplacental passage of poliovirus and Coxsackie virus has been reported [298], infection usually occurs with contact with the virus during passage through the birth canal, and postnatal exposure [299]. Jenista et al. cultured nonpolio enterovirus from 12.8% of infants during their first month of life; risk factors included lower SE status and bottle feeding [300]. Several nursery epidemics have been reported with different enteroviruses [298].

While most cases of enteroviral infection in the newborn are asymptomatic or mildly symptomatic, serious infection may occur [298, 299]. Symptoms of neonatal enterovirus infection vary widely. An extensive review of these potential symptoms by organ system and by virus has been written [298]. Abzug et al. identified 29 infants with culture-proven enterovirus infection in the first 14 days of life [301]. Fever, irritability, lethargy, and anorexia were noted in over half, while decreased perfusion, respiratory abnormalities, jaundice, and rash were also common. CNS involvement was found in 53% of the infants in whom CSF cultures were obtained. Severe multisystem disease (often called enterovirus sepsis) including hepatitis, coagulopathy, meningitis, and pneumonitis, may occur. The largest risk factor for symptomatic infection is absence of neutralizing antibody to the virus [299]. Other risk factors include infection in the first days of life and prematurity [299]. Echovirus 11 and Coxsackie viruses B2–5 are also reported to be risk factors for severe disease [298, 299].

Diagnosis

Because of the fact that results can be obtained much more quickly, PCR testing for enteroviruses has become the preferred diagnostic test [299, 302]. Enterovirus can be isolated by PCR from stool specimens or rectal swabs, throat swabs, nasopharyngeal aspirates, and other body fluids and tissues [302]. Cerebrospinal fluid can be positive in infants with meningitis. The large number of potential serotypes makes antibody detection impractical.

Hematologic Manifestations of Neonatal and Congenital Enterovirus Infection

Disseminated intravascular coagulation is a common feature of enteroviral hepatitis with multiorgan involvement. In a series of patients who, by definition, had hepatitis and coagulopathy, thrombocytopenia and increased partial thromboplastin and thrombin times were seen in 100%, and prolonged prothrombin times, elevated fibrin split products, and decreased fibrinogen concentrations were seen in over 85%. Two-thirds had anemia and 60% had peripheral leukocytosis [303]. In another series of infants diagnosed with enteroviral infection in the first 14 days of life but not limited to those with hepatitis and coagulopathy, 17% were noted to have thrombocytopenia [301]. Bleeding complications occur and may be severe [304, 305]. Intraventricular hemorrhage may result [306]. Leukocytosis, neutrophilia, and increased numbers of band forms are often noted [307]. One case report of a newborn with bone marrow failure presumably due to echovirus 11 infection has been published [308]. In a 3-day-old baby an enterovirus infection apparently precipitated hemophagocytic (macrophage activation) syndrome [309].

Treatment

From the hematologic perspective, supportive care consists of platelet, RBC, and plasma transfusion. Vitamin K may be useful in patients with bleeding and hepatic dysfunction [298]. The management of DIC is outlined in Chapter 18. Intravenous gammaglobulin has been tried with variable results, likely indicating the need for high titers of antibody against the infecting virus [305]. Although there are no approved antiviral agents that treat enteroviral infection, a recent double-blind study showed improved 2-month survival for infants with neonatal enterovirus sepsis treated with pleconaril [310].

Human Parvovirus B19

Human parvovirus B19 is a small, non-enveloped, single-stranded DNA virus that propagates in the human erythrocyte precursor. It enters the cell through the P antigen [311]; hence individuals whose RBCs lack the P antigen are not susceptible to infection. The common childhood illness erythema infectiosum, also known as "fifth disease," is caused by parvovirus B19.

Parvovirus B19 is transmitted mainly by respiratory droplets, although percutaneous exposure to blood or blood products and vertical maternal–fetal transmission have also been documented [302]. Infection is often asymptomatic. Common symptoms include fever, rash, and arthralgia. Symptoms of the joints may be difficult to distinguish from rheumatoid arthritis, especially in adults. In rare instances, vasculitis, myocarditis, and neurologic disease have been reported [312]. In immunocompromised individuals, pancytopenia or chronic anemia may result. Pregnant women may have asymptomatic infection.

While most people are infected with parvovirus B19 in childhood [313], and thus immune, susceptibility rates in pregnant women varies. For example one study from five European countries found the range of susceptibility to this infection in women of childbearing age to be 26%–44% [314]. The risk of seroconversion during pregnancy is about 1% during endemic periods but may be up to 13% during outbreaks [313], with an approximate vertical transmission rate of 35% [315].

Diagnosis

Gestational parvovirus screening is not routinely performed. Diagnosis of parvovirus B19 infection can be made serologically through a four-fold increase in IgG titers or by the presence of parvovirus-specific IgM. Parvovirus-specific IgM testing is available commercially and has a sensitivity of 90%–97% with a specificity of 88%–96% in adults [316]. Alternatively, PCR can be used to identify parvovirus DNA, but does not indicate the timing of the infection [302]. IgM may be absent, especially if the infant is infected early in gestation. Koch and colleagues [317] studied infants from 43 women with primary parvovirus B19 infection during pregnancy. Using a combination of IgG, IgM, IgA, and PCR, they identified 22 infected infants. Of these, 10 were positive for

IgA, 11 were positive for IgM, and 11 were positive by PCR. Only 22% of the infants infected in the first trimester were positive for IgM. Ideally, serology and B19 DNA PCR should be performed on both the mother and the fetus or infant. Giant pronormoblasts may be identified in the marrow of individuals infected with parvovirus B19 [318].

Hematologic Manifestations of Congenital Parvovirus B19 Infection

Fetal hydrops is a complication of maternal infection with parvovirus B19 [312, 319]. The risk of fetal demise is highest with early pregnancy primary infection in the mother while fetal hydrops appears to be highest with mid-pregnancy infection [313]. The outcome has been reported to be related to the presence or absence of fetal hydrops. If fetal hydrops was present there was a higher rate of intrauterine transfusion, fetal loss, abnormal brain imaging, and abnormal neurodevelopmental outcomes as well as lower rates of spontaneous resolution of the infection, although numbers were too small to reach statistical significance [320].

If a woman is diagnosed with acute parvovirus during pregnancy, the fetus should be monitored for anemia by MCA-PSV. Intrauterine transfusions have been performed for severe anemia. Consideration should be given for fetal thrombocytopenia as may occur with intrauterine parvovirus B19 infection. Intrauterine IVIg has also been attempted [321]. One study showed a survival rate for intrauterine exchange transfusions to be similar to that of intrauterine simple transfusions [322].

In addition to fetal anemia, severe fetal thrombocytopenia (defined as platelet count <50,000/mcL) is seen in 38%–46% or moderate (platelet count 50,000–99,000/mcL) in 35%–40% of fetal blood samples obtained in infected women whose fetal US demonstrated hydrops or anemia [323, 324]. Those fetuses with severe thrombocytopenia had lower hemoglobin levels, lower reticulocyte counts and earlier gestational age at diagnosis. A higher fetal death rate within 48 hours of fetal blood sampling was noted in infants with severe thrombocytopenia, suggesting an increased risk of the procedure [324].

The long-term outlook, however, is quite good. In a long-term follow-up study of 129 congenitally infected infants, Miller and colleagues found two instances of transient iron deficiency, one case of transient idiopathic thrombocytope-nic purpura, and one case of transient eosinophi-lia [325]. While there was not a control group, there did not appear to be an increase in non-hematologic long-term issues. Other long-term outcome studies have also shown good outcomes [315, 326]. Outcomes in babies who developed fetal hydrops and required intrauterine transfu-sion are less salutary; of 16 such survivors, five had developmental delays, which were severe in two [59].

Treatment

Red blood cell transfusions may be necessary in the newborn with parvovirus-induced anemia. Chronic hypoproliferative anemia may respond to intravenous gammaglobulin [315, 327, 328].

Human Immunodeficiency Virus

Despite intensive research, education, and the development of new effective therapies, human immunodeficiency virus (HIV) infection remains a problem of massive worldwide proportions. Natural perinatal transmission rates from infected mothers range from 13% to 40%. Current transmission rates in the United States have been reduced to approximately 2% or less. Transmission rates are higher in Africa because prevention requires an infrastructure that has been difficult to establish [329].

Hematologic Manifestations of Human Immunodeficiency Virus

Human immunodeficiency virus infection affects virtually every aspect of hematology in the infected host. While hepatomegaly and/or spleno-megaly may be present, most neonates are asymp-tomatic, and the clinical manifestations occur later in infancy and childhood. The hematologic aspects of HIV in older infants and children have been reviewed elsewhere [330]. The immunologic effects of congenital HIV infection are discussed in Chapter 5.

Combination anti-retroviral therapy (cART) has been effective in reducing maternal-to-child transmission of HIV, but is not universally avail-able to pregnant women. This topic has been recently reviewed [331]. Neonates at high risk are now given combination antiretroviral therapy rather than zidovudine monotherapy. Mild ane-mia is not uncommon in neonates born to mothers treated with combination antiretroviral

therapy, whether the neonates are HIV-infected or not. While studies show that infants exposed to cART therapy have lower mean Hb concentra-tions in the first few months of life, clinically significant anemia is uncommon [332–334].

Neutropenia has been seen in HIV-exposed infants treated with antiretrovirals. Smith et al. noted relatively severe neutropenia for age in 12% of infants receiving a 3-drug antiretroviral regimen [334]. Pacheco et al. found statistically but not clinically significant lower neutrophil counts in infants exposed to antiretroviral treat-ment and very infrequent severe hematologic toxicity [333]. Other studies have also documen-ted neutropenia occurring more frequently in babies exposed to combination perinatal antire-troviral therapy [332, 335]. No clinical conse-quence of neutropenia in HIV-exposed but uninfected babies has been demonstrated in these studies. A case report of a baby who devel-oped severe paronychia of the great toes at age 4 weeks has been reported; the baby was both ane-mic and neutropenic, and both conditions resolved with cessation of AZT therapy [336].

Thrombocytosis is common in infants; HIV-exposed infants while clinically significant thrombcytopenia is rare [332]. Both anemia and neutropenia are less common with more recent antiretrovirals than they were when mothers were taking older agents [337]. The addition of prophy-lactic co-trimoxazole may not increase the risk of severe anemia or neutropenia [338]. In one study, low absolute neutrophil counts persisted as long as 8 months [332].

Management

The general and antiviral management of the infant with congenital HIV is complex and beyond the scope of this chapter; it is discussed in Chapter 5. A bone-marrow examination should be considered in HIV-infected infants with depressed hematopoiesis to rule out marrow inva-sion or infection by opportunistic organisms.

Nutritional and other potential causes of ane-mia as described in other sections of this textbook should be considered in any HIV-exposed infant with significant anemia. Red blood cell transfu-sion may be necessary occasionally for severe or symptomatic anemia. Anemia due to chronic infection may be ameliorated with appropriate antimicrobial therapy. Intravenous gammaglobu-lin has been beneficial for HIV-infected patients with chronic human parvovirus B19 infection [339]. Relatively low doses of granulocyte colony-stimulating factor can increase the neutrophil count to normal in children with HIV-induced neutropenia [340].

Severe thrombocytopenia can cause clinical bleeding. Microangiopathic changes on the peripheral blood smear suggest the diagnosis of hemolytic uremic syndrome/thrombotic thrombocytopenic purpura or DIC. The management of DIC begins with appropriate therapy for the underlying cause. Platelet and/or plasma transfusion may be necessary to treat severe bleeding.

References

1. Rivers A, Slayton WB. Congenital cytopenias and bone marrow failure syndromes. *Semin Perinatol* 2009;**33**(1):20–8.

2. Roberts I, Stanworth S, Murray NA. Thrombocytopenia in the neonate. *Blood Rev* 2008;**22**(4):173–86.

3. Aher S, Malwatkar K, Kadam S. Neonatal anemia. *Semin Fetal Neonatal Med* 2008;**13**(4):239–47.

4. Christensen RD, Calhoun DA. Congenital neutropenia. *Clin Perinatol* 2004;**31**(1):29–38.

5. Crane JM, van den Hof MC, Dodds L, Armson BA, Liston R. Neonatal outcomes with placenta previa. *Obstet Gynecol* 1999;**93**(4):541–4.

6. Faxelius G, Raye J, Gutberlet R, et al. Red cell volume measurements and acute blood loss in high-risk newborn infants. *J Pediatr* 1977;**90**(2):273–81.

7. McShane PM, Heyl PS, Epstein MF. Maternal and perinatal morbidity resulting from placenta previa. *Obstet Gynecol* 1985;**65**(2):176–82.

8. Lubin B. Neonatal anaemia secondary to blood loss. *Clin Haematol* 1978;**7**(1):19–34.

9. Gagnon R. No. 231: Guidelines for the management of vasa previa. *J Obstet Gynaecol Can.* 2017;**39**(10):e415–e21.

10. Walker C, Ward J. Intrapartum umbilical cord rupture. *Obstet Gynecol* 2009;**113**(2 Pt 2): 552–4.

11. Tabor A, Bang J, Norgaard-Pedersen B. Fetomaternal haemorrhage associated with genetic amniocentesis: results of a randomized trial. *Br J Obstet Gynaecol* 1987;**94**(6):528–34.

12. Linderkamp O, Versmold HT, Strohhacker I, et al. Capillary-venous hematocrit differences in newborn infants. I. Relationship to *blood* volume, peripheral blood flow, and acid base parameters. *Eur J Pediatr* 1977;**127**(1):9–14.

13. Jorgensen J. Fetomaternal bleeding. During pregnancy and at delivery. *Acta Obstet Gynecol Scand* 1977;**56**(5):487–90.

14. Sebring ES, Polesky HF. Fetomaternal hemorrhage: Incidence, risk factors, time of occurrence, and clinical effects. *Transfusion* 1990;**30**(4):344–57.

15. Huissoud C, Divry V, Dupont C, Gaspard M, Rudigoz RC. Large fetomaternal hemorrhage: prenatal predictive factors for perinatal outcome. *Am J Perinatol* 2009;**26**(3):227–33.

16. Christensen RD, Lambert DK, Baer VL, et al. Severe neonatal anemia from fetomaternal hemorrhage: Report from a multihospital healthcare system. *J Perinatol* 2013;**33**(6):429–34.

17. Stefanovic V. Fetomaternal hemorrhage complicated pregnancy: Risks, identification, and management. *Curr Opin Obstet Gynecol* 2016;**28**(2):86–94.

18. Laube DW, Schauberger CW. Fetomaternal bleeding as a cause for unexplained fetal death. *Obstet Gynecol* 1982;**60**(5):649–51.

19. Catalano PM, Capeless EL. Fetomaternal bleeding as a cause of recurrent fetal morbidity and mortality. *Obstet Gynecol* 1990;**76**(5 Pt 2):972–3.

20. Downing GJ, Kilbride HW, Yeast JD. Nonimmune hydrops fetalis caused by a massive fetomaternal hemorrhage associated with elevated maternal serum alpha-fetoprotein levels. *A case report. J Reprod Med* 1990;**35**(4):444–6.

21. Duckett JR, Constantine G. The Kleihauer technique: An accurate method of quantifying fetomaternal haemorrhage? *Br J Obstet Gynaecol* 1997;**104**(7):845–6.

22. Davis BH, Olsen S, Bigelow NC, Chen JC. Detection of fetal red cells in fetomaternal hemorrhage using a fetal hemoglobin monoclonal antibody by flow cytometry. *Transfusion* 1998;**38**(8):749–56.

23. Fernandes BJ, von Dadelszen P, Fazal I, Bansil N, Ryan G. Flow cytometric assessment of fetomaternal hemorrhage: A comparison with Betke-Kleihauer. *Prenat Diagn* 2007;**27**(7):641–3.

24. Savithrisowmya S, Singh M, Kriplani A, et al. Assessment of fetomaternal hemorrhage by flow cytometry and Kleihauer-Betke test in Rh-negative pregnancies. *Gynecol Obstet Invest* 2008;**65**(2):84–8.

25. Kim YA, Makar RS. Detection of fetomaternal hemorrhage. *Am J Hematol* 2012;**87**(4):417–23.

26. Kennedy MS. Perinatal issues in transfusion medicine. In Robock ND, Grossman BJ, Harris T, Hillyer CD, eds. *AABB Technical Manual* (Bethesda, MD.: AABB; 2011).

27. Kim A, Economidis MA, Stohl HE. Placental abruption after amnioreduction for polyhydramnios caused by chorioangioma. *BMJ Case Rep* 2018;2018.

28. Alter BP, Weiner MA, Harris MB. Erythrocyte characteristics in childhood acute leukemia. *Am J Pediatr Hematol Oncol* 1989;**11**(1):8–15.

29. Schenone MH, Mari G. The MCA Doppler and its role in the evaluation of fetal anemia and fetal growth restriction. *Clin Perinatol* 2011;**38**(1):83–102, vi.

30. Tsuda H, Matsumoto M, Sutoh Y, et al. Massive fetomaternal hemorrhage. *Int J Gynaecol Obstet*.1995;**50**(1):47–9.

31. Whitecar PW, Moise KJ, Jr. Sonographic methods to detect fetal anemia in red blood cell alloimmunization. *Obstet Gynecol Surv* 2000;**55**(4):240–50.

32. Cosmi E, Rampon M, Saccardi C, Zanardo V, Litta P. Middle cerebral artery peak systolic velocity in the diagnosis of fetomaternal hemorrhage. *Int J Gynaecol Obstet* 2012;**117**(2):128–30.

33. Rubod C, Deruelle P, Le Goueff F, et al. Long-term prognosis for infants after massive fetomaternal hemorrhage. *Obstet Gynecol* 2007;**110**(2 Pt 1):256–60.

34. Kecskes Z. Large fetomaternal hemorrhage: Clinical presentation and outcome. *J Matern Fetal Neonatal Med* 2003;**13**(2):128–32.

35. Tollenaar LSA, Slaghekke F, Middeldorp JM, et al. twin anemia polycythemia Sequence: Current views on pathogenesis, diagnostic criteria, perinatal management, and outcome. *Twin Res Hum Genet* 2016;**19**(3):222–33.

36. Habli M, Lim FY, Crombleholme T. Twin-to-twin transfusion syndrome: A comprehensive update. *Clin Perinatol* 2009;**36**(2):391–416, x.

37. Djaafri F, Stirnemann J, Mediouni I, Colmant C, Ville Y. Twin-twin transfusion syndrome – What we have learned from clinical trials. *Semin Fetal Neonatal Med* 2017;**22**(6):367–75.

38. Emery SP, Bahtiyar MO, Dashe JS, et al. The North American Fetal Therapy Network Consensus Statement: Prenatal management of uncomplicated monochorionic gestations. *Obstet Gynecol* 2015;**125**(5):1236–43.

39. Lopriore E, Oepkes D. Fetal and neonatal haematological complications in monochorionic twins. *Semin Fetal Neonatal Med* 2008;**13**(4):231–8.

40. Senat MV, Deprest J, Boulvain M, et al. Endoscopic laser surgery versus serial amnioreduction for severe twin-to-twin transfusion syndrome. *N Engl J Med* 2004;**351**(2):136–44.

41. Slaghekke F, Lopriore E, Lewi L, et al. Fetoscopic laser coagulation of the vascular equator versus selective coagulation for twin-to-twin transfusion syndrome: An open-label randomised controlled trial. *Lancet* 2014;**383**(9935):2144–51.

42. Robyr R, Lewi L, Salomon LJ, et al. Prevalence and management of late fetal complications following successful selective laser coagulation of chorionic plate anastomoses in twin-to-twin transfusion syndrome. *Am J Obstet Gynecol* 2006;**194**(3):796–803.

43. Slaghekke F, Zhao DP, Middeldorp JM, et al. Antenatal management of twin-twin transfusion syndrome and twin anemia-polycythemia sequence. *Expert Rev Hematol* 2016;**9**(8):815–20.

44. Verbeek L, Slaghekke F, Sueters M, et al. Hematological disorders at birth in complicated monochorionic twins. *Expert Rev Hematol* 2017;**10**(6):525–32.

45. Fesslova V, Villa L, Nava S, Mosca F, Nicolini U. Fetal and neonatal echocardiographic findings in twin-twin transfusion syndrome. *Am J Obstet Gynecol* 1998;**179**(4):1056–62.

46. Scott F, Evans N. Distal gangrene in a polycythemic recipient fetus in twin-twin transfusion. *Obstet Gynecol* 1995; **86** (4 Pt 2): 677–9.

47. Dawkins RR, Marshall TL, Rogers MS. Prenatal gangrene in association with twin-twin transfusion syndrome. *Am J Obstet Gynecol* 1995;**172**(3):1055–7.

48. Broadbent RS. Recipient twin limb ischemia with postnatal onset. *J Pediatr* 2007;**150**(2):207–9.

49. Bowden JB, Hebert AA, Rapini RP. Dermal hematopoiesis in neonates: Report of five cases. *J Am Acad Dermatol* 1989;**20**(6):1104–10.

50. Schwartz JL, Maniscalco WM, Lane AT, Currao WJ. Twin transfusion syndrome causing cutaneous erythropoiesis. *Pediatrics* 1984;**74**(4):527–9.

51. Koenig JM, Hunter DD, Christensen RD. Neutropenia in donor (anemic) twins involved in the twin-twin transfusion syndrome. *J Perinatol* 1991;**11**(4):355–8.

52. Pietrantoni M, Stewart DL, Ssemakula N, et al. Mortality conference: twin-to-twin transfusion. *J Pediatr* 1998;**132**(6):1071–6.

53. Rainey KE, DiGeronimo RJ, Pascual-Baralt J. Successful long-term peritoneal dialysis in a very low birth weight infant with renal failure secondary to feto-fetal transfusion syndrome. *Pediatrics* 2000;**106**(4):849–51.

54. Sirotkina M, Douroudis K, Papadogiannakis N, Westgren M. Clinical outcome in singleton and multiple pregnancies with placental chorangioma. *PloS One* 2016;**11**(11):e0166562.

55. Abiramalatha T, Sherba B, Joseph R, Thomas N. Unusual complications of placental chorioangioma: consumption coagulopathy and hypertension in a preterm newborn. *BMJ Case Rep* 2016;2016.

56. Wu Z, Hu W. Clinical analysis of 26 patients with histologically proven placental chorioangiomas. *Eur J Obstet Gynecol Reprod Biol* 2016;**199**:156–63.

57. Ozer EA, Duman N, Kumral A, et al. Chorioangiomatosis presenting with severe anemia and heart failure in a newborn. *Fetal Diagn Ther* 2008;**23**(1):5–6.

58. Sirotkina M, Douroudis K, Wahlgren CF, Westgren M, Papadogiannakis N. Exploring the association between chorangioma and infantile haemangioma in singleton and multiple pregnancies: A case-control study in a Swedish tertiary centre. *BMJ Open.* 2017;**7**(9):e015539.

59. Nagel HT, de Haan TR, Vandenbussche FP, Oepkes D, Walther FJ. Long-term outcome after fetal transfusion for hydrops associated with parvovirus B19 infection. *Obstet Gynecol* 2007;**109**(1):42–7.

60. Jiao L, Ghorani E, Sebire NJ, Seckl MJ. Intraplacental choriocarcinoma: Systematic review and management guidance. *Gynecol Oncol* 2016;**141**(3):624–31.

61. Dance LR, Patel AR, Patel MC, Cornejo P, Pfeifer CM. Cutaneous metastases of infantile choriocarcinoma can mimic infantile hemangioma both clinically and radiographically. *Pediatr Radiol* 2018;**48**(8):1167–71.

62. Halliday HL. Neonatal management and long-term sequelae. *Best Pract Res Clin Obstet Gynaecol* 2009;**23**(6):871–80.

63. Poryo M, Wissing A, Aygun A, et al. Reference values for nucleated red blood cells and serum lactate in very and extremely low birth weight infants in the first week of life. *Early Hum Dev* 2017;**105**:49–55.

64. Christensen RD, Henry E, Andres RL, Bennett ST. Reference ranges for blood concentrations of nucleated red blood cells in neonates. *Neonatology* 2011;**99**(4):289–94.

65. Martinelli S, Francisco RP, Bittar RE, Zugaib M. Hematological indices at birth in relation to arterial and venous Doppler in small-for-gestational-age fetuses. *Acta Obstet Gynecol Scand* 2009;**88**(8):888–93.

66. Baschat AA, Harman CR, Gembruch U. Haematological consequences of placental insufficiency. *Arch Dis Child Fetal Neonatal Ed* 2004;**89**(1):F94.

67. Baschat AA, Gungor S, Kush ML, et al. Nucleated red blood cell counts in the first week of life: A critical appraisal of relationships with perinatal outcome in preterm growth-restricted neonates. *Am J Obstet Gynecol* 2007;**197**(3):286e1-8.

68. Baschat AA, Kush M, Berg C, et al. Hematologic profile of neonates with growth restriction is associated with rate and degree of prenatal Doppler deterioration. *Ultrasound Obstet Gynecol* 2013;**41**(1):66–72.

69. Cordero L, Landon MB. Infant of the diabetic mother. *Clin Perinatol* 1993;**20**(3):635–48.

70. Hay WW, Jr. Care of the infant of the diabetic mother. *Curr Diab Rep* 2012;**12**(1):4–15.

71. Cowett RM, Schwartz R. The infant of the diabetic mother. *Pediatr Clin North Am* 1982;**29**(5):1213–31.

72. Mimouni F, Miodovnik M, Siddiqi TA, et al. Neonatal polycythemia in infants of insulin-dependent diabetic mothers. *Obstet Gynecol* 1986;**68**(3):370–2.

73. Cordero L, Treuer SH, Landon MB, Gabbe SG. Management of infants of diabetic mothers. *Arch Pediatr Adolesc Med* 1998;**152**(3):249–54.

74. Green DW, Khoury J, Mimouni F. Neonatal hematocrit and maternal glycemic control in insulin-dependent diabetes. *J Pediatr* 1992; **120** (2 Pt 1): 302–5.

75. Stonestreet BS, Goldstein M, Oh W, Widness JA. Effects of prolonged hyperinsulinemia on erythropoiesis in fetal sheep. *Am J Physiol* 1989; **257** (5 Pt 2): R1199-204.

76. Perrine SP, Greene MF, Lee PD, Cohen RA, Faller DV. Insulin stimulates cord blood erythroid progenitor growth: Evidence for an aetiological role in neonatal polycythaemia. *Br J Haematol* 1986;**64**(3):503–11.

77. Widness JA, Teramo KA, Clemons GK, et al. Direct relationship of antepartum glucose control and fetal erythropoietin in human type 1 (insulin-dependent) diabetic pregnancy. *Diabetologia* 1990;**33**(6):378–83.

78. Widness JA, Susa JB, Garcia JF, et al. Increased erythropoiesis and elevated erythropoietin in infants born to diabetic mothers and in hyperinsulinemic rhesus fetuses. *J Clin Investi* 1981;**67**(3):637–42.

79. Green DW, Mimouni F. Nucleated erythrocytes in healthy infants and in infants of diabetic mothers [see comments]. *J Pediatr* 1990;**116**(1):129–31.

80. Green DW, Mimouni F, Khoury J. Decreased platelet counts in infants of diabetic mothers. *Am J Perinatol* 1995;**12**(2):102–5.

81. Perrine SP, Greene MF, Faller DV. Delay in the fetal globin switch in infants of diabetic mothers. *N Engl J Med* 1985;**312**(6):334–8.

82. Bard H, Prosmanne J. Relative rates of fetal hemoglobin and adult hemoglobin synthesis in cord blood of infants of insulin-dependent diabetic mothers. *Pediatrics* 1985;**75**(6):1143–7.

83. Cetin H, Yalaz M, Akisu M, Kultursay N. Polycythaemia in infants of diabetic mothers: beta-hydroxybutyrate stimulates erythropoietic activity. *J Int Med Res* 2011;**39**(3):815–21.

84. Van Allen MI, Jackson JC, Knopp RH, Cone R. In utero thrombosis and neonatal gangrene in an infant of a diabetic mother. *Am J Med Genet* 1989;**33**(3):323–7.

85. Darmency-Stamboul V, Chantegret C, Ferdynus C, et al. Antenatal factors associated with perinatal arterial ischemic stroke. *Stroke* 2012;**43**(9):2307–12.

86. Hathaway WE, Mahasandana C, Makowski EL. Cord blood coagulation studies in infants of high-risk pregnant women. *Am J Obstet Gynecol* 1975;**121**(1):51–7.

87. Stuart MJ, Elrad H, Graeber JE, et al. Increased synthesis of prostaglandin endoperoxides and platelet hyperfunction in infants of mothers with diabetes mellitus. *J Lab Clin Med* 1979;**94**(1):12–26.

88. Stuart MJ, Sunderji SG, Allen JB. Decreased prostacyclin production in the infant of the diabetic mother. *J Lab Clin Med* 1981;**98**(3):412–16.

89. Sarkar S, Hagstrom NJ, Ingardia CJ, Lerer T, Herson VC. Prothrombotic risk factors in infants of diabetic mothers. *J Perinatol* 2005;**25**(2):134–8.

90. Easa D, Coen RW. Coagulation studies in infants of diabetic mothers. *Am J Dis Child* 1979;**133**(8):851–2.

91. Ambrus CM, Ambrus JL, Courey N, et al. Inhibitors of fibrinolysis in diabetic children, mothers, and their newborn. *Am J Hematol* 1979;**7**(3):245–54.

92. Fonseca VA, Reynolds T, Fink LM. Hyperhomocysteinemia and microalbuminuria in diabetes. *Diabetes Care* 1998;**21**(6):1028.

93. Mehta R, Petrova A. Neutrophil function in neonates born to gestational diabetic mothers. *J Perinatol* 2005;**25**(3):178–81.

94. Lapolla A, Sanzari MC, Zancanaro F, et al. A study on lymphocyte subpopulation in diabetic mothers at delivery and in their newborn. *Diabetes Nutr Metab* 1999;**12**(6):394–9.

95. Roll U, Scheeser J, Standl E, Ziegler AG. Alterations of lymphocyte subsets in children of diabetic mothers. *Diabetologia* 1994;**37**(11):1132–41.

96. American College of Obstetricians and Gynecologists. Report of the American College of Obstetricians and Gynecologists' Task Force on Hypertension in Pregnancy. *Obstet Gynecol* 2013;**122**(5):1122–31.

97. Manroe BL, Weinberg AG, Rosenfeld CR, Browne R. The neonatal blood count in health and disease. I. Reference values for neutrophilic cells. *J Pediatr* 1979;**95**(1):89–98.

98. Engle WD, Rosenfeld CR. Neutropenia in high-risk neonates. *J Pediatr* 1984;**105**(6):982–6.

99. Mouzinho A, Rosenfeld CR, Sanchez PJ, Risser R. Effect of maternal hypertension on neonatal neutropenia and risk of nosocomial infection. *Pediatrics* 1992;**90**(3):430–5.

100. Koenig JM, Christensen RD. Incidence, neutrophil kinetics, and natural history of neonatal neutropenia associated with maternal hypertension. *N Engl J Med* 1989;**321**(9):557–62.

101. Doron MW, Makhlouf RA, Katz VL, Lawson EE, Stiles AD. Increased incidence of sepsis at birth in neutropenic infants of mothers with preeclampsia. *J Pediatr* 1994;**125**(3):452–8.

102. Christensen RD, Henry E, Wiedmeier SE, Stoddard RA, Lambert DK. Low blood neutrophil concentrations among extremely low birth weight neonates: Data from a multihospital health-care system. *J Perinatol* 2006;**26**(11):682–7.

103. Teng RJ, Wu TJ, Garrison RD, Sharma R, Hudak ML. Early neutropenia is not associated with an increased rate of nosocomial infection in very low-birth-weight infants. *J Perinatol* 2009;**29**(3):219–24.

104. Bolat A, Gursel O, Kurekci E, Atay A, Ozcan O. Blood parameters changes in cord blood of newborns of hypertensive mothers. *Eur J Pediatr* 2013;**172**(11):1501–9.

105. Christensen RD, Yoder BA, Baer VL, Snow GL, Butler A. Early-onset neutropenia in small-for-gestational-age infants. *Pediatrics* 2015;**136**(5): e1259-67.

106. Bizerea TO, Stroescu R, Rogobete AF, Marginean O, Ilie C. Pregnancy induced hypertension versus small weight for gestational age: Cause of neonatal hematological Disorders. *Clin Lab* 2018;**64**(7):1241–8.

107. Sharma G, Nesin M, Feuerstein M, Bussel JB. Maternal and neonatal characteristics associated with neonatal neutropenia in hypertensive pregnancies. *Am J Perinatol* 2009;**26**(9):683–9.

108. Gray PH, Rodwell RL. Neonatal neutropenia associated with maternal hypertension poses a

risk for nosocomial infection. *Eur J Pediatr* 1999;**158**(1):71–3.

109. Saini H, Puppala BL, Angst D, Gilman-Sachs A, Costello M. Upregulation of neutrophil surface adhesion molecules in infants of pre-eclamptic women. *J Perinatol* 2004;**24**(4):208–12.

110. Stoll BJ, Hansen N. Infections in VLBW infants: Studies from the NICHD Neonatal Research Network. *Semin Perinatol* 2003;**27**(4):293–301.

111. Makhlouf RA, Doron MW, Bose CL, Price WA, Stiles AD. Administration of granulocyte colony-stimulating factor to neutropenic low birth weight infants of mothers with preeclampsia. *J Pediatr* 1995;**126**(3):454–6.

112. Carr R, Modi N, Dore C. G-CSF and GM-CSF for treating or preventing neonatal infections. *Cochrane Database Syst Rev* 2003(**3**):CD003066.

113. Chakravorty S, Murray N, Roberts I. Neonatal thrombocytopenia. *Early Hum Dev* 2005;**81**(1):35–41.

114. Baschat AA, Gembruch U, Reiss I, et al. Absent umbilical artery end-diastolic velocity in growth-restricted fetuses: A risk factor for neonatal thrombocytopenia. *Obstet Gynecol* 2000;**96**(2):162–6.

115. Brazy JE, Grimm JK, Little VA. Neonatal manifestations of severe maternal hypertension occurring before the thirty-sixth week of pregnancy. *J Pediatr* 1982;**100**(2):265–71.

116. Bhat YR, Cherian CS. Neonatal thrombocytopenia associated with maternal pregnancy induced hypertension. *Indian J Pediatr* 2008;**75**(6):571–3.

117. McPherson RJ, Juul S. Patterns of thrombocytosis and thrombocytopenia in hospitalized neonates. *J Perinatol* 2005;**25**(3):166–72.

118. Christensen RD, Henry E, Wiedmeier SE, et al. Thrombocytopenia among extremely low birth weight neonates: data from a multihospital healthcare system. *J Perinatol* 2006;**26**(6):348–53.

119. Raval DS, Co S, Reid MA, Pildes R. Maternal and neonatal outcome of pregnancies complicated with maternal HELLP syndrome. *J Perinatol* 1997;**17**(4):266–9.

120. Singhal N, Amin HJ, Pollard JK, et al. Maternal haemolysis, elevated liver enzymes and low platelets syndrome: Perinatal and neurodevelopmental neonatal outcomes for infants weighing less than 1250 g. *J Paediatr Child Health* 2004;**40**(3):121–6.

121. Dotsch J, Hohmann M, Kuhl PG. Neonatal morbidity and mortality associated with maternal haemolysis elevated liver enzymes and low platelets syndrome. *Eur J Pediatr* 1997;**156**(5):389–91.

122. Tsao PN, Wei SC, Su YN, et al. Excess soluble fms-like tyrosine kinase 1 and low platelet counts in premature neonates of preeclamptic mothers. *Pediatrics* 2005;**116**(2):468–72.

123. Tsao PN, Teng RJ, Chou HC, Tsou KI. The thrombopoietin level in the cord blood in premature infants born to mothers with pregnancy-induced hypertension. *Biol Neonate* 2002;**82**(4):217–21.

124. Kalagiri RR, Choudhury S, Carder T, et al. Neonatal thrombocytopenia as a consequence of maternal preeclampsia. *AJP Rep* 2016;**6**(1):e42-7.

125. Kurlat I, Sola A. Neonatal polycythemia in appropriately grown infants of hypertensive mothers. *Acta Paediatr* 1992;**81**(9):662–4.

126. Silverman ED, Laxer RM. Neonatal lupus erythematosus. *Rheum Dis Clin North Am* 1997;**23**(3):599–618.

127. Zuppa AA, Fracchiolla A, Cota F, et al. Infants born to mothers with anti-SSA/Ro autoantibodies: neonatal outcome and follow-up. *Clin Pediatr (Phila)* 2008;**47**(3):231–6.

128. Zuppa AA, Riccardi R, Frezza S, et al. Neonatal lupus: Follow-up in infants with anti-SSA/Ro antibodies and review of the literature. *Autoimmun Rev* 2017;**16**(4):427–32.

129. Hariharan D, Manno CS, Seri I. Neonatal lupus erythematosus with microvascular hemolysis. *J Pediatr Hematol Oncol* 2000;**22**(4):351–4.

130. Kanda K, Sato A, Abe D, Nishijima S, Ishigami T. The unique coexistence of anti-SS-A/Ro antibodies in a neonate with symptomatic ischemic stroke. *Pediatr Neurol* 2016;**62**:47–50.

131. Gotestam Skorpen C, Hoeltzenbein M, Tincani A, et al. The EULAR points to consider for use of antirheumatic drugs before pregnancy, and during pregnancy and lactation. *Ann Rheum Dis* 2016;**75**(5):795–810.

132. Brewster JA, Shaw NJ, Farquharson RG. Neonatal and pediatric outcome of infants born to mothers with antiphospholipid syndrome. *J Perinat Med* 1999;**27**(3):183–7.

133. Contractor S, Hiatt M, Kosmin M, Kim HC. Neonatal thrombosis with anticardiolipin antibody in baby and mother. *Am J Perinatol* 1992;**9**(5–6):409–10.

134. Tabbutt S, Griswold WR, Ogino MT, et al. Multiple thromboses in a premature infant associated with maternal phospholipid antibody syndrome. *J Perinatol* 1994;**14**(1):66–70.

135. Boffa MC, Lachassinne E. Infant perinatal thrombosis and antiphospholipid antibodies: a review. *Lupus* 2007;**16**(8):634–41.

136. Motta M, Chirico G, Rebaioli CB, et al. Anticardiolipin and anti-beta2 glycoprotein I antibodies in infants born to mothers with antiphospholipid antibody-positive autoimmune disease: A follow-up study. *Am J Perinatol* 2006;**23**(4):247–51.

137. Berkun Y, Simchen MJ, Strauss T, et al. Antiphospholipid antibodies in neonates with stroke: A unique entity or variant of antiphospholipid syndrome? *Lupus* 2014;**23** (10):986–93.

138. Ngu S-F, Hgan HYS. Chemotherapy in pregnancy. *Best Pract Res Clin Obstet Gynaecol* 2016;**33**:86–101.

139. Azim HA, Jr., Pavlidis N, Peccatori FA. Treatment of the pregnant mother with cancer: a systematic review on the use of cytotoxic, endocrine, targeted agents and immunotherapy during pregnancy. Part II: Hematological tumors. *Cancer Treat Rev* 2010;**36**(2):110–21.

140. Azim HA, Jr., Peccatori FA, Pavlidis N. Treatment of the pregnant mother with cancer: a systematic review on the use of cytotoxic, endocrine, targeted agents and immunotherapy during pregnancy. Part I: Solid tumors. *Cancer Treat Rev* 2010;**36**(2):101–9.

141. Waalen J. Pregnancy poses tough questions for cancer treatment [news]. *J Natl Cancer Inst* 1991;**83**(13):900–2.

142. Cordeiro CN, Gemignani ML. Gynecologic malignancies in pregnancy: Balancing fetal risks with oncologic safety. *Obstet Gynecol Surv* 2017;**72**(3):184–93.

143. Esposito S, Tenconi R, Preti V, Groppali E, Principi N. Chemotherapy against cancer during pregnancy: A systematic review on neonatal outcomes. *Medicine (Baltimore)* 2016;**95**(38): e4899.

144. Lishner M, Avivi I, Apperley JF, et al. Hematologic malignancies in pregnancy: Management guidelines From an international consensus meeting. *J Clin Oncol* 2016;**34**(5):501–8.

145. Doll DC, Ringenberg QS, Yarbro JW. Antineoplastic agents and pregnancy. *Semin Oncol* 1989;**16**(5):337–46.

146. Zemlickis D, Klein J, Moselhy G, Koren G. Cisplatin protein binding in pregnancy and the neonatal period. *Med Pediatr Oncol* 1994;**23** (6):476–9.

147. Amant F, Vandenbroucke T, Verheecke M, et al. Pediatric outcome after maternal cancer diagnosed during pregnancy. *N Engl J Med* 2015;**373**(19):1824–34.

148. de Haan J, Verheecke M, Van Calsteren K, et al. Oncological management and obstetric and neonatal outcomes for women diagnosed with cancer during pregnancy: a 20-year international cohort study of 1170 patients. *Lancet Oncol* 2018;**19**(3):337–46.

149. Buekers TE, Lallas TA. Chemotherapy in pregnancy. *Obstet Gynecol Clin North Am* 1998;**25**(2):323–9.

150. Achtari C, Hohlfeld P. Cardiotoxic transplacental effect of idarubicin administered during the second trimester of pregnancy. *Am J Obstet Gynecol* 2000;**183**(2):511–2.

151. Udink ten Cate FE, ten Hove CH, Nix WM, et al. Transient neonatal myelosuppression after fetal exposure to maternal chemotherapy. Case report and review of the literature. *Neonatology* 2009;**95** (1):80–5.

152. Chakravarty EF, Murray ER, Kelman A, Farmer P. Pregnancy outcomes after maternal exposure to rituximab. *Blood* 2011;**117**(5):1499–506.

153. Cardonick E, Usmani A, Ghaffar S. Perinatal outcomes of a pregnancy complicated by cancer, including neonatal follow-up after in utero exposure to chemotherapy: Results of an international registry. *Am J Clin Oncol* 2010;**33** (3):221–8.

154. Cardonick E, Dougherty R, Grana G, et al. Breast cancer during pregnancy: Maternal and fetal outcomes. *Cancer J* 2010;**16**(1):76–82.

155. Luis SA, Christie DR, Kaminski A, Kenny L, Peres MH. Pregnancy and radiotherapy: Management options for minimising risk, case series and comprehensive literature review. *J Med Imaging Radiat Oncol* 2009;**53**(6):559–68.

156. Mayr NA, Wen BC, Saw CB. Radiation therapy during pregnancy. *Obstet Gynecol Clin North Am* 1998;**25**(2):301–21.

157. Brent RL. The effect of embryonic and fetal exposure to x-ray, microwaves, and ultrasound: Counseling the pregnant and nonpregnant patient about these risks. *Semin Oncol* 1989;**16** (5):347–68.

158. Pentheroudakis G, Pavlidis N. Cancer and pregnancy: Poena magna, not anymore. *Eur J Cancer* 2006;**42**(2):126–40.

159. Needleman S, Powell M. Radiation hazards in pregnancy and methods of prevention. *Best Pract Res Clin Obstet Gynaecol* 2016;**33**:108–16.

160. Sebire NJ, Jauniaux E. Fetal and placental malignancies: prenatal diagnosis and

management. *Ultrasound Obstet Gynecol* 2009;**33**(2):235–44.

161. Walker JW, Reinisch JF, Monforte HL. Maternal pulmonary adenocarcinoma metastatic to the fetus: First recorded case report and literature review. *Pediatr Pathol Mol Med* 2002;**21**(1):57–69.

162. Hurley TJ, McKinnell JV, Irani MS. Hematologic malignancies in pregnancy. *Obstet Gynecol Clin North Am* 2005;**32**(4):595–614.

163. Mountain KR, Hirsh J, Gallus AS. Neonatal coagulation defect due to anticonvulsant drug treatment in pregnancy. *Lancet* 1970;**1**(7641):265–8.

164. Hey E. Effect of maternal anticonvulsant treatment on neonatal blood coagulation. *Arch Dis Child Fetal Neonatal Ed* 1999;**81**(3):F208-10.

165. Howe AM, Oakes DJ, Woodman PD, Webster WS. Prothrombin and PIVKA-II levels in cord blood from newborn exposed to anticonvulsants during pregnancy. *Epilepsia* 1999;**40**(7):980–4.

166. Chong DJ, Lerman AM. Practice update: Review of anticonvulsant therapy. *Current Neurol Neurosci Rep* 2016;**16**(4):39.

167. Harden CL, Pennell PB, Koppel BS, et al. Management issues for women with epilepsy–focus on pregnancy (an evidence-based review): III. Vitamin K, folic acid, blood levels, and breast-feeding: Report of the Quality Standards Subcommittee and Therapeutics and Technology Assessment Subcommittee of the American Academy of Neurology and the American Epilepsy Society. *Epilepsia* 2009;**50**(5):1247–55.

168. Albisetti M, Monagle P. Bleeding disorders. In de Alarcón PA, Werner EJ, Christensen RD, eds. *Neonatal Hematology Pathogenesis, Diagnosis and Management of Hematologic Problems* (New York: Cambridge University Press, 2013), pp. 286–301.

169. Greinacher A, Eckhardt T, Mussmann J, Mueller-Eckhardt C. Pregnancy complicated by heparin associated thrombocytopenia: management by a prospectively in vitro selected heparinoid (Org 10172]. *Thromb Res* 1993;**71**(2):123–6.

170. Konkle BA. Diagnosis and management of thrombosis in pregnancy. *Birth Defects Res C Embryo Today* 2015;**105**(3):185–9.

171. D'Souza R, Ostro J, Shah PS, et al. Anticoagulation for pregnant women with mechanical heart valves: A systematic review and meta-analysis. *Eur Heart J* 2017;**38**(19):1509–16.

172. Haghikia A, Langer-Gould A, Rellensmann G, et al. Natalizumab use during the third trimester of pregnancy. *JAMA Neurol* 2014;**71**(7):891–5.

173. Barak M, Cohen A, Herschkowitz S. Total leukocyte and neutrophil count changes associated with antenatal betamethasone administration in premature infants. *Acta Paediatr* 1992;**81**(10):760–3.

174. Anday EK, Harris MC. Leukemoid reaction associated with antenatal dexamethasone administration. *J Pediatr* 1982;**101**(4):614–6.

175. Juul SE, Haynes JW, McPherson RJ. Evaluation of neutropenia and neutrophilia in hospitalized preterm infants. *J Perinatol* 2004;**24**(3):150–7.

176. Calhoun DA, Kirk JF, Christensen RD. Incidence, significance, and kinetic mechanism responsible for leukemoid reactions in patients in the neonatal intensive care unit: A prospective evaluation. *J Pediatr* 1996;**129**(3):403–9.

177. WHO Guidelines Approved by the Guidelines Review Committee. *WHO Recommendations on Antenatal Care for a Positive Pregnancy Experience* (Geneva: World Health Organization, 2016).

178. Achebe MM, Gafter-Gvili A. How I treat anemia in pregnancy: Iron, cobalamin, and folate. *Blood* 2017;**129**(8):940–9.

179. Breymann C. Iron deficiency anemia in pregnancy. *Semin Hematol* 2015;**52**(4):339–47.

180. Rahman MM, Abe SK, Rahman MS, et al. Maternal anemia and risk of adverse birth and health outcomes in low- and middle-income countries: Systematic review and meta-analysis. *Am J Clin Nutr* 2016;**103**(2):495–504.

181. Milman N, Bergholt T, Byg KE, Eriksen L, Graudal N. Iron status and iron balance during pregnancy. A critical reappraisal of iron supplementation. *Acta Obstet Gynecol Scand* 1999;**78**(9):749–57.

182. Werner EJ, Stockman JA, 3rd. Red cell disturbances in the fetomaternal unit. *Semin Perinatol* 1983;**7**(3):139–58.

183. Lesser KB, Schoel SB, Kling PJ. Elevated zinc protoporphyrin/heme ratios in umbilical cord blood after diabetic pregnancy. *J Perinatol* 2006;**26**(11):671–6.

184. Rao R, Georgieff MK. Iron in fetal and neonatal nutrition. *Semin Fetal Neonatal Med* 2007;**12**(1):54–63.

185. American College of Obstetricians and Gynecologists. ACOG Practice Bulletin No. 95: Anemia in pregnancy. (Reaffirmed in 2017.) *Obstet Gynecol* 2008;**112**(1):201–7.

186. Siu AL, USPS Task Force. Screening for iron deficiency anemia and iron supplementation in pregnant women to improve maternal health and birth outcomes: US Preventive Services Task

Force recommendation statement. *Ann Intern Med* 2015;**163**(7):529–36.

187. Lee S, Guillet R, Cooper EM, et al. Prevalence of anemia and associations between neonatal iron status, hepcidin, and maternal iron status among neonates born to pregnant adolescents. *Pediatr Res* 2016; **79** (1–1): 42–8.

188. Pena-Rosas JP, De-Regil LM, Garcia-Casal MN, Dowswell T. Daily oral iron supplementation during pregnancy. *Cochrane Database Syst Rev* 2015(7):CD004736.

189. Rukuni R, Bhattacharya S, Murphy MF, et al. Maternal and neonatal outcomes of antenatal anemia in a Scottish population: A retrospective cohort study. *Acta Obstet Gynecol Scand* 2016;**95**(5):555–64.

190. O'Brien KO, Ru Y. Iron status of North American pregnant women: An update on longitudinal data and gaps in knowledge from the United States and Canada. *Am J Clin Nutr* 2017;**106**(Suppl6):1647s–54s.

191. Levy S, Schapkaitz E. The clinical utility of new reticulocyte and erythrocyte parameters on the Sysmex XN 9000 for iron deficiency in pregnant patients. *Int J Lab Hematol* 2018;**40**(6):683–90.

192. Allen LH. Anemia and iron deficiency: Effects on pregnancy outcome. *Am J Clin Nutr* 2000;**71**(5 Suppl):1280S-4S.

193. Chaparro CM. Setting the stage for child health and development: Prevention of iron deficiency in early infancy. *J Nutr* 2008;**138**(12):2529–33.

194. Siddappa AM, Rao R, Long JD, Widness JA, Georgieff MK. The assessment of newborn iron stores at birth: A review of the literature and standards for ferritin concentrations. *Neonatology* 2007;**92**(2):73–82.

195. Preziosi P, Prual A, Galan P, et al. Effect of iron supplementation on the iron status of pregnant women: Consequences for newborns. *Am J Clin Nutr* 1997;**66**(5):1178–82.

196. McDonald SJ, Middleton P, Dowswell T, Morris PS. Effect of timing of umbilical cord clamping of term infants on maternal and neonatal outcomes. *Cochrane Database Syst Rev* 2013(7):Cd004074.

197. Andersson O, Hellstrom-Westas L, Andersson D, Domellof M. Effect of delayed versus early umbilical cord clamping on neonatal outcomes and iron status at 4 months: A randomised controlled trial. *BMJ* 2011;**343**:d7157.

198. Basnet S, Schneider M, Gazit A, Mander G, Doctor A. Fresh goat's milk for infants: Myths and realities: A review. *Pediatrics* 2010;**125**(4):e973-7.

199. Watkins D, Whitehead VM, Rosenblatt DS. Megaloblastic anemia. In Orkin SH, Nathan DG, Ginsburg D, et al. eds. *Nathan and Oski's Hematology and Oncology of Infancy and Childhood*, 8th ed. (Philadelphia, PA: Elsevier, 2015).

200. Watkins S, Yunge M, Jones D, Kiely E, Petros AJ. Prolonged use of tissue plasminogen activator for bilateral lower limb arterial occlusion in a neonate. *J Pediatr Surg* 2001;**36**(4):654–6.

201. US Preventive Services Task Force. Folic acid for the prevention of neural tube defects: US Preventive Services Task Force recommendation statement. *Ann Intern Med* 2009;**150**(9):626–31.

202. Obeid R, Oexle K, Rissmann A, Pietrzik K, Koletzko B. Folate status and health: Challenges and opportunities. *J Perinat Med* 2016;**44**(3):261–8.

203. Pritchard JA, Scott DE, Whalley PJ, Haling RF, Jr. Infants of mothers with megaloblastic anemia due to folate deficiency. *JAMA* 1970;**211**(12):1982–4.

204. Green R. Vitamin B12 deficiency from the perspective of a practicing hematologist. *Blood* 2017;**129**(19):2603–11.

205. Watkins D, Rosenblatt DS. Update and new concepts in vitamin responsive disorders of folate transport and metabolism. *J Inherit Metab Dis* 2012;**35**(4):665–70.

206. Stabler SP. Clinical practice. Vitamin B12 deficiency. *N Engl J Med* 2013;**368**(2):149–60.

207. Obeid R, Murphy M, Sole-Navais P, Yajnik C. Cobalamin Status from pregnancy to early childhood: Lessons from global experience. *Adv Nutr* 2017;**8**(6):971–9.

208. Chanarin I. Folate and cobalamin. *Clin Haematol* 1985;**14**(3):629–41.

209. Bjorke Monsen AL, Ueland PM, Vollset SE, et al. Determinants of cobalamin status in newborns. *Pediatrics* 2001;**108**(3):624–30.

210. Finkelstein JL, Layden AJ, Stover PJ. Vitamin B-12 and perinatal health. *Adv Nutr* 2015;**6**(5):552–63.

211. Pawlak R, Lester SE, Babatunde T. The prevalence of cobalamin deficiency among vegetarians assessed by serum vitamin B12: A review of literature. *Eur J Clin Nutr* 2014;**68**(5):541–8.

212. Rosenblatt DS, Whitehead VM. Cobalamin and folate deficiency: Acquired and hereditary disorders in children. *Semin Hematol* 1999;**36**(1):19–34.

213. Lampkin BC, Shore NA, Chadwick D. Megaloblastic anemia of infancy secondary to maternal pernicious anemia. *N Engl J Med* 1966;**274**(21):1168–71.

214. Quentin C, Huybrechts S, Rozen L, et al. Vitamin B12 deficiency in a 9-month-old boy. *Eur J Pediatr* 2012;**171**(1):193–5.

215. Pappo AS, Fields BW, Buchanan GR. Etiology of red blood cell macrocytosis during childhood: impact of new diseases and therapies. *Pediatrics* 1992; **89** (6 Pt 1): 1063–7.

216. Kamoun F, Guirat R, Megdich F, et al. Frequent infections, hypotonia, and anemia in a breastfed infant. *J Pediatr Hematol Oncol* 2017;**39**(2):141–2.

217. American Academy of Pediatrics, Kimberlin DW, Brady MT, Jackson MA, Long SS, eds. *Red Book®: 2018–2021 Report of the Committee on Infectious Diseases*, 31st ed. (Itasca, IL: American Academy of Pediatrics, 2018).

218. Remington JS, McLeod R, Thulliez P, Desmonts G. Toxoplasmosis. In Remington JS, Klein JO, eds. *Infectious Disease of the Fetus and Newborn* (Philadelphia, PA: W. B. Saunders Company, 2001).

219. Petersen E. Toxoplasmosis. *Semin Fetal Neonatal Med* 2007;**12**(3):214–23.

220. Peyron F, Mc Leod R, Ajzenberg D, et al. Congenital toxoplasmosis in France and the United States: One parasite, two diverging approaches. *PLoS Neg Trop Dis* 2017;**11**(2): e0005222.

221. Foudrinier F, Marx-Chemla C, Aubert D, Bonhomme A, Pinon JM. Value of specific immunoglobulin A detection by two immunocapture assays in the diagnosis of toxoplasmosis. *Eur J Clin Microbiol Infect Dis* 1995;**14**(7):585–90.

222. Hohlfeld P, Daffos F, Costa JM, et al. Prenatal diagnosis of congenital toxoplasmosis with a polymerase-chain-reaction test on amniotic fluid. *N Engl J Med* 1994;**331**(11):695–9.

223. Romand S, Wallon M, Franck J, et al. Prenatal diagnosis using polymerase chain reaction on amniotic fluid for congenital toxoplasmosis. *Obstet Gynecol* 2001;**97**(2):296–300.

224. Lukens JN. Neonatal haematological abnormalities associated with maternal disease. *Clin Haematol* 1978;**7**(1):155–73.

225. Alford CA, Jr., Stagno S, Reynolds DW. Congenital toxoplasmosis: Clinical, laboratory, and therapeutic considerations, with special reference to subclinical disease. *Bull NY Acad Med* 1974;**50**(2):160–81.

226. Koskiniemi M, Lappalainen M, Hedman K. Toxoplasmosis needs evaluation. An overview and proposals. *Am J Dis Child* 1989;**143**(6):724–8.

227. Barron SD, Pass RF. Infectious causes of hydrops fetalis. *Semin Perinatol* 1995;**19**(6):493–501.

228. Hohlfeld P, Forestier F, Kaplan C, Tissot JD, Daffos F. Fetal thrombocytopenia: a retrospective survey of 5,194 fetal blood samplings. *Blood* 1994;**84**(6):1851–6.

229. Hohlfeld P, Forestier F, Marion S, et al. Toxoplasma gondii infection during pregnancy: T lymphocyte subpopulations in mothers and fetuses. *Pediatr Infect Dis J* 1990;**9**(12):878–81.

230. Ingall D, Sanchez PJ. Syphilis. In Remington JW, Klein JO, eds. *Infectious Diseases of the Fetus and Newborn Infant* (Philadelphia, PA: W. B. Saunders Company; 2001), pp. 643–81.

231. Hurtig AK, Nicoll A, Carne C, et al. Syphilis in pregnant women and their children in the United Kingdom: Results from national clinician reporting surveys 1994–7. *BMJ (Clinical research ed)* 1998;**317**(7173):1617–9.

232. Korenromp EL, Mahiane SG, Nagelkerke N, et al. Syphilis prevalence trends in adult women in 132 countries: Estimations using the Spectrum Sexually Transmitted Infections model. *Sci Rep* 2018;**8**(1):11503.

233. American Academy of Pediatrics. Syphilis. In Kimberlin DW, Brady MT, Jackson MA, Long SS, eds. *Red Book®: 2018–2021 Report of the Committee on Infectious Diseases*, 31st ed. (Itasca, IL: American Academy of Pediatrics,2018), pp. 773–88.

234. Kollmann TR, Dobson S. Syphilis. In Remington JW, Kleinhauer E, Wilson CB, Nizet V, Maldonado YA, eds. *Infectious Diseases of the Fetus and Newborn Infant*, 7th ed. (Philadelphia, PA: Elsevier Saunders, 2011).

235. Woods CR. Congenital syphilis-persisting pestilence. *Pediatr Infect Dis J* 2009;**28**(6):536–7.

236. Mavrov GI, Goubenko TV. Clinical and epidemiological features of syphilis in pregnant women: The course and outcome of pregnancy. *Gynecol Obstet Invest* 2001;**52**(2):114–8.

237. Chhabra RS, Brion LP, Castro M, Freundlich L, Glaser JH. Comparison of maternal sera, cord blood, and neonatal sera for detecting presumptive congenital syphilis: Relationship with maternal treatment. *Pediatrics* 1993;**91** (1):88–91.

238. Whitaker JA, Sartain P, Shaheedy M. Hematologic aspects of congenital syphilis. *J Pediatr* 1965;**66**:629.

239. Freiman I, Super M. Thrombocytopenia and congenital syphilis in South African Bantu infants. *Arch Dis Child* 1965;**41**:87–90.

240. Karayalcin G, Khanijou A, Kim KY, Aballi AJ, Lanzkowsky P. Monocytosis in congenital syphilis. *Am J Dis Child* 1977;**131**(7):782–3.

241. Shah AA, Desai AB. Paroxysmal cold hemoglobinuria (case report). *Indian Pediatr* 1977;**14**(3):219–21.

242. Pohl M, Niemeyer CM, Hentschel R, et al. Haemophagocytosis in early congenital syphilis. *Eur J Pediatr* 1999;**158**(7):553–5.

243. Brown HL, Abernathy MP. Cytomegalovirus infection. *Semin Perinatol* 1998;**22**(4):260–6.

244. Nelson CT, Demmler GJ. Cytomegalovirus infection in the pregnant mother, fetus, and newborn infant. *Clin Perinatol* 1997;**24**(1):151–60.

245. Stagno S. Cytomegalovirus. In Remington JS, Klein JO, eds. *Infectious Diseases of the Fetus and Newborn Infant* (Philadelphia, PA: W.B Saunders Company, 2001), pp. 389–424.

246. Adler SP. Transfusion-acquired CMV infection in premature infants. *Transfusion* 1989;**29** (3):278–90.

247. Yeager AS, Palumbo PE, Malachowski N, Ariagno RL, Stevenson DK. Sequelae of maternally derived cytomegalovirus infections in premature infants. *J Pediatr* 1983;**102**(6):918–22.

248. Fowler KB, Stagno S, Pass RF, et al. The outcome of congenital cytomegalovirus infection in relation to maternal antibody status. *N Engl J Med* 1992;**326**(10):663–7.

249. Pass RF, Fowler KB, Boppana SB, Britt WJ, Stagno S. Congenital cytomegalovirus infection following first trimester maternal infection: Symptoms at birth and outcome. *J Clin Virol* 2006;**35**(2):216–20.

250. Britt W. Cytomegalovirus. In Remington JW, Kleinhauer E, Wilson CB, Nizet V, Maldonado YA, eds. *Infectious Diseases of the Fetus and Newborn Infant*, 7th ed. (Philadelphia, PA: Elsevier Saunders, 2011).

251. Hittner HM, Desmond M M, Montgomery JR. Optic nerve manifestations of human congenital cytomegalovirus infection. *Am J Ophthalmol* 1976;**81**(5):661–5.

252. Boppana SB, Fowler KB, Britt WJ, Stagno S, Pass RF. Symptomatic congenital cytomegalovirus infection in infants born to mothers with preexisting immunity to cytomegalovirus. *Pediatrics* 1999;**104**(1 Pt 1):55–60.

253. Schopfer K, Lauber E, Krech U. Congenital cytomegalovirus infection in newborn infants of mothers infected before pregnancy. *Arch Dis Child* 1978;**53**(7):536–9.

254. Lazzarotto T, Varani S, Gabrielli L, Spezzacatena P, Landini MP. New advances in the diagnosis of congenital cytomegalovirus infection. *Intervirology* 1999;**42**(5–6): 390–7.

255. Rivers A, Slayton W. Development of the immune system. In de Alarcón PA, Werner EJ, Christensen RD, eds. *Neonatal Hematology Pathogenesis, Diagnosis and Management of Hematologic Problems* (New York: Cambridge University Press; 2013), pp. 25–36.

256. Revello M G, Zavattoni M, Baldanti F, et al. Diagnostic and prognostic value of human cytomegalovirus load and IgM antibody in blood of congenitally infected newborns. *J Clin Virol* 1999;**14**(1):57–66.

257. Hughes BL, Gyamfi-Bannerman C. Diagnosis and antenatal management of congenital cytomegalovirus infection. *Am J Obstet Gynecol* 2016;**214**(6):B5-B11.

258. Goegebuer T, Van Meensel B, Beuselinck K, et al. Clinical predictive value of real-time pcr quantification of human cytomegalovirus DNA in amniotic fluid samples. *J Clin Microbiol* 2009;**47**(3):660–5.

259. Boppana SB, Ross SA, Shimamura M, et al. Saliva polymerase-chain-reaction assay for cytomegalovirus screening in newborns. *N Engl J Med* 2011;**364**(22):2111–8.

260. Yamamoto AY, Mussi-Pinhata MM, Marin LJ, et al. Is saliva as reliable as urine for detection of cytomegalovirus DNA for neonatal screening of congenital CMV infection? *J Clin Virol* 2006;**36** (3):228–30.

261. Arav-Boger R, Reif S, Bujanover Y. Portal vein thrombosis caused by protein C and protein S deficiency associated with cytomegalovirus infection. *J Pediatr* 1995;**126**(4):586–8.

262. Hathaway WE, Mull MM, Pechet GS. Disseminated intravascular coagulation in the newborn. *Pediatrics* 1969;**43**(2):233–40.

263. Mizutani K, Azuma E, Komada Y, et al. An infantile case of cytomegalovirus induced idiopathic thrombocytopenic purpura with predominant proliferation of CD10 positive lymphoblast in bone marrow. *Acta Paediatr Jpn* 1995;**37**(1):71–4.

264. Crapnell K, Zanjani ED, Chaudhuri A, et al. In vitro infection of megakaryocytes and their precursors by human cytomegalovirus. *Blood* 2000;**95**(2):487–93.

265. Liesner RJ. Non-immune neonatal anemias. In Lilleyman JS, Hann IM, Blanchette VS, eds. *Pediatric Hematology* (London: Churchill Livingstone, 1999), pp. 185–202.

266. Murray JC, Bernini JC, Bijou HL, Rossmann SN, Mahoney DH, Jr., Morad AB. Infantile cytomegalovirus-associated autoimmune hemolytic anemia. *J Pediatr Hematol Oncol.* 2001;**23**(5):318–20.

267. Maciejewski JP, Bruening EE, Donahue RE, Mocarski ES, Young NS, St Jeor SC. Infection of hematopoietic progenitor cells by human cytomegalovirus. *Blood* 1992;**80**(1):170–8.

268. Leruez-Ville M, Ville Y. Fetal cytomegalovirus infection: *Best Prac Res Clin Obstet Gynaecol* 2017;**38**:97–107.

269. Cole FS. Viral infections of the fetus and newborn. In Taeusch HW, Ballard RA, eds. *Avery's Diseases of the Newborn*, 7th ed. (Philadelphia, PA: W. B. Saunders Co., 1998), pp. 467–89.

270. Mace AO, Carter T, Rueter K, Bowen AC. Congenital cytomegalovirus and infantile neutropenia: A causal relationship? *J Paediatr Child Health* 2018;**54**(1):88–92.

271. Lambert N, Strebel P, Orenstein W, Icenogle J, Poland GA. Rubella. *Lancet* 2015;**385** (9984):2297–307.

272. American Academy of Pediatrics. Rubella. In Kimberlin DW, Brady MT, Jackson MA, Long SS, eds. *Red Book: 2018–2021 Report of the Committee on Infectious Diseases*, 31st ed. (Itasca, IL: American Academy of Pediatrics; 2018), pp. 705–11.

273. Coulter C, Wood R, Robson J. Rubella infection in pregnancy. *Commun Dis Intell* 1999;**23**(4):93–6.

274. Robinson J, Lemay M, Vaudry WL. Congenital rubella after anticipated maternal immunity: Two cases and a review of the literature. *Pediatr Infect Dis J* 1994;**13**(9):812–5.

275. Peckham CS. Clinical and serological assessment of children exposed in utero to confirmed maternal rubella. *Br Med J* 1974;**1**(5902):259–61.

276. Plotkin SA, Reef SE, Cooper LZ, Alford CA, Jr. Rubella. In Remington JW, Kleinhauer E, Wilson CB, Nizet V, Maldonado YA, eds. *Infectious Diseases of the Fetus and Newborn Infant*, 7th ed. (Philadelphia, PA: Elsevier Saunders, 2011).

277. Thomas HI, Morgan-Capner P, Cradock-Watson JE, et al. Slow maturation of IgG1 avidity and persistence of specific IgM in congenital rubella: Implications for diagnosis and immunopathology. *J Med Virol* 1993;**41** (3):196–200.

278. Bosma TJ, Corbett K M, Eckstein MB, et al. Use of PCR for prenatal and postnatal diagnosis of congenital rubella. *J Clin Microbiol* 1995;**33** (11):2881–7.

279. Bayer WL, Sherman FE, Michaels RH, Szeto IL, Lewis JH. Purpura in congenital and acquired rubella. *N Engl J Med* 1965;**273**(25):1362–6.

280. Zinkham WH, Medearis DN, Jr., Osborn JE. Blood and bone-marrow findings in congenital rubella. *J Pediatr* 1967;**71**(4):512–24.

281. Cooper LZ, Green RH, Krugman S, Giles JP, Mirick GS. Neonatal thrombocytopenic purpura and other manifestations of rubella contracted in utero. *Am J Dis Child* 1965;**110**:416–27.

282. Rausen AR, Richter P, Tallal L, Cooper LZ. Hematologic effects of intrauterine rubella. *JAMA* 1967;**199**(2):75–8.

283. Cooper LZ. The history and medical consequences of rubella. *Rev Infect Dis* 1985;**7** Suppl 1:S2-10.

284. Lafer CZ, Morrison AN. Thrombocytopenic purpura progressing to transient hypoplastic anemia in a newborn with rubella syndrome. *Pediatrics* 1966;**38**(3):499–501.

285. Gutierrez K M, Whitley RJ, Arvin AM. Herpes Simplex. In Remington JW, Kleinhauer E, Wilson CB, Nizet V, Maldonado YA, eds. *Infectious Diseases of the Fetus and Newborn Infant*, 7th ed. (Philadelphia, PA: Elsevier Saunders, 2011).

286. Anderson NW, Buchan BW, Ledeboer NA. Light microscopy, culture, molecular, and serologic methods for detection of herpes simplex virus. *J Clin Microbiol* 2014;**52**(1):2–8.

287. Scott LL, Hollier L M, Dias K. Perinatal herpesvirus infections. Herpes simplex, varicella, and cytomegalovirus. *Infect Dis Clin North Am* 1997;**11**(1):27–53.

288. American Academy of Pediatrics . Herpes simplex. In Kimberlin DW, Brady MT, Jackson MA, Long SS, eds. *Red Book®: 2018–2021 Report of the Committee on Infectious Diseases*, 31st ed. (Itasca, IL: American Academy of Pediatrics, 2018), pp. 437–49.

289. Koch LH, Fisher RG, Chen C, et al. Congenital herpes simplex virus infection: Two unique cutaneous presentations associated with probable intrauterine transmission. *J Am Acad Dermatol* 2009;**60**(2):312–5.

290. Kohl S. Neonatal herpes simplex virus infection. *Clin Perinatol* 1997;**24**(1):129–50.

291. Douglas J, Schmidt O, Corey L. Acquisition of neonatal HSV-1 infection from a paternal source contact. *J Pediatr* 1983;**103**(6):908–10.

292. Kimberlin DW, Lakeman FD, Arvin AM, et al. Application of the polymerase chain reaction to the diagnosis and management of neonatal herpes simplex virus disease. National Institute of

Allergy and Infectious Diseases Collaborative Antiviral Study Group. *J Infect Dis.* 1996;**174**(6):1162–7.

293. Greenes DS, Rowitch D, Thorne GM, et al. Neonatal herpes simplex virus infection presenting as fulminant liver failure. *Pediatr Infect Dis J* 1995;**14**(3):242–4.

294. Shershow LW, Ekert H, Swanson VL, Wright HT, Jr., Gilchrist GS. Intravascular coagulation in generalized herpes simplex infection of the newborn. *Acta Paediatr Scand* 1969;**58**(5):535–9.

295. Ekert H. Coagulation abnormalities in generalised herpes-simplex infection of newborn. *Lancet* 1970;**2**(7676):775–6.

296. Miller DR, Hanshaw JB, O'Leary DS, Hnilicka JV. Fatal disseminated herpes simplex virus infection and hemorrhage in the neonate. Coagulation studies in a case and a review. *J Pediatr* 1970;**76**(3):409–15.

297. Cherry JD. Enteroviruses. In Remington JS, Klein JO, eds. *Infectious Diseases of the Fetus and Newborn Infant* (Philadelphia, PA: W. B. Saunders Company, 2001), pp. 477–518.

298. Cherry JD, Krogstad P. Enterovirus and parechovirus infections. In Remington JW, Kleinhauer E, Wilson CB, Nizet V, Maldonado YA, eds. *Infectious Diseases of the Fetus and Newborn Infant*, 7th ed. (Philadelphia, PA: Elsevier Saunders, 2011).

299. Harik N, DeBiasi RL. Neonatal nonpolio enterovirus and parechovirus infections. *Semin Perinatol* 2018;**42**(3):191–7.

300. Jenista JA, Powell KR, Menegus MA. Epidemiology of neonatal enterovirus infection. *J Pediatr* 1984;**104**(5):685–90.

301. Abzug MJ, Levin MJ, Rotbart HA. Profile of enterovirus disease in the first two weeks of life. *Pediatr Infect Dis J.* 1993;**12**(10):820–4.

302. American Academy of Pediatrics. Parvovirus B19. In Kimberlin DW, Brady MT, Jackson MA, Long SS, eds. *Red Book®: 2018–2021 Report of the Committee on Infectious Diseases*, 31st ed. (Itasca, IL: American Academy of Pediatrics, 2018), pp. 602–6.

303. Abzug MJ. Prognosis for neonates with enterovirus hepatitis and coagulopathy. *Pediatr Infect Dis J* 2001;**20**(8):758–63.

304. Modlin JF. Fatal echovirus 11 disease in premature neonates. *Pediatrics* 1980;**66**(5):775–80.

305. Abzug MJ. The enteroviruses: Problems in need of treatments. *J Infect* 2014;**68** Suppl 1:S108-14.

306. Abzug MJ, Johnson SM. Catastrophic intracranial hemorrhage complicating perinatal viral infections. *Pediatr Infect Dis J* 2000;**19**(6):556–9.

307. Lake AM, Lauer BA, Clark JC, Wesenberg RL, McIntosh K. Enterovirus infections in neonates. *J Pediatr* 1976;**89**(5):787–91.

308. Tarcan A, Ozbek N, Gurakan B. Bone marrow failure with concurrent enteroviral infection in a newborn. *Pediatr Infect Dis J* 2001;**20**(7):719–21.

309. Barre V, Marret S, Mendel I, Lesesve JF, Fessard CI. Enterovirus-associated haemophagocytic syndrome in a neonate. *Acta Paediatr* 1998;**87**(4):469–71.

310. Abzug MJ, Michaels M G, Wald E, et al. A randomized, double-blind, placebo-controlled trial of pleconaril for the treatment of neonates with enterovirus sepsis. *J Pediatric Infect Dis Soc* 2016;**5**(1):53–62.

311. Brown KE, Anderson SM, Young NS. Erythrocyte P antigen: Cellular receptor for B19 parvovirus. *Science* 1993;**262**(5130):114–7.

312. Brown KE, Young NS. Parvovirus B19 in human disease. *Annu Rev Med* 1997;**48**:59–67.

313. Bonvicini F, Bua G, Gallinella G. Parvovirus B19 infection in pregnancy-awareness and opportunities. *Curr Opin Virol* 2017;**27**:8–14.

314. Mossong J, Hens N, Friederichs V, et al. Parvovirus B19 infection in five European countries: seroepidemiology, force of infection and maternal risk of infection. *Epidemiol Infect* 2008;**136**(8):1059–68.

315. Neu N, Duchon J, Zachariah P. TORCH infections. *Clin Perinatol* 2015;**42**(1):77–103, viii.

316. Markenson GR, Yancey MK. Parvovirus B19 infections in pregnancy. *Semin Perinatol* 1998;**22**(4):309–17.

317. Koch WC, Harger JH, Barnstein B, Adler SP. Serologic and virologic evidence for frequent intrauterine transmission of human parvovirus B19 with a primary maternal infection during pregnancy. *Pediatr Infect Dis J* 1998;**17**(6):489–94.

318. Gallagher PG, Forget BG, Lux SE. Disorders of the erythrocyte membrane. In Nathan DG, Orkin SH, eds. *Nathan and Oski's Hematology of Infancy and Childhood*, 5th ed. (Philadelphia, PA: W.B. Saunders Company, 1998), pp. 544–664.

319. Katz VL, Chescheir NC, Bethea M. Hydrops fetalis from B19 parvovirus infection. *J Perinatol* 1990;**10**(4):366–8.

320. Bascietto F, Liberati M, Murgano D, et al. Outcome of fetuses with congenital parvovirus B19 infection: systematic review and meta-analysis. *Ultrasound Obstet Gynecol* 2018;**52**(5):569–76.

321. Matsuda H, Sakaguchi K, Shibasaki T, et al. Intrauterine therapy for parvovirus B19 infected symptomatic fetus using B19 IgG-rich high titer gammaglobulin. *J Perinat Med* 2005;**33**(6):561–3.

322. Vanspranghels R, Houfflin-Debarge V, Vaast P, et al. Does an intrauterine exchange transfusion improve the fetal prognosis in parvovirus infection cases? *Transfusion* 2019;**59**(1):185–90.

323. de Haan TR, van den Akker ES, Porcelijn L, et al. Thrombocytopenia in hydropic fetuses with parvovirus B19 infection: incidence, treatment and correlation with fetal B19 viral load. *BJOG* 2008;**115**(1):76–81.

324. Melamed N, Whittle W, Kelly EN, et al. Fetal thrombocytopenia in pregnancies with fetal human parvovirus-B19 infection. *Am J Obstet Gynecol* 2015;**212**(6):793e1–8.

325. Miller E, Fairley CK, Cohen BJ, Seng C. Immediate and long-term outcome of human parvovirus B19 infection in pregnancy [see comments]. *Br J Obstet Gynaecol* 1998;**105** (2):174–8.

326. Rodis JF. Parvovirus infection. *Clin Obstet Gynecol*.1999;**42**(1):107–20; quiz 74–5.

327. Lejeune A, Cremer M, von Bernuth H, et al. Persistent pure red cell aplasia in dicygotic twins with persistent congenital parvovirus B19 infection-remission following high dose intravenous immunoglobulin. *Eur J Pediatr* 2014;**173**(12):1723–6.

328. Kurtzman G, Frickhofen N, Kimball J, et al. Pure red-cell aplasia of 10 years' duration due to persistent parvovirus B19 infection and its cure with immunoglobulin therapy. *N Engl J Med* 1989;**321**(8):519–23.

329. The Working Group on Mother-To-Child Transmission of HIV. Rates of mother-to-child transmission of HIV-1 in Africa, America, and Europe: Results from 13 perinatal studies. *J Acquir Immune Defic Syndr Hum Retrovirol* 1995;**8**(5):506–10.

330. Owen WC, Werner EJ. Hematologic problems. In Zeichner SL, Read JS, eds. *Handbook of Pediatric HIV Care* (Philadelphia, PA: Lippencott Williams and Wilkens; 1999), pp. 403–13.

331. Lynch NG, Johnson AK. Congenital HIV: Prevention of maternal to child transmission. *Adv Neonatal Care* 2018;**18**(5):330–40.

332. Feiterna-Sperling C, Weizsaecker K, et al. Hematologic effects of maternal antiretroviral therapy and transmission prophylaxis in HIV-1-exposed uninfected newborn infants. *J Acquir Immune Defic Syndr* 2007;**45**(1):43–51.

333. Pacheco SE, McIntosh K, Lu M, et al. Effect of perinatal antiretroviral drug exposure on hematologic values in HIV-uninfected children: An analysis of the Women and Infants Transmission Study. *J Infect Dis* 2006;**194** (8):1089–97.

334. Smith C, Forster JE, Levin MJ, et al. Serious adverse events are uncommon with combination neonatal antiretroviral prophylaxis: A

335. Bae WH, Wester C, Smeaton LM, et al. Hematologic and hepatic toxicities associated with antenatal and postnatal exposure to maternal highly active antiretroviral therapy among infants. *AIDS* 2008;**22**(13):1633–40.

336. Russo F, Collantes C, Guerrero J. Severe paronychia due to zidovudine-induced neutropenia in a neonate. *J Am Acad Dermatol* 1999;**40**(2 Pt 2):322–4.

337. Rovira N, Noguera-Julian A, Rives S, et al. Influence of new antiretrovirals on hematological toxicity in HIV-exposed uninfected infants. *Eur J Pediatr* 2016;**175**(7):1013–7.

338. Dryden-Peterson S, Jayeoba O, Hughes MD, et al. Cotrimoxazole prophylaxis and risk of severe anemia or severe neutropenia in HAART-exposed, HIV-uninfected infants. *PloS One* 2013;**8**(9):e74171.

339. Brown KE, Green SW, Antunez de Mayolo J, et al. Congenital anaemia after transplacental B19 parvovirus infection. *Lancet* 1994;**343** (8902):895–6.

340. Kuritzkes DR. Neutropenia, neutrophil dysfunction, and bacterial infection in patients with human immunodeficiency virus disease: The role of granulocyte colony-stimulating factor. *Clin Infect Dis* 2000;**30** (2):256–60.

Chapter 24

Reference Intervals in Neonatal Hematology

Robert D. Christensen

The Reference Interval Concept

"Normal ranges" for hematologic values of neonates are not available. This is because blood is not drawn on healthy normal neonates to establish such ranges, as is done with the consent of healthy adult volunteers. Instead, neonatal hematology utilizes "reference intervals." These consist of 5th to 95th percentile values compiled from laboratory tests that were performed on neonates thought to have minimal pathology relevant to the specific laboratory test under consideration, or with pathology unlikely to significantly affect that test result. The premise on which the reference interval concept is based is that these values approximate normal ranges, although they were admittedly obtained for a clinical reason and not from healthy volunteers. Basically, reference intervals are the best tools we have to interpret a neonate's complete blood count (CBC), and they likely will continue to be the best we will have for several years to come [1].

Establishing reference intervals for the various parameters in the neonatal CBC is complicated by the fact that values obtained from term infants often do not apply to preterm infants, and values obtained from low birthweight preterm infants can be very different from ranges obtained from extremely low birthweight infants. As an example, a venous hematocrit of 38% of a 24 week gestation preterm neonate on the day of birth would be well within the reference interval of 30%–52%, and thus would be "normal." However, a hematocrit of 38% of a term neonate on the day of birth is low, in the anemic range, because the reference interval for hematocrit at term is 42%–64%.

Reference intervals at birth are not static, but change over the first days, weeks, and months following birth. Therefore one set of reference intervals, at birth, is not sufficient for judging normalcy over the entire neonatal period. Another problem encountered in defining reference intervals in neonatal hematology is that unstable, sick neonates may have values within the reference interval, yet those values may not be optimal for patient care. As an example, a neonate born at 24 weeks' gestation, now 4 weeks old, has a hematocrit of 24%, which is within the reference interval. However, if that patient develops an infection and becomes hypoxemic and tachycardic, the hematocrit of 24% might be too low for optimal patient care. A higher hematocrit might facilitate better tissue oxygenation, diminish the heart rate, and permit better caloric utilization for growth. Therefore, just because a value falls within the reference interval does not assure that it is optimal for the clinical circumstance.

Determining whether a hematologic value is normal often requires cognizance of the gestational age, the age (hours after delivery) when the sample was obtained, any illnesses involved, the level of intensive care support, and the anatomical site of the blood sampling (venous, arterial, capillary). Sometimes knowledge of other factors is pertinent, such as whether delayed clamping of the umbilical cord, or "cord milking" was performed. This chapter describes the reference intervals published for use in neonatology, and provides information needed to avoid pitfalls in interpreting these values.

Neonatal Hematology, Pathogenesis, Diagnosis, and Management of Hematologic Problems, 3rd edition, ed. Pedro A. de Alarcón, Eric J. Werner, Robert D. Christensen, and Martha C. Sola-Visner. Published by Cambridge University Press. © Cambridge University Press 2021.

Erythrocytes

Hemoglobin Concentration

The concentration of hemoglobin in the blood and the hematocrit are among the most commonly performed of all clinical laboratory tests. The hemoglobin can be quantified by manual or automated techniques. The standard assay for hemoglobin determination, approved by the World Health Organization, is simple but highly reproducible [2]. It involves the conversion of the several forms of hemoglobin in the blood, including oxyhemoglobin, carboxyhemoglobin, and the minor quantities of other hemoglobin species present, to a single compound, hemoglobincyanide, which is then determined spectrophotometrically. The hemoglobin concentration and the hematocrit are for the most part different measurements of the same biologic variable. However, because the hemoglobin concentration is a direct measurement but the hematocrit is usually calculated, as explained later, the hemoglobin concentration has sometimes been a slightly preferred method.

Reference ranges for hemoglobin values of newborn infants 22 to 42 weeks' gestation [3] are shown in Fig. 24.1. In keeping with the reference range concept, values were not included in the figure if the mother had a diagnosis of placenta previa, abruptio placenta, or any antenatal hemorrhage, or if the patient had a diagnosis of hemorrhage at birth. No differences occur on the basis of gender. Postmature infants do not have higher hemoglobin concentrations than those delivered at term, unless chronic hypoxemia has occurred.

Reference ranges for hemoglobin over the first 28 days after birth are shown in Fig. 24.2 for patients 35–42 weeks' gestation at birth, and in Fig. 24.3 for patients 29–34 weeks' gestation. Hemoglobin values for patients <29 weeks were not included in the report because virtually all had repeated phlebotomy and erythrocyte transfusions, thus confounding the slope of the hemoglobin reference range.

Hematocrit

In 1929, Dr. Maxwell M. Wintrobe described a clinical laboratory test that he called the *volume of packed red blood cells* (VPRC) [4]. The test was performed by centrifuging blood in a specifically designed glass tube called a *hematocrit*. Originally, "hematocrit" was the name of the tube used in the measurement, not the measurement itself. However, usage subsequently changed, and the term hematocrit now typically indicates the measurement, and the term VPRC is rarely used.

The hematocrit measurement is the proportion of the blood sample occupied by erythrocytes. The units for hematocrit are usually given as either a percentage or a decimal fraction (liters of red blood cells/liter of blood). Because neonates and young children do not have a liter of blood in their entire circulation, children's hospital laboratories sometimes choose to express the hematocrit as a percentage not as liters per liter.

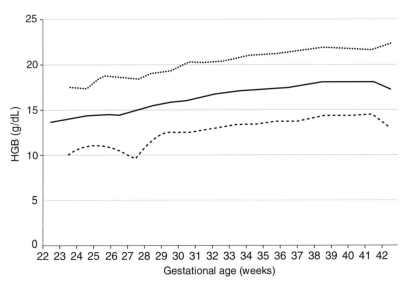

Fig. 24.1 Reference range for blood hemoglobin concentration on the day of birth (*n* = 24 416 patients) at 22 to 42 weeks' gestation. The solid line shows the mean value and the dashed lines show the 5% and 95% reference range. (From [3], Jopling et al. Reference ranges for hematocrit and blood hemoglobin concentration during the neonatal period: Data from a multihospital healthcare system. *Pediatrics* 2009;**123**; e333–77.)

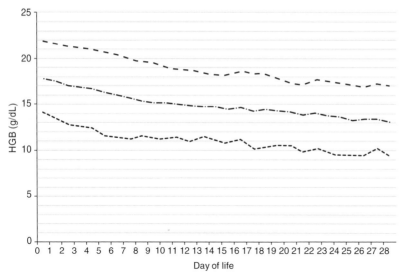

Fig. 24.2 Reference range for blood hemoglobin concentration during the 28 days after birth for neonates 35 to 42 weeks' gestation. The solid line shows the mean value and the dashed lines show the 5% and 95% reference range. (From [3], Jopling et al. Reference ranges for hematocrit and blood hemoglobin concentration during the neonatal period: Data from a multihospital healthcare system. *Pediatrics* 2009;**123**: e333–77.)

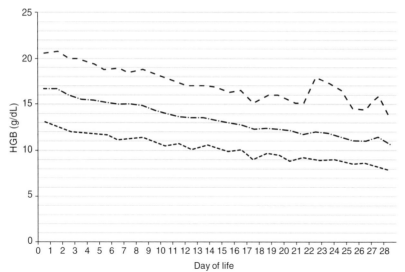

Fig. 24.3 Reference range for blood hemoglobin concentration during the 28 days after birth for neonates 29 to 34 weeks' gestation. The solid line shows the mean value and the dashed lines show the 5% and 95% reference range. (From [3], Jopling et al. Reference ranges for hematocrit and blood hemoglobin concentration during the neonatal period: Data from a multihospital healthcare system. *Pediatrics* 2009;**123**: e333–77.)

Originally, the result of the hematocrit test was read directly from the tube, after a standardized centrifugation, as the proportion of the height of the total column of blood occupied by red cells. Although an extremely simple concept, this test constituted a significant advance in clinical medicine. It was highly successful and became widely used, probably because the results were very reproducible and useful in patient care and because the test could be performed without complicated or expensive instrumentation. Subsequent modifications of the hematocrit test to permit using small blood samples led to its applicability to neonates. Ten years after it was described for testing adults, Waugh and colleagues reported that the hematocrit of normal infants, averaging 51.3%, was higher than that of normal adults [5].

Most hospital laboratories no longer use centrifugation methods for hematocrit determinations; instead, aperture-impedance instruments calculate the hematocrit. This is done by electronically measuring the mean red blood cell volume and multiplying this number by the erythrocyte concentration, also measured electronically. The mean volume of the erythrocytes multiplied by their number per microliter yields the volume of red blood cells per microliter, or the hematocrit.

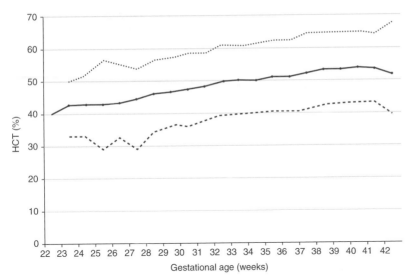

Fig. 24.4 Reference range for hematocrit on the day of birth ($n = 25\,464$ patients) at 22 to 42 weeks' gestation. The solid line shows the mean value and the dashed lines show the 5% and 95% reference range. (From [3], Jopling et al. Reference ranges for hematocrit and blood hemoglobin concentration during the neonatal period: Data from a multihospital healthcare system. *Pediatrics* 2009;**123**: e333–77.)

Other types of cell counters calculate the hematocrit using laser optics, correlating the magnitude of a light pulse generated by passing a red blood cell through a laser with the cell's volume.

Many neonatologists have noticed that when manual and electronic methods for hematocrit determination are used on an individual neonate, a consistent difference occurs between the two, a difference usually not seen in testing older children and adults. Neonates tend to have a slightly higher spun hematocrit than automated hematocrit. The reason for this involves the phenomenon of trapped plasma in the spun hematocrit determinations. When blood is centrifuged in a hematocrit tube, a small amount of plasma is always "trapped" between the erythrocytes, slightly elevating the spun hematocrit value. The amount of trapped plasma is insignificant in most cases, usually in the range of 1% to 3% of the plasma volume, as determined by radioiodinated serum albumin labeling experiments [6]. However, in samples with a very high hematocrit, more plasma becomes trapped when the cells are centrifuged. Because term neonates have considerably higher hematocrits than adults, this additional plasma trapping tends to make the spun hematocrit a higher value than the automated, calculated value (which is not subject to the plasma trapping pitfall). Few spun hematocrits are used in modern neonatology, but in any neonatal intensive care units (NICUs) doing so, this difference between spun and automated hematocrit values should be recognized.

Reference intervals for hematocrits of neonates 22 to 42 weeks' gestation are shown in Fig. 24.4 [3]. As with hemoglobin values, no differences occur on the basis of gender. Reference intervals for hematocrit over the first 28 days after birth are shown in Fig. 24.5 for patients 35–42 weeks' gestation at birth, and in Fig. 24.6 for patients 29–34 weeks' gestation.

The hematocrit, like the hemoglobin concentration and the erythrocyte count, normally increases during the first 4 hours after birth. The increase, as shown in Fig. 24.7, might not occur in preterm infants. Gairdner et al. first reported this consistent postnatal increase in hematocrit during the hours following birth, and speculated that it was the result of the intravascular concentration of blood received by placental transfusion [7]. Its absence in preterm infants might be due to early phlebotomy losses for laboratory studies, lack of a placental transfusion (because of the desire to rapidly hand the patient to the neonatology team), or other reasons.

Erythrocyte Count

The erythrocyte count is the number of erythrocytes in a volume of blood, usually expressed as cells per micro-liter, or cells per liter. Older methods for determining the erythrocyte count used a counting chamber viewed from a microscope, but modern methods use an electronic particle counter, sampling many logs more cells than the previous methods.

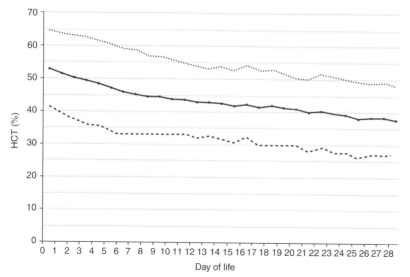

Fig. 24.5 Reference range for hematocrit during the 28 days after birth for neonates 35 to 42 weeks' gestation. The solid line shows the mean value and the dashed lines show the 5% and 95% reference range. (From [3], Jopling et al. Reference ranges for hematocrit and blood hemoglobin concentration during the neonatal period: Data from a multihospital healthcare system. *Pediatrics* 2009;**123**: e333–77.)

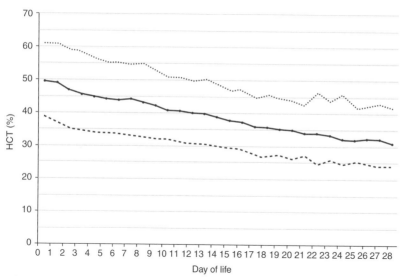

Fig. 24.6 Reference range for hematocrit during the 28 days after birth for neonates 29 to 34 weeks' gestation. The solid line shows the mean value and the dashed lines show the 5% and 95% reference range. (From [3], Jopling et al. Reference ranges for hematocrit and blood hemoglobin concentration during the neonatal period: Data from a multihospital healthcare system. *Pediatrics* 2009;**123**:e333–77.)

Erythrocyte Indices

In addition to devising the hematocrit, Dr. Wintrobe introduced the concept of erythocyte indices and described methods for their calculation. Virtually every CBC includes a report of these indices. The original manual methods for making the measurements with which the erythrocyte indices were calculated have been replaced by automated instruments, which provide measurements that are more precise and reproducible. Although sometimes overlooked, these indices can provide the neonatologist with valuable information not otherwise available.

The mean corpuscular volume (MCV) is a measure of the average size of circulating erythrocytes, expressed in femtoliters (fL, 10^{-15} L). Most modern automated cell counters, using laser optics or aperture impedance, measure the MCV of erythrocytes directly. However, as originally described, the MCV was calculated after measuring the hematocrit and the erythrocyte count by the formula:

$$MCV(fL) = \frac{Hematocrit\ (L/L) \times 1000}{Erythrocyte\ count\ (\times 10^{12}/L)}.$$

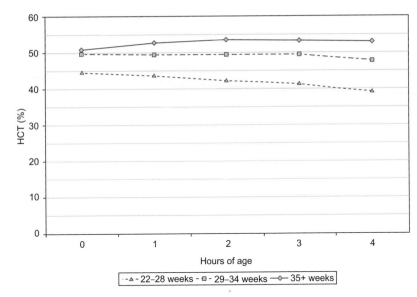

Fig. 24.7 Reference range for hematocrit over the 4 hour period following birth (*n* = 23,534 patients). Three groups are shown based on gestational age. (From [3], Jopling et al. Reference ranges for hematocrit and blood hemoglobin concentration during the neonatal period: Data from a multihospital healthcare system. *Pediatrics* 2009;**123**: e333–77.)

The mean corpuscular hemoglobin (MCH) is a measure of the amount of hemoglobin in an average circulating erythrocyte. It is expressed in picograms of hemoglobin (pg, 10^{-12} gram) and is given by the formula:

$$MCV(pg) = \frac{Hemoglobin\ (g/L)}{Erythrocyte\ count\ (\times 10^{12}/L)}.$$

The mean corpuscular hemoglobin concentration (MCHC) is a measure of the concentration of hemoglobin in an average circulating erythrocyte, and is expressed as units of grams of hemoglobin per deciliter of packed red blood cells (g/dL):

$$MCHC(g/dL) = \frac{Hemoglobin\ (g/dL)}{Hematocrit\ (L/L)}.$$

Reference ranges for MCV and MCH from 22 to 42 weeks' gestation are shown in Fig. 24.8 [8]. A fetus at 22–24 weeks' gestation, and similarly an extremely preterm neonate at 22–24 weeks' gestation, has erythrocytes that are exceedingly large, in comparison to those of adults. The MCV and MCH fall immediately when a preterm neonate receives an erythrocyte transfusion, because the MCV and MCH of the blood donor will be much lower. By 3 to 4 months after birth, the MCV and MCH of a neonate have diminished gradually to that of the level of a normal adult (88 ± 8 fL). Thereafter, the MCV continues to decline, reaching nadir levels during the fourth to sixth months and then slowly increasing to adult values after the

first year. When a newborn infant has an MCV of less than 94 fL, α-thalassemia trait or iron deficiency should be considered. Erythrocyte indices of central African neonates do not differ from those of neonates from other parts of the world, although the hematocrits of these neonates are somewhat lower [9].

Unlike the MCV and MCH, the MCHC does not change, either during gestation or after delivery. A reference range for MCHC of 34±1 g/dL is appropriate to all ages [8]. An elevated MCHC can be a useful screen for hereditary spherocytosis. Michaels and associates compared automated MCHC measurements from 112 children with hereditary spherocytosis who had not undergone splenectomy with 112 matched healthy children and observed that the MCHC of the group with hereditary spherocytosis was 35.9 g/dL, significantly higher than the controls (34.3 g/dL, *P* <0.001) [10]. Similarly, newborn infants with hereditary spherocytosis have a higher MCHC than do neonates with similar peak serum bilirubin concentrations that do not have hereditary spherocytosis (see Table 24.1).

Red Blood Cell Distribution Width

The red cell distribution width (RDW) and the hemoglobin distribution width (HDW) are commonly reported on automated CBCs. The RDW is a measure of the homogeneity of red

Table 24.1 An elevated mean corpuscular hemoglobin concentration (MCHC) in a neonate can suggest the possibility of hereditary spherocytosis

	N	MCHC (g/dL)
Non-transfused neonates <12 hrs since birth	17,624	34.0 (33.0–35.1)
Neonates with Coombs (−) jaundice	1,592	34.4 (33.2–35.5)
Neonates with Coombs (+) jaundice	363	34.7 (33.3–36.0)
Neonates with hereditary spherocytosis	15	36.9 + 0.7
P (Coombs (+) vs. Coombs (−) neonates)		<0.001
P (Hereditary spherocytosis vs. Coombs (−) neonates)		<0.001
P (Hereditary spherocytosis vs. Coombs (+) neonates)		<0.001

Note: Values are shown as mean and 95% confidence intervals or mean + SD (when too few values were present to calculate confidence intervals).

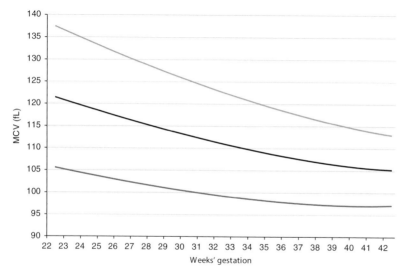

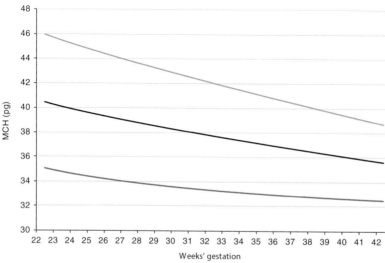

Fig. 24.8 Reference range for mean corpuscular volume (MCV) and mean corpuscular hemoglobin (MCH) for neonates on the first day after birth for neonates 22 to 42 weeks' gestation. The lower line shows the 5th percentile values, the middle line shows the mean values and the upper line shows the 95th percentile values. (From [8], Christensen et al. The erythrocyte indices of neonates, defined using data from over 12,000 patients in a multihospital healthcare system. *J Perinatol* 2008; **28**:24–8.)

blood cell size, and the HDW is a measure of the homogeneity of red blood cell hemoglobin. The RDW is expressed as a percentage, meaning the percent of erythrocytes that fall outside (smaller or larger) the standard gated population of erythrocytes. An elevated RDW value reflects an abnormal divergence of erythrocyte size [11]. The RDW begins to increase in cases

of iron deficiency before any other change in erythrocyte indices or concentrations.

The HDW is expressed in grams per deciliter (g/dL) and provides an index of divergence of hemoglobin concentration within erythrocytes. The RDW provides a numeric assessment of anisocytosis, and the HDW provides a numeric assessment of anisochromasia. Figure 24.9 shows

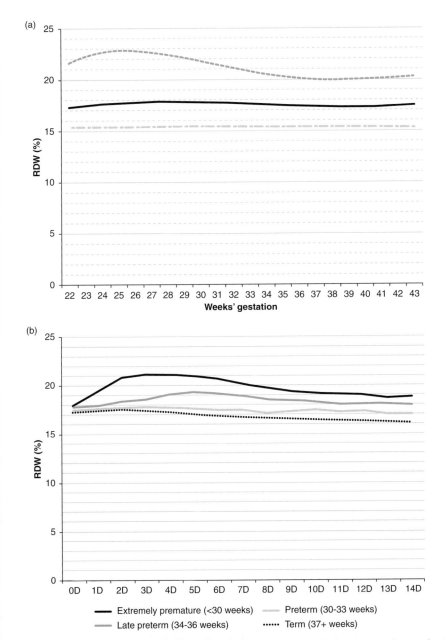

Fig. 24.9 Reference interval for red blood cell distribution width (RDW%). (a) Shows values on the day of birth as a function of gestational age. (b) Shows values over the first two weeks as related to gestational age at birth. The lower line shows the 5th percentile values, the middle line shows the mean values and the upper line shows the 95th percentile values. (From [11], Christensen et al. Red blood cell distribution width: reference intervals for neonates. *J Matern Fetal Neonatal Med.* 2015;28:883–8.)

the reference intervals for RDW (%) on the day of birth, according to gestational age in panel A, and RDW (%) over the first 14 days following birth, according to gestational age group.

Reticulocyte Count

As the erythroid precursor cells clonally mature within the bone marrow their nucleus becomes pyknotic and is extruded (usually at the ortho-chromatic normoblast stage), and the cells are thereafter released into the blood. Cytoplasmic organelles, such as ribosomes, mitochondria, and the Golgi complex, generally persist for some time after the erythrocytes have reached the circulation. Supravital stains, such as new methylene blue and brilliant cresyl blue, stain the nucleic acid within these organelles (new methylene blue is a distinct chemical stain; regular methylene blue stains reticulocytes poorly). The circulating erythrocytes that contain organelles and thus have a reticulum of blue stain, are termed reticulocytes [12]. Reticulocytes have generally been in the circulation for 24 hours or less and thereafter they lose organelles and fail to stain as reticulocytes. The quantity of reticulum (i.e., nucleic acid) in an erythrocyte diminishes as it matures, thus in the youngest reticulocytes the reticulum is densely packed while in the oldest ones only a few scattered threads are found. Reticulocytes are on average about 20% larger than mature erythrocytes [13]. Scanning electron microscopy has shown that reticulocytes are not generally bilaterally indented disks like mature erythrocytes, but rather are irregularly shaped and polylobulated.

A neonatologist usually orders a reticulocyte count to assess the level of erythrocyte production, because high reticulocyte counts signify increased erythropoiesis and counts of 0 signify a low level of effective erythropoiesis. Reticulocytes can be reported in at least three different ways, which can sometimes be confusing: (1) as a percentage, (2) as an absolute number, or (3) as a corrected value. The immature reticulocyte fraction (IRF) is also gaining popularity among neonatologists [14].

A reticulocyte percentage is the percentage of erythrocytes that stain as reticulocytes. An obvious limitation of this method is that it fails to account for differences in the absolute number of erythrocytes. For example, each of two neonates may have a reticulocyte count of 5%. The neonatologist may be tempted to conclude

that the two patients have similar levels of erythrocyte production. However, the first patient is anemic, with an erythrocyte count of $2 \times 10^6/\mu L$, and the other is not anemic, with an erythrocyte count of $4 \times 10^6/\mu L$. The anemic infant actually has only one-half the number of reticulocytes in the circulation (5% of 2×10^6, or 100,000 reticulocytes/μL of blood) as does the normal infant (5% of 4×10^6, or 200,000 reticulocytes/μL). Failure to recognize this pitfall can give the neonatologist the false impression that the anemic patient is mounting an appropriate increase in erythrocyte production. Reporting the reticulocyte count as an absolute number appears to be gaining popularity in neonatal intensive care units. In reporting the results of clinical trials of recombinant erythropoietin administration to preterm neonates, it has been more common to report a percentage because it gives a clearer comparison of effective erythropoiesis between groups, despite differences in hematocrit.

A third method of reporting reticulocytes is by using one or two corrections. One type of correction is for hematocrit. The reticulocyte percentage is adjusted to a standard hematocrit (hct), usually 45% (0.45 L/L) and the correction is applied as follows:

corrected reticulocyte count =

$$\frac{\text{patient's reticulocyte count (\%)} \times \text{patient's hct (L/L)}}{0.45 \text{ (L/L)}}.$$

This correction is usually appropriate for neonatal patients and provides a better framework for assessing the level of effective erythropoiesis, because it normalizes all values to a standard hematocrit.

Another type of correction is sometimes made for "shift" reticulocytes. This correction accounts for the observation that whereas reticulocytes generally survive in the circulation for about 1 day, during increased erythropoiesis even younger reticulocytes can be released from the marrow to the blood (i.e., shifted). These shift reticulocytes, prematurely released from the marrow into the blood, survive longer than 1 day in the blood before losing their organelles, giving the false impression that the reticulocyte count is higher than it actually is. When reticulocytes survive in the circulation for 2 days, rather than 1 day, the correction for shift reticulocytes is made by reducing the percentage reported by half. To apply this correction, the degree of shift is assumed to be related to the intensity of stimulation of the marrow by erythropoietin. The examiner assumes that the maturation time of the reticulocyte in the circulation is 1 day when the hematocrit is normal, 1.5 days when the hematocrit is reduced moderately, and 2.0 days when the hematocrit is reduced markedly. With a hematocrit of 20%, the physician assumes a marked erythropoietic effort, causing a shift in premature reticulocytes that survive 2 days in the circulation:

corrected reticulocyte count =

$$\frac{\text{patient's reticulocyte count\%}}{2.0}.$$

The shift reticulocyte count correction is rarely used by neonatologists. The correction for shift reticulocytes is only appropriate when the anemia is the result of hemorrhage or hemolysis, because it assumes that erythrocyte production has increased in response to the anemia. If the anemia is the result of hypoproduction of erythrocytes the reticulocyte count correction for shift reticulocytes would not be valid. Because relative hypoproduction of erythrocytes is thought to be a common component of anemia in preterm infants, the use of this correction might be misleading.

On the day of birth, normal term infants have reticulocyte values of 4% to 7% and absolute reticulocyte counts of 200,000 to 400,000/μL [15]. Infants delivered prematurely have somewhat higher reticulocyte counts; values of 6% to 10% and absolute counts of 400,000 to 500,000/μL are common [16]. In healthy neonates, reticulocyte levels fall markedly over the first few days of life. By the fourth day the reticulocytes can be 0% to 1%, with an absolute count of 0 to 50,000/μL.

Immature Reticulocyte Fraction and RET-He

The immature reticulocyte fraction (IRF) is a measure of the proportion of reticulocytes with intense reticulum staining. A threshold is set, and the fraction of reticulocytes staining above that threshold reflects the "young" reticulocytes. Thus, a high IRF is used as a parameter of brisk erythropoiesis. Thus, after erythropoietin treatment, the IRF might increase; contrariwise after an erythrocyte transfusion the IRF might fall.

The reticulocyte hemoglobin content (RET-He) is a quantification of the hemoglobin in reticulocytes. This parameter gives information about the availability of iron for hemoglobin synthesis in the days immediately before the specimen was collected [17, 18]. The RET-He has been used in the assessment of iron deficiency. With limited iron stores, subnormal amounts of iron are available to developing erythrocytes in the marrow for incorporation into hemoglobin, and therefore the amount of hemoglobin in reticulocytes, the RET-He parameter, is low. The RET-He remains at the same values in erythrocytes from the time they enter the blood until they are removed from the circulation. Figure 24.10 shows reference intervals for reticulocytes, the IRF, and the RET-He over the first 90 days following birth.

Nucleated Red Blood Cells

Nucleated red blood cells (NRBC) are often observed in the blood of term and preterm neonates [19–22]. A high concentration of NRBC at birth has been associated with an increased risk of developing intraventricular hemorrhage and or retinopathy of prematurity [22]. Circulating NRBCs are rarely observed in healthy adults and non-neonatal children, because the nucleus of a developing normoblast is almost always extruded before the cell exits the marrow. Enucleation is so efficient that finding NRBC in the blood of older children raises the suspicion of hematopathology such as a myeloproliferative disorder.

Reference ranges for NRBC using a dataset of over 30,000 neonates, on the day of birth, are shown in Fig. 24.11 as a function of gestational age [19]. In this large study, no relationships were observed between the highest first-day NRBC and the cord pH or the 1 minute or 5 minute Apgar score, but if the NRBC count on the day of birth was above the 95th percentile, the odds of developing severe intraventricular hemorrhage (IVH) were 4.28 (95% CI; 3.17–5.77) and the odds of developing severe retinopathy of prematurity (ROP) were 4.18 (2.74–6.38).

Fragmented Red Cells

The CBC parameter "fragmented red cells" (FRC) was developed for certain automated cell counters using technology similar to flow cytometry. A "gate" is set to quantify cells just smaller than

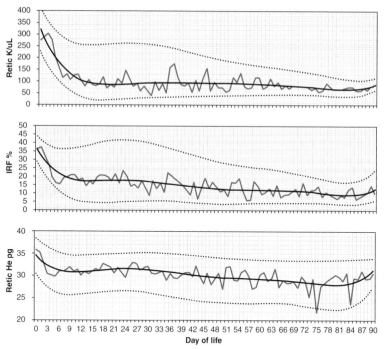

Fig. 24.10 Reference intervals for reticulocytes per microliter blood, immature reticulocyte fraction (IRF) (%), and RET-He (pg) over the first 90 days following birth. The lower line shows the 5th percentile values, the middle line shows the mean values and the upper line shows the 95th percentile values. (From [17], Christensen et al. Reference intervals for reticulocyte parameters of infants during their first 90 days after birth. *J Perinatol* 2016; **36**:61–66.) (See plate section for color version.)

those in the red blood cell gate. The FRC parameter can be expressed either as a percent (the percent of the red blood cells that fall within the gate, just smaller in size than red blood cells) or as an absolute number of these cells per microliter of blood. In neonates the FRC parameter is generally composed of schistocytes, but cells in this gate also include microcytes and other red blood cell subspecies that are smaller than those within the normal red blood cell gate. Figure 24.12 shows FRC/μL over the first 90 days after birth [23].

were discocytes, only about 40% of the erythrocytes of neonates had this characteristic shape. Morphologic abnormalities of erythrocytes of neonates have also been reported using other methods. For instance, interference-contrast microscopy shows pits or craters on the surface of about 2.6% of erythrocytes of healthy adults. In contrast, about 25% of the erythrocytes of term infants and about one-half of the erythrocytes of preterm infants have pits [25]. It is believed that these pits are cytoplasmic vacuoles and represent hypofunction of the spleen or reticuloendothelial system, but their significance is not clear.

Site of Sampling

The hematocrit, hemoglobin concentration, and erythrocyte concentration of newborn infants vary, somewhat predictably, according to the vascular source from which the sample is obtained (see Table 24.2) [26–34]. In general, erythrocyte values are higher (i.e., more concentrated) when samples are obtained by lancing capillary beds than when drawn from an artery or a vein or obtained from an indwelling arterial or venous catheter. The specific anatomic site of the vein, artery, or capillary bed sampled appears not to affect the results. For instance, values obtained from a femoral vein are equivalent to those obtained from a scalp vein [28, 29], and values from an umbilical artery are equivalent to those from a radial artery. Similarly, values from a capillary bed, such as from a heel, toe, or finger, are also equal if perfusion of those sites is similar [29].

As a general rule, capillary blood obtained from a neonate's poorly perfused extremity is a poor source on which to base clinical decisions. The erythrocyte values from such a source are about 15% (range of 5% to 25%) above those of simultaneously obtained venous or arterial blood. Capillary values obtained from a poorly perfused extremity can erroneously indicate the diagnosis of polycythemia and can erroneously exclude anemia. The amount that a capillary hematocrit is elevated above a venous or arterial hematocrit cannot be accurately predicted in individual cases, but in general it appears to vary with perfusion of the extremity.

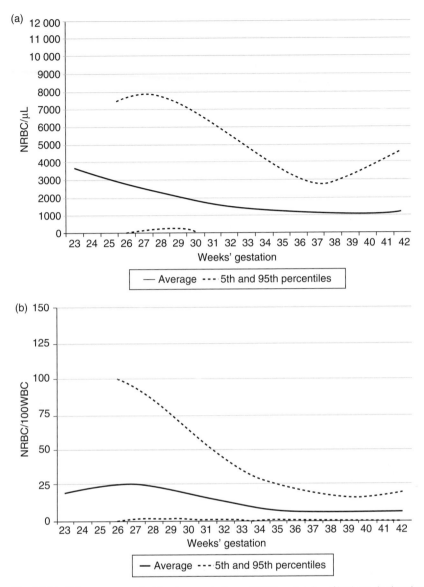

Fig. 24.11 Reference ranges for blood concentrations of NRBC on the day of birth are displayed according to gestational age. The lower and upper lines represent the 5% and 95% limits and the middle line represents the mean value. (a) Shows the data expressed as "NRBC/μL" and (b) shows the data expressed as "NRBC/100WBC." (From [19], Christensen et al. Neonatal reference ranges for blood concentrations of nucleated red blood cells. *Neonatology* 2010;**99**:289–94.)

When a CBC is obtained from a sick neonate with poor skin perfusion, the neonatologist interpreting the value should realize that a capillary hematocrit is less informative and less reproducible than a venous or an arterial hematocrit. Oh and Lind [27] and Lindercamp and colleagues [29] found that infants of the shortest gestation generally have the largest difference in capillary and venous hematocrits (Table 24.2). Studies by Oh and Lind [27] and by Moe [28] indicate that warming the extremity before lancing the capillary bed can result in a better correlation between capillary and venous hematocrits. However, when a neonatologist feels it important to detect changes in serial hematocrit samples, it should likewise be important to keep a uniform site of sampling (i.e., all venous or all arterial). When comparing serial hematocrits of an ill neonate, it is useful to have the sample site documented.

Table 24.2 The effect of site of blood sampling on hematocrit or blood hemoglobin concentrations of neonates

Anatomic sites of comparison	Average difference	Author	Year
Capillary vs. femoral vein	Capillary 10% higher	Vahlquist [31]	1941
Great toe vs. internal jugular	Capillary 21% higher	Oettinger & Mills [26]	1949
Capillary vs. venous	Capillary 5% higher	Mollision [32]	1951
Heel vs. scalp or femoral vein	Capillary 15% higher*	Oh & Lind [27]	1966
Patients with erythroblastosis fetalis; heel vs. umbilical vessel	Capillary 25% higher	Moe [28]	1967
Capillary vs. umbilical vessel	Capillary 10%–21% higher	Linderkamp et al. [29]	1977
Heel vs. antecubital vein	Capillary 12%–20% higher	Rivera & Rudolph [33]	1982
Heel vs. UAC	Capillary 15% higher	Thurlbeck & McIntosh [34]**	1987

Notes: UAC, umbilical artery catheter.

* The capillary hematocrit was only 5% higher when the heel was warmed.

** Preterm infants, 24 to 32 weeks' gestation, with respiratory distress.

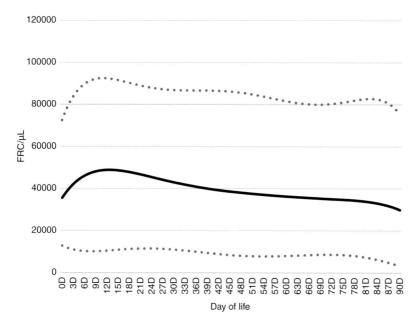

Fig. 24.12 Reference intervals for fragmented red cells/μL blood over the first 90 days after birth. The lower and upper lines represent the 5% and 95% limits and the middle line represents the mean value. (From [23], Judkins et al. Automated quantification of fragmented red blood cells: Neonatal reference intervals and clinical disorders of neonatal intensive care unit patients with high values. *Neonatology* 2018;**115**:5–12.)

Blood Sampling Relative to Delivery

About 100 mL of blood can usually be withdrawn from the placental vessels at term by using the technique of catheterizing the vessels and washing out the blood [27]. Direct venipuncture of the placental end of the umbilical vein after cord clamping generally yields somewhat less blood (50 to 60 mL). The blood within the umbilical cord and placenta constitute about one-third of the entire circulating blood volume of the fetus. About 15 to 20 mL/kg can be transferred, at birth,

from placenta to neonate when cord clamping is delayed 120 to 180 seconds [35].

Normally, after a term fetus is delivered, the umbilical arteries constrict in response to the increasing PO$_2$, retarding the flow of blood from the neonate into the placenta. The umbilical vein, however, fails to significantly constrict, permitting blood to flow in a direction partly controlled by gravity from the placenta to the neonate or vice versa. The effect may have little clinical consequence, as position of the neonate, relative to the mother, after birth but before cord clamping, seems to have little effect on the neonate's hematocrit/hemoglobin [36]. Delayed clamping of the umbilical cord, or cord "milking" of blood toward the neonate before the cord is clamped and cut, have positive effects on the short- and long-term outcome and one or the other technique is a common practice at delivery [37].

Leukocytes

The 1972 edition of Holt's *Pediatrics* stated, "the blood count is of relatively little help in the diagnosis of sepsis neonatorum" [38]. This was a prevalent teaching of the time, and when the first cases of group B streptococcal infection were reported, no mention was made of blood leukocyte counts or differential cell counts in these neonates. The notion that the CBC was not a useful test to perform on neonatal patients was based on the extreme variability of neutrophil counts in neonates, and the apparent lack of correlation between the blood neutrophil findings and the presence of infection.

Attitudes about the utility of CBCs of neonates began to change after publications of Xanthou [39], Akenzua and associates [40], and Manroe and coworkers [41]. These reports showed differences in blood neutrophil concentrations in groups of infected compared with noninfected neonates, and they pointed out that neutropenia, accompanied by a high ratio of immature neutrophils (bands and metamyelocytes) to total neutrophils (segmented neutrophils and band neutrophils and metamyelocytes) was particularly common in neonates with sepsis.

Site of Sampling

Neutrophil concentrations are lower in blood drawn from an umbilical artery catheter than in blood drawn by venipuncture or capillary stick [42]. Arterial values are about 75% of venous or capillary values. After moderate exercise in the form of chest physical therapy, leukocyte counts increase to about 115% of baseline, but this is not accompanied by a change in the differential count. Lower neutrophil concentrations in arterial blood are also observed in mice [43]. The explanation appears to be related to the differences in blood flow of arterial vs. capillary or venous blood. The pulsatile flow of arterial blood appears to "push" the larger cells toward the periphery of the vessel.

Leukocyte Counts in Term Infants

In 1979, Manroe and associates from the University of Texas Southwestern Medical Center in Dallas published reference ranges for blood neutrophil concentrations in neonates and for the proportion of circulating neutrophils that were immature (nonsegmented) (Figs. 24.13 and 24.14). They reported values for neonates of 26 to 44 weeks' gestation and with birthweights of 660 to 5,000 g [41]. The data were obtained from 1974 to 1976, when the survival of very low birth weight (VLBW) infants was 42% (compared with 79% a decade later) [44]. Although the number of VLBW infants represented in the Manroe study was limited, the publication constituted a landmark. For the first time neonatologists could determine with some confidence whether their patient had a blood neutrophil count that was low, normal, or high [41].

Neonates at high altitude, such as those in the NICUs of Colorado [45], Utah [46], and New Mexico [47] have a higher range of neutrophil counts than do those reported from near sea level (Dallas) [41, 44]. Figure 24.15 shows the reference range of blood neutrophils among neonates at altitude and Fig. 24.16 shows the altitude and sea level ranges superimposed to directly compare the differences.

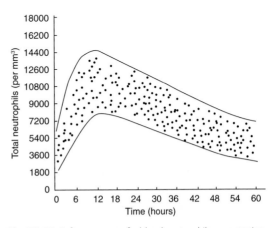

Fig. 24.13 Reference range for blood neutrophil concentration of normal newborn infants in Dallas, Texas during the first 60 hours after birth. Dots represent single values and numbers represent the number of values at that same point. (From [41], Manroe, et al. The neonatal blood count in health and disease. 1. Reference values for neutrophilic cells. *J Pediatr* 1979;**95**:89–98.)

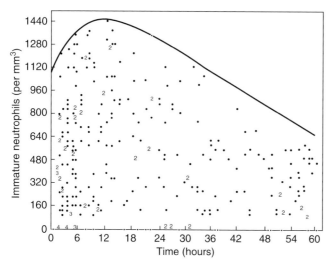

Fig. 24.14 Reference range for immature neutrophils of normal newborn infants in Dallas, Texas, during the first 60 hours after birth. Dots represent single values and numbers represent the number of values at that same point. (From [41], Manroe, et al. The neonatal blood count in health and disease. 1. Reference values for neutrophilic cells. *J Pediatr* 1979;**95**:89–98.)

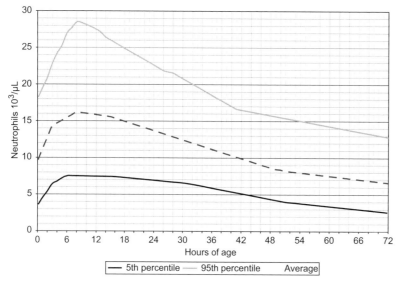

Fig. 24.15 Reference range for blood neutrophil concentrations during the first 72 hours after birth of term and near term (>36 weeks' gestation) neonates. A total of 12,149 values were used in this analysis. The 5th percentile, mean, and 95th percentile values are shown. (From [46], Schmutz et al. Expected ranges for blood neutrophil concentrations of neonates: The Manroe and Mouzinho charts revisited. *J Perinatol* 2008;**28**:275–81.)

Leukocyte Counts in Preterm Infants

Several studies suggested that the normal values reported by Manroe might not be applicable to VLBW infants. One of the first of these was a report by Coulombel and coworkers of 132 neonates with CBCs obtained during their first 12 hours of life [48]. Blood was sometimes obtained from capillary samples and other times from umbilical venous or arterial catheters. All 132 infants had a clinical reason for obtaining a CBC, although this report excluded those with culture-positive evidence of bacterial infection. The researchers observed an inverse relationship between gestational age and blood neutrophil concentration.

In 1982, Lloyd and Oto reported serial leukocyte counts from 24 preterm infants, all less than 33 weeks' gestation [49]. They observed that the group's blood neutrophil concentrations were lower than those reported by Manroe (predominantly term infants). In 1994, Mouzinho and colleagues reported the results of 1799 blood leukocyte and differential counts obtained from 193 VLBW infants [44]. After excluding counts from neonates with perinatal and/ or neonatal complications, values from normal VLBW neonates were displayed and compared with the Manroe reference ranges (Fig. 24.17).

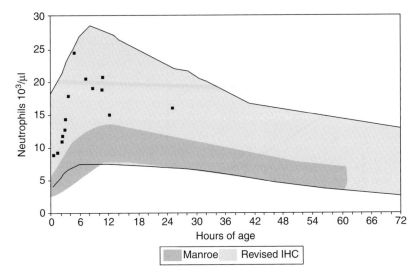

Fig. 24.16 Reference range for blood neutrophil concentrations, superimposed Manroe and Schmutz curves. (From [46], Schmutz et al. Expected ranges for blood neutrophil concentrations of neonates: The Manroe and Mouzinho charts revisited. *J Perinatol* 2008;**28**:275–81.)

Infants of younger gestations had reference ranges for blood neutrophils that differed significantly from those of larger, older neonates. The VLBW infants had the same upper limit boundary for absolute neutrophil count of the larger, older infants, but their lower limit boundary was significantly less than the boundary of the older infants. Reference ranges for neonates 28 to 36 weeks' gestation are shown in Fig. 24.18 and for neonates <28 weeks' gestation in Fig. 24.19.

Automated Leukocyte Differentials

The automated leukocyte differential cell count is a relatively new innovation in neonatal clinical laboratory science [50]. This parameter enumerates large numbers of leukocytes, using flow cytometric techniques, according to their size and cytoplasmic and nuclear characteristics. The immature granulocyte percent (IG%) and the immature granulocyte count (IG/µL blood) include promyelocytes, myelocytes, and metamyelocytes in the circulating blood. The IG% and IG/µL can be thought of as somewhat analogous to the I/T ratio and the absolute band count, which are reported only when a manual differential cell count is performed as part of the CBC.

Automated leukocyte differential cell counts have some advantages over manual methods. Specifically, automated counts do not require a blood smear or the technician time to perform a manual differential cell count. Automated methods

count logs more cells than do typical manual counts, and they also eliminate human error in discriminating between cell types and transcribing values from a tally device to the medical record. Reference intervals for IG% and IG/µL over the first week after birth are shown in Fig. 24.20.

Eosinophils

Eosinophilia is not a rare finding in the neonatal intensive care unit. In growing preterm infants a nonspecific low-grade eosinophilia is so common as to warrant the label "eosinophilia of prematurity" [51, 52]. Despite its relatively frequent occurrence, the causes and significance of this condition are uncertain.

Eosinophils in the blood can increase to very high concentrations without a concomitant increase in the concentration of other leukocytes. This attests to a unique controlling mechanism. The mechanisms regulating eosinophil concentrations in blood are reviewed in Chapter 16 and the material given here relates only to reference ranges for eosinophils.

Defining the normal range of eosinophils in the blood of neonates has been attempted in relatively few studies. Medoff and Barbero reported that during the first 12 hours of life, absolute blood eosinophil concentrations range from 20 to 850/µL [53]. On the basis of this report, eosinophilia on the first day of life would be defined as an absolute blood eosinophil count of more than

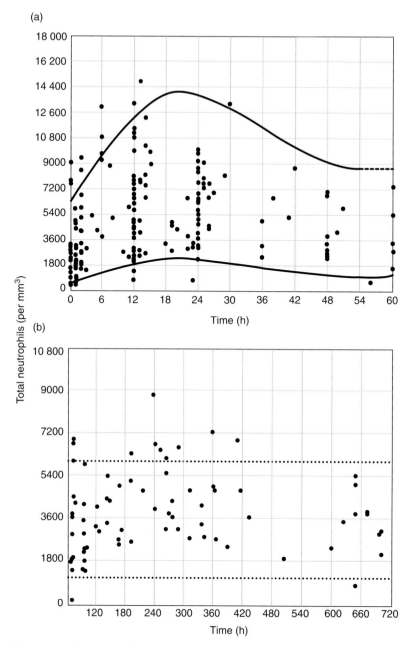

Fig. 24.17 Reference range for absolute blood neutrophil concentration of very low birthweight infants. Dots represent single values. (From [44], Mouzinho et al. Revised reference ranges for circulating neutrophils in very low birthweight neonates. *Pediatrics* 1994;**94**:76.)

850/μL. Xanthou reported that, by the fifth day of life, eosinophil concentrations had a much greater range than on the first day, with values of 100 to 2,500/μL [54]. By day five, eosinophilia would be diagnosed if the count was more than 2,500/μL. It is not clear whether these numbers should be used to define eosinophilia in preterm infants.

According to the reports of Medoff and Xanthou, absolute eosinophil counts of less than 20/μL on the first day of life and less than 100/μL after the first 5 days should define eosinopenia. However, the diagnosis of eosinopenia in the neonatal intensive care unit is made rarely, because so many apparently normal infants have no eosinophils identified on individual differential cell counts. In contrast to this

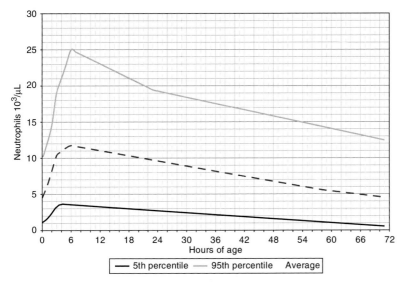

Fig. 24.18 Reference range for blood neutrophil count during the first 72 hours after birth of neonates 28 to 36 weeks' gestation. A total of 8,896 values were used in this analysis. The 5th percentile, mean, and 95th percentile values are shown. (From [46], Schmutz et al. Expected ranges for blood neutrophil concentrations of neonates: The Manroe and Mouzinho charts revisited. *J Perinatol* 2008;**28**:275–81.)

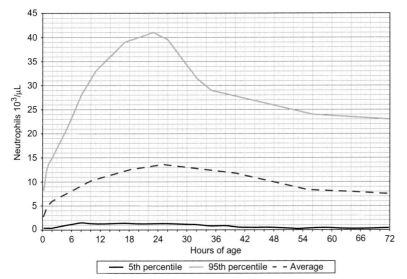

Fig. 24.19 Reference interval for blood neutrophil count during the first 72 hours after birth of neonates <28 weeks' gestation. A total of 8,896 values were used in this analysis. The 5th percentile, mean, and 95th percentile values are shown. (From [46], Schmutz et al. Expected ranges for blood neutrophil concentrations of neonates: The Manroe and Mouzinho charts revisited. *J Perinatol* 2008;**28**:275–81.)

statement, Burell suggested that a complete lack of eosinophils in neonates should be considered an abnormality [55]. He found that a complete absence of eosinophils was common in infants who fared poorly and subsequently died. He reported that on the day of death there was generally a complete absence of blood eosinophils. Bass reported that blood eosinophil concentrations declined rapidly in the presence of bacterial infection [56].

By defining eosinophilia as blood concentration of more than 700/μL (a definition of eosinophilia sometimes used in adult medicine), Gibson and coworkers found that about 75% of preterm infants develop eosinophilia [57]. They also observed that this eosinophilia of prematurity generally occurs during a period in which an anabolic state is established. This anabolic state and the accompanying eosinophilia are usually seen in the second or third week of life, and the eosinophilia persists for many days and sometimes for weeks. Portuguez-Molavasi reported that at least one episode of eosinophilia (defined as an absolute eosinophil count of more than 1,000/μL) occurred in 35% of all infants admitted to an intensive care nursery [58]. Craver reported that eosinophils can be seen in the cerebrospinal fluid

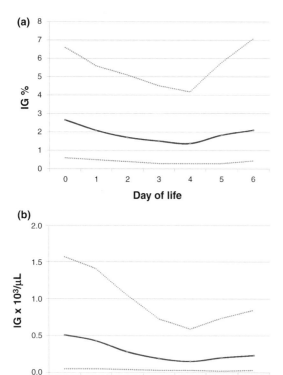

Fig. 24.20 Reference interval in the first week of life after birth (a) for immature granulocytes (%) and (b) immature granulocytes per microliter blood. (From [50], MacQueen et al, Comparing automated vs manual leukocyte differential counts for quantifying the "left shift" in the blood of neonates. *J Perinatol* 2016;**36**:843–8.)

weeks after intraventricular hemorrhage [59], but the significance of this finding is not clear, and this finding did not correlate with blood eosinophil counts.

Reference ranges for eosinophil counts on the day of birth, using a dataset of over 60,000 neonates are shown in Fig. 24.21 [60]. Reference ranges during the first 28 days following birth are shown in Fig. 24.22. Now that a reference range exists for eosinophil counts of neonates, additional study is needed regarding groups that fall outside the range. Before the reference range study [60], it was not clear whether abnormally low concentrations of eosinophils could be identified. Specifically, it was not clear whether a result of zero/μL was within the reference range. It is now clear that zero is not generally within the reference range, with the exception of eosinophils in neonates less than 24 weeks' gestation. Therefore neonates with a persistent eosinophil count of zero should be considered to have an abnormality.

Monocytes

Monocytes are part of the reticuloendothelial system, which is composed of granulocytic precursors, circulating monocytes, and tissue macrophages [60]. Like other granulocytes, monocytes generally reside in the blood for less than 1 day ($T_{1/2}$ 8.4 hours) after which they transmigrate to tissues and become mononuclear phagocytes in lung, kidney, peritoneum, gastrointestinal tract, or reproductive tract, or become Langerhans cells, Kupffer

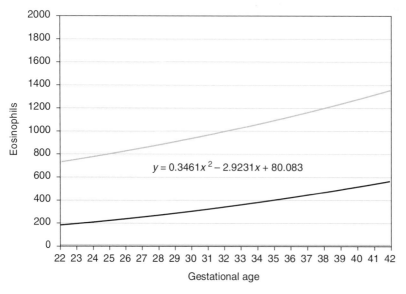

$$y = 0.3461x^2 - 2.9231x + 80.083$$

Fig. 24.21 Reference range for blood concentration of eosinophils (eosinophils/μL blood) on the day of birth, displayed according to gestational age. The lower and upper lines represent the 5% and 95% limits and the middle line represents the mean value. (From [60], Christensen et al. Reference ranges for blood concentrations of eosinophils and monocytes during the neonatal period defined from over 63,000 records in a multihospital healthcare system. *J Perinatol* 2010;**30**:540–5.)

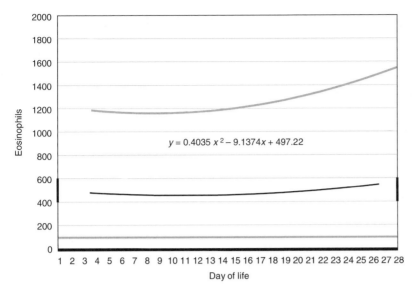

Fig. 24.22 Reference range for blood concentration of eosinophils (eosinophils/μL blood) during the first 28 days following birth. The lower and upper lines represent the 5% and 95% limits and the middle line represents the mean value. (From [60], Christensen et al. Reference ranges for blood concentrations of eosinophils and monocytes during the neonatal period defined from over 63,000 records in a multihospital health-care system. *J Perinatol* 2010;**30**:540–5.)

$y = 0.4035\,x^2 - 9.1374x + 497.22$

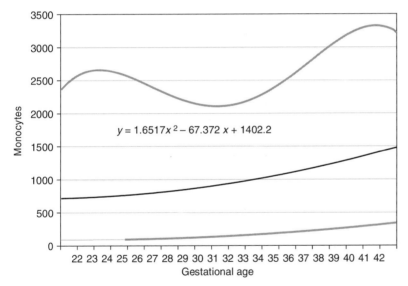

Fig. 24.23 Reference range for blood concentration of monocytes (monocytes/μL blood) on the day of birth, displayed according to gestational age. The lower and upper lines represent the 5% and 95% limits and the middle line represents the mean value. (From [60], Christensen et al. Reference ranges for blood concentrations of eosinophils and monocytes during the neonatal period defined from over 63,000 records in a multihospital healthcare system. *J Perinatol* 2010;**30**:540–5.)

$y = 1.6517x^2 - 67.372\,x + 1402.2$

cells, microglial cells, or osteoclasts. Blood concentrations of monocytes on the day of birth increase as a function of gestational age (Fig. 24.23). This is consistent with the kinetic information from human fetal studies showing a maturational increase in the number of monocyte precursors. Monocytes constitute 2%–4% of all hemic cells during the first trimester, 3%–7% at 30 weeks, and they continue to increase through the third trimester. Monocyte counts remain low in fetal blood until the fifth month of gestation and increase gradually once the marrow becomes the predominant site of hematopoiesis. Monocyte

concentrations generally increase during the first 2 weeks before beginning a downward trend in the third postnatal week (Fig. 24.24) [60].

Platelets

Site of Sampling

Thurlbeck and McIntosh reported no difference in the platelet counts drawn from umbilical arterial lines, venipunctures, or heel stick [34]. Therefore, unlike the case for neutrophils and erythrocytes, it does not appear to matter what vascular source is used for drawing a platelet

459

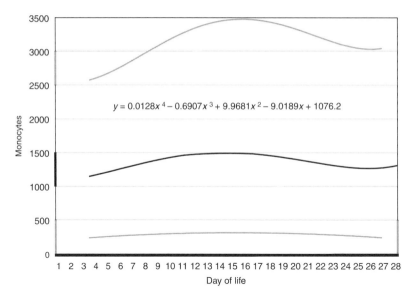

$$y = 0.0128x^4 - 0.6907x^3 + 9.9681x^2 - 9.0189x + 1076.2$$

Fig. 24.24 Reference range for blood concentration of monocytes (monocytes/μL blood) during the first 28 days following birth. The lower and upper lines represent the 5% and 95% limits and the middle line represents the mean value. (From [60], Christensen et al. Reference ranges for blood concentrations of eosinophils and monocytes during the neonatal period defined from over 63,000 records in a multihospital healthcare system. *J Perinatol* 2010;**30**:540–5.)

count. On that basis, it is common practice to obtain platelet counts of neonates from the most convenient sampling site, without concern about a potential sampling site difference.

Reference Ranges for Platelet Counts and Mean Platelet Volume on Day of Birth

In adults, the reference range for platelet count is about >150,000/μL and <450,000/μL [61]. This same range has been used to define thrombocytopenia and thrombocytosis in neonates. However, the data suggest a more complex situation. The reference range for platelet count at birth, between 22 and 42 weeks' gestation, is shown in Fig. 24.25 [62]. Platelet counts as low as 100,000/μL can be normal for neonates <29 weeks' gestation and counts above 350,000/μL are high for neonates <29 weeks. While the blood concentration of platelets increases gradually between 22 and 42 weeks, the mean platelet volume (MPV) does not. The MPV averages 8 fL, with a range of about 7 to 9.5 fL.

Following birth, the platelet count gradually increases. As shown in Fig. 24.26a, the reference range over the first 90 days after birth has the appearance of a sine-wave. We speculate that the first wave is the result of thrombopoietin (and perhaps other megakaryopoietic stimulators) surging after birth. The explanation for the second and third wave of peak platelet counts is not clear. Accompanying the increase in platelet count after

birth is an increase in MPV (shown in Fig. 24.26b). At 2 weeks after birth, the reference range for platelet count is about 7.5 to 12 fL, but platelet size gradually falls to that at birth at a month or two.

Reticulated Platelets, Immature Platelet Fraction, and Immature Platelet Count

Additional information on platelet characteristics can sometimes be useful in managing a thrombocytopenic neonate. Relatively new tests include the reticulated platelet count, which requires flow cytometric capability, and the platelet distribution width and plateletcrit (PCT), which can be performed on routine hematology analyzers (Beckman Coulter Inc.), and the immature platelet fraction (IPF), which can be performed on other hematology analyzers (Sysmex, Inc.).

Newly synthesized platelets generally have a higher content of ribonucleic acid than platelets that have been circulating for several days. These newly produced platelets can be recognized by flow cytometric analysis after RNA staining with thiazole orange. Such platelets have been called reticulated platelets to reflect their similarity to reticulocytes [63]. Between 3% and 5% of the circulating platelets of healthy term neonates and LBW infants are recognized as reticulated platelets. Peterec and colleagues reported that infants of less than 30 weeks' gestation had reticulated platelet percentages about twice those of term infants, although with a very large variation (8.8% ±5.1%) [63]. Joseph and

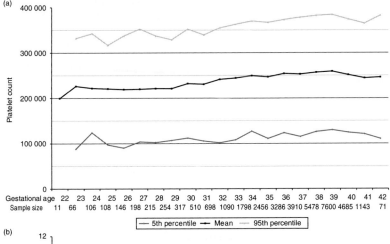

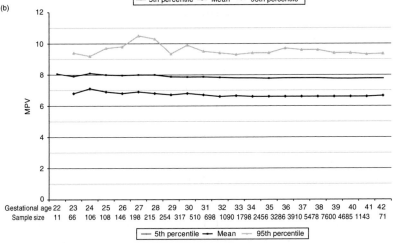

Fig. 24.25 Reference intervals for platelet count (a) and mean platelet volume (b) on the day of birth, for neonates delivered at 22 to 42 weeks' gestation. Values are shown for the 5th percentile, mean, and 95th percentile. (From [62], Wiedmeier, et al. Platelet reference ranges for neonates, defined using data from over 47,000 patients in a multihospital healthcare system. *J Perinatol* 2009: **29**;130–6.)

associates observed that adults ($n = 18$) had a slightly but significantly higher percentage of reticulated platelets than did healthy term neonates ($n = 42$) [64]. They observed no difference in reticulated platelet count between infants depending on mode of delivery.

As with the reticulocyte count, the IPF can be reported as either immature fraction percent, or an absolute number of immature platelets per microliter of blood. There are no apparent differences in IPF between male and female neonates [65]. In thrombocytopenic neonates, high IPF values are typical for those with consumptive varieties of neutropenia and normal values are typical for those with hyporegenerative varieties of thrombocytopenia [65–67]. Reference intervals for immature platelet fraction (%) and for immature platelet count (×1,000/μL) on the day of birth are shown in Fig. 24.27 and reference intervals over the first 90 days following birth are shown in Fig. 24.8.

The platelet distribution width, like the erythrocyte distribution width, is a measure of the distribution of various sized platelets in the circulation.

Template Bleeding Time

The template bleeding time is a method of assessing an important aspect of primary hemostatic capacity [68, 69]. It measures the time required to produce a functional platelet plug in vivo, which plug occurs through the interaction of platelets with the subendothelial structures of a damaged vessel, leading to the arrest of bleeding. Accordingly, the bleeding time is a means of investigating quantitative and qualitative platelet disorders and hemostatically defective blood vessels. Unfortunately, a pitfall in the bleeding time involves poor inter-operator agreement [68, 69]. This error can be remedied, at least in part, by

(a)

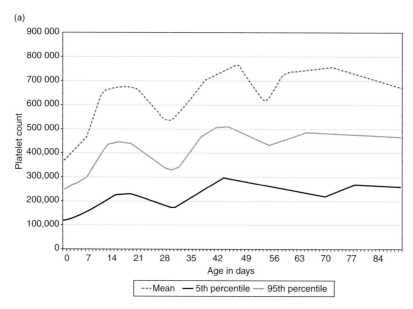

(b)

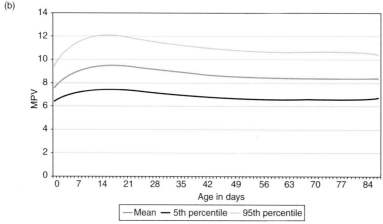

Fig. 24.26 Reference range for platelet count (a) and mean platelet volume (b) during the first 90 days following birth. Values are shown for the 5th percentile, mean, and 95th percentile. (From [62], Wiedmeier, et al. Platelet reference ranges for neonates, defined using data from over 47,000 patients in a multihospital healthcare system. *J Perinatol* 2009:**29**;130–6.)

having a limited number of technicians performing the test and assuring that only experienced technicians are utilized.

The largest study of bleeding time in neonates involved a single technician (Dr. Antonio DelVecchio) in Brindisi, Italy, who studied 240 neonates each on three occasions: on the day of birth, 10 days later, and at 1 month [69]. On the first day of life, preterm neonates had bleeding times about twice that measured in term and late preterm neonates. Figure 24.29 shows the relationship between gestational age and bleeding time on the first day after birth. When restudied on day of life 10 the bleeding times had diminished to the same range as term neonates. Another finding of that study

was mild thrombocytopenia, platelet counts between 100,000/μL and 150,000/μL, did not result in prolonged bleeding times. On that basis it is proposed that giving prophylactic platelet transfusions to stable neonates with mild thrombocytopenia is of no benefit.

Platelet Function Analyzer Closure Time

The platelet function analyzer (PFA)-100® test was developed as a way to quantify platelet dysfunction in vitro, using relatively small volumes of whole blood. Test results are reported in seconds, which is the time required for platelets to plug a standard collagen-coated aperture through which a blood sample is drawn. The terminology used is "closure time," indicating the time for a platelet plug to close or occlude the aperture.

For PFA-100® tests in neonates, blood samples are generally obtained by central line or by a clean venipuncture. Samples drawn by heel stick, or those obtained after a non-ideal line draw or venipuncture often give ambiguous or faulty results, or fail to generate a result. The test is usually done using two cartridges, one containing epinephrine and the other containing ADP. When PFA-100® studies are done on neonates, in order to minimize phlebotomy losses, sometimes only the epinephrine cartridge is used, and thus only half the usual blood sample is needed. When using this modification it is critical to maintain the recommended ratio of blood to citrate (9:1).

PFA-100® studies from umbilical cord blood generally have a shorter closure time than from adult blood [70, 71], but the reason for this is not clear. Few PFA-100® studies have been reported from blood drawn from newborn infants after birth. In approximately 40 neonates, PFA-100® values in the first day or two after birth did not vary significantly between preterm and term neonates, as shown in Table 24.3. Mean values were about 120 seconds with a range of about 90 to 140 seconds. Saxonhouse et al. found PFA-100® values were longer among neonates with shortest

Table 24.3 PFA-100® times drawn from newborn infants by central line or venipuncture on the first day after birth

Gestational age	Birth weight	PFA-100 mean and 95% CI
23–30 weeks	<1,500 grams	119 (90–148) seconds
33–41 weeks		123 (96–149) seconds

Note: Only the epinephrine cartridge (not the ADP cartridge) was used in these studies to minimize phlebotomy volume for study purposes.

(a)

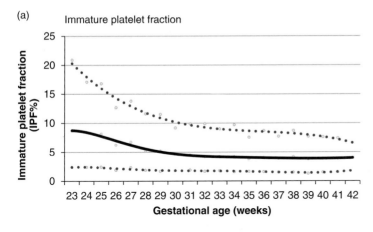

(b)

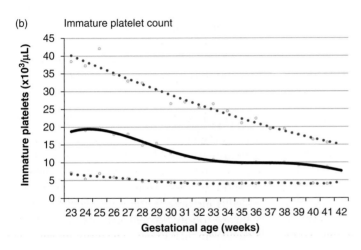

Fig. 24.27 Reference intervals for (a) immature platelet fraction (%) and (b) immature platelets/μL blood, on the day of birth, arranged according to gestational age. (From [65], MacQueen et al. The immature platelet fraction: creating neonatal reference intervals and using these to categorize neonatal thrombocytopenias. *J Perinatol* 2017;**37**:834–8.)

(a) Immature platelet fraction

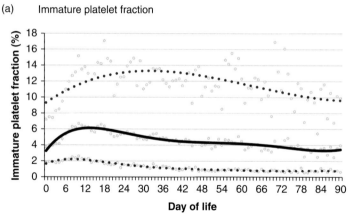

(b) Immature platelet count

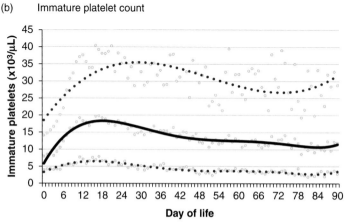

Fig. 24.28 Reference intervals of (a) immature platelet fraction (%) and (b) immature platelets/μL blood, over the first 90 days following birth. (From [65], MacQueen et al. The immature platelet fraction: creating neonatal reference intervals and using these to categorize neonatal thrombocytopenias. *J Perinatol* 2017;**37**:834–8.) (See plate section for color version.)

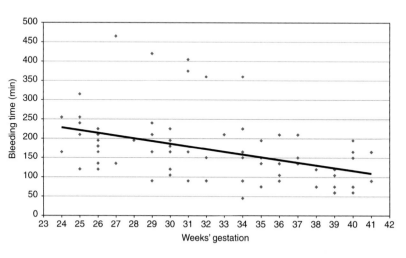

Fig. 24.29 Relationship of gestational age (weeks) to template bleeding time (seconds) measured during the first 24 hours after delivery. (From [69], Del Vecchio et al. Template bleeding times of 240 neonates born at 24–41 weeks' gestation. *J Perinatol* 2008:**28**;427–31.)

gestation, with an inverse relationship between closure time and gestational age [71]. They also found PFA-100® closure times of preterm infants shortened over the first week. Medications known to increase the bleeding time of neonates, such as indomethacin, ampicillin (particularly in high doses), or ibuprofen, also prolong the PFA-100® time [72, 73].

Bone Marrow

A bone marrow aspirate or biopsy is occasionally useful in providing information not otherwise available. In cases of a persistent cytopenia, a neonatologist might want information relating to the state of production. For example, a persistent thrombocytopenia could be the result of decreased platelet production or of increased platelet destruction or use. A marrow examination can sometimes help differentiate these conditions because in cases of decreased platelet production the marrow contains few megakaryocytes, but in cases of increased platelet use, the proportion of megakaryocytes should be increased.

Unfortunately, bone marrow aspirates of neonates are often diluted with peripheral blood, which can lead to misinterpretations about the state of production. This limitation can be minimized by taking care to withdraw the smallest possible marrow sample, thereby not over diluting the specimen with blood. The limitation can be further minimized by using a biopsy technique [74].

Marrow is accessible from essentially any bone in the neonate. We have found that the flat part of the proximal tibia is a simple and reliable site from which to obtain a marrow sample, because this site is easy to stabilize, the landmarks are obvious, and the amount of tissue between the skin and the bone is small. The (right-handed) operator holds the tibia firmly in a gloved left hand, while the right hand is used to prepare and sterilely drape the area and then to inject 1% lidocaine as a local anesthetic. Lidocaine (typically 0.1 mL without epinephrine) is injected subcutaneously, holding the needle in place for several seconds, after the needle is advanced to the bone and another 0.1 mL is injected into the periosteum. A few minutes later, the operator holds the 19-gauge, 1/2-inch needle (Osgood marrow needle fitted with a trocar) in the right hand and twists it carefully through the anesthetized periosteum with the mid-tibia clearly marked directly between the left thumb and forefinger. The needle is directed toward the middle of the tibial shaft to enter the middle of the marrow cavity. The needle is correctly positioned when it is solidly in place and when, on aspiration, marrow enters the aspirating syringe [74].

If only a microscopic analysis of the bone marrow cells is to be accomplished, only a few drops of marrow should be aspirated. If flow cytometry, a karyotype analysis, or a hematopoietic progenitor cell culture is needed, more cells are needed, and up to 0.25 mL of marrow can sometimes be aspirated. Volumes exceeding this amount, particularly in very small preterm infants, essentially always draw significant amounts of peripheral blood through

the marrow and result in a dilute specimen, which may be difficult to interpret.

Little information is available on bone marrow biopsies in neonates. Although the issue of cellularity is much more accurately assessed with a biopsy specimen than with an aspirate, neonatologists have been reluctant to perform this somewhat more invasive procedure, particularly on very small and ill neonates. We have found success in obtaining marrow needle biopsies, even in the smallest preterm infants in our neonatal intensive care unit, by using a modification of the aspiration method [74].

After the operator feels the Osgood needle penetrating the cortex of the tibia, the stylet (trocar) is withdrawn. The hollow needle is then advanced into the marrow space an additional 3 to 5 mm. Advancing the needle without a stylet cores a small segment of marrow into the needle. A syringe is then attached to the needle hub, and minimal suction is applied for about 1 second. This process helps secure the small core marrow biopsy specimen within the needle. The syringe and the attached needle are then withdrawn, and the core of marrow is pushed out of the needle by reintroducing the stylet. The core can be placed into fixative and subsequently sectioned and stained, or it can be smeared on cover glasses.

Anticipated results of bone marrow differential counts are shown in Table 24.4. Studies in 1941 and 1952 used marrow aspirates obtained from normal neonates. The normal values for marrow nucleated cell concentrations in neonates are available, but normal values for laboratory tests that were devised since 1952 (e.g., concentrations of hematopoietic progenitor cells) are not available [75, 76]. In modern practice, bone marrow aspirates are only performed on neonates if a clinical reason exists to do so or the patient is enrolled in a study that requires a bone marrow study. These subjects therefore are not strictly normal subjects, and the results should not be considered normal values.

References

1. Henry E, Christensen RD. Reference Intervals in neonatal hematology. *Clin Perinatol* 2015;42:483–97.

2. International Committee for Standardization in Haematology. Recommendations for reference method for haemoglobinometry in human blood. *J Clin Pathol* 1978;31:139–43.

Table 24.4 Differential cell counts of nucleated cells aspirated from the bone marrow of normal infants at term and from healthy adult men

Cell types	Term neonates (% [mean ± SD])	Healthy adult men (% [mean, 95% CI])
Nucleated erythroid		
Proerythroblast	0.1±0.1	0.6; 0.1–1.1
Basophilic erythroblast	0.2±0.2	1.4; 0.4–2.4
Polychromatic erythroblast	13.1±6.8	21.6; 13.1–30.1
Orthochromic erythroblast	0.7±0.7	2.0; 0.3–3.7
Neutrophil		
Promyelocytes	0.8±0.9	3.3; 1.9–4.7
Myelocytes	3.9±2.9	12.7; 8.5–16.9
Metamyelocytes	19.4±4.8	15.9; 7.1–24.7
Band neutrophils	28.9±7.6	12.4; 9.4–15.4
Segmented neutrophils	7.4±4.6	7.4; 3.8–11.0
Eosinophils	2.7±1.3	3.1; 1.1–5.2
Basophils	0.1±0.2	0.1
Other cells		
Monocytes	0.9±0.9	0.3; 0.0–0.6
Lymphocytes	14.4±5.5	16.2; 8.6–23.8
Megakaryocytes	0.1±0.1	0.1
Plasma cells	0.0 ±0.1	1.3; 0.0–3.5
Undifferentiated blasts	0.3 ±0.3	0.9:0.1–1.7
Unknown or damaged cells	6.0±3.2	
Myeloid:erythroid ratio	4.3:1	3.1:1; 1.1–5.2:1

Note: Data for term neonates from Rosse et al. 1977 [75], Shapiro & Bassen 1941 [76].

3. Jopling J, Henry E, Wiedmeier SE, Christensen RD. Reference ranges for hematocrit and blood hemoglobin concentration during the neonatal period: data from a multihospital healthcare system. *Pediatrics* 2009;**123**;e333–77.

4. Wintrobe MM. A simple and accurate hematocrit. *J Lab Clin Med* 1929;**15**:287–94.

5. Waugh TF, Merchant FT, Maugham GB. Blood studies on newborn: Determination of hemoglobin, volume of packed red cells, reticulocytes and fragility of erythrocytes over 9 day period. *Am J Med Sci* 1939;**198**:646–9.

6. Perkins SL. Principles of hematologic examination. In Greer JP, Foerster J, Rodgers GM, et al. eds. *Wintrobe's Clinical Hematology.* (Philadelphia, PA: Lippincott, Williams & Wilkins, 2009), p. 3.

7. Gairdner D, Marks J, Bosco JD. Blood formation in infancy: The normal bone marrow. *Arch Dis Child* 1952;**27**:124–32.

8. Christensen RD, Jopling J, Henry E, et al. The erythrocyte indices of neonates, defined using data from over 12,000 patients in a multihospital healthcare system. *J Perinatol* 2008;**28**:24–8.

9. Scott-Emuakpor AB, Okolo M, Omene JA, Ukpe SI. Normal hematological values of the African neonate. *Blut* 1985;**51**:11–18.

10. Michaels LA, Cohen AR, Zhao H, et al. Screening for hereditary spherocytosis by use of automated erythrocyte indexes. *J Pediatr* 1997;**130**:57–61.

11. Christensen RD, Yaish HM, Henry E, Bennett ST. Red blood cell distribution width: reference intervals for neonates. *J Matern Fetal Neonatal Med.* 2015;**28**:883–8.

12. Dessypris EN, Sawyer ST. Erythropoiesis. In Greer JP, Foerster J, Rodgers GM, et al. eds. *Wintrobe's Clinical Hematology.* (Philadelphia, PA: Lippincott, Williams & Wilkins, 2009), pp. 108,109.

13. Killman SA. On the size of normal human reticulocytes. *Acta Med Scand* 1964;**176**:529–31.

14. Warwood TL, Ohls RK, Lambert DK, et al. Urinary excretion of darbepoetin after intravenous vs. subcutaneous administration to preterm neonates. *J Perinatol* 2006;**26**:636–9.

15. Wegelius R. On changes in peripheral blood picture of newborn infant immediately after birth. *Acta Paediatr* 1948;**35**:1–6.

16. Humbert JR, Abelson H, Hathaway WE, et al. Polycythemia in small for gestational age infants. *J Pediatr* 1969;75:812–18.

17. Christensen RD, Henry E, Bennett ST, Yaish HM. Reference intervals for reticulocyte parameters of infants during their first 90 days after birth. *J Perinatol* 2016;36:61–66.

18. Al-Ghananim RT, Nalbant D, Schmidt RL, et al. Reticulocyte hemoglobin content during the first month of life in critically ill very low birth weight neonates differs from term infants, children, and adults. *J Clin Lab Anal* 2016;30:326–34.

19. Christensen RD, Henry E, Andres RL, Bennett ST. Neonatal reference ranges for blood concentrations of nucleated red blood cells. *Neonatology* 2010;99:289–94.

20. Perrone S, Vezzosi P, Longini M, et al. Nucleated red blood cell count in term and preterm newborns: Reference values at birth. *Arch Dis Child Fetal Neonatal Ed* 2005;90:F174–5.

21. Buonocore G, Perrone S, Gioia D, et al. Nucleated red blood cell count at birth as an index of perinatal brain damage. *Am J Obstet Gynecol* 1999;181:1500–5.

22. Green DW, Hendon B, Mimouni FB. Nucleated erythrocytes and intraventricular hemorrhage in preterm neonates. *Pediatrics* 1995;96:475–8.

23. Judkins AJ, MacQueen BC, Christensen RD, et al. Automated quantification of fragmented red blood cells: neonatal reference intervals and clinical disorders of neonatal intensive care unit patients with high values. *Neonatology* 2018;115:5–12.

24. Zipursky A. Erythrocyte morphology in newborn infants: A new look. *Pediatr Res* 1977;11:843–8.

25. Pearson EA, McIntosh S, Rooks Y, et al. Interference phase microscopic enumeration of pitted RBC and splenic hypofunction in sickle cell anemia. *Pediatr Res* 1978;12:471–5.

26. Oettinger L Jr., Mills WE. Simultaneous capillary and venous hemoglobin determinations in the newborn infant. *J Pediatr* 1949;35:362–70.

27. Oh W, Lind J. Venous and capillary hematocrit in newborn infants and placental transfusion. *Acta Paediatr Scand* 1966;55:38–42.

28. Moe PJ. Umbilical cord blood and capillary blood in the evaluation of anemia in erythroblastosis fetalis. *Acta Paediatr Scand* 1967;56:391–400.

29. Linderkamp O, Versmold HT, Strohhacker I, et al. Capillary–venous hematocrit differences in newborn infants.1. Relationship to blood volume, peripheral blood flow, and acid-base parameters. *Eur J Pediatr* 1977;127;9–14.

30. Turner CW, Luzins J, Hutcheson C. A modified harvest technique for cord blood hematopoietic stem cells. *Bone Marrow Transpl* 1992;10:89–92.

31. Vahlquist B. Das Serumeisen. Eine padiatrischklinische und experimentelle Studie. *Acta Paediatr* 1941;28:1–9.

32. Mollision PL. *Blood transfusion in clinical medicine*, 3rd ed. (Oxford: Blackwell, 1951).

33. Rivera LM, Rudolph N. Postnatal persistence of capillary-venous differences in hematocrit and hemoglobin values in low-birth-weight and term infants. *Pediatrics* 1982;70:956.

34. Thurlbeck SM, McIntosh N. Preterm blood counts vary with sampling site. *Arch Dis Child* 1987;62:74–9.

35. Carroll PD, Christensen RD. New and underutilized uses of umbilical cord blood in neonatal care. *Matern Health Neonatol Perinatol.* 2015;16;1–16.

36. Vain NE, Satragno DS, Gorenstein AN, et al. Effect of gravity on volume of placental transfusion: a multicentre, randomised, non-inferiority trial. *Lancet* 2014;384:235–40.

37. Katheria A, Garey D, Truong G, et al. A randomized clinical trial of umbilical cord milking vs delayed cord clamping in preterm infants: neurodevelopmental outcomes at 22–26 months of corrected age. *J Pediatr* 2018;194:76–80.

38. Barnett HL, Einhorn AH, eds. and Holt LE (author). *Pediatrics* 15th ed. (New York: Appleton Century-Crofts, 1972), p. 597.

39. Xanthou M. Leukocyte blood picture in healthy full term and premature babies during the neonatal period. *Arch Dis Child* 1970;45:242–7.

40. Akenzua GI, Hui IT, Milner R, et al. Neutrophil and band counts in the diagnosis of neonatal infection. *Pediatrics* 1974;54:38–43.

41. Manroe BL, Weinberg AG, Rosenfeld CR, et al. The neonatal blood count in health and disease. 1. Reference values for neutrophilic cells. *J Pediatr* 1979;95:89–98.

42. Christensen RD, Rothstein G. Pitfalls in the interpretation of leukocyte counts of newborn infants. *Am J Clin Path* 1979;72:608–12.

43. Chervenick PA, Boggs DR, March JC, et al. Quantitative studies of blood and bone marrow neutrophils in normal mice. *Am J Physiol* 1968;215:353–9.

44. Mouzinho A, Rosenfeld CR, Sanchez PJ, Risser R. Revised reference ranges for circulating neutrophils in very-low-birth-weight neonates. *Pediatrics* 1994;94:76–81.

45. Maynard EC, Reed C, Kircher T. Neutrophil counts in newborn infants at high altitude. *J Pediatr* 1993;**122**:990–1.

46. Schmutz N, Henry E, Jopling J, Christensen RD. Expected ranges for blood neutrophil concentrations of neonates: The Manroe and Mouzinho charts revisited. *J Perinatol* 2008;**28**:275–81.

47. Carballo C, Foucar K, Swanson P, et al. Effect of high altitude on neutrophil counts in newborn infants. *J Pediatr* 1991;**119**:464–6.

48. Coulombel L, Dehan M, Tehernia G, et al. The number of polymorphonuclear leukocytes in relation to gestational age in the newborn. *Acta Padeiatr Scand* 1979;**68**:709–12.

49. Lloyd BW, Oto A. Normal values for mature and immature neutrophils in very preterm babies. *Arch Dis Child* 1982;**57**:233–6.

50. MacQueen BC, Christensen RD, Yoder BA, et al. Comparing automated vs manual leukocyte differential counts for quantifying the "left shift" in the blood of neonates. *J Perinatol.* 2016;**36**:843–8.

51. Calhoun DA, Sullivan SE, Lunoe M, et al. Granulocyte-macrophage colony stimulating factor and interleukin-5 concentrations in premature neonates with eosinophilia. *J Perinatol* 2000;**26**:166–71

52. Sullivan SE, Calhoun DA. Eosinophils in the neonatal intensive care unit. *Clin Perinatol* 2000;**27**:603–9.

53. Medoff HS, Barbero GJ. Total blood eosinophil counts in the newborn period. *Pediatrics* 1950;**6**:737–50.

54. Xanthou M. Leukocyte blood picture in ill newborn babies. *Arch Dis Child* 1972;**47**:741–7.

55. Burell JM. A comparative study of the circulating eosinophil levels in babies. *Arch Dis Child* 1952;**27**:337–40.

56. Bass DA. Behavior of eosinophil leukocytes in acute inflammation. II. Eosinophil dynamics during acute inflammation. *J Clin Invest* 1975;**56**:870–6.

57. Gibson JG Jr., Vaucher Y, Corrigan JJ. Eosinophils in premature infants: Relationship to weight gain. *J Pediatr* 1979;**95**:99–104.

58. Portuguez-Molavasi A, Cote-Boileau T, Aranda JV. Eosinophilia in the newborn, possible role in adverse drug reactions. *Pediatr Res* 1980;**14**:537–41.

59. Craver RD. The cytology of cerebrospinal fluid associated with neonatal intraventricular hemorrhage. *Pediatr Pathol Lab Med* 1996;**16**:713–18.

60. Christensen RD, Jensen J, Maheshwari A, Henry E. Reference ranges for blood concentrations of eosinophils and monocytes during the neonatal period defined from over 63,000 records in a multihospital health-care system. *J Perinatol* 2010;**30**:540–5.

61. Rogers GM. In Greer JP, Forester J, Rodgers GM, et al., eds. *Wintrobe's Clinical Hematology* (Philadelphia: Lippincott, Williams & Wilkins, 2009), p. 1277.

62. Wiedmeier SE, Henry E, Sola-Visner MC, Christensen RD. Platelet reference ranges for neonates, defined using data from over 47,000 patients in a multihospital healthcare system. *J Perinatol* 2009;**29**:130–6.

63. Peterec SM, Brennan SA, Tinder EM, et al. Reticulated platelet values in normal and thrombocytopenic neonates. *J Pediatr* 1996;**12**:269–73.

64. Joseph MA, Adams D, Maragos J, Saving KL. Flow cytometry of neonatal platelet RNA. *J Pediatr Hematol Oncol* 1966;**17**:277–81.

65. MacQueen BC, Christensen RD, Henry E, et al. The immature platelet fraction: Creating neonatal reference intervals and using these to categorize neonatal thrombocytopenias. *J Perinatol.* 2017;**37**:834–8.

66. Cremer M, Weimann A, Szekessy D, et al. Low immature platelet fraction suggests decreased megakaryopoiesis in neonates with sepsis or necrotizing enterocolitis. *J Perinatol* 2013;**33**:622–6.

67. Cremer M, Paetzold J, Schmalisch G, et al. Immature platelet fraction as novel laboratory parameter predicting the course of neonatal thrombocytopenia. *Br J Haematol* 2009;**144**:619–621.

68. Andrew M, Castle v, Mitchell L, Paes B. Modified bleeding time in the infant. *Am J Hematol* 1989;**30**:190–1.

69. DelVecchio A, Latin G, Henry E, Christensen RD. Template bleeding times of 240 neonates born at 24–41 weeks' gestation. *J Perinatol* 2008;**28**;427–31.

70. Boudewins M. Raes M, Pteters V, et al. Evaluation of platelet function on cord blood in 80 healthy term neonates using the Platelet Function Analyser (PFA-100); Shorter in vitro bleeding times in neonates than adults. *Eur J Pediatr* 2003;**162**:212–13.

71. Saxonhouse MA, Garner R, Mammel L, et al. Closure times measured by the platelet function analyzer PFA-100 are longer in neonatal blood

compared to cord blood samples. *Neonatol* 2010;**97**:242–9.

72. Sheffield MS, Schmutz N, Lambert DK, Henry E, Christensen RD. Ibuprofen lysine administration to neonates with a patent ductus arteriosus: Effect on platelet plug formation assed by in vivo and in vitro measurements. *J Perinatol* 2009;**29**:39–43.

73. Sheffield MJ, Lambert DK, Henry E, Christensen RD. Effect of ampicillin on the bleeding time of neonatal intensive care unit patients. *J Perinatol* 2010;**30**:527–30.

74. Sola MC, Rimsza LM, Christensen RD. A bone marrow biopsy technique suitable for use in neonates. *Br J Haematol* 1999;**107**: 458–60.

75. Rosse C, Kraemer MJ, Dillon TL, et al. Bone marrow cell populations of normal infants: the predominance of lymphocytes. *J Lab Clin Med* 1977;**89**:1228–32.

76. Shapiro LM, Bassen FA. Sternal marrow changes during first week of life. *Am J Med Sci* 1941:**202**;341–54.

Index